HEAD AND NECK MANIFESTATIONS OF SYSTEMIC DISEASE

HEAD AND NECK MANIFESTATIONS OF SYSTEMIC DISEASE

EDITED BY

JEFFREY P. HARRIS
University of California, San Diego
VA San Diego Healthcare System
San Diego, California, USA

MICHAEL H. WEISMAN
Cedars-Sinai Medical Center
Los Angeles, California, USA

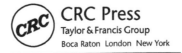

CRC Press
Taylor & Francis Group
Boca Raton London New York

CRC Press is an imprint of the
Taylor & Francis Group, an **informa** business

CRC Press
Taylor & Francis Group
6000 Broken Sound Parkway NW, Suite 300
Boca Raton, FL 33487-2742

First issued in paperback 2019

© 2007 by Taylor & Francis Group, LLC
CRC Press is an imprint of Taylor & Francis Group, an Informa business

No claim to original U.S. Government works

ISBN-13: 978-0-8493-4050-5 (hbk)
ISBN-13: 978-0-367-38880-5 (pbk)

A CIP record for this book is available from the British Library.

Library of Congress Cataloging-in-Publication Data available on application

**Visit the Taylor & Francis Web site at
http://www.taylorandfrancis.com**

**and the CRC Press Web site at
http://www.crcpress.com**

Foreword

This book provides a great wealth of the most current information for today's readers and will serve as a respected resource for decades to come.

The two editors, one from otolaryngology-head and neck surgery and the other from rheumatology, are distinguished scientist-clinicians who have made important contributions to our knowledge of basic and clinical immunology. They have designed a work with a unique perspective: First, to present the fundamental information on a multitude of diseases that have manifestations in the head and neck, and, second, to relate commonly encountered head and neck symptoms and signs to an array of diseases and disorders that should be considered in the differential diagnosis. In the first instance, the diseases are grouped under the broad rubrics of immune disorders, infections, and neoplasia, with immunology as the underlying basic theme and emphasis on pathophysiology and molecular medicine. In the second instance, the clinical approach to problem-solving analyzes the possible causes of the patient's symptoms and signs, and presents evidence-based therapeutic options. Both come together under the editors' guidance to make fascinating reading and to produce a treasure-trove of knowledge. Both are equally rewarding to specialists in neurology, rheumatology, infectious diseases, oncology, dermatology, and otorhinolaryngology-head and neck surgery, and generalists in pediatrics, internal medicine, and family practice. This important book provides an outstanding educational experience for students, residents, fellows, and practitioners of both groups.

The authors of the chapters have been selected for their preeminence in clinical management, as well as having made seminal contributions through research to their topics, thus assuring authoritative presentation of them.

The readers become active members of the team and are involved in the intellectual process that states that everything in medicine is related to everything else in medicine, each one illuminating the others. The reader's role is reminiscent of my role in a little game I used to enjoy playing with the residents, which was occasioned by an offhand remark that I was dwelling on a subject that was not germane to the specialty of otorhinolaryngology-head and neck surgery. At this, I would challenge them to name any other topic in the basic or clinical sciences of medicine that was not related to otorhinolaryngology-head and neck surgery and let me try to mention an important connection of it to their specialty; and, no matter what they chose, I would, with very few exceptions, be able to relate it in a meaningful way to their principal interest. This book provides the same scholarly satisfaction in the unity of medicine.

The design, organization, and execution of this book make it reader-friendly, and its intellectual tone ensures an informative and enjoyable educational experience.

James B. Snow, Jr., M.D., F.A.C.S.
Professor Emeritus, University of Pennsylvania School of Medicine
Philadelphia, Pennsylvania, U.S.A.
Former Director, National Institute on Deafness
and Other Communication Disorders
National Institutes of Health
Bethesda, Maryland, U.S.A.

Preface

In thinking about a contribution we could make to the modern practice of medicine that had not yet been achieved by others, we remembered what constituted the complete physician at the time of Sir William Osler: A working knowledge of multiple disciplines and of disease processes that affect many organ systems. This was perhaps even more important in that era of medicine when laboratory and imaging modalities were essentially nonexistent, forcing physicians to use their powers of history-taking, physical examination, keen observation, and even sense of smell to enable them to come to a correct diagnosis. Further, Osler's famous and oft-quoted comment, "To know syphilis is to know medicine," was especially meaningful at the time because of that particular disease's possible presentation in so many different organ systems. Osler clearly understood that a physician must know the manifestation of a systemic disease in every region of the body.

We have spent our respective careers caring for challenging patients and investigating diseases in the laboratory, as well as serving as teachers of young physicians and medical students. As a result, we can confirm that one must strive to enlarge the base of knowledge of one's own specialty to a broader knowledge of systemic diseases. Because of the enormous expansion of medical knowledge over the past several decades, it is natural to find comfort in a subspecialty area. However, it is still apparent that the very accomplished physician must know more than his or her own specialty area and be well-versed in multiple disciplines.

It is in this spirit we have assembled this textbook, *Head and Neck Manifestations of Systemic Disease*. We recognize that while we have made every effort to include common as well as somewhat esoteric entities that affect the head and neck, this list is not complete or exhaustive and is somewhat limited by what is practical and timely for the life of this textbook. We have selected disorders that a specialist or primary-care practitioner working in this area of the body should keep in mind when seeing an ailment or a complaint. We have divided this book into two sections. The first section, Systemic Disorders with Head and Neck Manifestations, includes chapters that deal with specific disease classifications: rheumatic diseases, infectious diseases, malignant diseases, and other systemic diseases. The second section, Differential Diagnosis and Treatment of Clinical Presentations in the Head and Neck, covers common signs and symptoms in the head and neck region and is intended to give a perspective of the differential diagnosis that would be compiled by an expert practicing in the field. In this way we have presented our topics both from a traditional didactic approach and a practical hands-on point of view.

We wish to thank the many individuals who have contributed their time, expertise, and energy to this effort. Additionally, we want to thank our students, who have taught us the value of our own knowledge and the need to keep current by prodding and questioning what we teach them. Finally, we wish to thank our mentors and professors, who imbued in us the intellectual curiosity and ethical responsibility to become well-rounded physicians. We both acknowledge that much of the joy we get from practicing our profession is enhanced by the interactions we have with our colleagues in sharing these difficult clinical problems and challenging patients.

Jeffrey P. Harris
Michael H. Weisman

Acknowledgment

The authors and editors would like to thank Melanie L. Ariessohn of the Department of Surgery, Division of Otolaryngology-Head and Neck Surgery, University of California, San Diego, for her hard work and fine editorial assistance in the preparation of this book.

Contents

SECTION 1 SYSTEMIC DISORDERS WITH HEAD AND NECK MANIFESTATIONS

PART A ■ RHEUMATIC DISEASES

PART B ■ INFECTIOUS DISEASES

SECTION 2 DIFFERENTIAL DIAGNOSIS AND TREATMENT OF CLINICAL PRESENTATIONS IN THE HEAD AND NECK

Contributors

Maria T. Abreu Department of Medicine, Division of Gastroenterology, Inflammatory Bowel Disease Center, Mount Sinai School of Medicine, New York, New York, U.S.A.

Kedar K. Adour Department of Head and Neck Surgery, Kaiser Permanente Medical Center, Oakland, California, U.S.A.

Brian T. Andrews Department of Otolaryngology-Head & Neck Surgery, University of Iowa College of Medicine, Iowa City, Iowa, U.S.A.

Robert W. Baloh Department of Neurology, David Geffen School of Medicine, University of California, Los Angeles, California, U.S.A.

Ben J. Balough Department of Otolaryngology, Naval Medical Research Command, Naval Medical Center, San Diego, California, U.S.A.

Antoanella Bardan Division of Dermatology, University of California, San Diego, California, U.S.A.

Gregory C. Barkdull Department of Surgery, Division of Otolaryngology-Head and Neck Surgery, University of California, San Diego, California, U.S.A.

Tim Bongartz Division of Rheumatology, Mayo Clinic College of Medicine, Rochester, Minnesota, U.S.A.

Jane C. Burns Department of Pediatrics, School of Medicine, University of California and Rady Children's Hospital, San Diego, California, U.S.A.

Troy E. Daniels The Sjögren's Syndrome Clinic and Department of Orofacial Sciences, School of Dentistry, University of California, San Francisco, California, U.S.A.

Terence M. Davidson Department of Surgery, Division of Otolaryngology-Head and Neck Surgery, University of California and VA San Diego Healthcare System, San Diego, California, U.S.A.

Kevin Deane Division of Rheumatology, University of Colorado and Health Sciences Center, Denver, Colorado, U.S.A.

Joel A. Goebel Department of Otolaryngology-Head and Neck Surgery, Washington University School of Medicine, St. Louis, Missouri, U.S.A.

Quinton Gopen Department of Otology and Laryngology, Harvard Medical School, Boston, Massachusetts, U.S.A.

Joel Guss Department of Otorhinolaryngology: Head and Neck Surgery, University of Pennsylvania School of Medicine, Philadelphia, Pennsylvania, U.S.A.

Jeffrey P. Harris Department of Surgery, Division of Otolaryngology-Head and Neck Surgery, University of California and VA San Diego Healthcare System, San Diego, California, U.S.A.

Tissa Hata Division of Dermatology, University of California, San Diego, California, U.S.A.

Michelle Hernandez Department of Medicine, Division of Rheumatology, Allergy, and Immunology, University of California, San Diego, California, U.S.A.

Michael E. Hoffer Department of Otolaryngology, Naval Medical Research Command, Naval Medical Center, San Diego, California, U.S.A.

Gary S. Hoffman Lerner College of Medicine, Center for Vasculitis Care and Research, Cleveland Clinic Foundation, Cleveland, Ohio, U.S.A.

Henry T. Hoffman Department of Otolaryngology-Head & Neck Surgery, University of Iowa College of Medicine, Iowa City, Iowa, U.S.A.

Peter R. Holman Division of Blood and Marrow Transplant, Moores Cancer Center, University of California, San Diego, California, U.S.A.

Timothy E. Hullar Department of Otolaryngology-Head and Neck Surgery and Department of Anatomy and Neurobiology, Washington University School of Medicine, St. Louis, Missouri, U.S.A.

Darrell Hunsaker Department of Otolaryngology, Naval Medical Research Command, Naval Medical Center, San Diego, California, U.S.A.

Jacob Husseman Department of Surgery, Division of Otolaryngology-Head and Neck Surgery, University of California, San Diego, California, U.S.A.

Christy M. Jackson Department of Neurosciences and School of Medicine, University of California, San Diego, California, U.S.A.

Romaine F. Johnson Department of Pediatric Otolaryngology, University of Texas, Dallas, Texas, U.S.A.

Theodoros F. Katsivas Owen Clinic and Department of Medicine, Division of Infectious Diseases, University of California, San Diego, California, U.S.A.

Maihgan A. Kavanagh John Wayne Cancer Institute at Saint John's Health Center, Santa Monica, California, U.S.A.

Sharon L. Kolasinski Department of Medicine, Division of Rheumatology, Hospital of the University of Pennsylvania, Philadelphia, Pennsylvania, U.S.A.

Junsuke Maki Department of Medicine, Division of Gastroenterology, Inflammatory Bowel Disease Center, Mount Sinai School of Medicine, New York, New York, U.S.A.

Eric L. Matteson Division of Rheumatology, Mayo Clinic College of Medicine, Rochester, Minnesota, U.S.A.

Rex M. McCallum Department of Medicine, Division of Rheumatology, Duke University School of Medicine and Medical Center, Durham, North Carolina, U.S.A.

Edwin M. Monsell Department of Otolaryngology-Head and Neck Surgery, Wayne State University School of Medicine, Detroit, Michigan, U.S.A.

Donald L. Morton John Wayne Cancer Institute at Saint John's Health Center, Santa Monica, California, U.S.A.

Charles M. Myer III Department of Pediatric Otolaryngology, Cincinnati Children's Hospital and Department of Otolaryngology, University of Cincinnati, Cincinnati, Ohio, U.S.A.

Quyen Nguyen Department of Surgery, Division of Otolaryngology-Head and Neck Surgery and School of Medicine, University of California, San Diego, California, U.S.A.

Andrew K. Patel   Department of Surgery, Division of Otolaryngology-Head and Neck Surgery, University of California, San Diego, California, U.S.A.

Phillip K. Pellitteri   Geisinger Health System, Danville, Pennsylvania, U.S.A.

Michael J. Ruckenstein   Department of Otorhinolaryngology-Head and Neck Surgery, University of Pennsylvania School of Medicine, Philadelphia, Pennsylvania, U.S.A.

David R. Salley   Department of Otolaryngology-Head and Neck Surgery, Virginia Commonwealth University Medical Center, Richmond, Virginia, U.S.A.

Anderson S. Santos   Hospital Municipal de Lagoa, Secretaria Municipal de Saúde do Rio de Janeiro, Rio de Janeiro, Brazil

Mark J. Shikowitz   Albert Einstein School of Medicine and Department of Otolaryngology and Communicative Disorders, Long Island Jewish Medical Center, New Hyde Park, New York, U.S.A.

Aristides Sismanis   Department of Otolaryngology-Head and Neck Surgery, Virginia Commonwealth University Medical Center, Richmond, Virginia, U.S.A.

E. William St. Clair   Department of Medicine, Division of Rheumatology, Duke University School of Medicine and Medical Center, Durham, North Carolina, U.S.A.

Geetha Subramanian   Department of Otolaryngology-Head and Neck Surgery, Wayne State University School of Medicine, Detroit, Michigan, U.S.A.

Apurva Thekdi   Department of Surgery, Division of Otolaryngology-Head and Neck Surgery, University of California, San Diego, California, U.S.A.

Douglas K. Trask   Department of Otolaryngology-Head & Neck Surgery, University of Iowa College of Medicine, Iowa City, Iowa, U.S.A.

Shyan Vijayasekaran   Department of Pediatric Otolaryngology, Ear Science Institute, University of Western Australia, Perth, Australia

Erik S. Viirre   Department of Surgery, Division of Otolaryngology-Head and Neck Surgery and School of Medicine, University of California, San Diego, California, U.S.A.

Alexandra Villa-Forte   Vasculitis Clinic, Universidade do Estado do Rio de Janeiro, Rio de Janeiro, Brazil and Center for Vasculitis Care and Research, Cleveland Clinic Foundation, Cleveland, Ohio, U.S.A.

Stephen I. Wasserman   Department of Medicine, Division of Rheumatology, Allergy, and Immunology, University of California, San Diego, California, U.S.A.

Robert A. Weisman   Division of Otolaryngology, Head and Neck Oncology Program, Moores Cancer Center, University of California, San Diego, California, U.S.A.

Sterling West   Division of Rheumatology, University of Colorado Health Sciences Center, Denver, Colorado, U.S.A.

John P. Whitcher   The Sjögren's Syndrome Clinic and The Francis I. Proctor Foundation for Research in Ophthalmology, University of California, San Francisco, California, U.S.A.

Joseph C. Whitt   Oral and Maxillofacial Pathology, School of Dentistry, University of Missouri, Kansas City, Kansas, U.S.A.

Gayle E. Woodson   Department of Surgery, Division of Otolaryngology, Southern Illinois University, Springfield, Illinois, U.S.A.

Ava J. Wu   The Sjögren's Syndrome Clinic and Department of Orofacial Sciences, School of Dentistry, University of California, San Francisco, California, U.S.A.

Section 1

Systemic Disorders with Head and Neck Manifestations

Part C ■ Malignant Diseases

Part D ■ Other Systemic Disorders

1

Systemic Lupus Erythematosus, Scleroderma, Dermatomyositis/ Polymyositis, and Rheumatoid Arthritis

Sharon L. Kolasinski
Department of Medicine, Division of Rheumatology, Hospital of the University of Pennsylvania, Philadelphia, Pennsylvania, U.S.A.

INTRODUCTION

The presentation and expression of multisystem disease is diverse. The onset of systemic diseases such as systemic lupus erythematosus (SLE), scleroderma, dermatomyositis (DM), polymyositis (PM), and rheumatoid arthritis (RA) may occur with symptoms in a variety of organ systems, sometimes typical and sometimes unusual. The eventual course of the disease may include involvement of yet other organ systems. While otorhinolaryngeal manifestations of systemic rheumatic diseases are not among the most common hallmarks of these diseases, they can be quite characteristic and their recognition and management can be of considerable importance (1).

DEFINITION

Systemic Lupus Erythematosus

SLE is the prototypical autoimmune disease characterized by the production of numerous autoantibodies and a wide variety of clinical manifestations. Features of SLE that are of diagnostic importance occur in the head and neck regions regularly. These include abnormalities of the skin and mucous membranes. Other disease features include arthritis and renal and central nervous system abnormalities.

Scleroderma

Scleroderma can involve limited or widespread changes in the skin, with a host of associated internal organ manifestations. In cases of limited skin involvement, the acronym CREST has been widely used to denote the characteristic features of calcinosis, Raynaud's phenomenon, esophageal dysmotility, sclerodactyly, and telangiectasias. In cases of widespread skin involvement, the term "systemic sclerosis" may be used. Additional features include fibrotic lung disease, pulmonary hypertension, and renal failure.

Dermatomyositis/Polymyositis

DM is an inflammatory disease of skin and muscle. A variety of rashes may occur, often on the head and neck. Muscle inflammation leading to weakness, especially in the proximal muscles, is a common feature. When myositis occurs in the absence of skin manifestations, the disorder is termed "polymyositis."

Rheumatoid Arthritis

RA is the most common cause of inflammatory arthritis. Inflammation of the synovium occurs in a distribution that often includes the proximal interphalangeal and metacarpophalangeal joints, along with the wrists and the analogous joints in the feet. Systemic manifestations can include abnormalities of the skin, eyes, lungs, and other organs.

It is important to recognize that discrete rheumatologic diseases share clinical features, and the individual patient may have evidence of more than one disease at a time. Thus, patients with SLE or scleroderma may have inflammatory myositis. Such overlap syndromes require diagnostic vigilance, but often result in therapeutic choices that are particular to the disease manifestation rather than the original diagnosis.

EPIDEMIOLOGY

Systemic Lupus Erythematosus

SLE is a disease of young women. The peak age of onset is between 15 and 40 and the female-to-male ratio is 6:1 to 10:1. SLE affects about 1 in 2000 individuals, but the incidence and severity of disease vary among different racial, ethnic, and socioeconomic groups.

Scleroderma
Scleroderma is rare in children and has its peak occurrence between ages 35 and 65. Female predominance is also seen in scleroderma, with a female-to-male ratio of about 7:1 to 12:1. Scleroderma is rare, affecting 20 to 75 individuals in 100,000.

Dermatomyositis/Polymyositis
Inflammatory myopathies have two peaks of onset. One occurs in children aged 10 to 15, with characteristic skin and muscle involvement, and the other in adults aged 45 to 60, often with muscle involvement alone. In adult disease, women may be affected twice as commonly as men. DM and PM are rare diseases.

Rheumatoid Arthritis
RA can occur at any age, although its incidence increases with increasing age. The peak age of onset is between 30 and 60, and there is a female-to-male ratio of 2.5:1. RA affects about 1% of the population.

PATHOGENESIS

Systemic Lupus Erythematosus
Manifestations of SLE occur through a variety of pathogenetic mechanisms. Lesional skin biopsies can demonstrate inflammation and degeneration of the dermo-epidermal junction. Granular deposits of immunoglobulins and complement components can be seen, often in a band-like pattern, under immunofluorescent microscopy. Frank vasculitis can affect small blood vessels as well. Whether otorhinolaryngeal manifestations such as autoimmune hearing loss seen in association with SLE result primarily from autoantibody-mediated events, or vasculitis, or a combination of inflammatory and immune events, is largely unknown. Some neurologic manifestations of SLE have been associated with antiphospholipid antibodies, giving risc to the possibility that pathogenesis could be linked to thrombosis.

Scleroderma
Sclerodermatous changes in skin and internal organs are characterized by a threefold pathogenic process of abnormal immune system activation, vasculopathy, and fibrosis. Autoantibodies present in patients with scleroderma have no known pathogenic role, but structural changes of the vasculature and replacement of normal tissue with excessive collagen uniquely characterize the pathogenic processes of scleroderma.

Dermatomyositis/Polymyositis
A variety of specific autoantibodies may be present in some patients with DM or PM, implicating the immune system in their pathogenesis. In DM, humoral immune mechanisms may be particularly important, given the predilection for inflammatory cellular infiltration in nonnecrotic muscle fibers and around blood vessels. Vasculopathy can be a particularly prominent feature of childhood disease, with deposition of immunoglobulins and complement components in blood vessels sometimes making skin biopsy specimens indistinguishable from those found in SLE patients. In PM, cell-mediated antigen-specific cytotoxicity appears to be more in pathogenesis, since increased expression of major histocompatibility class I molecules and increased numbers of T cells are found in the muscle in this disorder.

Rheumatoid Arthritis

Pathologic changes seen in the synovium in RA consist of nonspecific inflammation and increases in synoviocytes. Lymphocytes and macrophages infiltrate affected joints, and lymphoid follicles with germinal centers of proliferating B cells surrounding dendritic cells can be seen. These pathogenetic changes may be seen within rheumatoid nodules that can occur in any organ. Further neoangiogenesis and synovial lining hyperplasia lead to destruction of cartilage and bone. In other organs, inflammatory infiltrates, vasculopathy, and fibrosis may be present as well.

CLINICAL MANIFESTATIONS

Systemic Lupus Erythematosus

The most obvious lesions of the head and neck that can be seen in SLE are those involving the skin. The most characteristic dermatologic feature of lupus is the malar rash (Fig. 1). Also known as the "butterfly rash," because of its shape across the cheeks and bridge of the nose, the malar rash is an erythematous and edematous eruption that classically spares the nasolabial folds. A similar rash may be seen on the forehead and chin. It may or may not result from exposure to sunlight, but is often abrupt in onset and can last for days. Malar rashes occur in 30% to 60% of patients. Discoid lupus (Fig. 2) is less frequent, occurring in 15% to 30% of patients. It too may occur in a malar distribution; however, discoid lesions can occur anywhere on the face or scalp, in the pinnae, behind the ears, or on the neck. Discoid lesions tend to be discrete plaques, often erythematous with an adherent scale that extends into hair follicles. They can progress to lesions with indurated margins of erythema and hyperpigmentation, and central atrophic scarring. Discoid lesions have been reported to result in perforation of the pinna (2). Other rashes that can appear in the head and neck area include the photosensitive subacute

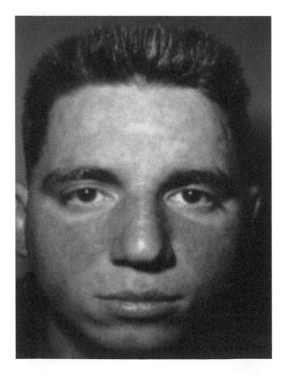

FIGURE 1   Systemic lupus erythematosus: butterfly rash. *Source*: American College of Rheumatology.

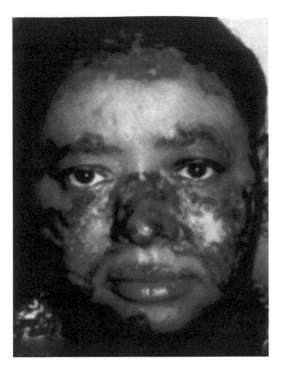

FIGURE 2 Discoid lupus. *Source*: American College of Rheumatology.

cutaneous lupus, tumid lupus (3), and lupus panniculitis. Panniculitis has been reported to occur in isolation on the pinna (4) and to lead to nasal septal perforation (5). Alopecia can occur diffusely or in patches. The oral mucosa (Fig. 3) may also be affected by shallow ulcerations, most typically on the hard palate, but also on the tongue and buccal mucosa. Hyperkeratotic, lichen planus–like plaques have been reported on the buccal mucosa and palate (6). One report of laryngeal inflammation in a lupus patient was associated with cricoarytenoid arthritis (7), although cricoarytenoid arthritis occurs substantially more frequently in RA than in any other rheumatic disease. The nasal mucosa may be affected by ulcerations, as well (8), with resultant perforation (9). Autoimmune hearing loss

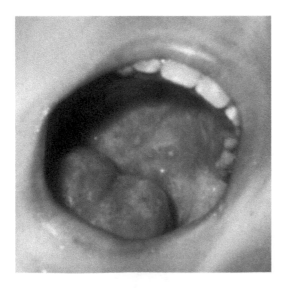

FIGURE 3 Systemic lupus erythematosus: oral ulcerations. *Source*: American College of Rheumatology.

(10,11) has uncommonly been reported to occur in SLE patients, as well as those with antiphospholipid antibodies. Case reports have suggested that inflammatory, autoimmune, or vasculitic mechanisms may play a role, but the precise pathophysiology involved remains obscure (12). Tinnitus may be a common symptom in lupus patients, with or without hearing loss (13). Rarely, nasal and auricular chondritis may be seen in patients with lupus (14). Spontaneous jugular vein thrombosis has very rarely been reported to occur in patients with discoid lupus and antiphospholipid antibodies (15). Central nervous system manifestations in SLE patients will occur from time to time, but a discussion of these events is beyond the scope of this chapter. It is important to note, however, that not all central nervous system events that take place in SLE patients can be due to the SLE itself; a diligent search for an infectious agent or hemorrhagic or thrombotic event should always be undertaken when an SLE patient presents with central nervous system manifestations such as seizures, severe headache, visual disturbance, or change in mood, personality, or cognition.

Scleroderma

As in SLE, changes in the skin are the most obvious manifestations of scleroderma in the head and neck. In systemic sclerosis, the skin changes can begin with a sometimes pruritic, edematous phase, as inflammatory cells and fibroblasts are activated and cytokines are released. The skin in the affected areas tightens, loses flexibility, and thickens. In systemic sclerosis, characteristic facies may be noted, with a pursed-lip appearance and reduction in the oral aperture (Fig. 4). After several years, thinning and atrophy occur. Pigmentation changes may occur as well, giving a "salt and pepper" appearance. The dramatic en coup de sabre lesion (Fig. 5) is rare and is a manifestation of localized scleroderma. A nondermatomal fibrotic band infiltrates skin, subcutaneous fat, fascia, and muscle in the midline of the face, giving the appearance of a sword wound. Telangiectasias may be prominent on the head and neck, including involvement of the palate, oral mucosa, and tongue (Fig. 6). Raynaud's phenomenon is a virtually universal feature of scleroderma and may transiently affect the tip of the nose and the pinnae. A variety of changes may occur in the nasal mucosa (16); nasal perforation can occur (17); and calcinosis has been reported rarely on the nose (18). Chondrodermatitis nodularis helicis has rarely been seen in

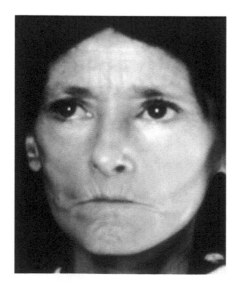

FIGURE 4 Scleroderma: characteristic facies.
Source: American College of Rheumatology.

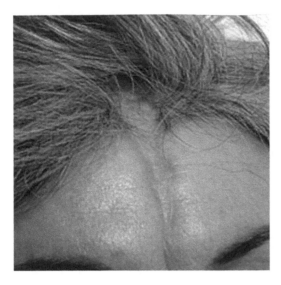

FIGURE 5 Scleroderma: En coup de sabre lesion. *Source*: American College of Rheumatology.

scleroderma (19). Sensorineural hearing loss has been reported to occur, but has not been found to correlate with other disease manifestations (20,21). Virtually the entire gastrointestinal tract can be affected in scleroderma. Swallowing dysfunction due to oropharyngeal involvement can occur (22) and increase the risk of aspiration. Esophageal dysmotility and nonobstructive dysphagia are seen in the majority of patients, making symptoms of gastroesophageal reflux very common.

Dermatomyositis/Polymyositis

DM also may include head and neck dermatologic manifestations that can have considerable diagnostic importance. Among these is the virtually pathognomonic heliotrope rash (Fig. 7). This lesion, which leads to edema and discoloration of the eyelids, takes its name from the deep purple flower of the heliotrope plant, although the lesion may vary in color from pink to red to brown. DM may also lead to an erythematous rash on many locations on the body, including the face and neck (Fig. 8). Nasal septal perforation has been

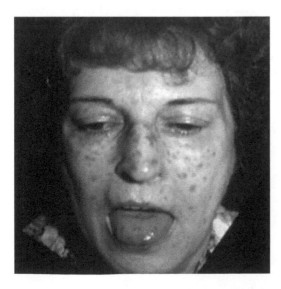

FIGURE 6 Scleroderma: telangiectasias. *Source*: American College of Rheumatology.

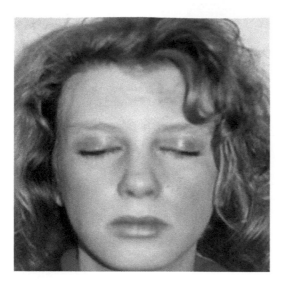

FIGURE 7 Dermatomyositis: heliotrope rash. *Source*: American College of Rheumatology.

reported in DM (23). Two case reports have been made of children with chondrodermatitis nodularis helicis and DM (24,25).

Inflammatory myositis in both DM and PM can prominently involve musculature in the head and neck area. About one-half of patients experience weakness of the neck flexors; ocular and facial muscles are virtually never involved. Weakness of the striated oropharyngeal muscles can result in dysphonia and difficulty swallowing. Dysphagia can also result from esophageal dysmotility or cricoarytenoid sphincter muscle hypertrophy leading to obstruction (26).

Rheumatoid Arthritis

RA can affect any diarthrodial joint. The temporomandibular and cricoarytenoid joints and ossicles of the ear may be among those affected. The temporomandibular joint (TMJ) is symptomatic in over half of patients with RA, and radiographic evidence of involvement may be even more common. The TMJ may be tender to palpation and crepitus may be present. Patients may experience an acute onset of pain and be unable to fully close the mouth. Over time, an overbite may develop if the mandibular condyle and temporal bone surfaces are eroded. In children with RA, TMJ growth centers may fail to develop normally, with resultant micrognathia (Fig. 9). Cricoarytenoid involvement may lead to hoarseness, aspiration and, if severe enough to immobilize the joint, inspiratory stridor. Rheumatoid nodules have been reported to occur on the vocal cords, mimicking laryngeal

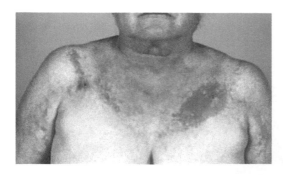

FIGURE 8 Dermatomyositis: diffuse erythematous rash. *Source*: American College of Rheumatology.

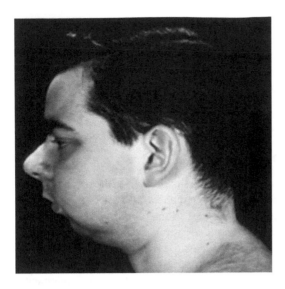

FIGURE 9 Juvenile rheumatoid arthritis: micrognathia. *Source*: American College of Rheumatology.

carcinoma. Keratoconjunctivitis sicca leads to symptoms of dry eyes and is commonly seen in RA, along with dry mouth.

Although not seen commonly today, vasculitic complications can take place in RA patients and have produced nasal septal perforations and even ulcerations on the external ear surfaces. Fortunately, these complications are rarely present in the modern era.

Cervical spine involvement in RA is of particular importance because of the potential for catastrophic neurological consequences. Extension of inflammation into the discovertebral area can lead to bone and cartilage destruction, with malalignment and subluxation. Early involvement may lead to occipital headache. However, the course of neck pain and myelopathy or other neurological symptoms do not always run parallel. Alternate presentations include progressive spastic quadriparesis with painless sensory loss in the hands or transient episodes of medullary dysfunction. Spinal cord compression can occur; and radiographs, including flexion and extension views of the cervical spine, should routinely be performed in any RA patient undergoing surgery with general anesthesia, particularly those with longstanding disease.

TREATMENT

Autoimmune disorders such as those discussed in this chapter are generally treated with immunosuppressive therapy. Corticosteroids are a mainstay of therapy in all of these disorders, but doses may vary widely, depending on the severity of disease manifestations. Among other immunosuppressives, those with more serious potential side effects are reserved for more severe disease manifestations. Often, however, the dermatologic manifestations of SLE and DM can be treated by hydroxychloroquine. This is a long-acting anti-inflammatory agent, not generally considered immunosuppressive, whose precise mechanism of action remains unclear. Hydroxychloroquine is frequently used alone or in combination with immunosuppressive therapy when skin rash is present; however, it is not effective for the skin changes of scleroderma or the myositis of DM/PM.

Certain immunosuppressive agents may be efficacious for particular manifestations of a disease, such as cyclophosphamide for diffuse proliferative glomerulonephritis in SLE or methotrexate for synovitis in RA, but may lack efficacy for other manifestations of the same disease. It is, therefore, difficult to generalize about choices of immunosuppressive agents, especially when confronted with an unusual manifestation in the head or neck. No randomized, controlled trials have specifically addressed the otorhinolaryngeal manifestations of these rheumatic diseases, in part because of their rarity.

The cricoarytenoid muscle hypertrophy associated with DM has been reported to be amenable to surgical treatment (27).

COMPLICATIONS, PROGNOSIS, AND OUTCOME

Observations on the wide array of head and neck manifestations seen in this group of rheumatic diseases have been published as case reports and short case series, and little is available from the literature to assess long-term outcomes. Some clinical events, such as the facial rashes in SLE, serve a diagnostic purpose and are rarely seen later as the disease is treated or as it unfolds. Many times, these head and neck manifestations are overlooked by both the patient and the physician because attention is drawn to the articular or life-threatening internal organ manifestations of these diseases. Awareness (and management) of these complications of the disease most certainly will benefit the quality of life and functional aspects of the patient's long-term outcome.

SUMMARY

Systemic rheumatic disease may present with a variety of manifestations in the head and neck regions. Especially important among these are the dermatologic findings of SLE, DM, and scleroderma. Rashes characteristic of these disorders may also arise later in the course of the diseases. Some of the more frequently reported manifestations to be aware of are autoimmune hearing loss, especially in SLE; esophageal dysmotility in scleroderma; oropharyngeal and esophageal involvement in DM/PM; and keratoconjunctivitis sicca and cervical spine involvement in RA.

REFERENCES

1. Papadimitraki ED, Kyrmizakis DE, Kritikos I, et al. Ear-nose-throat manifestations of autoimmune rheumatic diseases. Clin Exp Rheumatol 2004; 22(4):485–494.
2. Lucky PA. Lupus erythematosus with perforation of the pinna. Cutis 1983; 32(6):554–557.
3. Wan Ihm C, Ki Choi C, Il Suh J. Lupus tumidus involving facial skin, nasal cavity, throat and eye. Dermatologica 1983; 166(1):38–39.
4. Sardana K, Menditta V, Koranne RV, et al. Lupus erythematosus profundus involving the ear lobe. J Eur Acad Dermatol Venereol 2003; 17(6):727–729.
5. Lerner DN. Nasal septal perforation and carotid cavernous aneurysm: unusual manifestations of systemic lupus erythematosus. Otolaryngol Head Neck Surg 1996; 115(1):163–166.
6. Burge SM, Frith PA, Juniper RP, et al. Mucosal involvement in systemic and chronic cutaneous lupus erythematosus. Br J Dermatol 1989; 121(6):727–741.
7. Smith GA, Ward PH, Berci G. Laryngeal involvement by systemic lupus erythematosus. Trans Sect Otolaryngol Am Acad Ophthalmol Otolaryngol 1977; 84(1):124–128.
8. Bruno E, Russo S, Nucci R, et al. Nasal mucosal involvement in systemic lupus erythematosus: histopathologic and immunopathologic study. Int J Immunopathol Pharmacol 2000; 13(1):39–42.
9. Rahman P, Gladman DD, Urowitz MB. Nasal-septal perforation in systemic lupus erythematosus—time for a closer look. J Rheumatol 1999; 26(8):1854–1855.
10. Ruckenstein MJ. Autoimmune inner ear disease. Curr Opin Otolaryngol Head Neck Surg 2004; 12 (5):426–430.

11. Kastanioudakis I, Ziavra N, Voulgari PV, et al. Ear involvement in systemic lupus erythematosus patients: a comparative study. J Laryngol Otol 2002; 116(2):103–107.

12. Sone M, Schachern PA, Paparella MM, et al. Study of systemic lupus erythematosus in temporal bones. Ann Otol Rhinol Laryngol 1999; 108(4):338–344.

13. Sperling NM, Tehrani K, Liebling A, et al. Aural symptoms and hearing loss in patients with lupus. Otolaryngol Head Neck Surg 1998; 118(6):762–765.

14. Kitridou RC, Wittmann AL, Quismorio FP Jr. Chondritis in systemic lupus erythematosus: clinical and immunopathologic studies. Clin Exp Rheumatol 1987; 5(4):349–353.

15. Kale US, Wight RG. Primary presentation of spontaneous jugular vein thrombosis to the otolaryngologist–in three different pathologies. J Laryngol Otol 1998; 112(9):888–890.

16. Elwany S, Talaat M, Kamel N, et al. Further observations on nasal mucosal changes in scleroderma. A histochemical and electron microscopic study. J Laryngol Otol 1984; 98(9):879–886.

17. Willkens RF, Roth GJ, Novak A, et al. Perforation of nasal septum in rheumatic diseases. Arthritis Rheum 1976; 19(1):119–121.

18. Temekonidis TI, Drosos AA. Subcutaneous calcification on the nose in a patient with scleroderma. Clin Exp Rheumatol 2001; 19(5):560.

19. Bottomley WW, Goodfield MD. Chondrodermatitis nodularis helicis occurring with systemic sclerosis–an under-reported association? Clin Exp Dermatol 1994; 19(3):219–220.

20. Berrettini S, Ferri C, Pitaro N, et al. Audiovestibular involvement in systemic sclerosis. ORL J Otorhinolaryngol Relat Spec 1994; 56(4):195–198.

21. Kastanioudakis I, Ziavra N, Politi EN, et al. Hearing loss in progressive systemic sclerosis patients: a comparative study. Otolaryngol Head Neck Surg 2001; 124(5):522–525.

22. Montesi A, Pesaresi A, Cavalli ML, et al. Oropharyngeal and esophageal function in scleroderma. Dysphagia 1991; 6(4):219–223.

23. Martinez-Cordero E, Lasky D, Katona G. Nasal septal perforation in dermatomyositis. J Rheumatol 1986; 13(1):231–232.

24. Sasaki T, Nishizawa H, Sugita Y. Chondrodermatitis nodularis helicis in childhood dermatomyositis. Br J Dermatol 1999; 141(2):363–365.

25. Rogers NE, Farris PK, Wang AR. Juvenile chondrodermatitis nodularis helicis: a case report and literature review. Pediatr Dermatol 2003; 20(6):488–490.

26. Ertekin C, Secil Y, Yuceyar N, et al. Oropharyngeal dysphagia in polymyositis/dermatomyositis. Clin Neurol Neurosurg 2004; 107(1):32–37.

27. Bachmann G, Streppel M, Krug B, et al. Cricopharyngeal muscle hypertrophy associated with florid myositis. Dysphagia 2001; 16(4):244–248.

2

Sjögren's Syndrome

Ava J. Wu
The Sjögren's Syndrome Clinic and Department of Orofacial Sciences, School of Dentistry, University of California, San Francisco, California, U.S.A.

John P. Whitcher
The Sjögren's Syndrome Clinic and The Francis I. Proctor Foundation for Research in Ophthalmology, University of California, San Francisco, California, U.S.A.

Troy E. Daniels
The Sjögren's Syndrome Clinic and Department of Orofacial Sciences, School of Dentistry, University of California, San Francisco, California, U.S.A.

INTRODUCTION

Sjögren's syndrome (SS) is a chronic systemic autoimmune disease that initially presents in the head and neck region, affecting the lacrimal and salivary glands. Clinically, the patient will have objective findings of lacrimal and salivary dysfunction with subjective complaints of dry eyes and dry mouth.

Diagnosing SS is a challenge, as there are many conditions associated with dry eyes and dry mouth that can mimic the ocular and oral components (Tables 1 and 2). Documentation of objective tests of ocular and salivary dysfunction (Schirmer I test; ocular surface staining with a vital dye; labial salivary gland biopsy) is the most reliable for diagnosis of this syndrome.

SS may be the second most common autoimmune disease after rheumatoid arthritis, yet recent data suggests that there is an average delay in diagnosis of 6.5 years and many individuals remain undiagnosed. SS represents a spectrum of disease with great diversity in its initial presentation and clinical course, but with common underlying themes of lacrimal and salivary gland dysfunction associated with an autoimmune process. The diagnostic process is complicated by the lack of any single diagnostic test for SS. The three components, ocular, salivary, and systemic, are often assessed independently; and conditions that can mimic each component must be ruled out (Table 3).

Reported ear, nose, and throat manifestations of SS include swallowing disorders, mucosal dryness, dysgeusia, anosmia, epistaxis, gastric reflux, major salivary gland swelling, and lymphoma.

DEFINITION

There are two forms of SS. Primary SS is a systemic autoimmune disease with early and progressive salivary and lacrimal dysfunction that can have associated extraglandular conditions (Table 4). Secondary SS develops in some patients with a preexisting auto-immune connective tissue disease, usually rheumatoid arthritis.

EPIDEMIOLOGY

Over the past three decades, many diagnostic/classification criteria have been proposed for SS. Some of these criteria use exclusively objective tests for evaluation of each SS

TABLE 1 Causes of Dry Eyes

Bacterial and viral infections of the eye (blepharitis, meibomitis, conjunctivitis)
Excessive blinking
The use of anticholinergic eye drops
The use of systemic anticholinergic medication
Allergic response to preservatives in eye drops
Excessive computer use
Cosmetic eyelid surgery
Corneal surgery
Menopause
Foreign body sensation
Anxiety/depression/stress
Contact lens wear
Dehydration
Congenitally missing lacrimal glands

TABLE 2 Causes of Dry Mouth

Mouth breathing
Continuous positive airway pressure for sleep apnea
Use of systemic anticholinergic medication
Dehydration
Congenitally missing salivary glands
Acute bacterial/viral illnesses affecting the salivary glands
Radiation therapy to the head and neck
Bell's palsy
Excessive thirst (i.e., diabetes)
Anxiety/depression/stress
Past treatment with I^{131}

component, while others also use subjective criteria. As a result of these differing criteria, the prevalence estimates of SS have ranged from 2 to 10 million persons in the United States, and it has remained undiagnosed in many. The disease affects primarily peri- or postmenopausal women, at a ratio of nine females to one male; however, it is being diagnosed with increased frequency in younger individuals. SS has also been described in a cohort of young persons under the age of 16 who presented with salivary gland swelling, positive antinuclear antibody, and an indolent course over a seven-year follow-up period (3).

Among individuals with rheumatoid arthritis, the prevalence of secondary SS is 30% to 50%. In patients with systemic lupus erythematosus (SLE), the prevalence has been estimated between 8% and 30%.

PATHOGENESIS

The cause of SS is unknown, but several stages of its pathogenesis are being elucidated. The initial event may be activation of ductal epithelial cells by an unknown antigen. Expression of co-stimulatory molecules [i.e., HLA-DR, CD80, CD86, intracellular adhesion molecule (ICAM)] by ductal epithelium highlights an unexpected role in the regulation of the immune response. Affected organs exhibit periductal lymphocytic infiltrates composed initially of CD4$^+$ T-cells, which can subsequently attract B-cells. The T-cells release cytokines

TABLE 3 Diseases That Can Share Signs and Symptoms with SS

Amyloidosis
Sarcoidosis
Graft vs. host disease
HIV disease (diffuse infiltrative lymphocytosis syndrome)
Hepatitis C
Reiter's syndrome
Wegener's granulomatosis
Diabetes (uncontrolled)
Bilateral chronic sialadenitis

Abbreviation: SS, Sjögren's syndrome.

TABLE 4 A Revised Classification Criteria for SS by the 2002 American–European Consensus Group

    I. Ocular symptoms: a positive response to at least one of the following questions
        a. Have you had daily, persistent, troublesome dry eyes for more than 3 mo?
        b. Do you have a recurrent sensation of sand or gravel in the eyes?
        c. Do you use tear substitutes more than three times a day?
    II. Oral symptoms: a positive response to at least one of the following questions
        a. Have you had a daily feeling of dry mouth for more than 3 mo?
        b. Have you had recurrent or persistently swollen salivary glands?
        c. Do you frequently drink liquids to aid in swallowing?
    III. Ocular signs: that is, *objective evidence* of ocular involvement as defined as a positive result for one of the following
        a. Schirmer I test performed without anesthesia ($\leq$5 mm in 5 min)
        b. Rose-bengal score or other ocular dye score ($\geq$4 according to van Bijsterveld's scoring system)
    IV. Histopathology: in minor salivary glands (obtained through normal appearing mucosa) focal lymphocytic sialadenitis, evaluated by an expert histopathologist with a focus score $\geq$1 (2)
    V. Salivary gland involvement: *objective evidence* of salivary gland involvement defined as a positive result for at least one of the following diagnostic tests
        a. Unstimulated whole salivary flow ($\leq$1.5 mL in 15 min or $\leq$0.10 mL in 1 min)
    VI. Autoantibodies: presence in the serum of the following autoantibodies:
        a. Autoantibodies to Ro(SSA) or La(SSB), or both
Rules for classification
  For primary SS
    In patients without any potentially associated disease, primary SS may be defined as follows:
    a. The presence of any four of the six items is indicative of primary SS, as long as either item IV (histopathology) or VI (serology) is positive
    b. The presence of any three of the four objective items (that is, items III, IV, V, VI)
    c. The classification tree procedure represents a valid alternative method for classification, although it is should be more properly used in clinico-epidemiological survey (not shown)
  For secondary SS
    In patients with a potentially associated disease (for instance, another well-defined connective tissue disease), the presence of item I or item II plus any two from items III, IV, and V may be considered as indicative of secondary SS
  Exclusion criteria
    Past head and neck radiation; hepatitis C infection, HIV infection, preexisting lymphoma, sarcoidosis, graft vs. host disease, use of anticholinergic medication

Abbreviation: SS, Sjögren's syndrome.
Source: Ref. 1.

including tumor necrosis factor-α (TNF-α), interferon-γ, transforming growth factor-β, interleukin 6, and interleukin 10.

The pathogenesis of SS also includes polyclonal B-cell activation with germinal centers developing in the T-cell organ infiltrates, elevated circulating immunoglobulins IgG, IgA, and IgM, circulating autoantibodies [anti–SS-A, anti–SS-B, rheumatoid factor (RF), and antinuclear antibody], and elevated levels of B-cell proliferation factors BAFF and APRIL. Antagonist muscarinic receptor (M3) antibodies have also been identified in patients with SS, which may offer an explanation for the clinical findings of decreased exocrine secretion in this population. The B-cell component, in a few patients, can progress to mucosa-associated lymphoid tissue (MALT) lymphoma or high-grade B-cell non-Hodgkin's lymphoma.

The predominance of women affected by SS raises questions of genetic and hormonal roles. The SS genotype has not been defined, but HLA-DR3 has been observed in Caucasian patients with primary SS, although not in Japanese patients. Current evidence suggests that clinically distinct autoimmune diseases may be controlled by a common set of susceptibility genes. The influence of environmental factors will likely complicate the ultimate search for an SS susceptibility gene. There has been very little research in the area of hormonal influence on the pathogenesis of SS; however, dehydroepiandrosterone, a steroid hormone that is a precursor to both estrogen and testosterone, has shown no efficacy in the treatment of primary SS (4).

CLINICAL MANIFESTATIONS

The majority of individuals ultimately diagnosed with SS initially present with dry eyes and/or dry mouth. A few will present with the result of a secretory deficiency such as increased dental decay at incisal edges or exposed root surfaces of the teeth, oral mucosal burning secondary to a fungal infection, and corneal ulceration or corneal scarring. Dryness complaints may be accompanied by involvement of a diverse array of other organ systems: Hashimoto's thyroiditis/Graves' disease, severe fatigue, increased sedimentation rate, fever of unknown origin, myositis, peripheral neuropathy, leukocytoclastic vasculitis-purpura, renal tubular acidosis, atrophic gastritis, arthritis, and positive test for antinuclear antibodies or RF in asymptomatic patients (2,5,6).

Ocular manifestations are associated with lacrimal gland dysfunction. Many patients with SS cannot cry. The symptoms of ocular dryness may manifest as itching, grittiness, a sandy sensation, photophobia, eye fatigue, decreased visual acuity, discharge, a sensation of film across the eye, photosensitivity, and conjunctival injection. Ocular symptoms may be exacerbated by air-conditioning, computer use, cigarette smoke, low humidity, and medication with anticholinergic effects. It should be noted that tear flow rates are often not correlated with ocular discomfort. That is, individuals with objective signs of severe dry eyes may have minimal complaints. Because tears contain antimicrobial components, the loss of tears predisposes to ocular infections, including blepharitis, bacterial keratitis, and conjunctivitis, which can further exacerbate the sensation of dryness. In addition to the decreased volume of tears, there is a change in the mucous component. Filamentary keratitis can occur with mucous filaments adhering to damaged sections of the ocular surface. Ocular complications include corneal ulceration/abrasion, corneal melt, vascularization, opacification, and, rarely, perforation with loss of vision. Enlargement of the lacrimal glands rarely occurs.

Oral manifestations are associated with salivary gland dysfunction (7). The patient may complain of difficulty in eating dry foods (e.g., crackers), oral soreness, hoarseness, lipstick adhering to the front teeth, increased dental decay, swollen salivary glands, and dry mouth. There will often be a history of carrying a water bottle and of needing fluid at mealtimes to aid swallowing. It is estimated that salivary gland swelling will occur in only 25% of those diagnosed with SS. Interestingly, the clinical oral examination can be within normal limits, as some individuals eventually diagnosed with SS will have normal or near-normal salivary flow rates. The oral findings will be distinctive in those with the most severe salivary gland dysfunction, including depapillation, fissuring, and erythema of the dorsal tongue, and/or generalized mucosal erythema, with or without burning symptoms (fungal infection); cloudy and/or viscous saliva expressible from the parotid or submandibular/sublingual ducts; multiple carious lesions located at the incisal or root surfaces of teeth; angular cheilitis; and a lack of salivary pooling in the floor of the mouth. There may be a "clicking" sound heard during speech, due to the tongue sticking to teeth.

While dryness is known to occur in the eyes and mouth, it can also occur in other organ systems including skin, vagina, ear, nose (blockage, dryness, and epistaxis are common; crusting and hyposmia are rare), and throat (hoarseness; chronic, nonproductive cough). A recent paper on otolaryngological examinations of 111 patients with primary SS and 26 patients with secondary SS reported that symptoms were common, but objective observations were rare and included dry mucosa, postnasal drip, and middle ear effusion (8). Sensorineural hearing loss of high-frequency hearing may be present and associated with autoimmunity, but is considered to be of limited clinical impact in SS (8–10).

Extraglandular manifestations of SS involve numerous organ systems listed in Table 5. These may be treated separately without recognition of the underlying process. The diversity of the manifestations, perhaps coupled with an insidious onset of the sicca complaints, may help explain delays in SS diagnosis.

DIAGNOSIS

Many different sets of classification criteria have been proposed for SS over the past 30 years. Depending on the stringency of criteria used, there can be up to a 10-fold difference in the number of individuals diagnosed. The classification criteria developed by an American–European consensus group are currently the most widely used (Table 4) (1).

Diagnosis of primary SS is more difficult than that of secondary SS because it requires objective findings of the *salivary* (histopathology, unstimulated whole salivary flow rate, sialography, or scintigraphy), *ocular* (Schirmer I test or staining with rose bengal or lissamine green), and *systemic* (anti–SS-B and/or anti–SS-A) components. Subjective findings of salivary and ocular symptoms via patient history can be unreliable (Table 4, points I and II) or can be the result of a disease process other than SS (Tables 1–3).

The ocular component of SS is termed "keratoconjunctivitis sicca" (KCS). The Schirmer I test is used to test tear production. Standardized Schirmer strips 35 mm long and 5 mm wide, composed of sterilized filter paper, are folded at the notched ends and placed over the lateral lid margin of both lower lids and allowed to remain for five minutes, or until the strips are saturated, if sooner. The Schirmer I is preferred because it tests the ability of the lacrimal gland to produce tears under normal conditions of relatively mild stimulation. Application of a topical anesthetic (Schirmer II) creates an artificial situation in which test values are abnormally low, even in some patients without KCS. In most circumstances, less than 5 mm of wetting in five minutes is considered abnormal. Low Schirmer values are also caused by other ocular conditions not associated with SS.

The tear break-up time (BUT) evaluates the stability of the tear film. A drop of 0.5% fluorescein, applied to both eyes, is allowed to equilibrate for three minutes, and then the

TABLE 5 Extraglandular Manifestations in Primary SS

Hashimoto's thyroiditis/Graves' disease
Interstitial nephritis/renal tubular acidosis
Autoimmune hepatitis/primary biliary cirrhosis
Peripheral neuropathies
Vasculitis-purpura
Interstitial lung disease
Atrophic gastritis
Non-Hodgkin's lymphoma (extraglandular or glandular)

Abbreviation: SS, Sjögren's syndrome.

ocular surface of both eyes is observed through the slit lamp using the cobalt blue filter. The amount of time between the last blink and the break-up of the fluorescein-stained precorneal tear film is determined by noting the first blue spot that appears on the surface of the cornea. A BUT of less than 10 seconds is suggestive of an aqueous or mucous tear deficiency, consistent with the ocular component of SS. Fluorescein is also used to assess the integrity of the corneal epithelium through the number of punctate epithelial erosions, their location, and presence or absence of confluence. Corneal filaments may be present in severe KCS.

Rose bengal or lissamine green can be used interchangeably to assess the integrity of the conjunctival epithelium. Both dyes stain devitalized, desiccated, and keratinized conjunctival cells, as well as goblet cells. Rose bengal is irritating to the eye, particularly in patients with moderate to severe disease, while lissamine green produces no irritation, even in extremely dry eyes. The staining pattern of the interpalpebral bulbar conjunctiva is equivalent to both. Ocular dryness symptoms can be exacerbated by various conditions unrelated to SS (Table 1) and this should be considered when evaluating a patient for the ocular component of SS.

Current diagnostic criteria for SS offer alternatives for assessing salivary function that need to be understood before applying them. The range of tests recommended for evaluation of the salivary component by the American–European Consensus criteria is not diagnostically equivalent (Table 4).

A labial salivary gland biopsy can provide the most disease-specific diagnosis of the salivary component of SS. The biopsy technique and specimen acquisition are critical to a successful outcome. Following local anesthetic infiltration of the lower labial mucosa, an approximately 1.5 cm incision is made through the epithelium, but no deeper (Fig. 1A). After blunt dissection of the incision margin, at the level of the lamina propia, approximately five minor salivary glands are dissected free from the underlying connective tissue, one at a time (Fig. 1B). Clear visualization of the field during dissection permits sensory nerves in the area to be preserved. The incision is then closed with approximately three interrupted, resorbable sutures. If histological examination reveals focal lymphocytic sialadenitis, the pathologist must then determine a focus score (11), which provides a diagnostic threshold and severity estimate. A punch or wedge biopsy is not recommended, as it is a blind procedure with a greater risk of missing the minor salivary glands and includes significant probability of sensory nerve damage.

Determination of unstimulated whole salivary flow rate is simple to perform in the outpatient office. Sialography is a technically difficult radiographic technique exhibiting anatomic changes in parotid or submandibular duct structure; this is somewhat

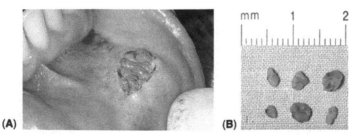

(A)   **(B)**

FIGURE 1   Minor salivary gland biopsy. (**A**) Incision is made to the right or left of midline of the inner lip halfway between the vermillion border and vestibule. Minor glands and nerves can be visualized. (**B**) Individual minor salivary glands are individually dissected.

uncomfortable for the patient and examines only one major gland at a time. If utilized, water-soluble contrast media are preferable to fat-soluble media in individuals with decreased salivary flow, because of the risk of medium retention in the salivary gland with subsequent foreign body reaction. In the case of scintigraphy, there are currently no clear guidelines to assess what constitutes delayed uptake, reduced concentration, and/or delayed excretion of the tracer. Assessment of the rate of uptake and release of the tracer by the salivary gland is a judgment that can vary from practitioner to practitioner.

RF and antinuclear antibody occur in about 90% of patients with SS, but lack specificity and have been deleted from the most recent classification criteria (1). Testing for the presence of autoantibodies directed toward two ribonuclear antigens (SS-A and SS-B) is the only serologic test used in current classification criteria. The prevalence of these autoantibodies in SS varies as a function of the diagnostic criteria used to define the study population as well as the sensitivity of the methodology used to detect the autoantibody. Neither anti–SS-A nor anti–SS-B is specific for SS, as approximately 50% of patients with SLE will be positive and a small percentage of normal adults will also have a low titer.

Diagnosis of SS also requires exclusion of other conditions that can mimic it. These include previous radiation therapy to the head and neck, amyloidosis, sarcoidosis, lymphoma, graft versus host disease, hepatitis C virus infection, HIV-diffuse infiltrative lymphocytosis syndrome, medication-induced dryness, and uncontrolled diabetes mellitus.

TREATMENT

Treatment of SS is complicated by its unique multiorgan involvement. Timely organ-specific treatment can effectively increase patient comfort and reduce potential damage to the corneas and teeth. Systemic complications of SS are secondary to autoimmune processes and potentially life-threatening, and are discussed below.

Ocular management of KCS has three goals: (*i*) replacing the aqueous tear film and restoring normal tear function through the use of preservative-free artificial tears; (*ii*) improving retention of the patient's diminished tear volume by closing lacrimal puncta, either temporarily or permanently; and (*iii*) treating various ocular complications that can lead to scarring of the cornea, such as persistent epithelial erosions, exposure keratitis, corneal ulceration, and chronic staphylococcus infection of the lid margins.

There are many forms of artificial tears that can be used for tear replacement, but those in multi-dose containers should be avoided. Multi-dose bottles contain preservatives to which many patients develop hypersensitivity reactions that may eventually lead to conjunctival scarring and a further decrease in tear production. Preservative-free single-unit-dose eye drops such as Refresh®, Cellufresh®, and Celluvics® are the most effective artificial tears, and do not cause chronic ocular irritation or damage to the cornea and conjunctiva. Artificial tears in multi-dose containers that claim to be preservative-free because the preservative is ephemeral can nevertheless cause irritation because of residual irritants, and should be avoided. Topical steroid preparations should not be used routinely in patients with KCS. If they are required in cases where inflammation is severe, they should be used judiciously with frequent careful follow-up examinations by an ophthalmologist. Commercially available topical preparations of 0.05% cyclosporine (Restasis®) improve symptoms in some patients with mild KCS, but in general they have very little effect on SS patients with severe KCS. Cyclosporine in 1% or 2% concentrations may prove to be more effective. Alternatives to commercially available preservative-free artificial tears include 1.25% gum cellulose drops, low molecular weight dextran, hyaluronic acid, fibronectin, and autologous human serum albumin.

When punctal occlusion does not lead to marked improvement of ocular symptoms, many patients find the use of moisture chamber glasses helpful. Wearing moisture chambers, soft rubber swim goggles, or saran wrap over the eyes while sleeping can increase ocular comfort for a few hours during the day. Environmental changes such as humidifying the bedroom can also be helpful. In extreme cases, a temporary tarsorrhaphy can be preformed to prevent corneal thinning, melting, and perforation while the underlying problem, whether it be infection or exposure, can be effectively addressed.

Treatment of the salivary and oral component of SS has four goals: (*i*) ongoing dental caries prevention through patient education about diet, oral hygiene, and the role of fluoride supplements; professionally applied and patient applied topical fluoride preparations; and dental restoration with procedures and materials appropriate to an oral environment of chronic salivary hypofunction; (*ii*) salivary flow stimulation with systemically administered drugs, such as pilocarpine or cevimeline, and physiological stimulation using sugar-free lozenges or gum; (*iii*) recognition of chronic erythematous candidiasis, which occurs in about one-third of SS patients, and its treatment with appropriate antifungal drugs which greatly reduce oral symptoms, even with continuing salivary hypofunction; and (*iv*) selective use of saliva substitutes, which remain in the mouth for a relatively short time and do not replace the functions of normal saliva, but can be helpful for patients with fairly severe chronic hyposalivation (7).

Topical fluoride application is critical for caries prevention in this susceptible population. Typically, the patient is stratified into a low, medium, or high risk caries group, and the use of the following types of fluoride, either alone or in combination, is considered: professionally-applied high-concentration fluoride solutions (e.g., 1.23% fluoride in acidulated phosphate fluoride gel for four minutes, four times per year; or a 2.26% fluoride varnish applied directly to the teeth, four times per year); patient-applied sodium fluoride gel (0.5% fluoride) in a custom-fitted tray for five minutes daily (to supplement professionally-applied fluoride); or a daily rinse with a 0.05% sodium fluoride, which is another useful addition to professionally-applied fluorides. Neutral sodium fluoride preparations are generally preferred to stannous fluoride preparations because patients tolerate them better. Chlorhexidine rinses may be used to control the quantity of mutans streptococci in the flora. This can be in the form of a patient-applied 0.12% chlorhexidine gluconate rinse, one minute daily for two weeks.

All currently available "oral" topical antifungal drugs contain substantial amounts of sucrose or glucose (i.e., brands of clotrimazole oral troches, nystatin oral pastilles, and nystatin oral suspension), which creates significant risk for supporting dental caries development when used as directed. Systemic antifungals may not be fully effective in those with severe salivary dysfunction, as the medication is delivered to the oral cavity through saliva. Therefore, the best topical antifungal drug to use with patients at high risk for dental caries is nystatin vaginal tablets. These do contain lactose, which is a potentially cariogenic carbohydrate, but much less so than either sucrose or glucose. They must be dissolved slowly in the mouth for 15 to 20 minutes, two or three times per day. Such patients usually must take frequent sips of water to allow the tablet to dissolve in that time. The treatment end-point for erythematous candidiasis should be resolution of all the mucosal erythema, return of filiform papillae to the dorsal tongue, and resolution of associated oral symptoms (i.e., burning sensation). Dentures will also need to be treated for fungus to decrease the risk of reinfection.

Organ-specific manifestations that require treatment are diverse and can be managed by a series of medical specialists (2,5,6). Those conditions can include chronic low-grade problems such as myalgias, polyarthralgias, fatigue, and Raynaud's phenomenon, or organ-specific diseases such as chronic interstitial lung disease, atrophic gastritis, peripheral neuropathies, primary biliary cirrhosis, and renal tubular acidosis, or hematological diseases such as nonthrombocytopenic purpura, leukopenia, and hyper-gammaglobulinemia, or non-Hodgkin's lymphoma. Systemic therapy for SS is currently limited to a few classes of drugs. Cholinergic agonists (i.e., pilocarpine, cevimeline) can be prescribed to stimulate salivary and lacrimal secretion. Vasculitic skin lesions or visceral involvement is usually treated with a corticosteroid alone or in combination with methotrexate, cyclphosphamide, or chlorambucil. Arthritis is usually managed, depending on the severity, with nonsteroidal anti-inflammatory drugs (NSAIDs), hydroxylcholoroquine, or methotrexate. TNF inhibitors (i.e., etanercept, infliximab) have not been effective for SS in clinical trials. Long-term immunosuppressive therapy should be used with caution in this population with a chronic, nonfatal disease process. A monoclonal antibody, Rituximab, is available for treatment of $CD20^+$ B-cell non-Hodgkin's lymphoma.

COMPLICATIONS AND PROGNOSIS

Existing longitudinal studies of persons with SS show that the clinical course of SS is slowly progressive and is life altering, rather than life threatening, for most patients. One study found no overall increased mortality in a population of individuals with SS when compared to controls (12). Those with SS also do not have increased cardiovascular mortality, as do individuals with SLE, despite the apparent overlap in signs and symptoms. Salivary glands in SS begin with focal lymphocytic infiltrates but can progress to a lymphoepithelial lesion (lymphoepithelial sialadenitis). This is often associated with chronic clinical enlargement of major salivary glands, occurring in about one-third of patients. Rarely, it may progress to a MALT lymphoma, an indolent tumor progressing for years, or become a high-grade B-cell non-Hodgkin's lymphoma. Various studies have shown a significantly higher prevalence of lymphoma in SS patients than in the general population. Lymphomas occur most frequently in the salivary glands, but also can occur in the gastrointestinal tract, thyroid gland, lung, kidney, lacrimal glands, or lymph nodes. Clinical predictors for lymphoma development in SS include low C4 level, persistently enlarged salivary glands, regional or general lymphadenopathy, hepatosplenomegaly, pulmonary infiltrates, vasculitis in a setting of hypergammaglobulinemia, high erythrocyte sedimentation rate associated with hypergammaglobulinemia, and a monoclonal immunoglobulinemia.

SUMMARY

Sjögren's syndrome is a chronic disease, primarily affecting women, with significant morbidity. Signs and symptoms of this disease often occur in the head and neck area. The identification and diagnosis of this disease is complicated by its multiorgan involvement, the presence of several sets of diagnostic criteria, and the lack of a single identifying test. However, there is the underlying theme that SS comprises three components: ocular, salivary, and systemic. The use of recently published criteria by the American–European consensus group is the current standard for the diagnosis of SS.

While there is no treatment available for the underlying pathogenesis of SS, there are useful treatments for symptom relief and complication prevention that can significantly stabilize or improve patients' quality of life.

REFERENCES

1. Vitali C, Bombardieri S, Jonsson R, et al. Classification criteria for Sjögren's syndrome: a revised version of the European criteria proposed by the American-European Consensus Group. Ann Rheum Dis 2002; 61(6):554–558.
2. Derk CT, Vivino FB. A primary care approach to Sjögren's syndrome. Helping patients cope with sicca symptoms, extraglandular manifestations. Postgrad Med 2004; 116(3):49–54,59,65. http://www.postgradmed.com/issues/2004/09_04/derk.html (accessed October 2005).
3. Cimaz R, Casadei A, Rose C, et al. Primary Sjögren's syndrome in the paediatric age: a multicentre survey. Eur J Pediatr 2003; 162(10):661–665.
4. Pillemer SR, Brennan MT, Sankar V, et al. Pilot clinical trial of dehydroepiandrosterone (DHEA) versus placebo for Sjögren's syndrome. Arthritis Rheum 2004; 51(4):601–604.
5. Kassan SS, Moutsopoulos HM. Clinical manifestations and early diagnosis of Sjögren's syndrome. Arch Intern Med 2004; 164(12):1275–1284.
6. Fox RI. Sjögren's syndrome. Lancet 2005; 366(9482):321–331.
7. Daniels TE, Wu AJ. Xerostomia—clinical evaluation and treatment in general practice. J Calif Dent Assoc 2000; 28(12):933–941. http://www.cda.org/cda_member/pubs/journal/jour1200/xero.html (accessed October 2005).
8. Freeman SR, Sheehan PZ, Thorpe MA, et al. Ear, nose, and throat manifestations of Sjögren's syndrome: retrospective review of a multidisciplinary clinic. J Otolaryngol 2005; 34(1):20–24.
9. Boki KA, Ioannidis JP, Segas JV, et al. How significant is sensorineural hearing loss in primary Sjögren's syndrome? An individually matched case–control study. J Rheumatol 2001; 28(4): 798–801.
10. Ziavra N, Politi EN, Kastanioudakis I, et al. Hearing loss in Sjögren's syndrome patients. A comparative study. Clin Exp Rheumatol 2000; 18(6):725–728.
11. Vivino FB, Gala I, Hermann GA. Change in final diagnosis on second evaluation of labial minor salivary gland biopsies. J Rheumatol 2002; 29(5):938–944.
12. Theander E, Manthorpe R, Jacobsson LT. Mortality and causes of death in primary Sjögren's syndrome: a prospective cohort study. Arthritis Rheum 2004; 50(4):1262–1269.

3

Adamantiades-Behçet's Disease

Kevin Deane
Division of Rheumatology, University of Colorado and Health Sciences Center, Denver, Colorado, U.S.A.

INTRODUCTION

Adamantiades-Behçet's disease is a systemic inflammatory disorder classically character-ized by recurrent oral and genital ulcerations along with inflammatory eye disease, although multiple manifestations of the disease have been described, involving virtually every organ system. The disease has likely been present since antiquity, with a description of an ulcerative disease similar to what we now call Adamantiades-Behçet's appearing in the writings of Hippocrates (1). The medical community turned its attention to this disease again in the early 1900s, when there were several case reports of patients with recurrent mucocutaneous ulcers, but it was not until the 1930s that the disease triad of oral and genital ulcers with inflammatory eye disease was attributed to a single syndrome, initially by the Greek ophthalmologist Benedict Adamantiades (2), and soon thereafter by Hulusi Behçet, a Turkish dermatologist whose name has since become synonymous with this disease (3). Because of Adamantiades's description of the same syndrome prior to Behçet's, many physicians feel the disease is most appropriately named Adamantiades-Behçet's disease, and although this title has not yet been widely accepted, the disease will be referred to by this name throughout the remainder of this chapter.

EPIDEMIOLOGY

Adamantiades-Behçet's disease is seen in virtually every country, but the region with the highest prevalence stretches from the Mediterranean across Asia to Japan—the so-called "Silk Route." Along this route, the disease is most common in Turkey, with prevalence rates approaching 370 cases per 100,000 (4). The disease becomes less prevalent as distance from the Silk Route increases, with prevalence rates in Europe and North America between 1 in 15,000 and 1 in 500,000 (4).

Typically, patients present with symptoms in their second or third decades, although a wide range of age-of-onset has been described, including childhood disease. In contrast to many other autoimmune diseases, Adamantiades-Behçet's tends to occur equally in males and females; however, disease in males seems to predominate in the Mediterranean area, while disease in females is more common in Europe and North America (5). Additionally, disease in males of Mediterranean and Asian ancestry tends to be more severe than that seen in patients of European descent.

PATHOGENESIS

Multiple aspects of the immune system have been shown to be abnormal in Adamantiades-Behçet's, including lowered neutrophil and endothelial cell activation thresholds, abnor-mal T-cell responses (including $\gamma\delta$ T-cells), increased cytokine expression and immune complex formation, increased Fas-ligand expression, abnormal complement activation proteins, and disrupted coagulation pathways (4,6). The driving process behind these multiple abnormalities is unknown. Infections have been thought to lead to the disease, and various organisms have been implicated, including *Staphylococcus*, *Streptococcus*, and some Gram-negative bacterial species, as well as multiple viruses, including herpes simplex. In most models, infection would act as the initial trigger for disease, with downstream inflammation being caused by immune cross-reactivity (7). This model is attractive, but conclusive evidence for a pathogenic role of these or other organisms has not been found (7). Antibodies reactive against oral mucosa and antiendothelial cell antibodies have been found in patients with Adamantiades-Behçet's, but they lack specificity for disease, although a subset of these antibodies directed against α-enolase in the vascular wall may prove to be fairly specific markers for Adamantiades-Behçet's (6). Abnormalities of the clotting system, including elevated homocysteine levels, low levels of activated protein C, and antiphospholipid antibodies, also have been observed in patients with disease and are thought to lead to the endothelial damage and the thrombotic complications seen with this disease (8,9).

Adamantiades-Behçet's does have a significant association with the class I human leukocyte antigens B51 and B52, although interestingly, the strength of these associations depends on the geographic region of disease, with a relative risk of disease of 13.3 in carriers of the HLA-B51 gene in Turkey versus a relative risk of 1.3 in carriers of the gene in the United States (4,10). It is thought that the HLA-B51 and -B52 molecules may act to present antigenic peptides to CD8+ T-cells, initiating the immune response seen in Adamantiades-Behçet's; however, the specific peptide(s) has not been identified (7). HLA-B51 and -B52 molecules may also act as antigens themselves, becoming targets after similar proteins are released from immunologic sequestered sites in the body, perhaps by an initial infection (7). Other genes have also been implicated in disease, including polymorphisms in genes for intracellular adhesion molecule-1 (ICAM-1), endothelial nitric oxide synthase, pyrin, major histocompatibility complex class I (MICA), vascular endothelial growth factor (VEGF), interleukin-1A (IL-1A), and other proteins related to antigen processing, although further investigations are needed to define the pathways by which these specific genetic alterations lead to Adamantiades-Behçet's (4,11–13).

Histopathologic evaluation of early Adamantiades-Behçet's mucocutaneous lesions shows a neutrophilic vascular process involving the small vessels. Its appearance is similar to leukocytoclastic vasculitis with neutrophilic infiltrates, nuclear dust, and extravasation of red blood cells, with immune complex deposition and endothelial and neutrophil activation thought to play a role in initiation of this process (6). In late mucocutaneous lesions, lymphocytic infiltrate may predominate. In larger-vessel disease, similar vasculitic changes of the vasa vasorum are seen, with lymphocytic infiltration of these vessel lesions likely representing more chronic inflammation (5). It is this larger-vessel vasculitis that can lead to vessel wall damage and aneurysms that are prone to rupture.

In sum, while the exact etiology of the disease is unknown, it appears that in the appropriate genetic and immunologic background, after a trigger by perhaps an initial infection, the signs and symptoms of Adamantiades-Behçet's occur when trauma or other vascular injury, allows for the activation of already overly sensitive components of the innate immune system, including neutrophils, endothelial cells, and more primitive γδ T-cells, with the resulting robust cytokine response and recruitment of T- and B-cells playing a role in continued inflammation and tissue injury.

CLINICAL MANIFESTATIONS

Head and Neck

Oral. Oral ulcerations represent the most common finding of disease and are seen in over 95% of patients with Adamantiades-Behçet's. They are required for diagnosis (Table 1), although some argue that in rare cases, oral ulcers need not be present for the diagnosis to be made. The oral ulcerations seen in Adamantiades-Behçet's may be present on the tongue, lips, gingival surfaces, buccal mucosa, soft palate, or posterior pharynx (Fig. 1). In general, they are shallow and painful, resolving in one to three weeks, usually healing without scarring. The ulcers (<3 mm) can range in size from small, herpetiform lesions

TABLE 1 Clinical Manifestations of Behçet's Disease

Oral ulcers (96–100%)	Stroke
Genital ulcers (65–90%)	Demyelinating disease
Systemic manifestations	Vasculitic brain stem or cord lesions
Weight loss	Intracranial aneurysms
Anorexia	Venous thrombosis
Malaise	Peripheral neuropathy
Fever	*Gastrointestinal manifestations*
Lymphadenopathy	Mucosal ulcerations
Skin manifestations	Intestinal perforations
Folliculitis	Budd–Chiari syndrome
Erythema nodosum	*Pulmonary manifestations* (8%) (16)
Pathergy test	Thromboembolic disease
Acneiform lesions	Pleural disease
Superficial thrombophlebitis	Bronchiolitis obliterans/organizing
Articular manifestations	pneumonia
Arthralgias	Pulmonary hypertension
Arthritis (polyarticular or monoarticular)	Interstitial lung disease/fibrosis
Ocular manifestations (75%) (14)	Pulmonary artery aneurysms
Conjunctivitis/ulceration	*Cardiac manifestations*
Anterior uveitis	Conduction abnormalities
Posterior uveitis	Myocardial fibrosis
Panuveitis	Vasculitic infarction
Retinal vasculitis	Pericarditis
Optic neuritis	Aortic aneurysms
Venous thrombosis	*Other*
Glaucoma (secondary)	Nailfold capillary abnormalities
Retinal neovascularization	Epididymitis/orchitis
Vitreal bleeding	Glomerulonephritis
Neurologic manifestations (20%) (15)	Amyloid deposition
Headache	
Aseptic meningitis	

($<$2 mm) to larger lesions ($\geq$2 cm). They can be found in focal areas or diffusely throughout the oropharynx. Oral ulcers may develop or worsen after patients ingest hard substances such as nuts or crackers, likely representing an inflammatory process triggered by microtrauma, similar to the pathergy response described next, although in the case of English walnut ingestion, there may also be an immunomodulatory function of the nuts (18,19). Interestingly, cigarette smoking may decrease the frequency of oral ulcers (20).

    Ocular. Ocular disease is common in Adamantiades-Behçet's and in one series, occurred in some form in up to 75% of patients (14). Uveitis, the eye manifestation most commonly seen, is often bilateral and recurrent, and can involve the entire uveal tract, findings that are unusual in other autoimmune diseases of the eye. Severe anterior uveitis may lead to hypopyon, with inflammatory cells accumulating in the anterior chamber and, this finding, assuming that infection is not present, can be very suggestive of Adamantiades-Behçet's disease (Fig. 2) (21). Isolated posterior uveitis, venous vascular occlusion, and optic neuritis may also occur and may rapidly progress to blindness if left untreated (Fig. 3). Other ocular changes seen include secondary cataracts and glaucoma from inflammation and corticosteroid use, adhesions of the iris to the lens, retinal neovascularization with vitreal bleeding, and conjunctival ulceration (Fig. 4). Eye disease usually appears at the same time as other manifestations of Adamantiades-Behçet's, but in some cases, can present late in the disease course, and subclinical inflammation may persist in between major flares, leading to progressive vision loss. Predictors for more severe vision loss include young age at onset,

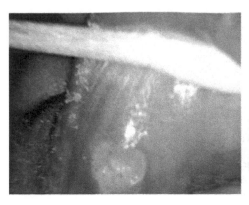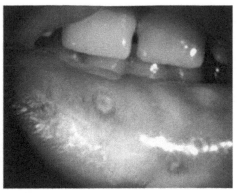

FIGURE 1   Oral ulcerations in Behçet's disease. *Source*: Courtesy of Pamela Chavis, MD. From Ref. 17.

male gender, bilateral disease, and panuveitis or retinal vasculitis; these patients should be treated aggressively to prevent blindness (14).

Systemic Manifestations

General Manifestations.   Patients with Adamantiades-Behçet's can experience any number of nonspecific symptoms including malaise, anorexia and weight loss, generalized weakness, fevers, lymphadenopathy, and headache (10). In some cases, these symptoms can predate the appearance of ulcerations, making initial diagnosis difficult.

Articular.   The arthritis seen in Adamantiades-Behçet's is variable, with polyarticular and monoarticular forms seen. The most commonly involved joints are the knees, wrists, ankles, and elbows. The arthritis is typically inflammatory but nonerosive. Sacroiliitis is not typically seen with Adamantiades-Behçet's and, if present, may represent HLA-B27–associated disease.

Cutaneous.   There are multiple skin lesions described in Adamantiades-Behçet's, including erythema nodosum, papular/pustular eruptions, folliculitis, and lesions similar to acne (Figs 4 and 5). The classic lesion is termed "pathergy," where a pustular lesion develops at a site of recent trauma (Figs 6 and 7). In the clinical setting, these lesions can occur at the site of needle punctures, and for diagnosis, are defined as the occurrence of a papular/pustular lesion at the site of oblique angle needle stick (20–25 gauge) 24 to 48 hours

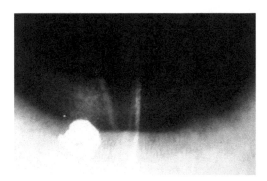

FIGURE 2   Anterior uveitis with hypopyon in Behçet's disease. *Source*: Courtesy of Pamela Chavis, MD. From Ref. 17.

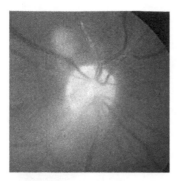

FIGURE 3 Retinal vasculitis with blurred disk margins and vascular abnormalities. *Source*: Courtesy of Pamela Chavis, MD. From Ref. 17.

later. Recurrent genital ulcerations also occur, with features similar to the oral ulcerations described above, although they tend to scar more frequently than the oral lesions (Fig. 8). Genital ulcerations can be located externally on the vulva, scrotal or penile tissue, or internally in the vaginal vault and on the cervix. They can also appear in the groin region and can rarely occur on the perineum and perianal area. A subset of Adamantiades-Behçet's that includes mouth and genital ulcers with inflamed cartilage has been termed the "MAGIC" syndrome and likely represents an overlap between Adamantiades-Behçet's and relapsing polychondritis (21).

Nervous System. Neurologic involvement in Adamantiades-Behçet's can be seen in up to 20% of patients (15). Multiple nervous system lesions have been described, including brain parenchymal disease, vasculitic brain stem or spinal tract involvement, aseptic meningitis, venous thrombosis, aneurysms, and peripheral neuropathy. Central nervous system involvement usually indicates a poorer prognosis, especially if abnormal cerebrospinal fluid is found or brain parenchymal disease is present (23).

Gastrointestinal. Patients with Adamantiades-Behçet's may have upper gastrointestinal (GI), gastric, small bowel, or large bowel involvement. GI ulcerations are similar in appearance to those seen in the orogenital regions and can lead to significant bleeding or intestinal perforation (4,5). If GI ulceration is present, evaluation for inflammatory bowel disease such as Crohn's disease or ulcerative colitis, both of which can mimic Adamantiades-Behçet's, should be considered.

Pulmonary. Lung manifestations may be present in up to 8% of patients with Adamantiades-Behçet's; these include thromboembolic events, inflammatory lung disease with pleuritis, bronchiolitis obliterans, vasculitic pneumonias, pulmonary hypertension, and

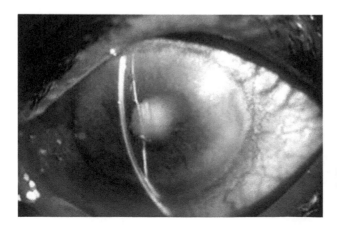

FIGURE 4 Cataract and posterior synechiae in Behçet's disease. *Source*: Courtesy of Pamela Chavis, MD. From Ref. 17.

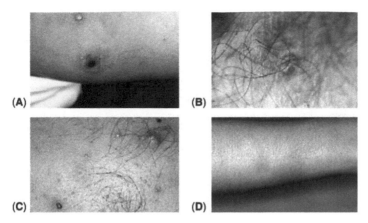

FIGURE 5   Skin lesions in Behçet's disease; (A) Ulcerative lesion; (B) pustular lesion; (C) Acneiform/pustular lesions; (D) erythema nodosum. *Source*: Courtesy of Pamela Chavis, MD. From Ref. 17.

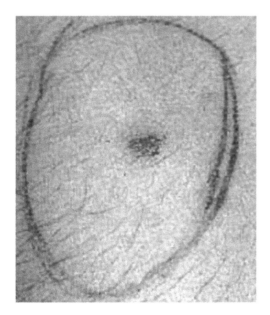

FIGURE 6   Mild pathergy in Behçet's disease. *Source*: Courtesy of Pamela Chavis, MD. From Ref. 17.

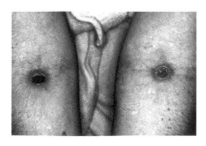

FIGURE 7   Severe pathergy in Behçet's disease. *Source*: Courtesy of NZ DermNet. From Ref. 22.

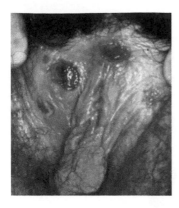

FIGURE 8 Vulvar ulcerations in Behçet's disease. *Source*: Courtesy of NZ DermNet. From Ref. 22.

fibrosis (16,24). One of the most feared, as well as most common, pulmonary complications of Adamantiades-Behçet's is the development of pulmonary artery aneurysms, which are due to vasculitis of the vaso vasorum of the pulmonary vasculature (24,25). Clinically, patients with aneurysms may present with mild hemoptysis, although massive fatal hemoptysis has been reported as a presenting symptom (16). As might be expected, rupture of these aneurysms is associated with significant mortality. In patients with Adamantiades-Behçet's who present with hemoptysis, a search for an underlying aneurysm should be performed. Computed tomography (CT), angiography, magnetic resonance imaging, and ventilation-perfusion scanning have been used to identify lesions which, if seen early and treated with immunosuppression, may regress, leading to improved outcomes (26). Pulmonary complications of Adamantiades–Behçet's usually occur in the setting of the complete syndrome, but can be seen without obvious systemic involvement, and it is suggested that the Hughes-Stovin syndrome of isolated pulmonary artery aneurysms may be a *forme fruste* of Adamantiades-Behçet's (27).

   Other.   Renal manifestations of Adamantiades-Behçet's are rare and are thought to be due to immune complex deposition (28). Cardiac involvement can include conduction abnormalities, endomyocardial fibrosis, vasculitic infarction or myocarditis, pericarditis, or cardiac or aortic aneurysm formation, with histopathology similar to the lesions seen in pulmonary arterial aneurysms. Epididymitis and orchitis may occur in conjunction with genital ulcerations. Nailfold capillary abnormalities are present in a subset of patients with Adamantiades-Behçet's (29). Secondary amyloid deposition can occur with uncontrolled disease.

DIAGNOSIS

The diagnosis of Adamantiades-Behçet's is a clinical one, as there are not yet any specific biomarkers for disease available. Several sets of diagnostic criteria are available to assist in making the diagnosis of Adamantiades-Behçet's, each with varying sensitivity and specificity for disease classification. Perhaps the most commonly used set of criteria is the International Study Group's Criteria for the Diagnosis of Adamantiades-Behçet's Disease, established in 1990 (Table 2) (30). This set of criteria has a sensitivity of 91% and specificity of 96%, although some feel that its inclusion of acneiform lesions decreases specificity, and recommend that these lesions, if present, be biopsied to confirm vasculitis (4).

   Nonspecific tests including inflammatory anemia and markers such as elevated erythrocyte sedimentation rate and C-reactive protein can be present during flares. Serum-soluble ICAM-1, a marker of neutrophil activation, has been shown to be elevated in patients with active disease; however, its use in diagnosis is limited (31).

Antibodies against the endothelial cell component α-enolase may prove to be specific markers for disease activity, but further studies are needed (9,10). Antinuclear antibodies, antineutrophil cytoplasmic antibodies, and rheumatoid factor are not associated with disease, and, if present, may indicate that another autoimmune process is present. Testing for the Adamantiades-Behçet's–associated HLA-B51 or -B52 alleles is not commonly performed for diagnostic purposes.

Further evaluation for involvement of specific organ systems should be performed as symptoms and signs dictate, although due to potentially catastrophic consequences if lung aneurysms are missed, some advocate pulmonary imaging in all cases of Adamantiades-Behçet's (16).

DIFFERENTIAL DIAGNOSIS

Multiple diseases can present with findings similar to those seen with Adamantiades-Behçet's disease and should be considered when a patient presents with recurrent oral or genital ulcers, inflammatory eye disease, or other manifestations of vasculitis. Included in the differential diagnosis are systemic lupus erythematosus (Chapter 1), seronegative spondyloarthropathies, inflammatory bowel disease (Crohn's or ulcerative colitis) (Chapter 20), herpes or other viral infections (Chapter 10), other forms of vasculitis (Chapter 8), and inflammatory skin diseases such as pemphigus vulgaris or pemphigoid lesions (Chapter 37). All patients presenting with oral and genital ulcerations should undergo testing for herpes simplex virus using culture or polymerase chain reaction methods, to ensure that viral infection is not present.

TABLE 2   International Study Group Criteria for the Diagnosis of Behçet's Disease[a]

Recurrent oral ulceration
  Minor aphthous, major aphthous, or herpetiform ulceration observed by a physician or
    patient that recurred at least three times in one 12-mo period
Plus, two of the following criteria
Recurrent genital ulceration
  Aphthous ulceration or scarring observed by physician or patient
Eye lesions
  Anterior uveitis, posterior uveitis, or cells in vitreous on slit-lamp examination
    Or
  Retinal vasculitis observed by ophthalmologist
Skin lesions
  Erythema nodosum observed by a physician or patient, pseudofolliculitis, or
    papulopustular lesions
    Or
  Acneiform nodules observed by a physician in postadolescent patients not on corticosteroid
    treatment
Positive result on pathergy testing[b]
  Read by a physician at 24–48 hr

[a]Findings applicable only in the absence of other clinical explanations (systemic lupus erythematosus, inflammatory bowel disease, seronegative spondyloarthropathies, and viral infections).
[b]Pathergy testing is performed by pricking the skin with a 20–25 gauge needle. A positive test is defined as a papular/ pustular lesion >2 mm that appears at the site 24–48 hr later.
Source: From Ref. 30.

TREATMENT

Treatment depends on organ involvement and severity of disease (Table 3). Mild orogenital ulcerative disease can be treated on a periodic basis; however, severe systemic disease may require chronic immunosuppressive therapy. For mild oral or genital ulcerations, topical anesthetics or corticosteroids can be used. Oral colchicine (0.6–1.8 mg/day) and dapsone are also effective. For more severe mucocutaneous disease, oral corticosteroids, azathioprine, or methotrexate can be used. Thalidomide has also been shown to be effective for more severe mucocutaneous disease, but due to its association with birth defects, its use in the United States requires adherence to the federally mandated drug use pathway (32). Interferon-α (IFN-α) therapy has also been used for severe mucocutaneous and systemic manifestations of disease (33). Additionally, antitumor necrosis factor-α (INF-α) therapy with etanercept or infliximab has been shown to improve mucocutaneous lesions and features of systemic disease (34).

For ocular disease, past treatment algorithms included the use of high-dose corticosteroids, cyclosporine, and cytotoxics such as chlorambucil and cyclophosphamide. However, there is growing evidence that anti–TNF-α therapy can lead to rapid resolution of uveitis and retinal vasculitis, and its early use in severe ocular disease should be considered (34,35). The anti–TNF-α agent best studied for ocular Adamantiades-Behçet's is infliximab. Although some have seen improvement in disease with a single infusion, to maintain disease control, infliximab is usually dosed at 5 mg/kg at four- to eight-week intervals once drug loading at weeks 0, 2, and 6 has been performed (35,36). The duration of therapy needed for control of eye disease is unknown, but many propose that immunosuppressive therapy be continued for at least one year after resolution of inflammation, although many patients may require prolonged therapy to control disease, as well as concomitant use of other immunosuppressive agents to ensure control.

For nervous system disease, treatment with potent immunosuppressive agents, including use of high-dose corticosteroids and antimetabolite or cytotoxic therapies, is needed. The use of anti–TNF-α agents in nervous system manifestation of disease is not well studied, but may also be beneficial (37).

For superficial thrombophlebitis, local therapy including heat and cold along with aspirin or other nonsteroidal anti-inflammatory therapy may be adequate. If deep venous thrombosis is present, full anticoagulation should be considered.

Determining who to screen for pulmonary aneurysms is difficult. Some advocate evaluating all patients with Adamantiades-Behçet's for pulmonary aneurysms, but this is costly and may not be necessary for all patients. Certainly, if a patient presents with hemoptysis, further imaging should be performed, with contrasted CT imaging being the preferred initial diagnostic test. If pulmonary embolism is suspected, evaluation for the presence of aneurysms should also be performed, as there have been cases of death reported in patients who are anticoagulated for presumed embolus, with resultant severe pulmonary hemorrhage from undiagnosed aneurysms (16,25). If pulmonary artery aneurysms are identified, combinations of cytotoxic therapy and high-dose corticosteroids, followed by long-term immunosuppressive therapy, are recommended, although no controlled trials have been performed (16). The role of anti–TNF-α therapy in the treatment of arterial aneurysms is unknown. For patients with active bleeding from an aneurysm, methylprednisolone dosed at 1000 mg intravenously daily for three to five days, along with pulse-dose cyclophosphamide, should be administered, with consideration of embolization or surgical intervention if symptoms are not controlled (16).

TABLE 3 Treatment of Behçet's Disease

Mild mucocutaneous disease
  Topical anesthetics
  Topical or intralesional corticosteroids
  Topical tacrolimus
  Topical tetracycline solutions
  Oral tetracycline or macrolide agents
  Topical amlexanox (paste)
  Sucralfate
  Oral colchicine
  Oral dapsone (25–200 mg daily)
  Antimalarials
  Rebamipide (mucoprotective agent)
Severe mucocutaneous disease
  Thalidomide
  Oral corticosteroids (0.5–1.0 mg/kg/day)
  Methotrexate
  Azathioprine
  Interferon-α
  Anti-TNF-α agents
Systemic disease
  Systemic corticosteroids
  Intravenous immunoglobulin
  Sulfasalazine
  Methotrexate
  Azathioprine
  Cyclophosphamide
  Chlorambucil
  Cyclosporine
  Anti–TNF-α agents
Ocular disease
  Corticosteroids (including intraocular injection)
  Cyclophosphamide
  Chlorambucil
  Azathioprine
  Cyclosporine
  Consideration of early use of anti–TNF-α agents (infliximab)
Pulmonary or thrombotic disease
  Pulmonary or aortic aneurysms—systemic corticosteroids, cytotoxic agents
  Superficial thrombophlebitis—local therapies, aspirin, nonsteroidal anti-inflammatory agents
  Deep venous thrombosis—heparin, warfarin

Abbreviation: TNF, tumor necrosis factor.

COMPLICATIONS AND PROGNOSIS

The disease course in Adamantiades-Behçet's is characterized by exacerbations and remissions, with a decrease in severity as patients become older (38). Patients should be counseled that while in some cases, the disease remits after a few years, in others, longer-term medications are required to control symptoms. The most severe disease is seen in younger males of Mediterranean descent, but even in this group, disease tends to be less damaging as patients age (38). Oral or genital ulcerations are usually the initial findings of disease, with other manifestations including ocular and nervous system involvement occurring simultaneously, although in some cases, eye and neurologic disease may occur years after ulcerations first appear. In addition, chronic uveal inflammation can lead to significant vision loss or blindness in over 50% of patients with untreated eye disease (39) and requires close ophthalmologic follow-up to ensure that inflammation is controlled.

Mortality occurs usually from rupture of pulmonary artery aneurysms, large-vessel thrombosis, severe GI involvement with perforations or the development of the Budd-Chiari syndrome, or infections as a result of immunosuppressive therapy. Mortality is highest in young male patients of Turkish descent, with standardized mortality rates in this group up to 10 times greater than normal, with decreases in these ratios as age at diagnosis increases and as duration of follow-up continues (39). Mortality rates from Adamantiades-Behçet's are lower for patients of European descent, although exact rates are difficult to determine, due to the rarity of disease.

IFN-α2a has been used in a number of trials, and some data regarding remission rates in Adamantiades-Behçet's are available. In one study of patients with panuveitis, IFN-α2a was used for a mean duration of 40 months with remission in 9/10 subjects (40). There is little data regarding the long-term remissions of other manifestations of disease with IFN-α2a, however. A review published in 2004 showed that the use of IFN-α2a resulted in improvement of articular disease and mucocutaneous disease in 95% and 86% of treated patients, respectively (41), but long-term data regarding efficacy with neurologic and vascular disease and overall mortality need to be obtained. The more recent use of anti-TNF agents, specifically infliximab, in Adamantiades-Behçet's will likely alter the morbidity and mortality seen in the past with this disease, but further studies are needed.

SUMMARY

Adamantiades-Behçet's disease is a systemic vasculitis of unclear etiology, with a worldwide distribution but more commonly seen in Mediterranean and Asian countries. The diagnosis of Adamantiades-Behçet's should be considered in patients presenting with orogenital ulcerations, skin disease, and inflammatory eye disease. Diagnosis can be difficult and requires a high index of suspicion, especially when not all diagnostic features are present. Treatment depends on the severity of disease manifestations, weighing the toxicity of medications with risk of adverse disease outcomes. Special attention should be paid to treatment of ocular disease, to prevent long-term morbidity from vision loss, and to identification of occult arterial aneurysms. Anti–TNF-α agents are proving to be effective therapies for disease and may reduce the need for cytotoxic therapy with Adamantiades-Behçet's in the future.

REFERENCES

1. Cheng TO. Some historical notes on Behçet's disease. Chest 2001; 119:667–668.
2. Adamantiades B. A case of relapsing iritis with hypopyon (in Greek). Archia Iatrikis Etairias (Proceedings of the Medical Society of Athens) 1930; 586–593.
3. Behçet H. Uber rezidivierende, aphthose durch ein virus verursachte geschwure am mund, am auge und an der genitalen. Dermatologische Wochenschrift 1937; 105:1152–1157.
4. Sakane T, Takeno M, Suzuki N, et al. Behçet's disease. N Engl J Med 1999; 341(17): 1284–1291.
5. Garton RA, Ghate JV, Jorizzo JL. Behçet's disease. In: Harris ED, Budd RC, Firestein GS, et al., eds. Kelly's Textbook of Rheumatology. 7th ed. Philadelphia: Elsevier Science, 2005: 1396–1401.
6. Zouboulis CC, May T. Pathogenesis of Adamantiades-Behçet's disease. Adv Exp Med Biol 2003; 528:161–171.
7. Direskeneli H. Behçet's disease: infectious aetiology, new autoantigens, and HLA-B51. Ann Rheum Dis 2001; 60:996–1002.
8. Navarro S, Ricart JM, Medina P, et al. Activated protein C levels in Behçet's disease and risk of venous thrombosis. Br J Haematol 2004; 126(4):550–556.
9. Musabak U, Baylan O, Cetin T, et al. Lipid profile and anticardiolipin antibodies in Behçet's disease. Arch Med Res 2005; 36(4):387–392.

10. Yurdakul S, Hamuryudan V, Yazici H. Behçet syndrome. Curr Opin Rheumatol 2004; 16(1):38–42.
11. Atagunduz P, Ergun T, Direskeneli H. MEFV mutations are increased in Behçet's disease (BD) and are associated with vascular involvement. Clin Exp Rheumatol 2003; 21(4 suppl 30):S35–S37.
12. Salvarani C, Boiardi L, Casali B, et al. Vascular endothelial growth factor gene polymorphisms in Behçet's disease. J Rheumatol 2004; 31(9):1785–1789.
13. Salvarani C, Boiardi L, Casali B, et al. Endothelial nitric oxide synthase gene polymorphisms in Behçet's disease. J Rheumatol 2002; 29(3):535–540.
14. Kansu T, Kadayifcilar S. Visual aspects of Behçet's disease. Curr Neurol Neurosci Rep 2005; 5(5):382–388.
15. Serdaroglu P. Behçet's disease and the nervous system. J Neurol 1998; 245(4):197–205.
16. Erkan F, Gul A, Tasali E. Pulmonary manifestations of Behçet's disease. Thorax 2001; 56(7): 572–578. [Comment in Thorax 2002; 57(5):469–470.]
17. www.eyetext.net
18. Kikuchi I. The effects of walnuts on Behçet's syndrome in two sisters. J Dermatol 1985; 12(3):290–291.
19. Marquardt JL, Snyderman R, Oppenheim JJ. Depression of lymphocyte transformation and exacerbation of Behçet's syndrome by ingestion of English walnuts. Cell Immunol 1973; 9(2): 263–272.
20. Soy M, Erken E, Konca K, et al. Smoking and Behçet's disease. Clin Rheumatol 2000; 19(6): 508–509.
21. Firestein GS, Gruber HE, Weisman MH, et al. Mouth and genital ulcers with inflamed cartilage: MAGIC syndrome. Five patients with features of relapsing polychondritis and Behçet's disease. Am J Med 1985; 79(1):65–72.
22. http://www.dermnetnz.org
23. Akman-Demir G, Serdaroglu P, Tasci B. Clinical patterns of neurological involvement in Behçet's disease: evaluation of 200 patients. The Neuro-Behçet Study Group. Brain 1999; 122(11):2171–2182.
24. Raz I, Okon E, Chajek-Shaul T. Pulmonary manifestations in Behçet's syndrome. Chest 1989; 95:585–589.
25. Uzun O, Akpolat T, Erkan L. Pulmonary vasculitis in Behçet disease: a cumulative analysis. Chest 2005; 127(6):2243–2253.
26. Tunaci M, Ozkorkmaz B, Tunaci A, et al. CT findings of pulmonary artery aneurysms during treatment for Behçet's disease. Am J Roentgenol 1999; 172(3):729–733.
27. Erkan D, Yazici Y, Sanders A, et al. Is Hughes–Stovin syndrome Behçet's disease? Clin Exp Rheumatol 2004; 22(4 suppl 34):S64–S68.
28. Kaklamani VG, Nikolopoulou N, Sotsiou F, et al. Renal involvement in Adamantiades-Behçet's disease. Case report and review of the literature. Clin Exp Rheumatol 2001; 19(5 suppl 24): S55–S58.
29. Vaiopoulos G, Pangratis N, Samarkos M, et al. Nailfold capillary abnormalities in Behçet's disease. J Rheumatol 1995; 22(6):1108–1111.
30. International Study Group for Behçet's Disease. Criteria for the diagnosis of Behçet's Disease. Lancet 1990; 335(8697):1078–1080.
31. Saglam K, Yilmaz MI, Saglam A, et al. Levels of circulating intracellular adhesion molecule-1 in patients with Behçet's disease. Rheumatol Int 2002; 21(4):146–148.
32. Hamuryudan V, Mat C, Saip S, et al. Thalidomide in the treatment of the mucocutaneous lesions of Behçet's syndrome. A randomized double-blinded, placebo controlled trial. Ann Intern Med 1998; 128(6):443–450.
33. Zouboulis CC, Orfanos CE. Treatment of Adamantiades-Behçet disease with systemic interferon alpha. Arch Dermatol 1998; 134(8):1010–1016.
34. Sfikakis PP. Behçet's disease: a new target for anti-tumour necrosis factor treatment. Ann Rheum Dis 2002; 61 (suppl 2):ii51–ii53.
35. Tugal-Tutkun I, Mudun A, Urgancioglu M, et al. Efficacy of infliximab in the treatment of uveitis that is resistant to treatment with the combination of azathioprine, cyclosporine, and corticosteroids in Behçet's disease: an open-label trial. Arthritis Rheum 2005; 52(8):2478–2484.
36. Ohno S, Nakamura S, Hori S, et al. Efficacy, safety, and pharmacokinetics of multiple administration of infliximab in Behçet's disease with refractory uveoretinitis. J Rheumatol 2004; 31(7):1362–1368.
37. Sarwar H, McGrath H Jr, Espinoza LR. Successful treatment of long-standing neuro-Behçet's disease with infliximab. J Rheumatol 2005; 32(1):181–183.
38. Yazici H, Basaran G, Hamuryudan V, et al. The ten-year mortality in Behçet's syndrome. Br J Rheumatol 1996; 35(2):139–141.

39. Kural-Seyahi E, Fresko I, Seyahi N, et al. The long-term mortality and morbidity of Behçet syndrome: a 2-decade outcome survey of 387 patients followed at a dedicated center. Medicine (Baltimore) 2003; 82(1):60–76.
40. Deuter CM, Kotter I, Gunaydin I, et al. Ocular involvement in Behçet's disease: first 5-year results for visual development after treatment with interferon alpha-2a [German]. Opthalmologe 2004; 101 (2):129–134.
41. Kotter I, Gunaydin I, Zierhut M, et al. The use of interferon alpha in Behçet's disease: review of the literature. Semin Arthritis Rheum 2004; 33(5):320–335.

4

Giant Cell Arteritis and Polymyalgia Rheumatica

Tim Bongartz and Eric L. Matteson
Division of Rheumatology, Mayo Clinic College of Medicine, Rochester, Minnesota, U.S.A.

INTRODUCTION

Giant cell arteritis (GCA) and polymyalgia rheumatica (PMR) are relatively common diseases of the middle aged and elderly. Their cause is unknown, and their incidence increases with age (1). The two conditions are genetically and clinically linked, although there are differences in their pathophysiology (2). They are systemic diseases frequently associated with constitutional symptoms including fevers, malaise, and weight loss. Both conditions may present with pain and stiffness of the neck and shoulder girdle muscles. GCA may also present with ear, nose, and throat manifestations.

DEFINITIONS

PMR is a clinical syndrome whose cause is unknown. There is no universally accepted definition, but several classification criteria include patients over the age of 50 years, who have moderate-to-severe aching and stiffness of the neck, torso, shoulders, or proximal regions of the arms, hips, or thighs, of at least one-month duration, with morning stiffness and elevated markers of systemic inflammation such as erythrocyte sedimentation rate (ESR) (3).

PMR often occurs in association with GCA (temporal) and may be the initial clinical feature of GCA. About 50% of patients with GCA have PMR, and between 10% and 40% of patients with PMR have GCA as the underlying disease. GCA is a chronic vasculitis of medium and large arteries. Although a systemic disease, symptomatic arterial inflammation most typically involves the cranial branches of the arteries having their origin at the aortic arch, leading to its characteristic head and neck disease features. The American College of Rheumatology criteria for the classification of GCA separate it from other primary vasculitides on the basis of five essential features (4). These are age at onset of greater than 50 years, new onset of head pain, abnormality of the temporal artery with tenderness to palpation or decreased pulse not related to atherosclerosis, elevation of the ESR (generally greater than 50 mm in the first hour by Westergren method), and abnormal findings of vasculitis on biopsy of the temporal artery.

EPIDEMIOLOGY

The incidence of new cases of PMR occurring among individuals over the age of 50 is 52.5 cases per 100,000 persons per year (3). The prevalence of PMR is approximately 600 per 100,000 persons over the age of 50. It is principally a disease of Caucasians, although it does occur in persons of other ethnic backgrounds. Approximately 70% of cases are women.

GCA is the most frequent idiopathic vasculitis, with an incidence of approximately 18 new cases per 100,000 persons over the age of 50 per year (3). Its prevalence is approximately 200 cases per 100,000 persons over the age of 50. If viewed over decades, the incidence of GCA fluctuates in a cyclic pattern, suggesting an infectious etiology, although a specific infectious etiology has thus far not been demonstrated. Like PMR, the disease is most common in Caucasians, particularly those of Northern European origin, and it is more common in Northern Europe than in Southern Europe. The average age of onset is 73 years, and 70% of patients are women.

PATHOGENESIS

The etiology of PMR and GCA is unknown. They are autoimmune disorders that may be triggered by exogenous factors, particularly infection in genetically susceptible individuals. HLA-DR4 antigens are present in roughly twice as many patients with GCA as in controls, and there is evidence that HLA class II–restricted CD4 positive-activated helper cells drive the disease (2). CD8-positive T-lymphocyte counts appear to be lower in patients with PMR and GCA.

The cell-mediated, antigen-driven response in GCA occurs in the arterial wall. There is T-cell activation likely to an antigen in the arterial wall, although it is not known whether this is exogenous, such as a viral product, or a component of the artery itself. The result is a granulomatous inflammation with giant cells, particularly at the intima and medial junction, seen in about 50% of cases. The remaining 50% of patients have a panarteritis with a mixed cell inflammatory infiltrate of lymphocytic and mononuclear cells and some neutrophils and eosinophils, without giant cells being present.

Antigen is recognized in the adventitia by T-cells that undergo clonal expansion and produce interferon-γ. This results in the differentiation and migration of macrophages and formation of giant cells. In the adventitia, macrophages produce interleukin (IL)-1 and IL-6; in the media, macrophages produce metalloproteinases; and in the intima, nitric oxide along with platelet-derived growth factor and vascular endothelial growth factor repair efforts destroy the vessel wall. Resultant inflammation of the arteries of the aortic arch and the primary branches causes focal and segmental disruption of the internal elastic lamina. Some patients with GCA have minimal systemic inflammatory disease with primary ischemic manifestations, while others have mainly PMR-related symptoms. The clinical variations in disease are correlated with local expression of cytokine messenger RNA (4). Ischemic symptoms occur with high levels of interferon-γ and IL-1B. Patients with fever tend to have low levels of interferon-γ, and patients with PMR and large vessel arteritis including aortitis have higher levels of IL-2.

CLINICAL MANIFESTATIONS

The onset of GCA and PMR symptoms is usually gradual, although in some patients, the disease presents abruptly (1,3). Systemic symptoms including fever, fatigue, and weight loss occur in approximately half of the patients, and in some patients, the fever may be as high as 40°C. Patients with PMR have bilateral proximal limb discomfort, which may restrict movement. Typically, about one-third of patients will have systemic manifestations. Some patients with PMR develop a peripheral arthritis, especially of the knees and wrists, and also may develop pitting edema of the dorsum of the hands, feet, and ankles (5).

Like PMR, the onset of GCA is usually gradual. About 50% of patients have systemic features including fever. Two-thirds of patients complain of headache, which may be located over the temporal, parietal, or occipital area but may be more diffuse. Scalp tenderness often accompanies the headache. At presentation, about 25% of patients have symptoms of PMR, and about 15% of patients have fevers, while one-third of patients will have headache as the initial presenting feature (1,3,5). Larger artery involvement in GCA occurs in approximately 15% of patients.

Early manifestations of larger artery involvement can include arm, or less frequently, leg claudication with absent or markedly diminished extremity pulses. Aortic aneurysms are 17 times more frequent in patients with GCA than nonaffected controls, with an incidence of approximately 15% (1,3). Large artery stenosis frequently presents within the first year of disease, while aneurysms are a late complication occurring after a mean of approximately five years of disease (6). Tables 1 and 2 contain a summary of the frequency of GCA-related symptoms on presentation and their prevalence.

Head and Neck
A plethora of head and neck symptoms and signs are associated with GCA. These are summarized in Table 3.

TABLE 1   The Initial Clinical Manifestations in 100 Consecutive
Patients with GCA

Clinical feature	Percentage
Headache	32
Polymyalgia rheumatica	25
Fever	15
Visual symptoms without visual loss	7
Fatigue/malaise	5
Myalgias or tender artery	3
Weight loss/anorexia	2
Jaw claudication	2
Visual loss	1
Tongue claudication	1
Sore throat	1
Vasculitis on angiogram	1
Hand and wrist stiffness	1

Abbreviation: GCA, giant cell arteritis.
Source: From Ref. 7.

TABLE 2   Prevalence of Selected Clinical Features in
100 Patients with GCA

Clinical feature	Percentage
Gender (female/male)	69/31
Constitutional symptoms	
Weight loss or anorexia	50
Fever	42
Malaise, fatigue, or weakness	40
Polymyalgia rheumatica	39
Other musculoskeletal pains	30
Synovitis	15
Symptoms related to arteries	83
Headache	68
Visual disturbance	30
Permanent visual loss	14
Jaw claudication	45
Dysphagia or swallowing claudication	8
Tongue claudication	6
Limb claudication	4
Signs related to arteries	66
Artery tenderness	27
Decreased temporal artery pulse	46
Swollen, nodular, or erythematous scalp arteries	23
Large artery bruit	21
Diminished large artery pulse	7
Central nervous system abnormalities	3
Sore throat	15

a, duration of symptoms before diagnosis was 7 months (range 1–48 months).
Abbreviation: GCA, giant cell arteritis.
Source: From Ref. 7.

TABLE 3 Head and Neck Symptoms and Findings of GCA

Organ	Symptoms and findings
Vessels	Pulselessness, thickening, pain on palpation, painful arterial nodules
Skin	Erythema, facial swelling, facial pain, and ischemic changes with necrosis
Jaw and masticatory muscles	Intermittent claudication of the jaw muscles, trismus, temporal mandibular joint pain, and tooth and gum pain
Mouth, oral cavity, pharynx, and larynx	Swelling and pain of the oral and nasal mucosa, dysphagia, tongue pain, ischemic tongue discoloration, tongue necrosis, necrosis of the oral mucosa, ulcerating glossitis and pharyngitis, hoarseness, anosmia, and ageusia
Ear	Ear pain, nystagmus, dizziness, hearing loss, and tinnitus
Salivary glands	Swelling
Lymph nodes and tonsils	Swelling

Abbreviation: GCA, giant cell arteritis.

Vascular and Skin. Thickening, pulselessness, pain with palpation, and the appearance of painful nodules of the affected arteries occur typically in the temporal artery but also may occur in other branches of the external carotid artery, particularly the facial, maxillary, occipital, and posterior auricular arteries (Fig. 1). Typical skin changes include erythema and local or generalized facial swelling and pain. Soft-tissue swelling may occur, particularly in the periorbital and cheek areas. Ischemic changes and necrosis of the skin may occur and may even lead to local bone destruction, but this is rare, since the temporal artery generally has good collateral formation (Fig. 2). Biopsies of the affected skin generally reveal nonspecific inflammatory changes or endarteritic obliterative changes.

Mouth and Neck. Jaw claudication is almost pathognomonic for GCA and can be severe enough to cause trismus (7). Symptoms of GCA in the oral cavity and the oropharynx are characterized especially by swelling and pain, as well as dysphagia, with burning tongue pain, pale discoloration, and swelling, which, in extreme cases, may necessitate a tracheotomy.

Tongue necrosis likely occurs when both the right and the left lingual arteries are obliterated and the collaterals become stenotic. Toothache and/or gum pain may be constant and lead to initial evaluation by a dentist. Dysarthria, dysphagia, and myosis are relatively rarely reported (7–9).

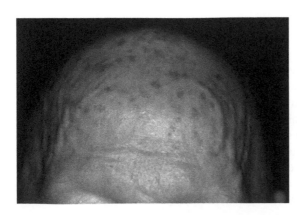

FIGURE 1 Markedly dilated temporal arteries in a 74-yr-old man with GCA. The arteries are visibly thickened and inflamed; palpation of the vessel is painful. *Abbreviation*: GCA, giant cell arteritis. *Source*: Courtesy of Lester Mertz, MD, Mayo Clinic Rochester, MN, U.S.A.

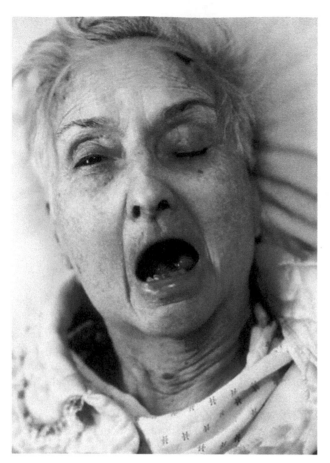

FIGURE 2 Scalp necrosis resulting from infarction of the temporal artery. There is also tongue necrosis and ptosis on the left. The patient had developed sudden hearing loss of the left ear as well. *Source*: Courtesy of Gene G. Hunder, MD, Mayo Clinic, Rochester, MN, U.S.A.

A disturbance in taste and smell with ageusia and anosmia are rarely described, likely due to vasculitis-related ischemia of the hippocampal or the uncinate gyrus. Rarely, salivary glands may become swollen and on biopsy reveal perivascular lymphocytic infiltrates. Some patients develop sicca symptoms, although the etiology of these changes is uncertain (9).

Audiovestibular Manifestations.   Ear pain may be due to involvement of the tympanic artery and may be associated with inner ear disease. Patients may develop dizziness with nystagmus and hearing loss, which may be profound. These symptoms are due to involvement of the labyrinth or the central regions of the cochleovestibular nucleus. Tinnitus may appear.

Up to two-thirds of patients with GCA may complain of subjective hearing loss at diagnosis, while about 16% have hearing loss after three months of treatment (10,11). This compares with approximately 10% of patients who may develop subjective hearing loss with PMR (based on a small number of patients studied for this outcome, $N = 10$), while patients with PMR do not develop tinnitus, vertigo, dizziness, or disequilibrium (10). On audiometry, parameters of hearing may improve in approximately 30% of patients but further deteriorate at three-month follow-up in approximately 7% of patients (10). Subjective hearing loss occurs in about 60% of patients, irrespective of vestibular function. The hearing loss may be refractory to treatment. A study of 44 patients (66%) showed no significant change in hearing after three months of glucocorticosteroid treatment, while hearing was improved in 27%. This improvement was unilateral in two-thirds of cases, and hearing declined in 7% of patients (10).

A retrospective study of 271 patients with GCA revealed only four patients with concomitant sensorineural hearing loss (12). In clinical practice, significant hearing loss from GCA is likely the exception. Vestibular dysfunction may be asymptomatic but on formal vestibular testing may be present in close to 90% of patients with GCA (10). The hearing loss and vestibular symptoms may be steroid-responsive when treated early. When detected prior to onset of therapy and tested after initiation of therapy, these changes are found to be frequently reversible. After three months of glucocorticosteroid therapy, vestibular dysfunction was noted in about 30% of 44 patients studied for this outcome (10). Patients with vestibular dysfunction were more likely to have associated persistent head-shaking nystagmus, noted in 73% of patients with biopsy-proven GCA (10).

Neck. Thyroid disease has been associated with PMR/GCA in over 50 patients. In one review of 43 patients, 19 (44%) were found to have hypothyroidism, which was secondary to thyroiditis in five. Seventeen patients (40%) had thyrotoxicosis (9). Thyroid disease preceded or appeared simultaneously with GCA/PMR. However, at least two other studies evaluating these findings from a literature review of cases were not duplicated in studies specifically evaluating thyroid disease in GCA (9). Swelling of the cervical lymph glands may sometimes occur in the acute phase of GCA. Histology reveals nonspecific, inflammatory, hyperplastic changes.

Airways and Lungs

Respiratory tract symptoms may occur in about 9% of patients with GCA and are the initial manifestation in 4% of patients (13). GCA should be considered in an elderly patient with new onset of cough, hoarseness, or throat pain without obvious cause. In a series of 16 patients with respiratory tract manifestations, cough was noted in 11 patients, while 15 patients had a sore or tender throat, 3 had hoarseness, 1 had a sensation of choking, 4 had a sore tongue, and 2 complained of chest pain (13).

Eye

Visual symptoms and signs are common in GCA, and blindness is one of its most feared complications. These symptoms may be the initial manifestation of GCA, and in 20% of patients with visual findings, visual loss is the only or initial symptom (3,14,15). Most patients, however, have had complaints consistent with GCA, including headache and jaw pain, as well as fevers, for several weeks or months prior to the onset of visual loss. Ultimately, permanent partial or complete loss of vision in one or both eyes occurs in 20% of patients, with a range according to series of 10% to 60% (3,14,15). Most patients with GCA-related visual loss have an elevated sedimentation rate and often have thrombocytosis.

Partial loss of vision may be transient or permanent. Patients may describe a sensation of "a shade covering one eye," proceeding to complete blindness. Transient monocular visual loss (amaurosis fugax) precedes permanent visual loss in approximately 44% of patients. This pattern of visual loss resembles that seen in patients with atherosclerotic, cerebrovascular, or heart disease, except that in GCA the visual loss may be transient, bilateral, and postural, and related to a change in body position (3,14,15). Diplopia and visual hallucinations (Charles Bonnet syndrome) rarely may occur. In patients presenting with unilateral symptoms that are left untreated, the other eye frequently is affected within one to two weeks.

The visual loss is caused by ischemia of the optic nerve or optic tracks. It may be due to an arteritis of the ophthalmic or posterior ciliary artery branches and less often is due to occlusion of the retinal arterials. GCA, however, is an unusual cause of retinal artery occlusion, and only about 5% to 10% of patients with this complication have GCA. Branch retinal artery occlusion is less frequent, with vasculitis-related hypoperfusion of the ophthalmic or central retinal arteries. Retinal arterials are not directly affected in GCA. Patients with retinal ischemia have findings of "cotton wool" spots and intraretinal hemorrhages. Postural change, such as bending over or standing up from a sitting position, may result in sludging of blood, detected on funduscopic examination, with return to normal in the supine position.

Anterior ischemic optic neuropathy (AION) is the most common cause of vision loss in GCA (3,14,15). It is usually unilateral but may be bilateral with the second eye involved simultaneously or some days to many weeks following involvement of the first eye. Up to 50% of patients presenting with unilateral blindness will develop blindness in the opposite eye without treatment (3,7,15). The funduscopic findings are of a pale swelling and occasional hyperemia, cotton wool spots, and intraretinal hemorrhages (Fig. 3A and B). Arteritic AION is caused by vasculitic occlusion of the short posterior ciliary arteries to the retrolaminar and laminar portions of the optic disc.

AION due to vasculitis, like GCA must be differentiated from that due to nonarteritic, atherosclerotic disease. Patients with this complication are predominantly female, the sedimentation rate is elevated, and there are constitutional symptoms and other typical symptoms of GCA (16). Improvement is rare, even with high-dose glucocorticosteroid treatment (3,15,17). In patients with nonarteritic anterior ischemic neuropathy similar in age to those with GCA, the sedimentation rate is normal, and there are no constitutional symptoms (14,15). There is hyperemic disc swelling. Symptoms often occur upon awakening, and in 40% of patients, there may be improvement.

Posterior ischemic optic neuropathy (PION) is a much less common cause of visual loss in patients with GCA than in those with AION (7,14,15). It is frequently confused with retrobulbar optic neuropathy, and visual loss is often not profound. It is caused by disruption of blood flow to the retrolaminar portion of the optic nerve, with infarction of the posterior orbital or intracranial portion of the nerve and vasculitis of the ophthalmic and short posterior ciliary arteries. Both AION and PION can be associated with sectorial choroidal ischemia.

Bitemporal visual loss may also occur when the arteries of the optic chiasm are affected. Occipital lobe infarction from inflammatory disease in the vestibular basilar arteries can lead to bilateral homonymous deficits and cortical blindness. Diplopia is caused by damage to the brain stem. Some of these patients may have strabismus.

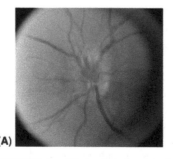
(A)
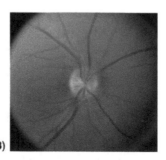
(B)

FIGURE 3 (A) Ischemic anterior optic neuropathy in a patient with GCA and sudden, nonprogressive visual loss. Left eye with pallid swelling affecting the optic disk. The superior pole is primarily affected with superficial retinal hemorrhages and nerve fiber layer edema. An afferent pupillary defect and an inferior altitudinal visual field defect were present. (B) The unaffected right eye with normal-appearing optic disc. *Abbreviation*: GCA, giant cell arteritis. *Source*: Courtesy of James Garrity, MD, Mayo Clinic Rochester, MN, U.S.A.

TABLE 4 Eye Disease in GCA

	Number of Patients	Percent
Visual manifestations	42	26.1
Permanent visual loss	24	14.9
Unilateral	16	9.9
Bilateral	8	5.0
Without amaurosis fugax	12	7.5
After amaurosis fugax	12	7.5
Transient visual loss	23	14.3
Diplopia	9	5.6

Abbreviation: GCA, giant cell arteritis.
Source: From Ref. 15.

Ischemic damage to the optic nerve or retina can cause unilateral or bilateral tonic pupils, usually with dilatation. Horner's syndrome has also been described in patients with GCA as the result of paralysis of the ocular motor or abducens nerve, ischemia of the cavernous sinus, or as a central process in the brain stem (14). Other ocular symptoms can include swelling about the eye with proptosis and periorbital swelling. Rarely, ocular hypotony may occur, as may marginal corneal ulcerations.

A retrospective study of eye disease occurring in 161 patients over a 17-year period provides a useful perspective of this complication (15). Visual manifestations occurred in about 26% of patients, and loss of vision in at least one eye occurred in about 15% (Table 4). Twenty-four patients had permanent vision loss; in 92% of these, anterior ischemic optic neuritis was the cause. Central retinal artery occlusion occurred in 8.3% of patients as the cause of permanent visual loss, and occipital infarction caused by vertebral basilar stroke occurred in one patient (4.2%). These authors noted that patients positive for HLA-DRB1 * 04 had visual manifestations more commonly than those who did not: the phenotype was found in 42% of patients versus 26% of controls (15).

DIAGNOSIS

The diagnosis of PMR/GCA is based upon typical clinical signs and symptoms, including shoulder and hip girdle aching and an elevated sedimentation rate in patients older than 50 years, and in GCA, new onset of localized headache with temporal artery tenderness, positive ESR, and an abnormal temporal artery biopsy.

GCA occasionally can occur with a low sedimentation rate. In a population-based study of 167 patients diagnosed between 1950 and 1998, 11% had an ESR of less than 50 mm in the first hour, and nine (5%) had ESRs of less than 40 mm per hour (17). These patients were less likely to have constitutional symptoms than patients with elevated ESRs. However, a review of 941 patients with biopsy-proven GCA found that only 4% had a normal ESR, underlining the sensitivity of an elevated sedimentation rate in the initial diagnosis of this condition (18).

A temporal artery biopsy should be performed in all patients in whom a diagnosis of GCA is suspected (19). Biopsies reveal medial and intimal inflammation and disruption of the internal elastic lamina. Lymphocytic and macrocytic infiltrates are typical, causing disruption of the arterial wall (Fig. 4). Multinucleated giant cells are frequently but not invariably present. Luminal occlusion and ischemia may result. The sensitivity of a temporal artery biopsy is 58% for diagnosis of GCA (20). A negative temporal artery biopsy has a high negative predictive value, 90%, so that if the temporal artery biopsy is negative, the patient may have GCA, but the probability is low (20). The predicting characteristics with which a

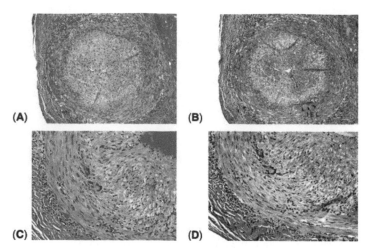

FIGURE 4 Photomicrographs of active arteritis in a temporal artery biopsy. (**A**) Transmural inflammation with marked intimal thickening (hematoxylin-eosin, 40X). (**B**) Elastic stain highlighting disruption of the IEL; arrows indicate a small segment of intact IEL (Verhoeff van Gieson, 40X). (**C**) Higher power view showing proliferation of intimal fibroblasts and transmural inflammation with multinucleated giant cells present at the media-intima junction (hematoxylin-eosin, 200X). (**D**) Elastic stain showing giant cells and complete loss of the IEL (Verhoeff van Gieson, 200X). *Abbreviations*: GCA, giant cell arteritis; IEL, internal elastic lamina. *Source*: Courtesy of Dylan Miller, MD, Mayo Clinic, Rochester, MN, U.S.A.

positive biopsy is associated are new headache, jaw claudication, abnormal temporal artery on examination, and high sedimentation rate and platelet count (21). Of patients who are suspected of having GCA and have no claudications and normal temporal arteries but who have synovitis, 95% are biopsy negative (21).

When performing a temporal artery biopsy, in general, a frozen section from the first side should be evaluated and if reported negative, and there is high suspicion of GCA, a second biopsy from the opposite side should be obtained. Prednisone therapy prior to biopsy may interfere with the results of the biopsy; however, 28% of patients who have received more than 14 days of standard treatment for GCA will have a positive biopsy, whereas, 31% of untreated patients had an initial positive biopsy in one series (22).

Vascular imaging techniques can be very helpful in evaluating patients with GCA. Particularly, conventional and MRI angiography may be helpful in visualizing typical abnormalities of the large- and medium-sized arteries and their walls, and stenotic narrowing, aneurysmal dilatation, particularly of the aortic root, ascending and/or descending aorta, may be seen (2,3). Ultrasonography has been advocated as a means of detecting evidence of inflammation in the temporal artery, and although attractive as a noninvasive and inexpensive method, the sensitivity and specificity have not been adequately established. Positron emission tomography may ultimately be found helpful in assessing disease activity. It has been suggested that it may have a sensitivity of 56% and a specificity of 98% in differentiating GCA from PMR (23).

The differential diagnosis of GCA includes other systemic inflammatory vasculitides, particularly polyarteritis nodosa and Wegener's granulomatosis (Chapter 8). Takayasu's arteritis typically is a GCA of patients less than 40 years of age. Subacute bacterial endocarditis, organ cancers, and systemic amyloidosis may also masquerade as GCA. Rheumatoid arthritis (RA) (the elderly onset RA), spondyloarthritis, and fibromyalgia, as well as solid organ cancers and other malignancies, may cause symptoms of PMR.

TREATMENT

Glucocorticosteroid therapy, usually with prednisone, is the treatment of choice for PMR and GCA (3). Initially, 10 to 20 mg of prednisone per day is used to manage PMR and generally results in prompt resolution of symptoms within a few days of initiation. The usual disease course for PMR averages between two and one-half and three years, although, in rare instances, patients may require some amount of treatment for periods of more than five years.

GCA should be treated with prednisone, 40 to 60 mg daily, given as a single dose or in divided doses (3). This initial dose is usually administered for two to four weeks and then is gradually reduced by about 10% of the total daily dose on a weekly to biweekly basis. As with PMR, the disease course may be protracted; GCA has an average disease duration of about three years. In most patients, glucocorticosteroid doses generally can be tapered over this period of time.

Patients with impending or acute visual loss may be treated with pulse IV methylprednisolone, usually at doses of 1000 mg daily for three days (3). Patients who have suffered visual loss usually do not recover vision, although it has been suggested that coadministration of low-dose aspirin may reduce the rate or severity of visual loss (24).

During treatment, patients should have followup every two to four weeks, particularly in the initial phase of treatment of clinical symptoms, with measurement of acute-phase reactants including the ESR or C-reactive protein. A clinical dilemma occurs when patients are asymptomatic but have an isolated increased ESR in the absence of other symptoms. There are, to date, no reliable predictors for duration of glucocorticosteroid therapy. At present, there are no universally agreed upon or proven adjunctive or alternative therapies to glucocorticosteroids for the management of GCA or PMR (25).

COMPLICATIONS AND PROGNOSIS

Patients with PMR generally will have resolution of symptoms with proper treatment and a self-limited course, although some patients subsequently develop signs and symptoms of GCA. Feared complications of GCA include stroke, loss of vision, and extremity ischemia. Aneurysms occur at a frequency of about 15 times the expected rate and are associated with increased risk of premature death (26).

Glucocorticosteroid treatment–related adverse events occur commonly among these elderly patients, and at least 65% of patients may have at least one adverse event (3). Patients are at a risk for diabetes mellitus and osteoporosis with osteoporotic fractures, which occur in this patient group at a rate two to five times higher than in age-matched controls. Complications are more frequent in patients over the age of 75 and patients receiving higher doses of steroids (3). All patients should receive calcium and vitamin D supplementation and appropriate treatment for osteoporosis including bisphosphonates.

SUMMARY

GCA and PMR are common diseases in the elderly, particularly in patients of European descent. GCA has pleomorphic symptoms related to the systemic inflammation; and compromise of arterial flow, by vasculitic lesions in particular, can lead to systemic as well as the characteristic head and neck manifestations. It must be distinguished from other systemic diseases including infections and cancer. With proper treatment, patients do well, although a substantial number of patients may suffer permanent visual impairment. Clinical judgment in assessing and in treating GCA is critical to favorable disease outcome.

REFERENCES

1. Evans J, Hunder GG. Polymyalgia rheumatica and giant cell arteritis. Rheum Dis Clin North Am 2000; 26:493–515.
2. Weyand C, Goronzy JJ. Giant-cell arteritis and polymyalgia rheumatica. Ann Intern Med 2003; 139:505–515.
3. Salvarani C, Cantini F, Boiardi L, et al. Polymyalgia rheumatica and giant-cell arteritis. New Engl J Med 2002; 347(4):261–271.
4. Hunder GG, Bloch DA, Michel BA, et al. The American College of Rheumatology 1990 criteria for the classification of giant cell arteritis. Arthritis Rheum 1990; 33:1122–1128.
5. Hunder GG. Clinical features of GCA/PMR. Clin Exp Rheumatol 2000; 18(4 suppl 20):S6–S8.
6. Nuenninghoff DM, Hunder GG, Christianson TJ, et al. Incidence and predictors of large-artery complication (aortic aneurysm, aortic dissection, and/or large-artery stenosis) in patients with giant cell arteritis: a population-based study over 50 years. Arthritis Rheum 2003; 48(12):3522–3531.
7. Calamia KT, Hunder GG. Clinical manifestations of giant cell (temporal) arteritis. Clin Rheum Dis 1980; 6:389–403.
8. Lee C, Su W, Hunder GG. Dysarthria associated with giant cell arteritis. J Rheumatol 1999; 26: 931–932.
9. Sonnenblick M, Nesher G, Rosin A. Nonclassical organ involvement in temporal arteritis. Semin Arthritis Rheum 1989; 19(3):183–190.
10. Amor-Dorado JC, Llorca J, Garcia-Porrua C, et al. Audiovestibular manifestations in giant cell arteritis: a prospective study. Medicine (Baltimore) 2003; 82:13–26.
11. Kramer MR, Nesher G, Sonnenblick M. Steroid-responsive hearing loss in temporal arteritis. J Laryngol Otol 1988; 102:524–525.
12. Hausch RC, Harrington T. Temporal arteritis and sensorineural hearing loss. Semin Arthritis Rheum 1998; 28:206–209.
13. Larson TS, Hall S, Hepper NG, et al. Respiratory tract symptoms as a clue to giant cell arteritis. Ann Intern Med 1984; 101:594–597.
14. Miller N. Visual manifestations of temporal arteritis. Rheum Dis Clin North Am 2001; 27: 781–797.
15. Gonzalez-Gay MA, Garcia-Porrua C, Llorca J, et al. Visual manifestations of giant cell arteritis. Trends and clinical spectrum in 161 patients. Medicine (Baltimore) 2000; 79:283–292.
16. Liozon E, Herrmann F, Ly K, et al. Risk factors for visual loss in giant cell (temporal) arteritis: a prospective study of 174 patients. Am J Med 2001; 111:211–217.
17. Salvarani C, Hunder GG. Giant cell arteritis with low erythrocyte sedimentation rate: frequency of occurrence in a population–based study. Arthritis Rheum 2001; 45:140–145.
18. Smetana GW, Shmerling RH. Does this patient have temporal arteritis? JAMA 2002; 287:92–101.
19. Brack A, Martinez-Taboada V, Stanson A, et al. Disease pattern in cranial and large-vessel giant cell arteritis. Arthritis Rheum 1999; 42:311–317.
20. Hall S, Persellin S, Lie JT, et al. The therapeutic impact of temporal artery biopsy. Lancet 1983; 2:1217–1220.
21. Gabriel SE, O'Fallon WM, Achkar AA, et al. The use of clinical characteristics to predict the results of temporal artery biopsy among patients with suspected giant cell arteritis. J Rheumatol 1995; 22: 93–96.
22. Achkar AA, Lie JT, Hunder GG, et al. How does previous corticosteroid treatment affect the biopsy findings in giant cell (temporal) arteritis? Ann Intern Med 1994; 120:987–992.
23. Blockmans D, Stroobants S, Maes A, et al. Positron emission tomography in giant cell arteritis and polymyalgia rheumatica: evidence for inflammation of the aortic arch. Am J Med 2000; 108 (3):246–249.
24. Nesher G, Berkun Y, Mates M, et al. Low-dose aspirin and prevention of cranial ischemic complications in giant cell arteritis. Arthritis Rheum 2004; 50(4):1332–1337.
25. Nuenninghoff DM, Matteson EL. The role of disease-modifying antirheumatic drugs in the treatment of giant cell arteritis. Clin Exp Rheumatol 2003; 21(16 suppl 32):S29–S34.
26. Nuenninghoff D, Hunder GG, Christiansen TJ, et al. Mortality of large-artery complication (aortic aneurysm, aortic dissection, and/or large-artery stenosis) in patients with giant cell arteritis: a population-based study over 50 years. Arthritis Rheum 2003; 48(12):3532–3537.

5

Autoimmune Inner Ear Disease

Quinton Gopen
Department of Otology and Laryngology, Harvard Medical School, Boston, Massachusetts, U.S.A.

Jeffrey P. Harris
Department of Surgery, Division of Otolaryngology-Head and Neck Surgery, University of California and VA San Diego Healthcare System, San Diego, California, U.S.A.

INTRODUCTION

Autoimmune inner ear disease (AIED) was first reported by Lehnhardt in 1958 when he theorized that anticochlear antibodies were the cause of progressive bilateral hearing loss in 13 patients (1). In 1979, McCabe described 18 patients with progressive bilateral sensorineural hearing loss, who responded to immunosuppressive therapy (2). Since then, substantial research efforts and clinical investigations have greatly enhanced our understanding of this disorder; however, AIED remains a difficult disorder to investigate for several reasons. The delicate inner ear structures are not amenable to biopsy and are often destroyed even by accessing the inner ear compartment. Additionally, the inner ear is encased in some of the densest bone in the body. Finally, its inherent size makes imaging of its functional components extremely difficult. For these reasons, the true pathogenesis of this disorder remains obscure. Much of our current understanding is based on animal models of the disease, which have definitively demonstrated the immune response itself as a cause of inner ear injury.

AIED can exist either in isolation or in combination with other systemic autoimmune disorders. Although uncommon, it remains one of the few reversible causes of sensorineural hearing loss. Timely administration of appropriate medication can stabilize or improve hearing as well as vestibulopathy in the majority of cases. Although active investigation into new agents is under way, high-dose corticosteroid therapy remains the treatment of choice for the disorder. Great progress has been made in our understanding of AIED, but much work is needed before its true nature is understood. This chapter will review the basic immunology of the inner ear, the pathogenesis of AIED based on animal models, the clinical manifestations and diagnostic features of the disorder, and its treatment.

DEFINITION

AIED can be defined as a fluctuating or rapidly progressing sensorineural hearing loss that is responsive to immunosuppressive therapy. Vestibular dysfunction may or may not be present. In some cases, a concurrent systemic autoimmune disorder exists at the time of diagnosis. Therefore, AIED can exist in isolation as an organ-specific disease (primary AIED) or can occur as a nonspecific injury as part of a systemic autoimmune disease (secondary AIED). Currently, there is no diagnostic laboratory test or imaging modality available to confirm the diagnosis with certainty.

EPIDEMIOLOGY

Both primary and secondary AIED are considered uncommon disorders. Although AIED can occur at any age, it is most often a disease of adults. A review of several large published studies of AIED, as listed in Table 1, reveals a wide range of affected ages (1–87 years), with mean ages ranging between 44 and 56 years. Men and women were affected equally. There is no known race predilection for AIED (Table 1).

PATHOGENESIS

Basic Inner Ear Immunology

Due to substantial research efforts, it is now well accepted that the inner ear is fully capable of generating an immune response and that this immune response can be destructive to the

TABLE 1   Epidemiology of AIED

Investigator	Year	Number of patients	Mean age (range)	Women	Men
Hughes et al. (3)	1988	52	44 (8–77)	34	18
Moscicki et al. (4)	1994	72	1–80	28	44
Rauch (5)	1997	61	47 (4–72)	29	32
Sismanis et al. (6)	1997	25	51 (27–77)	13	12
Lasak et al. (7)	2001	62	50 (5–87)	30	32
Harris et al. (8)	2003	116	49 (19–70)	53	63
Broughton et al. (9)	2004	42	50 (22–80)	20	22
Loveman (10)	2004	30	56	25	5
Cohen et al. (11)	2005	20	51	12	8
Matteson et al. (12)	2005	23	(27–76)	12	11
Total		503	(1–87)	256	247

Abbreviation: AIED, autoimmune inner ear disease.

delicate inner ear tissues. In 1982, Harris injected keyhole limpet hemocyanin (KLH) systemically and into the inner ears of guinea pigs. Measurements of antibodies within the serum, perilymph, and cerebrospinal fluids were quantified using radioimmunoassay. When intradermal KLH immunization was performed, antibodies to KLH were identified in the serum and, to a lesser extent, in the perilymph. When KLH was perfused into the inner ear, serum antibodies were once again detected, but the perilymphatic levels were found in a much greater concentration compared to the intradermal injections. The contralateral inner ear had the same amount of antibodies within the perilymph as did the injected ear. This experiment proved that the inner ear is able to respond to an antigen challenge and that it can produce a local as well as a systemic response to the antigen (13,14).

Further research has elucidated the basic steps in this inner ear response. Once an antigen enters the inner ear, it must be identified and processed by immunocompetent cells to initiate the cascade of events in the immune response. In the inner ear, the endolymphatic sac has been implicated as the main antigen-processing site, with blockage or destruction of the endolymphatic sac resulting in a decreased local and systemic immune response following inner ear antigen challenges (15,16). Once the antigen has been processed by cells within and around the endolymphatic sac, these immunocompetent cells release cytokines in order to upregulate the immune response. Of these cytokines, interleukin-1 (IL-1) and interleukin-2 (IL-2) have been identified early in the cascade of events within the inner ear. IL-1 is released by macrophages when they are activated. IL-1 then causes the release of IL-2 by T helper cells. IL-2 has widespread effects and has been shown to activate T cells, B cells, polymorphonuclear cells, monocytes, and lymphocytes. IL-2 is not found within the inner ear in its resting state, but upon antigen exposure, it can be identified as early as 6 hours after exposure, peaking at 18 hours with slow diminution over the ensuing 5 days (17).

Other cytokines released early in the inner ear immune response, such as tumor necrosis factor-α (TNF-α), have been implicated in the upregulation of intercelluar adhesion molecule-1 (ICAM-1) receptors along the spiral modiolar vein, turning this vein into a high endothelial venule (18–20). The spiral modiolar vein has been identified as the primary site for influx of immunocompetent cells into the inner ear from the systemic circulation (21).

In the inner ear's immune response, the first cells to arrive are the polymorphonuclear cells, followed by T cells and B cells. Antibodies specific to the antigen are released as a relatively late immune response (22). Concurrent with the ingress of immunocompetent cells into the inner ear is the production of an extracellular matrix likely produced by fibrocytes within the inner ear. This extracellular matrix often results in ossification, as the inner ear has an extremely limited capacity to clear this matrix. Ossification of the cochlea invariably results in profound hearing loss (23).

Animal Models for AIED

Animal models have definitively demonstrated that the immune response of the inner ear can lead to reversible or permanent damage to the delicate inner ear structures. One of the first animal models for AIED was developed by Beickert who immunized guinea pigs with homologous inner ear tissue. Although the guinea pigs developed cochlear lesions, hearing loss was not demonstrated and antibodies to inner ear antigens were not identified (24).

Yoo developed an animal model for AIED based on type II collagen. Rats were immunized with bovine type I and type II collagen. Rats immunized with type I collagen or with denatured collagen had no change in hearing, whereas rats immunized with type II collagen had hearing loss based on auditory brainstem recordings. High levels of antibodies to type II collagen were identified. Upon sacrifice, histologic findings were of cochlear nerve degeneration and perineural vasculitis (25).

Harris developed an animal model of AIED when he immunized guinea pigs with bovine inner ear antigen and found that the guinea pigs uniformly developed antibodies to the inner ear antigen in both their sera and perilymphatic fluids. Some of these animals (32%) developed hearing loss based on elevated cochlear action potentials. Interestingly, in the animals that developed hearing loss, roughly one-half had unilateral deficits only. When sacrificed, the animals with hearing loss had demonstrable loss of cochlear neurons, edema, hemorrhage, and a mononuclear cell infiltrate. The extent of these histopathologic changes was highly variable among the animals and was not correlated with the levels of antibodies found (26).

In 1991, Zajic et al. developed murine monoclonal antibodies against guinea pig cochlear epithelia. This was done by immunizing mice with inner ear homogenates extracted from guinea pigs. They identified three significant monoclonal antibodies: Kresge Hearing Research Institute (KHRI-1), an IgM antibody staining Hensen's cells; KHRI-2, an IgM antibody staining the tectorial membrane, spiral limbus, and Hensen's cells; and KHRI-3, an IgG antibody staining the phalangeal processes of outer pillar cells and the apical portions of Deiter's cells. A Western blot of the KHRI-3 monoclonal antibody against inner ear tissue bound to proteins at 70 to 75 kDa and 68 to 70 kDa. The KHRI-1 and KHRI-2 monoclonal antibodies did not bind to any proteins on Western blots (27). Subsequent experiments have taken KHRI-3 and infused it directly into the inner ears of guinea pigs via osmotic pumps. Half of these guinea pigs developed a 25 to 55 dB hearing loss. Control guinea pigs infused with irrelevant antibodies had no change in hearing (28). Further experiments have suggested that the inner ear antigen to which KHRI-3 monoclonal antibody is binding among the supporting cells is a choline transport protein, specifically, choline transporter-like protein-2 (CTL-2). These investigators suggest that CTL-2 is a possible target of autoimmune hearing loss in humans (29). Unfortunately, the KHRI-3 monoclonal antibody assay is not commercially available.

CLINICAL MANIFESTATIONS

The clinical manifestations of AIED are a consequence of injury to the delicate inner ear structures. As the inner ear is injured, patients sustain fluctuating or rapidly progressing sensorineural hearing loss, tinnitus, aural fullness, and vertigo attacks. Patients often complain of a decrease in hearing acuity or difficulty in understanding words. They may also have difficulty with balance.

The pattern of sensorineural hearing loss can vary, but the most common finding is a loss across all frequencies, or a flat pattern. Low frequency sensorineural hearing loss is also quite common. The hearing loss may be unilateral or bilateral. When the presentation is unilateral, symptoms often become bilateral over the course of days to weeks. Sometimes, however, there is a delay of many months to years before the contralateral ear becomes involved, and, in rare cases, the loss can be unilateral throughout the entire course of the illness.

Patients also note aural fullness, which may fluctuate along with the hearing loss. Tinnitus is a common complaint in patients with AIED. Depending on the frequencies involved in the hearing loss, patients will often complain of a constant tone or ringing at the frequencies lost. This is often described as an ocean roar, but is a nonspecific finding. The tinnitus is nonpulsatile. Relapses of the disease are often heralded by the return of loud roaring tinnitus, which precedes the hearing loss or vestibular symptoms and indicates the need for resumption of high-dose immunosuppressive therapy.

Acute episodes of vertigo are variably present in the disorder. The attacks usually last for several hours and are associated with severe nausea and vomiting. In between attacks, patients often complain of unsteadiness and have poor balance.

If the AIED is concurrent with a systemic autoimmune disorder (secondary AIED), patients will exhibit manifestations attributable to that disorder. Some of the more common systemic autoimmune disorders associated with AIED are listed in Table 2.

DIAGNOSIS

The diagnosis of AIED is made by a combination of the clinical presentation, audiometric testing (including test of vestibular function), laboratory evaluation, and response to immunosuppressive therapy. The clinical presentation is by far the most important of these parameters. Some patients note a preceding viral infection, although this is not always apparent. Patients typically present with fluctuating bilateral sensorineural hearing loss, which is progressive over several weeks, with or without vestibular symptoms. In some cases, hearing loss and tinnitus develop unilaterally without contralateral symptoms, thereby confounding the diagnosis. When followed, these patients may develop contralateral symptoms over time, although some do not.

The differential diagnosis includes Ménière's disease, sudden hearing loss, otosyphilis, and cerebellopontine angle masses. Otosyphilis (Chapter 15) is readily excluded by serum analysis, and cerebellopontine angle masses can be identified on magnetic resonance imaging with contrast administration. Sudden hearing loss (Chapter 28) is unilateral and does not fluctuate when followed over time. Ménière's disease is the most difficult diagnosis to differentiate from AIED, because no imaging modality or blood test can identify the disorder. These patients will often present with fluctuating hearing loss and vestibular attacks much akin to AIED; however, Ménière's disease is usually unilateral, whereas AIED is most often but not always bilateral. Most important, idiopathic Ménière's disease does not respond to immunosuppressive therapy (30).

Audiometric testing in such patients is crucial. A pure tone audiogram, tympanometry, speech discrimination testing, and acoustic reflexes are mandatory. Usually, a clear

TABLE 2 Common Systemic Autoimmune Diseases Associated with AIED

Polyarteritis nodosum	Rheumatoid arthritis
Systemic lupus erythematosus	Behçet's disease
Crohn's disease, ulcerative colitis (inflammatory bowel disease)	Temporal arteritis
	Sjögren's syndrome
Relapsing polychondritis	Scleroderma
Wegener's granulomatosis	Dermatomyositis/polymyositis

Abbreviation: AIED, autoimmune inner ear disease.

deterioration of the sensorineural levels in both ears can be documented on serial audiometry. Patients will also demonstrate a commensurate deterioration in speech discrimination along with their sensorineural hearing loss. This is important as speech discrimination will often improve after treatment (30a). Other audiometric tests can be helpful. Otoacoustic emissions are typically lost early in the disease course but remain a nonspecific finding. Electronystagmonography demonstrates findings consistent with a peripheral loss of vestibular function, specifically, a reduced caloric response; however, if both ears have degenerated to near the same level at the time of the evaluation, no asymmetry in caloric responses may be noted. Instead, testing to delineate bilateral vestibular loss, such as the rotational chair test, is needed. Patients with bilateral vestibular loss will often display a reduction in gain at lower rotational frequencies using this evaluation. Again, however, this is a nonspecific finding. There have been some patients with AIED who appear to develop oscillopsia and bilateral reduced caloric responses without a demonstrable hearing loss, but this is unusual. The response to immunosuppressives in this situation is unknown.

Laboratory testing is important. Screening for identification of a systemic autoimmune illness that may be undiagnosed at the time of presentation is warranted. It is also important to exclude syphilis as an etiology. A typical battery of tests might include rheumatoid factor, antinuclear antibodies, fluorescent test for treponemes (FTA-ABS), sedimentation rate (ESR), C-reactive protein (CRP), and cytoplasmic and perinuclear antineutrophil cytoplasmic antibodies (c-ANCA and p-ANCA).

Much effort has been expended toward developing a laboratory analysis for identification of AIED. The lymphocyte transformation test and the lymphocyte inhibition assay were used previously but were abandoned due to poor sensitivity and specificity. A Western blot for antibodies against inner ear antigens (Otoblot), particularly the 68 kDa protein, has been developed and is commercially available through Otoimmune Diagnostics, Inc. The Otoblot (Otoimmune Diagnostics, 60 Pineview Drive, Buffalo NY 14228, USA) is positive in a higher percentage of patients with rapidly progressive sensorineural hearing loss than in control patients (31,32). Specifically, in a study of 72 patients with AIED, the Otoblot was identified in 89% of patients with active disease but was not found in patients with inactive disease. This study also found that patients with a positive Otoblot had a 75% rate of hearing improvement when placed on corticosteroids, whereas patients with a negative Otoblot had only an 18% rate of hearing improvement when placed on corticosteroids (4). Another study, of 82 patients with rapidly progressive sensorineural hearing loss, reported the Otoblot test to have a 42% sensitivity and a 90% specificity for corticosteroid response, resulting in a positive predictive value of 91% (33). Kosaka used Western blot to evaluate the sera from 195 patients with sensorineural hearing loss and/or vertigo for reactivity to bovine inner ear antigen and found that 71.5% of patients with moderate or severe hearing loss had a positive reaction to the 68 kDa protein (34). Otoblot for the 68 kDa protein remains the most specific test for corticosteroid-responsive AIED. Other assays such as P0 myelin-associated antibody are currently being investigated as a potential identifying marker of this disease.

Using the clinical presentation, epidemiology, audiometric profile, laboratory tests, and response to immunosuppression as diagnostic factors, a classification for AIED has been developed by Harris and coworkers and is presented as a diagnostic scheme in Table 3.

TREATMENT

The treatment for AIED is high-dose oral or parenteral corticosteroids. Typically, treatment is initiated with oral prednisone at a dosing of 60 mg per day, as long as the patient does not have any contraindications to this therapy. A detailed list of possible side effects and complications of this therapy is given to the patient and includes hyperglycemia, insomnolence, hypertension, and mood disturbance, as well as sequelae of long-term usage such as moon facies, abdominal obesity, cataracts, and the low, but serious, risk of avascular necrosis of the femoral head. The high-dose steroid is continued for at least one month.

TABLE 3 Classification of AIED

Type	Conditions
1	*Organ (ear) specific*
	Rapidly progressive bilateral sensorineural hearing loss
	All age ranges, although middle age most common
	No other clinical evidence of systemic autoimmune disease
	Positive otoblot (Western blot 68 kDa)
	Negative serological studies (antinuclear antigen, sedimentation rate, rheumatoid factor, C1q binding assay, etc.)
	Greater than 50% response rate to high-dose steroids
2	*Rapidly progressive bilateral sensorineural hearing loss with systemic autoimmune disease*
	Rapidly progressive bilateral sensorineural hearing loss
	Hearing loss often worst with flare of autoimmune condition
	Other autoimmune condition is present (systemic lupus erythematosus, ulcerative colitis, polyarteritis nodosa, vasculitis, rheumatoid arthritis, Sjögren's disease)
	Otoblot may be positive or negative
	Serological studies will be positive in accordance with the illness (i.e., antinuclear antigen high titers, rheumatoid factor positive, circulating immune complexes)
	Steroid-responsive and may be managed with targeted therapies for underlying illness
3	*Immune-mediated Ménière's disease*
	Bilateral, fluctuating sensorineural hearing loss with vestibular symptoms that may predominate
	Subset of patients with delayed contralateral endolymphatic hydrops or recent instability of better hearing ear with burned out *Ménière's* disease
	Otoblot positive in 37–58%, may show presence of circulating immune complexes
	Steroid responsive, may require long-term immunosuppression due to relapses
4	*Rapidly progressive bilateral sensorineural hearing loss with associated inflammatory disease (chronic otitis media, Lyme disease, otosyphilis, serum sickness[a])*
	Evidence of profound drop in hearing with long-standing chronic otitis media
	May show inflammation of the tympanic membrane and perforations
	Hearing loss progresses despite treatment of the infectious agent (treponemal or rickettsial)
	Otoblot negative, serological tests for the underlying disease may be positive and should be evaluated for granulomatous disease and vasculitis by biopsy if tissue is available
	Steroid-responsive and may require long-term immunosuppression
5	*Cogan's Syndrome*
	Sudden onset of interstitial keratitis and severe vestibuloauditory dysfunction Otoblot negative for 68 kDa, but postive for 55 kDa
	Responds to high-dose steroids although becomes resistant over long term
6	*AIED-like*
	Young patients with idiopathic rapidly progressive bilateral sensorineural hearing loss leading to deafness
	Severe ear pain, pressure, and tinnitus
	Otoblot and all serology negative
	May have an unrelated, non-specific inflammatory event that initiates ear disease
	Not responsive to immunosuppressive drugs although they are tried
	May be related in some instances to ototoxicity from narcotics

[a]Has been reported after vaccinations although anecdotal.
Abbreviation: AIED, autoimmune inner ear disease.
Source: From Ref. 35.

Lower dosage or shorter-term therapy is fraught with exacerbations of AIED. If the patient has a good response, the steroid typically is slowly tapered. If an exacerbation occurs during the taper, full dose is resumed, with the hope of tapering at a later date. It is not uncommon for patients with AIED to require six or more months of high-dose steroids for adequate stabilization of their disease. If it appears that the hearing will be unstable with the tapering of prednisone, an adjuvant immunosuppressive is added to the regimen, as discussed below.

Plasmapheresis has also been advocated for refractory cases. Luetje studied 16 patients with AIED who underwent three sessions of plasmapheresis on alternate days. On long-term follow-up, roughly one-half of the patients required additional sessions of plasmapheresis, as they had initial benefit but relapsed later. Of the 16 patients, 8 had improved or stable hearing in one or both ears on long-term follow-up. Only four patients required immunosuppressive treatment on long-term follow-up (36,37). Further studies with this regimen have not been reported, however. Methotrexate showed initial promise for use in AIED, based on early case reports of efficacy, but a large, multi-institutional trial showed methotrexate to be no better than placebo (8). Etanercept (Enbrel), a TNF-α blocker, was effective in limiting hearing loss in AIED animal models, but unfortunately, studies have shown it to be no better than placebo in treating the disorder (11), although these results may have been dose dependant. Other TNF-α -blocking agents such as Remicade (infliximab) and Humira (adalimumab), as well as Rituxan (rituximab), a β-cell antagonist, are undergoing active clinical assessment for use in AIED.

Cyclophosphamide, a high-potency immunosuppressant, may be considered only for refractory cases with other serious rheumatological conditions such as polyarteritis nodosa or systemic lupus erythematosus in coexistence, but is contraindicated in children. Dosing is 1 to 2 mg orally per day, taken in the morning with copious fluids to minimize bladder toxicity. Side effects are substantial and include bone marrow and bladder toxicity with the risk of malignant transformation. Peripheral blood counts must be monitored closely for bone marrow suppression. Patients must be well informed of the risk of permanent sterility resulting from this medication.

Intratympanic therapy theoretically allows delivery of high levels of potent medications by diffusion through the round window membrane into the inner ear while obviating the systemic side effects. The pharmacokinetics of hydrocortisone, methylprednisolone, and dexamethasone was studied by Parnes, who documented that only limited amounts of corticosteroid were able to penetrate the blood-labyrinthine barrier and enter the inner ear with systemic administration in an animal model. Conversely, substantially increased levels of the corticosteroids were found within the perilymphatic as well as endolymphatic fluid upon intratympanic administration (38). Although intratympanic administration is promising, it is important to remember that much of the immune response within the inner ear is derived from recruited cells from the systemic circulation, which are not affected by intratympanic dosing. Currently, intratympanic steroid versus oral steroid treatment is being evaluated in a multi-institutional clinical trial for efficacy in sudden hearing loss.

COMPLICATIONS/PROGNOSIS

The prognosis for patients with AIED is quite variable. Part of this variability can be explained by the diverse nature of the disorder. Autoimmune injury in general can be from direct antibody injury toward specific epitopes, from immune complex deposits, or from cell-mediated attacks by T cells. Depending on the cause of the autoimmune process and the speed with which it is treated, the damage to the cochlea and vestibule can be reversible or permanent. Cogan's syndrome, for example, carries a poor prognosis leading to bilateral profound hearing loss in greater than 60% of cases, even with aggressive treatment (see

Chapter 6 for further discussion of Cogan's syndrome). However, primary AIED rarely progresses to such an endpoint and can usually be stabilized or improved with prolonged high-dose corticosteroid treatment. This might come at the expense of one dead ear, however.

Complications of AIED include deafness as well as oscillopsia. Cochlear implants are an excellent choice for rehabilitation of patients with AIED who have progressed to unaidable profound bilateral hearing loss. As the autoimmune process damages the inner ear, cochlear nerve function remains intact, allowing for excellent results upon cochlear implantation. There have been several patients with AIED in whom implants have been performed whose function deteriorates, but with the use of immunosuppressives, it has shown improvement. Whether this is due to continuing damage to the neuronal population is speculative but highly probable. Unfortunately, oscillopsia resulting from bilateral vestibular loss remains a much more difficult problem for rehabilitation. Currently, there are no vestibular implants clinically available. The recommended treatment is aggressive physical therapy to reinforce the visual and proprioceptive senses to accommodate for the loss of vestibular input. Fortunately, this remains a rare endpoint for most patients with AIED.

SUMMARY

AIED was first described by Lehnhardt in 1958. Since then, investigations have demonstrated that the inner ear is capable of participating in the immune response and that this immune response can cause autoimmune injury to the inner ear. AIED affects all ages but most commonly presents in the 45- to 55-year range. It has an equal male-to-female involvement. AIED presents as progressive bilateral sensorineural hearing loss over weeks to months, with or without vestibulopathy. In some cases, the presentation may be unilateral loss with substantial delay before contralateral involvement occurs. The most specific laboratory test remains a Western blot for antibodies to a 68 kDa antigen found in inner ear tissues, and, if positive, is predictive of a high likelihood of steroid responsive disease. Treatment is with high-dose corticosteroids for at least a month, as lower doses or shorter therapy durations are associated with a high incidence of disease exacerbation. Although significant improvements in the pathogenesis and treatment of AIED have occurred, it still remains a disease that is difficult to diagnose and treat.

REFERENCES

1. Lehnhardt E. Sudden hearing disorders occurring simultaneously or successively on both sides. Z Laryngol Rhinol Otol 1958; 37(1):1–16.
2. McCabe BF. Autoimmune sensorineural hearing loss. Ann Otol Rhinol Laryngol 1979; 88(5 Pt 1): 585–589.
3. Hughes GB, Barna BP, Kinney SE, et al. Clinical diagnosis of immune inner-ear disease. Laryngoscope 1988; 98(3):251–253.
4. Moscicki RA, San Martin JE, Quintero CH, et al. Serum antibody to inner ear proteins in patients with progressive hearing loss. Correlation with disease activity and response to corticosteroid treatment. JAMA 1994; 272(8):611–616.
5. Rauch SD. Clinical management of immune-mediated inner-ear disease. Ann NY Acad Sci 1997; 29 (830):203–210.
6. Sismanis A, Wise CM, Johnson GD. Methotrexate management of immune-mediated cochleovestibular disorders. Otolaryngol Head Neck Surg 1997; 116(2):146–152.
7. Lasak JM, Sataloff RT, Hawkshaw M, et al. Autoimmune inner ear disease: steroid and cytotoxic drug therapy. Ear Nose Throat J 2001; 80(11):808–811.
8. Harris JP, Weisman MH, Derebery JM, et al. Treatment of corticosteroid-responsive autoimmune inner ear disease with methotrexate: a randomized controlled trial. JAMA 2003; 290(14):1875–1883.
9. Broughton SS, Meyerhoff WE, Cohen SB. Immune-mediated inner ear disease: 10-year experience. Semin Arthritis Rheum 2004; 34(2):544–548.

10. Loveman DM, de Comarmond C, Cepero R, et al. Autoimmune sensorineural hearing loss: clinical course and treatment outcome. Semin Arthritis Rheum 2004; 34(2):538–543.
11. Cohen S, Shoup A, Weisman MH, et al. Etanercept treatment for autoimmune inner ear disease: results of a pilot placebo-controlled study. Otol Neurotol 2005; 26(5):903–907.
12. Matteson EL, Choi HK, Poe DS, et al. Etanercept therapy for immune-mediated cochleovestibular disorders: a multi-center, open-label, pilot study. Arthritis Rheum 2005; 53(3):337–342.
13. Harris JP. Immunology of the inner ear: response of the inner ear to antigen challenge. Otolaryngol Head Neck Surg 1983; 91(1):18–32.
14. Harris JP. Immunology of the inner ear: evidence of local antibody production. Ann Otol Rhinol Laryngol 1984; 93(2 Pt 1):157–162.
15. Tomiyama S, Harris JP. The endolymphatic sac: its importance in inner ear immune responses. Laryngoscope 1986; 96(6):685–691.
16. Tomiyama S, Harris JP. The role of the endolymphatic sac in inner ear immunity. Acta Otolaryngol 1987; 103(3–4):182–188.
17. Gloddek B, Harris JP. Role of lymphokines in the immune response of the inner ear. Acta Otolaryngol 1989; 108(1–2):68–75.
18. Suzuki M, Harris JP. Expression of intercellular adhesion molecule-1 during inner ear inflammation. Ann Otol Rhinol Laryngol 1995; 104(1):69–75.
19. Takasu T, Harris JP. Reduction of inner ear inflammation by treatment with anti-ICAM-1 antibody. Ann Otol Rhinol Laryngol 1997; 106(12):1070–1075.
20. Ichimiya I, Yoshida K, Suzuki M, et al. Expression of adhesion molecules by cultured spiral ligament fibrocytes stimulated with proinflammatory cytokines. Ann Otol Rhinol Laryngol 2003; 112(8):722–728.
21. Harris JP, Fukuda S, Keithley EM. Spiral modiolar vein: its importance in inner ear inflammation. Acta Otolaryngol 1990; 110(5–6):357–365.
22. Harris JP, Heydt J, Keithley EM, et al. Immunopathology of the inner ear: an update. Ann NY Acad Sci 1997; 830:166–178.
23. Keithley EM, Harris JP. Late sequelae of cochlear infection. Laryngoscope 1996; 106(3 Pt 1):341–345.
24. Beickert P. On the problem of perception deafness and autoallergy. Z Laryngol Rhinol Otol 1961; 40:837–842.
25. Yoo TJ, Tomoda K, Stuart JM, et al. Type II collagen-induced autoimmune sensorineural hearing loss and vestibular dysfunction in rats. Ann Otol Rhinol Laryngol 1983; 92(3 Pt 1):267–271.
26. Harris JP. Experimental autoimmune sensorineural hearing loss. Laryngoscope 1987; 97(1):63–76.
27. Zajic G, Nair TS, Ptok M, et al. Monoclonal antibodies to inner ear antigens: I. antigens expressed by supporting cells of the guinea pig cochlea. Hear Res 1991; 52(1):59–71.
28. Nair TS, Prieskorn DM, Miller JM, et al. In vivo binding and hearing loss after intracochlear infusion of KHRI-3 antibody. Hear Res 1997; 107(1–2):93–101.
29. Nair TS, Kozma KE, Hoefling NL, et al. Identification and characterization of choline transporter-like protein 2, an inner ear glycoprotein of 68 and 72 kDa that is the target of antibody-induced hearing loss. J Neurosci 2004; 24(7):1772–1779.
30. Harris JP, Gopen Q. Immunosuppression in Ménière's disease. Mini-symposium-4. Immune disorders of the inner ear. Proceedings of the 5th International Symposium on Ménière's disease and inner ear homeostasis disorders, Los Angeles, CA, Apr 2–5, 2005:79–81.
30a. Niparko JK, Wang N-Y, Rauch SD, et al. Serial Audiometry in a Clinical Trial of AIED Treatment. Otol Neurotol 2005; 26(5):908–918.
31. Harris JP, Sharp PA. Inner ear autoantibodies in patients with rapidly progressive sensorineural hearing loss. Laryngoscope 1990; 100(5):516–524.
32. Gottschlich S, Billings PB, Keithley EM, et al. Assessment of serum antibodies in patients with rapidly progressive sensorineural hearing loss and Ménière's disease. Laryngoscope 1995; 105(12 Pt 1):1347–1352.
33. Hirose K, Wener MH, Duckert LG. Utility of laboratory testing in autoimmune inner ear disease. Laryngoscope 1999; 109(11):1749–1754.
34. Kosaka K, Yamanobe S, Tomiyama S, et al. Inner ear autoantibodies in patients with sensorineural hearing loss. Acta Otolaryngol Suppl 1995; 519:176–177.
35. Harris JP, Keithley EM. Autoimmune inner ear disease. In: Snow JB, Ballenger JJ, eds. Ballenger's Otorhinolaryngology: Head and Neck Surgery. 16th ed. Ontario, Canada: BC Decker, 2002:396–407.
36. Luetje CM. Theoretical and practical implications for plasmapheresis in autoimmune inner ear disease. Laryngoscope 1989; 99(11):1137–1146.
37. Luetje CM, Berliner KI. Plasmapheresis in autoimmune inner ear disease: long-term follow-up. Am J Otol 1997; 18(5):572–576.
38. Parnes LS, Sun AH, Freeman DJ. Corticosteroid pharmacokinetics in the inner ear fluids: an animal study followed by clinical application. Laryngoscope 1999; 109(7 Pt 2):1–17.

6

Uveitis, Cogan's Syndrome, and Sarcoidosis

Rex M. McCallum and E. William St. Clair
Department of Medicine, Division of Rheumatology, Duke University School of Medicine and Medical Center, Durham, North Carolina, U.S.A.

*I*NTRODUCTION

Uveitis, Cogan's syndrome (CS), and sarcoidosis are inflammatory disorders in which the predominant manifestations often target the head and neck. However, the head and neck disease may only be a part of a systemic illness with a diverse array of signs and symptoms. The potential for these conditions to be associated with inflammatory disease beyond the head and neck must be taken into account, to ensure appropriate recognition of the full extent of organ system involvement. Uveitis, a type of inflammatory eye disease, may occur in isolation or be a sign of an underlying systemic illness such as ankylosing spondylitis, inflammatory bowel disease, or sarcoidosis. CS is a distinct, albeit rare, clinical entity characterized by inflammatory ocular and inner ear disease; however, it may also be associated with aortitis and systemic vasculitis, serious problems with potentially devastating consequences. Sarcoidosis affects not only the eye, ear, sinuses, oral cavity, parotid glands, and cervical lymph nodes, but also virtually any organ system in the body. While these three conditions affecting the head and neck are discussed separately in this chapter, they have overlapping clinical features and share many of the same principles of diagnosis and management.

*U*VEITIS

INTRODUCTION

Uveitis can occur alone, but is commonly the presenting feature of a systemic disease due to both infectious and noninfectious etiologies. It can be acute, recurrent, and chronic. Chronic uveitis in particular has a high incidence of vision-threatening complications (1). Approximately 10% of patients over 65 years of age with uveitis develop blindness. The number of people with blindness from uveitis is similar to that from diabetic retinopathy, despite the fact that uveitis is 250 times less common than diabetic retinopathy.

DEFINITION

Uveitis is a generic term for inflammation of the uveal tract, which includes the iris, ciliary body, and choroid. By definition, uveitis is chronic when it persists longer than three months. Acute uveitis may vary in its course, resolving completely without recurrence, recurring intermittently, or evolving into chronic uveitis. The anterior part of the uveal tract includes the iris and ciliary body. In most cases of anterior uveitis (also called iridocyclitis), inflammation is present at both of these sites. Iritis refers to inflammation of the iris alone and occurs only rarely. Among the patterns of anterior uveitis, the granulomatous type is characterized by large keratic precipitates (KP) on the corneal epithelium (Fig. 1A), while the nongranulomatous variety is associated with smaller KP, if they are noted at all. Intermediate uveitis principally affects the ciliary body, peripheral choroid, and retina, and uniformly is accompanied by cells or aggregates of cells in the anterior vitreous (called snowballs or snow banks) (Fig. 1B). Posterior uveitis refers to inflammation of the choroid and generally includes retinal inflammation (chorioretinitis or retinochoroiditis). Panuveitis refers to inflammation across all three of these areas. Inflammation of other ocular structures, such as the sclera, optic disc, and vitreous, is not uveitis, although they may be associated features of the same eye disease (1).

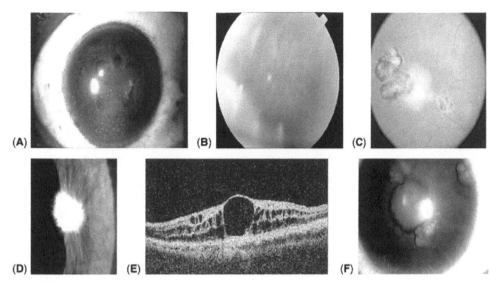

FIGURE 1 (**A**) Granulomatous anterior uveitis: Mutton-fat keratic precipitates (*large*) on the backside of the cornea and synechiae in a patient with sarcoidosis. (**B**) Intermediate uveitis: Snow bank and snow ball found at the periphery of the cornea in a patient with intermediate uveitis. (**C**) Recurrent toxoplasmosis: old and inactive pigmented retinal scars with cream-colored reactivation lesion at the edge. (**D**) Band keratopathy: corneal calcification in a patient with JRA. (**E**) Cystoid macular edema: CME imaged with OCT. Note cystic area in macula with thickened retina surrounding the macula. (**F**) Iris nodules: multiple iris nodules in a patient with sarcoidosis. *Abbreviations*: JRA, juvenile rheumatoid arthritis; CME, cystoid macular edema; OCT, ocular computerized tomography. *Source*: Courtesy of Dr. Glenn Jaffe, Duke University Eye Center.

EPIDEMIOLOGY

The prevalence of uveitis in the Western world has been estimated to be 38 to 714 per 100,000 persons, with an incidence of 17 to 52 per 100,000 persons per year. It is estimated that 2.3 million people in the United States have been diagnosed with uveitis. About 70% to 90% of patients with uveitis present between the ages of 20 and 60, including 50% in the third and fourth decades of life. The gender distribution may vary depending on the specific disease entity. Anterior uveitis is the most common form of uveitis and accounts for 50% to 60% of all cases. Intermediate uveitis represents 2% to 12% of the cases and is the least common. Posterior uveitis accounts for 15% to 50% of cases. Uveitis may signal an underlying systemic disease in 25% to 50% (2–4).

PATHOGENESIS

The uveal tract represents the vascular organ of the eye, providing a conduit for inflammatory cells to enter the eye. The ocular compartments, including the uveal tract, are relatively immune-privileged sites. As such, they are characterized by anatomical, cellular, and molecular factors that protect the eye from inflammation-induced visual loss. Similar to the brain, the eye has a blood–tissue barrier consisting of tight junctions between endothelial cells, as well as the ocular pigment epithelial layers. Although these barriers reduce the likelihood of a pathogen gaining entrance to the eye, they are not absolute, and viruses, bacteria, and parasites have evolved distinctive mechanisms to exploit these specialized properties. The eye has developed several strategies to modify the innate and adaptive immune system to create immune privilege: immunological ignorance, anterior-chamber-associated immune deviation (ACAID), and an intraocular immunosuppressive environment. In the eye, the absence of lymphatic drainage pathways is a means by which ocular antigens are shielded from the immune system. In addition, corneal cells lack MHC class II expression and show reduced class I major histocompatibility complex (MHC) expression, thwarting the ordinary process of antigen presentation and activation of $CD4^+$ and $CD8^+$ T-cells (5).

Antigens gaining access to the anterior chamber elicit a deviant systemic immune response termed ACAID. This response can prime $CD8^+$ T-cells and generate noncomplement-fixing antibodies, but a more robust stimulus is avoided through mechanisms that interfere with the activation of $CD4^+$ T helper 1 (T_H1) and T helper 2 (T_H2) cells, and activation of B-cells secreting complement-fixing antibodies. ACAID also is a feature of the immune response in the vitreous cavity and subretinal space.

The eye also produces both soluble and cell-surface factors that suppress the immune response. These soluble factors convey various anti-inflammatory and immuno-suppressive properties and include transforming growth factor-β2 (TGF-β2), α-melanocyte–stimulating hormone, vasoactive intestinal peptide, calcitonin gene-related peptide, thrombospondin, macrophage inhibitory factor, interleukin-1 (IL-1) receptor antagonist, inhibitors of complement activation, and CD95 ligand. Ocular cells also express molecules on their surface that promote apoptosis of $CD95^+$ T-cells, inhibit complement activation, and inhibit T-cell activation (5,6).

Despite its immune-privileged status, uveal inflammation may be stimulated by environmental antigens or autoantigens. Environmental triggers can be biological, physical, or chemical. Physical trauma in one eye may lead to delayed ocular inflammation in both the injured and contralateral eye; the inflammation in the noninjured eye is called "sympathetic ophthalmia." The occurrence of this syndrome has led to the concept that eye-restricted autoantigens can provoke an inflammatory response. In animal models, uveitis can be elicited by several means: injection of nonocular-derived antigens, injection of retinal autoantigens (e.g., experimental autoimmune uveoretinitis), and injection of ocular but nonretinal autoantigens. There is evidence for autoimmunity in humans with uveitis, but so far no causal link has been established between retinal autoantigens as triggers and the pathogenesis of uveitic conditions. In several studies, patients with uveitis have shown cellular responses to retinal antigens. Sera from patients with uveitis may also contain autoantibodies to retinal proteins (e.g., antiretinal antibodies) (6).

HLA associations have been found with certain types of uveitis. For example, HLA-B27 has been associated with acute anterior uveitis and HLA-A29 with Birdshot retinochoroidopathy. HLA-B27 is expressed by 70% to 90% of patients with acute anterior uveitis and spondyloarthropathy, and by about 50% of patients with acute recurrent anterior uveitis lacking features of a spondyloarthropathy. HLA-A29 is present in 80% to 98% of patients with Birdshot retinochoroidopathy, compared to only 7% of controls (7,8).

CLINICAL MANIFESTATIONS

The symptoms of uveitis derive from the site of involvement in the uveal tract. Patients with anterior uveitis complain mainly of painful, red, tearing eyes and photophobia. Posterior uveitis often produces symptoms of blurry vision, which can be diffuse or localized depending on its extent and the presence of an associated vitritis. In the absence of vitritis, localized posterior disease may lead to sharp demarcations in vision.

Uveitis occurs in a wide variety of systemic diseases including those described herein and in other chapters of this book. Several associated diseases are of primary clinical interest, although individually they are relatively uncommon or even rare in the usual practice of a head and neck specialist. Sarcoidosis is a common cause of anterior, intermediate, and posterior uveitis, which is covered in more detail later in this chapter. Other diseases causing uveitis are described in other chapters of this book and include Behçet's disease, relapsing polychondritis, syphilis, Lyme disease, cat-scratch disease, tuberculosis, fungal infection, and infection with the human immunodeficiency virus, cytomegalovirus, and herpes viruses.

Infectious Uveitis

Toxoplasmic chorioretinitis may be diagnosed as a congenital or postnatally acquired disease due to primary infection or reactivation of latent infection. Toxoplasmosis causes an acute focal retinitis in which the hallmark is a thickened cream-colored retina accompanied by an overlying intense vitreal inflammatory reaction ("headlight in the fog appearance"). Recurrent lesions are usually seen at the borders of chorioretinal scars (Fig. 1C). Primary ocular infections are less common than reactivation of old lesions. Based on seroprevalence data, the overall incidence of infection with *Toxoplasma gondii* ranges from 22.5% in the United States to 75% in El Salvador. In immunocompetent individuals, the primary infection is usually asymptomatic, although a small percentage of individuals will develop chorioretinitis, lymphadenitis, myocarditis, or polymyositis. An unfavorable, life-threatening course of toxoplasmosis would be expected only in persons with impaired T-cell–mediated immunity, such as those with acquired immunodeficiency syndrome, bone marrow transplant patients, and recipients of solid organ allografts. In immunocompromised patients, toxoplasmosis can result in fever, malaise, and severe central nervous system (CNS) disturbances, including confusion, seizures, focal neurologic deficits, and spinal cord myelopathy, as well as chorioretinitis as a presenting feature (9).

Whipple's disease is caused by rod-shaped bacteria called *Tropheryma whippelii*. This infection involves the eyes in about 5% of patients, causing uveitis and retinitis, as well as vitritis, papilledema, and direct involvement of the lens epithelium. Whipple's disease is extraordinarily rare. Lymphadenopathy is frequent and may involve the cervical nodes. Other common symptoms are fever, weight loss, diarrhea, and arthritis. Whipple's disease may also affect the cardiovascular, pulmonary, and CNSs, and produce anemia, hypo-albuminemia, and thrombocytosis (10).

Juvenile Rheumatoid Arthritis

The classification system for juvenile inflammatory arthritis (JRA) divides this form of childhood arthritis into three categories: systemic, pauciarticular (four or fewer affected joints), and polyarticular. Among children with JRA, the most important ocular disease is chronic, nongranulomatous anterior uveitis. It occurs in about 20% of children with pauciarticular JRA, 5% to 10% of children with polyarticular JRA, and rarely, if ever, in those with the systemic type. Young girls with the pauciarticular subtype of JRA and a positive test for serum antinuclear antibodies are at the highest risk for developing chronic anterior uveitis. Onset is usually insidious and the children are frequently asymptomatic; this type of uveitis is termed "white eye" because of its benign appearance to the causal observer. The uveitis may precede the arthritis by up to five years. In JRA, chronic anterior uveitis is bilateral in two-thirds of patients. Slit-lamp examination reveals cells and proteinaceous "flare" in the anterior chamber of the eye and/or KP on the posterior surface of the cornea. All children with JRA should be screened for anterior uveitis. According to the American Academy of Pediatrics, the frequency of subsequent examinations depends on the risk levels, ranging from every 3 to 4 months (high risk) to every 12 months (low risk) (11). In one study, asymptomatic uveitis continued into adulthood in almost half of the children (12). In the region of the head and neck, JRA may also cause cervical lymphadenopathy and micrognathia due to temporomandibular joint involvement and a bone growth disturbance.

Spondyloarthropathy

Spondyloarthropathies, including ankylosing spondylitis, are accompanied by acute anterior uveitis in about one-third of patients during the course of their disease. Anterior uveitis is typically acute in onset and unilateral; it lasts four to eight weeks, and subsides without sequelae, if treated early (13). Cervical spondylitis is the other common head and neck manifestation of spondyloarthropathy. Examination of the neck may reveal decreased range of motion in all planes. Temporomandibular joints are affected in about 10% of patients with spondyloarthropathy. Other sites of involvement often include the thoracic and lumbar spine, sacroiliac joints, hip, and shoulder; the smaller peripheral joints also can be affected. Spondyloarthropathy occurs in a subset of patients with psoriasis, inflammatory bowel disease, and reactive arthritis.

Multiple Sclerosis

Multiple sclerosis (MS) is associated with intermediate uveitis, which can antedate the diagnosis of MS.

Lymphoma

Ocular lymphoma can be extraordinarily difficult to diagnose because the clinical features are nonspecific and it often occurs without associated systemic symptoms and signs. Ocular involvement with Hodgkin's disease is unusual and can include iritis, chorioretinitis, and retinal vasculitis with an accompanying vitritis. Non-Hodgkin's lymphoma can also affect the eye with systemic or isolated CNS disease. Vitritis is the most common manifestation of a non-Hodgkin's lymphoma, followed by retinal lesions and anterior uveitis (14). Lymphoma of the head and neck is discussed in detail in Chapter 17.

Vogt-Koyanagi-Harada Disease

Vogt-Koyanagi-Harada (VKH), also known as an uveomeningoencephalitis, is characterized by a chronic granulomatous panuveitis affecting both of the eyes. Patients typically present with acute loss of vision and pain in one or both eyes. Inflammation can affect virtually any of the ocular structures. Early findings may include optic disc swelling, thickening of the posterior choroid with elevation of the peripapillary retinochoroidal layer, and exudative retinal detachments. Later findings may include extensive depigmentation of the fundus (called "sunset glow" fundus). The typical age of onset is 30 to 40 years of age; women are affected more frequently than men; and the disease occurs more frequently in pigmented ethnic groups.

Other head and neck symptoms may consist of tinnitus, vertigo, scalp sensitivity, and dysacousia. These symptoms, together with meningismus and headache, most frequently characterize the prodromal stage of VKH. Prodromal findings may also include low-grade fever, nausea, and vomiting. Cerebrospinal fluid analysis often reveals a lymphocytic pleocytosis indicative of meningeal inflammation. Other stages include the acute uveitic stage, the chronic stage when depigmentation occurs, and the chronic recurrent stage, characterized by mild panuveitis and recurrent episodes of anterior uveitis. Chronic stage depigmentation may also include perilimbal vitiligo ("Sugiura sign"); vitiligo symmetrically involving the face, hair, eyelids, and trunk; and poliosis (depigmentation of the eyelashes) (15).

Systemic Vasculitis

Systemic vasculitides frequently cause retinal vasculitis and can also be associated with retinochoroiditis, as well as other ocular nonuveitic inflammatory conditions, such as episcleritis, scleritis, ischemic optic neuropathy, and retro-orbital inflammatory disease. (See Chapter 8 for more detailed discussion of vasculitis.)

DIAGNOSIS

Specific uveitic diagnoses are made on the basis of disease patterns. Careful history, ocular examination, and a general physical examination, along with selected laboratory and imaging studies, may contribute to making the diagnosis. History is useful for distinguishing acute from chronic uveitis. Ocular examination, including slit-lamp biomicroscopy and indirect ophthalmoscopy, establishes the location and pattern of inflammation. These two features help to differentiate the various diagnostic possibilities (Table 1). All patients with uveitis should undergo a chest radiograph and serological testing for syphilis. Serum levels of angiotensin converting enzyme (ACE) may be elevated in patients with sarcoidosis, but the cost effectiveness of ACE testing in this clinical setting is unclear. Fundus photography may be used as a point of reference for comparison with the findings on future exams. Other ocular imaging studies, such as fluorescein angiography, indocyanine green angiography, ultrasound, and optical coherence tomography, may be warranted depending on the clinical picture (1,7,14). Vitrectomy coupled by analysis of the intraocular material by cytology, culture, immunophenotyping of cells, and polymerase chain reaction (PCR) for microbial pathogens may aid in the diagnosis of lymphoma and certain infections (14).

TREATMENT

Uveitis due to infection should be treated with the appropriate antimicrobial agent combined with judicious use of corticosteroids to modulate the inflammation. Antimicrobials are specific to the infecting agent, and are discussed in the relevant chapters in this book. Uveitis secondary to lymphoma should be referred to a hematologist-oncologist for treatment. (See Chapter 17 for further discussion of lymphoma.) Uveitis and other ocular inflammatory manifestations of systemic vasculitis should be treated according to the underlying illness.

The therapeutic aims for the patient with uveitis are to control symptoms, decrease inflammation, prevent visual loss, minimize long-term complications of the disease, and keep therapeutic side effects and complications to a minimum. Corticosteroids are the mainstay of treatment for uveitis. Anterior uveitis usually responds to topical corticosteroid therapy such as prednisolone acetate, and mydriatics to ensure the pupil is dilated and moving to limit synechiae formation. With acute attacks, hourly instillation of topical corticosteroids while awake, followed by a taper, may be necessary to achieve prompt control of symptoms. While topical therapy may have limited efficacy in intermediate uveitis, it does not penetrate to the posterior pole of the eye. Posterior uveitis and the common complication of cystoid macular edema (CME) may be treated with triamcinolone (or its equivalent) by injection via the posterior subtenons or the orbital floor. These injections are contraindicated in patients with glaucoma or a history of corticosteroid-induced intraocular pressure elevation. If corticosteroid injections are unsuccessful or

TABLE 1 Differential Diagnostic Considerations Based on Site of Ocular Inflammation

Location	Type	Differential diagnostic considerations
Anterior	Acute	Viral
		Spondyloarthropathy (often recurrent)
		HLA-B27–associated (often recurrent)
	Chronic	Juvenile rheumatoid arthritis
		Sarcoidosis
		Fuch's heterochromic cyclitis
		Herpetic keratouveitis
		Chronic idiopathic
		Masquerade syndromes[a]
Intermediate	Chronic	Multiple sclerosis
		Sarcoidosis
		Syphilis
		Lyme disease
		Lymphoma
		Pars planitis (idiopathic)
Posterior	Acute	Acute retinal necrosis (herpes-related)
		Toxoplasmosis (often recurrent)
		Cytomegalovirus (associated with HIV)
		Serpiginous choroiditis (often recurrent)
		Fungal endophthalmitis
	Chronic	Sarcoidosis
		Behçet's disease
		Vogt-Koyanagi-Harada syndrome
		Syphilis
		Lyme disease
		Tuberculosis
		Toxocara canis
		Birdshot choroidopathy
		Multifocal choroiditis with panuveitis
		Sympathetic ophthalmia
		Lymphoma

[a]Masquerade syndromes include lymphoma and low-grade infections, which are difficult to diagnose.

require a frequency greater than two to four per year, systemic corticosteroid therapy should be considered, particularly if the patient's visual acuity is decreased and CME is present. Treatment usually begins at 1 mg/kg/day of prednisone or equivalent for two weeks, with subsequent taper of the daily dose by 10 mg a week to the lowest dose possible, to minimize corticosteroid side effects (1).

If systemic corticosteroids are ineffective or unable to be tapered to 10 mg/day or less, then consideration should be given to initiation of other systemic immunosuppressive therapy (Table 2) (1,14,16). Surgery may be indicated for certain complications of uveitis such as glaucoma or cataracts. Vitrectomy may be needed to improve vision. Surgery should be performed when the eye is quiet and with a boost in the dose of corticosteroids, as surgery tends to increase uveitic inflammation (1,16).

COMPLICATIONS AND PROGNOSIS

Uveitis has numerous complications, which often cause visual loss. Treatment of uveitis can also contribute to these complications. Glaucoma may arise from a pressure response

TABLE 2 Immunosuppressive Therapy in Uveitis, Cogan's Syndrome, and Sarcoidosis

Drug	Dose	Major side effects
Hydroxychloroquine	100–400 mg daily	Retinopathy, nausea, rare neuromyopathy
Methotrexate	10–25 mg/wk	Nausea, mouth sores, hair loss, cytopenias, liver test abnormalities, rash, liver fibrosis, rare pneumonitis
Azathioprine	1–3 mg/kg daily	Nausea, infection, arthralgia, cytopenias, rash, rare lymphoreticular neoplasm
Mycophenolate mofetil	0.5–1 g twice daily	Diarrhea, nausea, constipation, dyspepsia, abdominal pain, anorexia, low blood counts, rash, risk of hematologic malignancy
Cyclosporine	2–4 mg/kg daily	Nephrotoxicity, hypertension, hirsutism, gingival hyperplasia, hypomagnesemia, infection, secondary malignancy
Cyclophosphamide	1–2 mg/kg daily	Low blood counts, nausea, infection, hemorrhagic cystitis, bladder cancer, hair loss, sterility, secondary malignancy, teratogenicity
Chlorambucil	0.1–0.2 mg/kg daily	Low blood counts, sterility, teratogenicity, secondary malignancy
Etanercept	50 mg SQ weekly	Injection site reactions, headaches, nasal and sinus congestion, risk of tuberculosis
Infliximab	200–800 mg every 8 wk	Headaches, nasal and sinus congestion, decrease in BP, rash, risk of tuberculosis, rare lymphoma
Adalimumab	40 mg SQ twice a month or weekly	Injection site reactions, headaches, nasal and sinus congestion, risk of tuberculosis

Abbreviation: SQ, subcutaneous.

to corticosteroid therapy; cataracts may develop from long-term use of these agents. Appropriate management of these complications provides the best opportunity for avoiding adverse visual outcomes. Band keratopathy is a complication specifically associated with JRA and is treated by chelation and excimer laser (Fig. 1D). CME is the most common cause of decreased visual acuity in patients with posterior uveitis (Fig. 1E). Finally, other complications may result from systemic treatments (1,14,16).

Prognosis is best in patients with anterior uveitis. In one study, 4% of patients with anterior uveitis lost at least 25% of visual acuity, while 43% and 40% of patients with posterior uveitis and panuveitis, respectively, developed this complication (2).

Cogan's syndrome

INTRODUCTION/DEFINITION

The principal features of CS are interstitial keratitis (IK) and vestibuloauditory neuronitis. This syndrome was reported in 1945 by David Cogan, an ophthalmologist at the Harvard Medical School, who meticulously described the medical history and findings of four patients with recurrent nonsyphilitic IK and Ménière's-like vestibuloauditory symptoms. The ocular component of CS subsequently expanded to include other types of eye inflammation, such as conjunctivitis, episcleritis, scleritis, and retinal vasculitis. Later cases also brought to light the association between CS and aortitis and systemic vasculitis, as well as the involvement of other organ systems.

EPIDEMIOLOGY

CS occurs rarely, with less than 250 patients reported in the scientific literature. The disease mainly affects young adults. Among the largest case series, the peak ages of onset range from 22 to 32 years of age (17–21); however, CS has been described in children as young as four years old and in elderly patients. Males and females are affected in equal proportions. Most of the reported cases of CS have occurred in Caucasians, but cases have been described infrequently in African Americans.

PATHOGENESIS

The cause of CS is unknown, but it has long been suspected to be triggered by infection. In approximately 40% of cases, the onset of CS is preceded by an infectious illness; however, numerous studies addressing this question have failed to uncover evidence of an inciting microbial agent. The clinical and pathological features of CS are compatible with a disease pathogenesis based on immune-mediated mechanisms. The ocular and vestibuloauditory manifestations of CS typically follow a relapsing-remitting course, which supports the concept of an immune-mediated process. In addition, CS has been associated with other immune-mediated systemic inflammatory diseases such as vasculitis. Moreover, patients with CS may improve using corticosteroid or other immunosuppressive therapies.

The histopathology of the IK lesions in CS reveals an infiltration of lymphocytes and plasma cells in the deeper layers of the cornea. The cornea and anterior chamber of the eye are usually considered immunologically privileged sites, as described previously. The insult in CS presumably revokes this immunological privilege by promoting corneal neovascularization, which, in turn, allows inflammatory cells to access these sites. In response to antigenic challenge or other "danger signals," corneal tissue has been shown to upregulate expression of proinflammatory cytokines such as tumor necrosis factor (TNF)-α and IL-1, which promotes trafficking of antigen-presenting cells from the intravascular space to the corneal tissue, as well as from the cornea to the regional lymph nodes (21). These mechanisms, together with upregulation of critical costimulatory molecules, prime naïve T-cells and elicit an adaptive immune response.

Although the blood–labyrinthine barrier was initially believed to protect the inner ear from an immune stimulus, subsequent work has shown that the inner ear is capable of eliciting a robust inflammatory response (22). Indeed, the inner ear has multiple routes of communication with the immune system, including a separate lymphatic drainage to the cervical lymph nodes (23). Experimentally, antigenic challenge in the inner ear can result in rapid accumulation of leukocytes (including activated T- and B-cells) that enter from the systemic circulation through the spiral modiolar veins. In animal studies, chronic inflammation of the inner ear, regardless of the nature of the insult, leads to accumulation of extracellular matrix and endolymphatic hydrops, and ultimately ossification. Further work in animals indicates that systemic activation of innate immunity (e.g., injection of lipopolysaccharide) can enhance the adaptive immune response to antigen challenge in the inner ear (24). The pathologic descriptions of the vestibuloauditory apparatus are limited to a few autopsy reports. Temporal bone specimens from these cases imply that the earliest lesions consist of lymphocytic and plasma cell infiltration of the spiral ligament, endolymphatic hydrops, degeneration of the Organ of Corti, and demyelination of the vestibular and cochlear branches of cranial nerve VIII (25). The specimens from patients with late disease showed extensive new bone formation, severe hydrops, and degeneration of the sensory receptors and supporting structures (26,27). Importantly, histopathological signs of vasculitis were absent in these specimens.

The eye and inner ear disease in CS has been postulated to result from organ-system-specific autoimmunity. While a few studies have described antibodies to corneal antigens, the most compelling evidence for organ-system autoimmunity in CS comes from recent work characterizing a putative autoantigen from the inner ear. In this study, antibodies in sera from eight patients with CS were shown to bind a peptide antigen sharing sequence homology with CD148 (cell-density enhanced protein tyrosine phosphatase-1) and connexin 26 (28), which are two proteins expressed in the inner ear. Interestingly, connexin 26 has been implicated in congenital deafness. These antibodies also cross-react with Ro/Sjögren's Syndrome A (Ro/SSA), a known autoantigen and the major core protein lambda 1 of Rheovirus III. They were not present in sera from 25 patients with rheumatoid arthritis, 25 patients with systemic lupus erythematosus, or 40 healthy controls. Moreover, affinity-purified antibodies to this peptide were also shown to react with human cochlear tissue, and to cause corneal pathology, hearing loss, and vasculitis when passively transferred to Balb/c mice (28).

CLINICAL MANIFESTATIONS

For patients with IK alone, the most common ocular complaints are pain, redness, and photophobia. Other eye symptoms may include excessive tearing, foreign body sensations, and blurry vision. Conjunctivitis, anterior uveitis, episcleritis, scleritis, and retinal vasculitis may be accompanied by eye pain, redness, photophobia, or reduced visual acuity. Acute angle glaucoma and proptosis have also been described in a few cases. The ophthalmological findings of IK may be relatively mild and evanescent and may consist of faint, peripheral, subepithelial corneal infiltrates. These lesions are similar to those of keratitis caused by adenovirus and chlamydia. The corneal lesions can evolve to a patchy granular infiltrate, localized predominately in the posterior cornea. The cornea can later vascularize and opacify with persistent inflammation, although such opacities occur in less than 5% of adequately treated patients.

The most common presenting vestibuloauditory complaints include Ménière's-like attacks with vertigo, nausea and vomiting, sudden hearing loss, and tinnitus. The vestibular component may be severe enough to warrant hospitalization. Sometimes, patients may present with a gradual decrease in hearing, of variable severity. Ataxia, nystagmus, and oscillopsia may also be present. The severe Ménière's-like attacks usually resolve within a few days. In one study, the mean interval between the onset of ocular and vestibuloauditory disease was three months (20).

The majority of patients with CS exhibit systemic manifestations. Cardiovascular disease develops in 10% to 15% of patients, with aortic value regurgitation developing in about 10% of these cases (29). Aortic valve insufficiency results from aortitis, with or without associated valvulitis. Other cardiac features observed in patients with CS include ostial coronary disease, coronary arteritis, myocardial infarction, pericarditis, and arrhythmias.

In CS, the most common type of vasculitis affects the large vessels and resembles Takayasu's arteritis. A large-sized vessel vasculitis, depending on the nature and severity of disease, may present with an asymptomatic bruit, intermittent limb claudication, severe hypertension, or constitutional complaints. Less frequently, CS may be associated with a medium-sized vessel vasculitis similar to polyarteritis nodosa. In these cases, the signs and symptoms will originate from the site of vessel involvement and may include purpura, multiple mononeuropathies, mesenteric ischemia, and glomerulonephritis.

Other manifestations associated with CS are fever, fatigue, weight loss, myalgias, arthralgia/arthritis, hepatomegaly, splenomegaly, lymphadenopathy, various types of rashes (urticaria, nodules, purpura ulcers, and pyoderma gangrenosum), pleuritis, lymphocytic meningitis, encephalitis, cerebral vascular accident, cerebellar syndrome, myelopathy, seizures, peripheral neuropathy, cranial neuropathies, and chondritis.

DIAGNOSIS

The diagnosis of CS is based on the presence of both ocular inflammation and vestibulo-auditory dysfunction. IK and other anterior ocular segment problems are diagnosed by slit-lamp examination, while posterior ocular segment disorders are recognized by ophthalmoscopy. Retinal vascular abnormalities may be revealed using fluorescein angiography.

Vestibuloauditory disease may result from a toxic/metabolic disturbance or a peripheral (labyrinth, vestibule, or cochlea) or central (brainstem, cerebellum, or cerebral cortex) lesion in the nervous system. The vestibuloauditory features of CS are due to a peripheral lesion, namely, in the inner ear. The examination should include a careful examination of the ear canal and tympanic membrane, a hearing test, and a neurological evaluation. In CS, nystagmus is only observed during the acute attack.

Several different tests can be used to diagnose vestibular dysfunction in the appropriate clinical setting. Electronystagmography (ENG) is the most useful and can identify vestibular asymmetry from various causes of vestibular neuronitis. If uncertainty about the location of the lesion exists after ENG, rotary chair testing can be performed to evaluate vestibular function. The hearing loss of CS is sensorineural in origin and comes from damage to the cochlear structures. These patients should undergo pure tone and speech audiometry to document the extent of hearing loss. In CS, the loss of hearing occurs preferentially at the low and high frequencies. Brain-stem auditory-evoked potentials (BAEPs) may be useful in difficult cases. A delay in wave I of the BAEP points toward a cochlear lesion and is compatible with the diagnosis of CS. Demyelinating diseases such as MS and cerebellopontine tumors also cause hearing loss and vertigo, and are excluded by magnetic resonance imaging (MRI) of the brain using gadolinium contrast.

Patients with systemic complaints should undergo further evaluation, depending on the nature of their symptoms or findings. Symptoms such as dyspnea, chest pain, or an abnormal heart examination (e.g., diastolic heart murmur) warrant a thorough cardiac examination, which may include chest X ray, electrocardiogram, echocardiogram, cardiac MRI scan, or coronary angiography. These studies may reveal aortic insufficiency, aortitis, or sites of coronary occlusion from ostial disease or arteritis. Bruits heard over a large peripheral artery suggest the presence of a large-sized vessel vasculitis and may be an indication for magnetic resonance angiography (MRA) or conventional angiography. Smooth tapered stenoses, dilatations, and aneurysms can be seen in large- and medium-sized vessel vasculitis.

The differential diagnosis of CS is broad and includes a diverse group of conditions with ocular and vestibuloauditory pathology, as well as systemic manifestations. These disorders are summarized in Table 3. Reliable assessment of disease in multiple organ systems is essential for appropriate management of CS and often requires a team of specialists, including ophthalmologists, otolaryngologists, audiologists, rheumatologists, and cardiologists.

TABLE 3 Differential Diagnosis of Cogan's Syndrome

Disorder	Eye manifestations	Ear manifestations	Other features
Chlamydia infection	Conjunctivitis, IK	Otitis media, CHL	Respiratory tract symptoms
Lyme disease	Conjunctivitis, episcleritis, uveitis, IK, choroiditis, retinitis, optic neuritis	—	Erythema, migraines, meningitis, carditis, arthritis
Congenital syphilis	IK	SNHL	+FTA-ABS
Whipple's disease	Uveitis, vitritis	SNHL	Diarrhea, weight loss, fever, arthritis, skin hyperpigmentation
Sarcoidosis	Conjunctivitis, IK, anterior uveitis, retinitis, keratoconjunctivitis sicca	SNHL	Hilar adenopathy, pulmonary fibrosis, CNS involvement, skin lesions, parotid gland enlargement
Vogt-Koyanagi-Harada	Panuveitis, iridocyclitis	Vertigo, SNHL	Aseptic meningitis, vitiligo, alopecia, poliosis
KID syndrome (congenital)	Keratoconjunctivitis, corneal vascularization	SNHL	Ichthyosis
Sjögren's syndrome	Keratoconjunctivitis sicca	SNHL	Xerostomia, parotid gland enlargement, serum ANA
Rheumatoid arthritis	Episcleritis, scleritis	SNHL	Arthritis, serum rheumatoid factor
SLE	Retinitis, optic atrophy	SNHL (mild)	Skin rash, arthritis, pleurisy, glomerulonephritis, cytopenias, serum ANA
APA	Retinal vascular occlusion	SNHL	Deep vein thrombosis, pulmonary emboli, arterial thrombosis, thrombocytopenia, serum APA
Polyarteritis nodosa	Retinal vasculitis	SNHL	Renal failure, hypertension, arthritis, skin lesions, neuropathy, CNS involvement, elevated ESR
Wegener's granulomatosis	Conjunctivitis, episcleritis scleritis, uveitis, retinitis	Otitis media (CHL), SNHL	Sinusitis, pulmonary infiltrates, glomerulonephritis, serum ANCA
Relapsing polychondritis	Conjunctivitis, IK, scleritis, uveitis	SNHL	Auricular, nasal, and laryngotracheal chondritis, systemic vasculitis
Behçet's syndrome	Anterior uveitis, episcleritis, IK, retinal vasculitis, chorioretinitis	Vertigo, SNHL	Oral and genital ulcers, CNS involvement, arthritis, skin lesions
Ulcerative colitis	Anterior uveitis	SNHL	Colitis
Crohn's disease	Anterior uveitis	SNHL	Enterocolitis
CNS lymphoma	Corneal, anterior chamber and vitreous opacities, sub-RPE infiltrates	SNHL	Cerebellopontine mass
CLL	Optic neuropathy	Otitis media, SNHL	CNS involvement, CSF lymphocytosis
Retinocochleocerebral vasculopathy	Retinal arteriolar occlusions	SNHL	CNS microangiopathy

Abbreviations: ANCA antineutrophil cytoplasmic antibodies; APA, antiphospholipid antibody; ANA, antinuclear antibodies; CHL, conductive hearing loss; CLL, chronic lymphocytic leukemia; CNS, central nervous system; CSF, cerebrospinal fluid; FTA-ABS, fluorescent treponemal antibody absorption; IK, interstitial keratitis; KID, keratitis, ichthyosis, and deafness; RPE, retinal pigment epithelial; SLE, systemic lupus erythematosus; SNHL, sensorineural hearing loss.

TREATMENT

In CS, IK is usually treated initially with topical ocular corticosteroid drops, such as prednisolone acetate 1%, and mydriatics. The IK usually responds within three to seven days. If IK fails to improve with topical corticosteroid therapy, then chlamydial infection should be considered as a possible alternative diagnosis. Only rarely does IK require systemic corticosteroid therapy. Conjunctivitis, anterior uveitis, and episcleritis/scleritis may also be treated initially with topical corticosteroids. Oral nonsteroidal anti-inflammatory drugs may benefit some patients with episcleritis/scleritis and may be added to the topical regimen. Refractory cases may be treated with systemic corticosteroids or other immunosuppressive agents.

Posterior segment inflammation should be treated with systemic corticosteroids beginning with prednisone 1 mg/kg/day. Other immunosuppressive drugs, such as methotrexate, cyclophosphamide, or cyclosporine, may be required for those patients who fail to respond adequately to two to three weeks of high-dose corticosteroid therapy (Table 2). Failure to taper the prednisone dose below 10 mg/day or the development of corticosteroid toxicity may also be an indication for using another immunosuppressive drug.

Vestibular dysfunction or a decrease in auditory acuity in a newly diagnosed patient with CS warrants a trial of systemic corticosteroid therapy. No clinical trials of any therapy have been done in CS, due to the rarity of this condition. Patients with hearing loss are usually treated initially with prednisone 1 to 2 mg/kg/day, often in divided doses for three to seven days before consolidating to a single daily dose. With improvement in hearing after two to three weeks, the dose of prednisone is tapered gradually over the next six to eight weeks to an every-other-day regimen. Further tapering of the prednisone dose depends on stability of auditory and vestibular function. Some patients may require long-term corticosteroid therapy to maintain hearing function. Decline in auditory function warrants an increase in prednisone dose to 0.5 to 1 mg/kg/day, depending on the severity of the hearing loss.

Treatment with a corticosteroid-sparing agent is often considered for patients who develop corticosteroid toxicity or require excessively high prednisone doses to control hearing loss. In these cases, consideration may be given to using cyclophosphamide, methotrexate, azathioprine, cyclosporine, or tacrolimus (Table 2). The evidence for the efficacy of these agents is only anecdotal.

The treatment of systemic vasculitis and other organ system manifestations is beyond the scope of this chapter. However, patients with systemic vasculitis, including aortitis, are usually treated with high doses of prednisone, 1 to 2 mg/kg/day, in combination with methotrexate, azathioprine, or cyclophosphamide. In addition, cyclosporine may be considered in patients with a Takayasu's-like arteritis.

COMPLICATIONS AND PROGNOSIS

Rarely, patients with chronic IK may develop progressive corneal opacification, which decreases visual acuity. Such patients may require corneal transplantation. Cataracts may also occur and require extraction. Serious posterior segment eye disease can lead to decreased visual acuity. The hearing decline is the major debilitating complication of CS. Progression to deafness is frequent and occurs in approximately 25% to 50% of patients. Many patients have benefited from a cochlear implant, which has dramatically improved their quality of life. Vestibular symptoms usually improve with time, but as many as 20% of patients may have persistent oscillopsia.

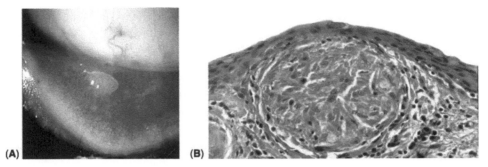

FIGURE 2 (**A**) Conjunctival nodule related to sarcoidosis. Note the circumscribed epithelioid inflammatory nodule, without necrosis (noncaseating). (**B**) Histopathology of a similar nodule. Note inflammation in surrounding areas, including plasma cells. There are no giant cells. *Source*: (**A**) Courtesy of Dr. Glenn Jaffe, Duke University Eye Center. (**B**) Courtesy of Dr. Alan Proia, Duke University School of Medicine, Department of Pathology.

SARCOIDOSIS

INTRODUCTION

Sarcoidosis, first described in 1877 by Jonathon Hutchinson, is a systemic granulomatous disease of uncertain etiology primarily affecting the lungs and lymph nodes. The disease can, however, involve virtually any organ system in the body, and has frequent head and neck manifestations.

DEFINITION

Sarcoidosis is a multisystem disease of unknown etiology characterized by noncaseating granulomatous inflammation of the affected tissue (Fig. 2B). The presence of bilateral hilar adenopathy, interstitial pulmonary infiltrates or fibrosis, inflammatory eye disease, and skin lesions suggests a diagnosis of sarcoidosis. Other commonly involved organs include the liver, lymph nodes, spleen, nervous system, bones, heart, muscles, salivary glands, and spleen. A diagnosis requires clinical and/or radiologic findings compatible with sarcoidosis in at least two sites combined with histological evidence of noncaseating granulomatous inflammation (30).

EPIDEMIOLOGY

Sarcoidosis is found throughout the world, affecting all races, all ages, and males as well as females, with a predilection for adults less than 40 years of age. The incidence of sarcoidosis peaks at the age of 20 to 25; in Scandinavian countries and Japan, a second peak is noted in women over 50 years of age. Women have a slightly higher rate of disease than men, 6.3 per 100,000 person-years for women and 5.9 per 100,000 person-years in men in the United States (31). Among the world population, Swedes, Danes, and African Americans have the highest prevalence of sarcoidosis. Analyses of clinical disease expression in various ethnic and racial groups reveal heterogeneity in disease presentation and severity. African Americans show greater severity of disease than Caucasian Americans. Certain manifestations are more common in specific ethnic groups: chronic uveitis in African Americans, erythema nodosum in Europeans, cardiac disease in Japan, and lupus pernio in Puerto Ricans. Mortality is secondary to respiratory failure, except in Japan, where myocardial disease is the most frequent cause of sarcoid-related death. The overall mortality due to sarcoidosis is 1% to 5%. Clusters of disease have been described in some studies, suggesting person-to-person transmission or shared environmental exposure; however, these etiologic hypotheses remain unproven. Sarcoidosis occurs more commonly in nonsmokers than in smokers (30).

PATHOGENESIS

While sarcoidosis has an unknown etiology, it is postulated to result from exposure to environmental agents in a genetically susceptible host. This hypothesis is supported by racial differences and clusters of disease, implying a genetic predisposition, and the immunophenotype of an antigen-driven response with restricted T-cell receptor usage. Studies throughout the world reveal different genetic associations depending on ethnicity; the most commonly associated genes are class I HLA-A1 and -B8 and class II HLA-DR3. The mode of inheritance is likely polygenic (30,32).

CLINICAL MANIFESTATIONS

Since sarcoidosis is a multisystem disease, its diverse manifestations lead patients to a variety of specialties. Constitutional manifestations occur in about one-third of patients and frequently include weight loss, fever, fatigue, and malaise. Constitutional symptoms are more frequent in African Americans and Asian Indians than in Caucasians and other Asians (30).

Head and Neck Manifestations

Painless enlargement of the salivary glands occurs in 4% to 6% of patients with sarcoidosis. The parotid glands are most commonly enlarged, but any of the salivary glands can be affected. Sarcoidosis may mimic Sjögren's syndrome by causing symptoms and signs of dry eyes and mouth. The constellation of parotid enlargement with facial palsy, fever, and anterior uveitis is called Heerfordt's syndrome (30,33).

Sarcoidosis targets the upper respiratory tract in up to 18% of patients and is probably more frequently seen in the nose than the sinuses (34). Sinonasal disease may occur in isolation or may accompany manifestations in other organ systems. Nasal obstruction, rhinorrhea, nasal crusts, epistaxis, anosmia, pain in maxillary teeth, facial pain, headache, and intermittent dysphagia are the most common symptoms (34,35). Examination most frequently reveals erythematous, edematous, friable, hypertrophied mucosa and nasal crusts with studding by small pale or erythematous nodules. Also seen may be polyps of the middle meatus, turbinoseptal synechiae, and a saddle nose deformity. Imaging studies with computerized tomography (CT) of the head and neck may show mucosal thickening, sinusitis, and nodular lesions of the septum and inferior turbinates; however, these findings are relatively nonspecific (34,35).

Tonsillar involvement with sarcoidosis is rare. Sarcoidosis was present in 0.08% of tonsil and adenoid cases seen at the Armed Forces Institute of Pathology over 59 years (36). Most patients with tonsillar sarcoid present with a sore throat, but other complaints may include dysphagia or nasal obstruction.

Laryngeal disease occurs in about 1% of patients with sarcoidosis. Symptoms are nonspecific and include dysphagia, dyspnea, throat pain, dysphonia, hoarseness, obstructive sleep apnea, and cough. The most common findings of laryngeal sarcoidosis are diffuse symmetric enlargement of the supraglottic structures and turban-like thickening of the epiglottis. The sites of laryngeal involvement in decreasing order of frequency are the epiglottis, aryepiglottic folds and arytenoids, false vocal cords, true vocal cords, and subglottis. Radiographic studies may demonstrate an enlarged epiglottis (37,38).

Neuro-otologic manifestations of sarcoidosis are rare and occur in less than 1% of patients. Symptoms include sudden, asymmetric, sensorineural hearing loss, tinnitus, aural fullness, and dizziness. A diagnosis of neuro-otologic sarcoidosis is generally inferred from evidence of sarcoidosis in other tissue (39).

Ocular involvement occurs in 20% to 30% of patients with sarcoidosis and can affect any part of the eye or orbit; this is the presenting problem in about 5% of patients with this disease. Uveitis is the most frequent and early ocular feature of sarcoidosis (40). Common ocular findings include anterior uveitis, posterior uveitis, retinal vasculitis, intermediate uveitis, vitritis, and keratoconjunctivitis sicca. Other ocular manifestations are conjunctival nodules (Fig. 2A), iris nodules (Fig. 1F), lacrimal gland enlargement, dacryocystitis, scleritis, and orbital muscle involvement (30,33,40). Corneal disease is extremely rare (40).

The prevalence of neurologic involvement is 5% to 10%. Sarcoidosis can produce basilar lymphocytic meningitis leading to cranial nerve palsies (41,42), central diabetes insipidus, hydrocephalus, and hypothalamic hypopituitarism. CNS lesions tend to occur early in the course of the disease (30,33).

One-third of patients with sarcoidosis have palpable peripheral lymph nodes. The most frequently involved are the cervical nodes, with posterior cervical triangle nodes more common than anterior cervical triangle nodes. Adenopathy is mobile, nontender, and discrete, without ulceration or drainage. Other frequent sites of lymphadenopathy are axillary, epitrochlear, and inguinal (30,33).

Skin disease occurs in 20% to 25% of patients with sarcoidosis, including lesions on the head and neck. Sarcoid skin lesions may appear as a maculopapular eruption of the alae nares, lips, eyelids, forehead, posterior neck, and at sites of trauma; pink nodular facial lesions; and plaque-like lesions, such as lupus pernio, a violaceous discoloration of the nose, cheeks, chin, and ears (30,33). Other cutaneous manifestations outside the head and neck region include erythema nodosum; changes in old scars; alopecia; subcutaneous nodules; and psoriaform, hypopigmented, morpheaform, and rosacea-like lesions (30,33). The simultaneous development of erythema nodosum, hilar adenopathy, migratory polyarthralgias, and fever is referred to as Lofgren's syndrome and occurs primarily in women.

Other Manifestations

A complete discussion of the clinical features of sarcoidosis is beyond the scope of this chapter. Briefly, sarcoidosis most commonly affects the lungs, where it may be asymptomatic or cause symptoms of dyspnea, dry cough, wheezing, and chest pain. Lung rales are heard in less than 20% of patients. The diagnosis may be aided by chest radiograph and high-resolution chest CT scan showing bilateral, symmetrical lymphadenopathy with or without pulmonary interstitial opacities. Sarcoidosis may also affect other organs (Table 4). Laboratory findings include anemia, leucopenia, thrombocytopenia, hypercalcemia, elevated erythrocyte sedimentation rate, hypergammaglobulinemia, and a positive test for rheumatoid factor (due to chronic immune stimulation). The serum levels of ACE are elevated in 75% of untreated patients with sarcoidosis, but a positive test is not diagnostically specific, and its value in monitoring disease activity is controversial (30,33).

TABLE 4   Other Organ Systems in Sarcoidosis

System	Frequency	Manifestations
Hepatic	>25%	Abnormal liver blood tests, hepatomegaly, rare portal hypertension or hepatic failure
Spleen	25%	Splenomegaly and less frequent pressure symptoms, anemia, leukopenia, thrombocytopenia
Cardiac	5%	Benign arrhythmias, palpitations, high-degree heart block, syncope, sudden death
Gastrointestinal	<1%	Mimic tumor, infection, or inflammatory bowel disease in the stomach, esophagus, appendix, rectum, and pancreas
Renal	<1%	Interstitial nephritis, membranous nephropathy, crescentic glomerulonephritis, tumor-like masses
Reproductive	<1%	Asymptomatic mass of uterus or testicle, epididymitis
Thyroid	<1%	Diffuse goiter, nodules, hypothyroidism, hyperthyroidism

DIAGNOSIS

The diagnosis of sarcoidosis is based on clinical grounds and a tissue biopsy showing noncaseating (without cheese-like necrosis) granulomatous inflammation, with exclusions of other diagnostic possibilities (e.g., infection). A definite diagnosis requires evidence of disease in at least two organ systems. Common biopsy sites include the lung (transbronchial biopsy is positive in 90% of patients with sarcoidosis), skin, labial salivary glands, lymph node, and conjunctival nodules.

TREATMENT

The mainstay of sarcoidosis treatment is corticosteroid therapy. Mild disease, such as cutaneous lesions, anterior uveitis, sinonasal disease, and cough, can be treated topically by direct application of a corticosteroid to the affected site (e.g., application of cream or drops, or inhaled form of corticosteroid). Additionally, local injections of corticosteroids can be used for the treatment of recalcitrant skin lesions. In addition to posterior segment ocular inflammation, systemic corticosteroid therapy may be warranted for severe sinus disease, progressive pulmonary disease, involvement of the heart or nervous system, and clinically significant hypercalcemia (30,33). The optimal dose, course, and duration of corticosteroid therapy have not been studied in randomized controlled trials. Dose and duration are individualized according to the clinical situation. For example, the initial treatment of pulmonary disease is 20 to 40 mg/day of prednisone; whereas, higher doses (e.g., 1 mg/kg/ day of prednisone or its equivalent) may be used for the treatment of neurologic, cardiac, and progressive ocular disease. With initial improvement, the corticosteroid dose is tapered to 5 to 10 mg daily or every other day. Treatment is usually given for 9 to 12 months. If a patient fails to respond to corticosteroid therapy in three months, it is unlikely that a longer course will be effective.

Patients with sarcoidosis who fail to improve adequately with corticosteroid therapy or who have significant corticosteroid side effects are candidates for treatment with other immunosuppressive drugs (Table 2). The effectiveness of immunosuppressive drugs has not been established in controlled trials, so the evidence for their efficacy is limited to case reports and small case series. Methotrexate is among the most widely used of these immunosuppressive agents. Some studies also suggest that TNF antagonists, etanercept, infliximab, and adalimumab provide clinical benefits for selected patients with treatment-refractory disease.

COMPLICATIONS AND PROGNOSIS

While sarcoidosis frequently pursues an unpredictable clinical course, its prognosis may correlate with specific types of disease onset and patterns of clinical manifestations. For example, acute onset of erythema nodosum with symptomatic bilateral hilar adenopathy usually has a self-limited course, while insidious onset of disease and extrapulmonary lesions are often followed by inexorable progression of pulmonary fibrosis (30). In the head and neck, complications of sarcoidosis include hearing loss, vestibular dysfunction, chronic sinusitis, infection, decreased visual acuity and blindness, hoarseness, upper respiratory obstruction, stridor, cranial nerve palsies, and pituitary dysfunction. The complications of the persistent ocular inflammation are described above, but it should be emphasized that sarcoidosis is a significant cause of blindness in the United States.

SUMMARY

Symptoms and signs referable to the head and neck often reveal a wealth of clues about underlying systemic disease. For example, eye inflammation, while a singular clinical event in many cases, may also herald an immunologic, infectious, or neoplastic process. Some diseases, such as CS, are the frequent domain of the head and neck specialist, while others, such as sarcoidosis, usually (but not always) come to the attention of the head and neck specialist through consultation. Regardless, the management of systemic disease with head and neck manifestations generally requires a multidisciplinary team of several subspecialists to diagnose the full extent of the disease, decide about therapy, and monitor its response.

REFERENCES

1. McCluskey P, Towler HM, Lightman S. Management of chronic uveitis. Br Med J 2000; 320 (7234):555–558.
2. Wakefield D, Chang JH. Epidemiology of uveitis. Int Opthalmol Clin 2005; 45(2):1–13.
3. Suttorp-Schulten MS, Rothova A. The possible impact of uveitis in blindness: a literature survey. Br J Ophthalmol 1996; 80(9):844–848.
4. Couto C, Merlo JL. Epidemiological study of patients with uveitis in Buenos Aires, Argentina. In: Dernouchamps JP, Verougstraete C, Casper-Velu L, et al., eds. Recent Advances in Uveitis: Proceedings of the Third International Symposium on Uveitis, Brussels, Belgium, May 24–27, 1992. Amsterdam, New York: Kugler Publications, 1993:171–174.
5. Streilein JW. Ocular immune privilege: therapeutic opportunities from an experiment of nature. Nat Rev Immunol 2003; 3(11):879–889.
6. Pras E, Neumann R, Zandman-Goddard G, et al. Intraocular inflammation in autoimmune diseases. Semin Arthritis Rheum 2004; 34(3):602–609.
7. Chan CC, Li Q. Immunopathology of uveitis. Br J Ophthalmol 1998; 82(1):91–96.
8. Gasch AT, Smith JA, Whitcup SM. Birdshot retinochoroidopathy. Br J Ophthalmol 1999; 83(2): 241–249.
9. Montoya JG, Liesenfeld O. Toxoplasmosis. Lancet 2004; 363(9425):1965–1976.
10. Dutly F, Altwegg M. Whipple's disease and *Tropheryma whippelli*. Clin Microbiol Rev 2001; 14 (3):561–583.
11. American Academy of Pediatrics Section on Rheumatology and Section on Ophthalmology: Guidelines for ophthalmologic examinations in children with juvenile rheumatoid arthritis. Pediatrics 1993; 92(2):295–296.
12. Kotaniemi K, Arkela-Kautiainen M, Haapasaari J, et al. Uveitis in young adults with juvenile idiopathic arthritis: a clinical evaluation of 123 patients. Ann Rheum Dis 2005; 64(12):871–874.
13. Monnet D, Breban M, Hudry C, et al. Ophthalmic findings and frequency of extraocular manifestations in patients with HLA-B27 uveitis: a study of 175 cases. Ophthalmology 2004; 111(4):802–809.
14. Zamiri P, Boyd S, Lightman S. Uveitis in the elderly—is it easy to identify the masquerade? Br J Ophthalmol 1997; 81(10):827–831.

15. Sheu SJ. Update on uveomeningoencephalitides. Curr Opin Neur 2005; 18(3):323–329.
16. Jabs DA, Akpek EK. Immunosuppression for posterior uveitis. Retina 2005; 25(1):1–18.
17. Haynes BF, Kaiser-Kupfer MI, Mason P, et al. Cogan syndrome: studies in thirteen patients, long-term follow-up, and a review of the literature. Medicine (Baltimore) 1980; 59(6):426–441.
18. Vollertsen RS, McDonald TJ, Younge BR, et al. Cogan's syndrome: 18 cases and a review of the literature. Mayo Clin Proc 1986; 61(5):344–361.
19. McCallum RM, Allen NB, Cobo LM, et al. Cogan's syndrome: clinical features and outcomes. Arthritis Rheum 1992; 35(suppl 9):S51.
20. Grasland A, Pouchot J, Hachulla E, et al. Typical and atypical Cogan's syndrome: 32 cases and review of the literature. Rheumatology (Oxford) 2004; 43(8):1007–1015.
21. Dana MR. Corneal antigen-presenting cells: diversity, plasticity, and disguise: the Cogan lecture. Invest Ophthalmol Vis Sci 2004; 45(3):722–727.
22. Harris JP, Heydt J, Keithley EM, et al. Immunopathology of the inner ear: an update. Ann NY Acad Sci 1997; 830:166–178.
23. Yimtae K, Song H, Billings P, et al. Connection between the inner ear and the lymphatic system. Laryngoscope 2001; 111(9):1631–1635.
24. Hashimoto S, Billings P, Harris JP, et al. Innate immunity contributes to cochlear adaptive immune responses. Audiol Neurootol 2005; 10(1):35–43.
25. Fisher ER, Hellstrom HR. Cogan's syndrome and systemic vascular disease. Analysis of pathologic features with reference to its relationship to thromboangiitis obliterans (Buerger). Arch Pathol 1961; 72:572–592.
26. Rarey KE, Bicknell JM, Davis LE. Intralabyrinthine osteogenesis in Cogan's syndrome. Am J Otolaryngol 1986; 7(6):387–390.
27. Schuknecht HF, Nadol JB. Temporal bone pathology in a case of Cogan's syndrome. Laryngoscope 1994; 104(9):1135–1142.
28. Lunardi C, Bason C, Leandri M, et al. Autoantibodies to inner ear and endothelial antigens in Cogan's syndrome. Lancet 2002; 360(9337):915–921.
29. Allen NB, Cox CC, Cobo M, et al. Use of immunosuppressive agents in the treatment of severe ocular and vascular manifestations of Cogans syndrome. Am J Med 1990; 88(3):296–301.
30. Statement on Sarcoidosis. Joint statement of the American Thoracic Society (ATS), the European Respiratory Society (ERS), and the World Association of Sarcoidosis and Other Granulomatous Disorders (WASOG) adopted by the ATS Board of Directors and by the ERS Executive Committee, February 1999. Am J Respir Crit Care Med 1999; 160(2):736–755.
31. Henke CE, Henke G, Elveback LR, et al. The epidemiology of sarcoidosis in Rochester, Minnesota: a population-based study of incidence and survival. Am J Epidemiol 1986; 123(5):840–845.
32. Grunewald J, Wahlstrom J, Berlin M, et al. Lung restricted T cell receptor AV2S3+ CD4+ T cell expansions in sarcoidosis patients with a shared HLA–DR beta chain conformation. Thorax 2002; 57 (4):348–352.
33. King TE. Overview of Sarcoidosis: UpToDate 2005, 13.2.
34. deShazo RD, O'Brien MM, Justice WK, et al. Diagnostic criteria for sarcoidosis of the sinuses. J Allergy Clin Immunol 1999; 103(5 Pt 1):789–795.
35. Braun JJ, Gentine A, Pauli G. Sinonasal sarcoidosis: review and report of fifteen cases. Laryngoscope 2004; 114(11):1960–1963.
36. Kardon DE, Thompson LDR. A clinicopathologic series of 22 cases of tonsillar granulomas. Laryngoscope 2000; 110(3 Pt 1):476–481.
37. Fortune S, Courey MS. Isolated laryngeal sarcoidosis. Otolaryngol Head Neck Surg 1998; 118(6):868–870.
38. Gerencer RZ, Keohane JD Jr, Russell L. Laryngeal sarcoidosis with airway obstruction. J Otolaryngol 1998; 27(2):90–93.
39. Shah UK, White JA, Gooey JE, et al. Otolaryngologic manifestations of sarcoidosis: presentation and diagnosis. Laryngoscope 1997; 107(1):67–75.
40. Rothova A. Ocular involvement in sarcoidosis. Br J Ophthalmol 2000; 84(1):110–116.
41. Adcock BB. Facial numbness: a manifestation of sarcoidosis. J Am Board Fam Pract 1999; 12(3):253–255.
42. Westlake, Heath JD, Spalton DJ. Sarcoidosis involving the optic nerve and hypothalamus. Arch Ophthalmol 1995; 113(5):669–670.

7

Relapsing Polychondritis

Sterling West
Division of Rheumatology, University of Colorado Health Sciences Center, Denver, Colorado, U.S.A.

INTRODUCTION

Relapsing polychondritis (RP) is an uncommon multisystem disorder characterized by recurrent episodes of inflammation and progressive destruction of cartilaginous tissues (1). The clinical course can range from a relatively benign disease to one that is fulminant, causing death within months of disease onset. There is no serologic test that is diagnostic or predictive of the severity of the clinical course. Treatment is empiric and tailored to the clinical presentation.

DEFINITION

RP is a systemic autoimmune disorder of unknown etiology, which causes inflammation and progressive destruction of cartilaginous tissues. It affects elastic cartilage of the ears and nose, hyaline cartilage of peripheral joints, fibrocartilage of the vertebrae, and tracheobronchial cartilage. Additionally, RP can involve the proteoglycan-rich structures of the eye, heart, blood vessels, or inner ear.

EPIDEMIOLOGY

RP is a rare disease with an estimated incidence of 3.5 per million population per year. It typically affects adults in the fifth decade (average age 47 years) but is well described in both children and the elderly (2). Caucasians are more commonly affected than other racial groups. Men and women are affected with equal frequency. RP is not a familial disease, although there may be a genetic predisposition.

PATHOGENESIS

Genetics

The etiology of RP is unknown. There appears to be a genetic susceptibility, with an association described with HLA-DR4 in Caucasian patients (56% patients vs. 26% healthy controls) (3). Unlike rheumatoid arthritis, however, no specific HLA-DR4 subtype allele has been found (4). A separate study of Caucasian patients with RP found additional associations with DQA1 * 0103, DQA1 * 0301, and DQB1 * 0601, with 59% of patients expressing one or more alleles compared with 38% of controls (5). No association with the HLA type I *MHC* gene or non-MHC genes has been demonstrated. The exact role these associated genes play in the pathogenesis is unclear, although transgenic mouse models expressing certain DQ Class II alleles develop severe RP following type II collagen immunization.

Associated Diseases

More than 30% of patients with RP have another associated systemic disease, including necrotizing vasculitis, autoimmune rheumatic disease (rheumatoid arthritis and others), hematologic disorders (especially myelodysplastic syndromes), endocrine disease (Graves' disease and others), inflammatory bowel disease, or another autoimmune disease (Table 1). Additionally, isolated cases have been described following ear piercing and intravenous substance abuse (6,7). How these associated conditions lead to RP is unknown. Tissue inflammation with release of sequestered connective tissue or cell membrane antigenic epitopes leading to an autoimmune response has been postulated.

TABLE 1 Diseases Associated with Relapsing Polychondritis

Autoimmune rheumatic diseases	*Hematological disorders*
Rheumatoid arthritis	Myelodysplastic syndromes
Juvenile idiopathic arthritis	Hodgkin's disease
Systemic lupus erythematosus	MALT-type lymphoma
Progressive systemic sclerosis	Non-Hodgkin's lymphomas
Sjögren's syndrome	Acute lymphoblastic leukemia
Mixed connective tissue disease	Pernicious anemia
Ankylosing spondylitis	
Psoriatic arthritis	*Endocrine diseases*
Reiter's syndrome	Diabetes mellitus type 1
RS3PE	Hashimoto's thyroiditis
	Graves' disease
Vasculitides	
Leucocytoclastic	*Gastrointestinal disease*
Wegener's granulomatosis	Crohn's disease
Polyarteritis nodosa	Ulcerative colitis
Microscopic polyangiitis	Primary biliary cirrhosis
Churg–Strauss syndrome	
Behçet's disease and MAGIC syndrome	*Other conditions*
Mixed cryoglobulinemia	Retroperitoneal fibrosis
	Myasthenia gravis
	Pyoderma gangrenosum
	Psoriasis vulgaris
	Chondrosarcoma

Abbreviations: MAGIC, mouth and genital ulcers with inflamed cartilage; MALT, mucosa-associated lymphoid tissue; RS3PE, remitting seronegative symmetrical synovitis with pitting edema.

Pathology

Biopsy of inflamed auricular tissue shows loss of basophilic staining of the cartilage matrix associated with perichondral inflammation at the cartilage–soft-tissue interface (8). The perichondral infiltrate is primarily lymphocytes (CD4+ more than CD8+ T cells), with variable numbers of polymorphonuclear cells, monocytes/macrophages, and plasma cells. Granular deposits of IgG and C3 can be found at the interface by direct immunofluorescence. Later, with disease progression, chondrocytes degenerate, the cartilage matrix becomes further depleted, and nonspecific granulation tissue invades the cartilage (Fig. 1). Eventually, there is a complete disruption of the cartilage architecture, with fibrosis and focal areas of calcification.

Pathophysiology

Patients with RP demonstrate both cell-mediated and humoral immunity against extracellular matrix components of cartilage, including type II, IX, and XI collagens, matrillin-1, cartilage oligomeric matrix protein, and proteoglycans. Evidence for cell-mediated autoimmunity includes demonstration of T cells directed against type II collagen in patients with RP. Additionally, T cell clones have been isolated from an RP patient which were specific for an immunodominant epitope of type II collagen and were restricted to HLA-DRB1*0101/0401 alleles (9). T cell responses to type IX and XI collagens and matrillin-1 have also been reported in individual RP patients (10,11).

Humoral autoimmunity is demonstrated by the presence of immunoglobulin and complement deposits in affected tissues (12). Additionally, circulating autoantibodies against native and denatured type II, IX, and XI collagens, as well as matrillin-1, are found in some patients with RP (13,14). The exact role that these autoantibodies play in the pathogenesis of RP is yet to be determined.

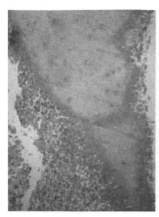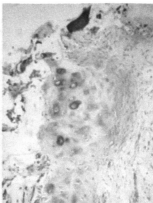

FIGURE 1 (*Left*) A section of ear from a patient with relapsing polychondritis showing necrosis of cartilage and inflammatory cell infiltration (hematoxylin-eosin, medium power). (*Right*) A marked loss of metachromasia is observed in cartilage from the ear, indicating disappearance or breakdown of chondroitin sulfate (azure A, medium power). *Source*: American College of Rheumatology.

The immunologic attack on cartilage matrix components helps to explain the distribution of tissue inflammation and clinical manifestations in patients with RP. Type II, IX, and XI collagens are only found in the fibrillar scaffolding of cartilage matrices found in the ear, nose, and joints. Furthermore, matrillin-1 is a matrix protein found only in auricular, nasal, tracheal, and costochondral cartilage. Finally, cartilage proteoglycans share potentially antigenic epitopes with a variety of tissues, including connective tissue of the aorta, anterior uveal tract, heart valves, endothelial cells, and synovium, among other sites. Primate and rodent animal models immunized with the various cartilage components develop a syndrome similar to RP. The clinical manifestations vary somewhat, depending on the matrix constituent used. For example, rats immunized with matrillin-1 were more likely to develop inspiratory stridor (15). This is notable, as matrillin-1 is found in significant amounts in the trachea. Interestingly, a recent study by Hansson et al. found that RP patients with laryngotracheal symptoms were more likely to have autoantibodies to matrillin-1 than patients without these symptoms (14).

The final result of the immunologic response to cartilage constituents is destruction of the cartilage matrix. Patients with RP have high serum levels of proinflammatory cytokines that are involved in the recruitment, accumulation, and activation of highly destructive cells (monocytes, macrophages, and neutrophils) to the local inflammatory sites (16). The neutrophils and macrophages can release oxygen metabolites, prostaglandins, and enzymes capable of destroying the cartilage matrix. Furthermore, interleukin-1 and tumor necrosis factor-α (TNF-α) from macrophages can induce chondrocytes to secrete matrix-degrading metalloproteinases (17).

Summary

Based on the current understanding of the pathogenesis of RP, a model can be proposed. The initial insult is unknown, but can include trauma, toxin, infection, or another systemic inflammatory disease. This insult results in injury to cartilage. Cartilage is avascular and consequently its tissue components can be viewed as hidden from the immune system ("immunologically privileged"). Therefore, injury to cartilage results in exposure of native or modified collagen/matrix protein antigens to the immune system. In the genetically predisposed host, a humoral and/or cell-mediated immune response could occur. The ensuing inflammatory response would result in further cartilage degradation and antigen release or modification. Due to epitope sharing with other connective tissue matrix constituents, the disease could become more widespread by affecting tissues at other sites such as the aorta and eye.

CLINICAL MANIFESTATIONS

Clinical manifestations usually have an acute onset. The severity and duration of the individual symptoms may vary during the course of the disease. Nonspecific symptoms such as fever, malaise, and weight loss may be the initial manifestation, or may occur during the disease course with exacerbations. Manifestations of RP at onset and during the course of the disease are listed in Table 2 (3,18–20).

Head and Neck Manifestations

Auricular chondritis is the most common presenting feature (40–50%) and eventually occurs in 83% to 95% of patients. The inflammation of the external ear occurs suddenly and can be unilateral or bilateral. Pain and tenderness are frequently severe. The cartilaginous portion of the pinna becomes red/violaceous and swollen while the noncartilaginous earlobe is spared. This helps to separate it from cellulitis. The auricular inflammation lasts a few days or can persist for weeks before subsiding spontaneously or with therapy. With sustained or recurrent episodes, the cartilage of the pinna is destroyed, and the ear can become soft and floppy or knobby and cauliflower-like in appearance (Fig. 2). Other areas of the ear can be affected, including the external auditory meatus. Audio and/or vestibular involvement from Eustachian tube obstruction with serous otitis, middle ear inflammation, or vasculitis of the internal auditory artery usually occurs later in the disease course, resulting in reduced hearing (17–46%) or vestibular dysfunction (13–53%).

Nasal chondritis is present at disease onset in 25% to 30% of patients, and occurs during the course of the disease in 48% to 72% of patients. Symptoms include rhinorrhea, crusting, epistaxis, and decreased olfaction. With sustained or recurrent episodes of inflammation, patients can develop a saddle nose deformity (17–29%) from destruction and collapse of the nasal bridge (Fig. 3).

TABLE 2 Clinical Manifestations of Relapsing Polychondritis

Manifestations	Disease onset (%)	Course of disease (%)
Auricular chondritis	40–50	83–95
Internal ear		
Reduced hearing		17–46
Vestibular dysfunction		13–53
Nasal chondritis	25–30	48–72
Saddle nose		17–29
Laryngotracheobronchial	20–25	30–67
Tracheal narrowing		14
Ocular inflammation	20–25	50–65
Arthritis	35–40	50–85
Cardiovascular		5–10
Valvular disease		2–8
Aneurysms		5
Vasculitis		15
Skin involvement	12–16	17–36
Kidney disease		5–10
Neurologic involvement		5–10
Death (8 yr)		6

Source: Adapted from Refs. 3,18–20.

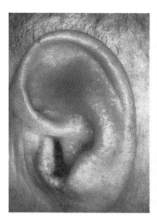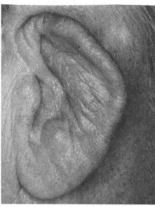

FIGURE 2 (*Left*) The ear of a patient with early relapsing polychondritis. The localized redness, swelling, tenderness, and warmth may be confused with an acute infection. (*Right*) Relapsing polychondritis that repeatedly recurs or progresses leads to cartilage destruction. The pinna thickens and collapses, resulting in a floppy ear. *Source*: American College of Rheumatology.

Laryngotracheobronchial involvement occurs in 20% to 25% of patients at disease onset and in 30% to 67% at some time during the disease (21,22). Notably, airway involvement may be the only manifestation, or it may be asymptomatic early in the disease course. Symptoms depend on the site of involvement and include hoarseness, nonproductive cough, and dyspnea. Luminal narrowing from inflammation or fibrosis can cause wheezing and inspiratory stridor. Tracheal tenderness may be present. With cartilage destruction, laryngeal collapse can occur during inspiration and tracheal collapse during expiration. Airway obstruction or collapse can lead to secondary infections.

Ocular inflammation affects 20% to 25% at disease onset and 50% to 65% during the disease course. Conjunctivitis, episcleritis, and scleritis are the most common manifestations (23). Nongranulomatous uveitis and keratitis can also occur and parallel other disease activities. Other eye manifestations include periorbital edema, chemosis, tarsitis, and proptosis from posterior choroiditis or a mucosa-associated lymphoid tissue (MALT) type lymphoma. Rarely, retinal vasculitis, retinal detachment, retinal artery or vein occlusion,

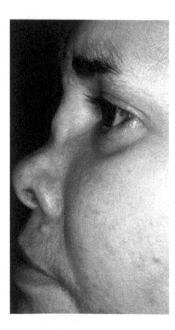

FIGURE 3 Patient with relapsing polychondritis with saddle-nose deformity caused by collapse of cartilaginous structures. *Source*: American College of Rheumatology.

optic neuritis/ischemic optic neuropathy, or corneoscleral perforation can cause diminished vision or blindness.

Systemic Manifestations

Joint involvement is the most common manifestation outside the head and neck. Arthritis is present in 35% to 40% of patients at the time of diagnosis and occurs in 50% to 85% during the course of RP (24). Joint involvement can consist of arthralgias or active synovitis. Peripheral arthritis involves the small and large joints and can be mono-, oligo-, or polyarticular. It is usually asymmetric but can be symmetric, resembling rheumatoid arthritis. Unlike rheumatoid arthritis, however, the arthritis of RP is seronegative, nonerosive, nondeforming, and associated with a noninflammatory synovial fluid. The joints most commonly involved are the metacarpophalangeal joints, proximal interphalangeal joints, wrists, and knees. Up to 25% can have involvement of the thoracic cage, including the sternoclavicular, costochondral, and manubriosternal joints. Joint symptoms typically resolve spontaneously or with therapy within days to weeks, but usually recur at variable intervals. Joint involvement is a poor prognostic sign, as it is usually associated with more widespread disease.

Cardiovascular involvement occurs in 5% to 10% of patients with RP. Aortic and/or mitral valvular insufficiency is the most common manifestation, occurring in 2% to 8% of patients, particularly males. It can occur within months to years after diagnosis and usually progresses insidiously (25). Therefore, any new or changing murmur must be investigated. The valvular insufficiency results from aortic root dilatation, aortic or mitral valvular annulus dilatation, or destruction of the valvular cusps, frequently with myxoid degeneration in the center of the valve (26). Less common manifestations include pericarditis, myocarditis, and variable degrees of heart block. Vasculitis involving small, medium, and large arteries can occur in up to 15% of patients, manifesting as leukocytoclastic vasculitis with palpable purpura, myocardial infarction from coronary arteritis, or thoracic/abdominal/subclavian aneurysms which can rupture (Fig. 4) (27).

Various skin manifestations can be a presenting symptom in 12% to 16% of patients and occur in up to 36% of patients during the course of the disease. None of the skin findings are pathognomonic, but can include mucosal ulcers, septal panniculitis with nodules, palpable purpura, ulcerations due to leukocytoclastic vasculitis, and superficial thrombophlebitis from thrombosis (28). Several other skin lesions have also been reported

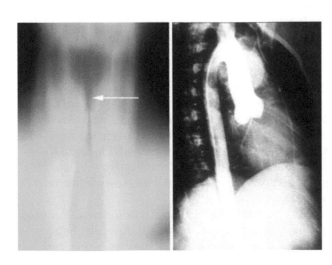

FIGURE 4 (*Left*) Tomogram of the trachea showing subglottic edema and tracheal narrowing in a patient with relapsing polychondritis. (*Right*) Aortogram demonstrates a large aneurysm of the ascending aorta in a patient with relapsing polychondritis. *Source*: American College of Rheumatology.

in RP patients. Patients with an associated myelodysplastic syndrome are particularly likely to have skin lesions. The combination of Behçet's-like features with RP has been called the "MAGIC syndrome" (mouth and genital ulcers with inflamed cartilage) (29).

Other systemic manifestations reported in RP patients include renal and neurologic diseases (30). Kidney disease occurs in 5% to 10% of patients and portends a worse prognosis. Up to 25% can have an abnormal urinalysis as evidenced by microscopic hematuria, proteinuria, or elevated creatinine. The most common renal biopsy findings are a mesangial glomerulonephritis with immune deposits and a segmental necrotizing glomerulonephritis with crescents. Tubulointerstitial disease and IgA nephropathy are also reported. Most renal disease in patients with RP is due to an associated vasculitis and not to RP itself. Similarly, neurologic manifestations in RP are usually due to a vasculitis. Neurologic disease may be acute or subacute and cause significant morbidity and mortality (31). The most common manifestation is a cranial neuropathy (cranial nerves II, VI, VII, VIII). Other manifestations include stroke syndromes, seizures, dementia, aseptic meningitis, and peripheral neuropathy.

Up to 30% of patients with RP will have a coexistent autoimmune, hematologic, or inflammatory disease which usually precedes RP by months to years. Importantly, many of the systemic manifestations listed above may be manifestations of the underlying associated disease and not directly due to RP.

DIAGNOSIS

The diagnosis of RP is best made by clinical manifestations, since there is no test diagnostic of RP. The diagnosis can be delayed for more than a year in up to two-thirds of patients, due to uncharacteristic symptoms. Diagnostic criteria have been proposed by McAdam et al. and modified by others (Table 3) (18,19,32).

Laboratory tests are nonspecific but can be supportive of the diagnosis. Anemia of chronic disease, mild leukocytosis, and thrombocytosis can be seen. Eosinophilia is seen in 10% of cases. Elevation of acute phase reactants (erythrocyte sedimentation rate, C-reactive protein), complement levels, and a polyclonal gammopathy are commonly seen. Urinalysis can show microscopic hematuria and proteinuria in up to 25% of patients. Although occasionally positive, tests for rheumatoid factor, antinuclear antibodies, antiphospholipid antibodies, and antineutrophil cytoplasmic antibodies are usually negative, unless the patient has another coexistent autoimmune disease. Antibodies to types II, IX, and XI collagen and matrillin-1 are found in less than 50% of patients (10,11,33). The titer of anticollagen II antibodies and levels of urinary type II collagen neoepitope reflecting catabolism of hyaline cartilage reportedly reflect disease activity, but are not routinely available (34).

Evaluation for upper and lower airway involvement should include a chest radiograph and pulmonary function testing with spirometry, including inspiratory and expiratory flow-volume loops (35). Computed tomography can identify lesions in the larynx, trachea, and lobar/segmental bronchi (Fig. 4) (36). Endobronchial ultrasound may show edema in the cartilage consistent with inflammation (37). Magnetic resonance imaging is useful to distinguish fibrosis from inflammation in the involved airways and the ascending aorta (38). Doppler echocardiography is used to assess the cardiac valves and function. Radio-nucleotide bone scan can show tracer accumulation in affected cartilaginous regions (39). Biopsy of the ear cartilage is not pathognomonic but can support a diagnosis; however, it is unnecessary if clinical manifestations are diagnostic of RP.

The differential diagnosis of patients presenting with auricular or nasal cartilage inflammation includes several important diseases that can mimic RP. Auricular inflammation may be secondary to an acute bacterial infection or a chronic infection such as

TABLE 3 Diagnostic Criteria for RP

For diagnosis of RP, patients must have one of the following

1. Three of the following clinical findings:
  Bilateral auricular chondritis
  Nonerosive, seronegative inflammatory polyarthritis
  Nasal chondritis
  Ocular inflammation
  Respiratory tract chondritis
  Cochlear and/or vestibular dysfunction
2. One or more of the above clinical findings with positive histologic confirmation
3. Chondritis at two or more separate anatomic sites with response to corticosteroid and/or dapsone

Abbreviation: RP, relapsing polychondritis.

tuberculosis, fungal disease, syphilis, or leprosy. Acute bacterial infections typically involve the earlobe in addition to the pinna and are associated with regional lymphadenopathy. Nasal cartilage inflammation and destruction (saddle nose deformity) can be due to chronic granulomatous infection, Wegener's granulomatosis, lymphomatoid granulomatosis, lethal midline granuloma, carcinoma, or cocaine abuse. Upper and lower airway lesions causing narrowing can be due to prolonged endotracheal intubation, Wegener's granulomatosis, sarcoidosis, localized amyloidosis, and chronic granulomatous infections, as well as other rarer diseases. Wegener's and other granulomatous diseases are discussed in detail in Chapter 8; sarcoidosis is discussed in Chapter 6.

TREATMENT

The low prevalence of RP prevents controlled clinical trials of drug therapy. Consequently, there is no standard medical therapy which remains empiric and varies with the extent and severity of disease manifestations. Some patients have milder disease, with symptoms limited to auricular or nasal chondritis with or without peripheral/axial arthritis. In these patients, nonsteroidal anti-inflammatory drugs, low-dose colchicine, and analgesics, either alone or in combination, may be effective in controlling symptoms (40). For patients who fail to respond within one to two weeks, dapsone should be initiated at 50 mg/day and increased by 25 mg every one to two weeks to a maximum dose of 200 mg/day. With control of symptoms and normalization of acute phase reactants, dapsone can be tapered to the lowest effective dose that maintains the response. Dapsone should not be used in patients with a sulfonamide allergy or glucose-6-phosphate dehydrogenase deficiency. Side effects include nausea, headaches, hemolytic anemia, severe rashes, peripheral neuropathy, hepatitis, and mental status changes.

Patients with minor manifestations that fail to respond to dapsone should be treated with low-dose corticosteroids (0.5 mg/kg/day prednisone equivalent). Patients who present with or later develop major disease manifestations including laryngotracheal, bronchial, or ocular involvement, systemic vasculitis, or cardiovascular, renal, or neurologic disease should be treated immediately with high-dose corticosteroids (1.0 mg/kg/day prednisone equivalent). Severe presentation such as acute airway obstruction should be treated with intravenous pulse methylprednisolone (1000 mg/day for three days) and nebulized racemic ephedrine (41,42).

Once the disease symptoms are controlled, corticosteroids should be tapered to the lowest dose that maintains control of visceral disease manifestations, to lessen the chance of side effects.

Several immunosuppressive drugs have been used empirically in patients who fail to respond to corticosteroids, have intolerable corticosteroid side effects, or would benefit from a corticosteroid-sparing regimen. Cyclophosphamide, methotrexate, azathioprine, chlorambucil, cyclosporin A, leflunomide, and plasmapheresis have all been used with reported success. Of these, the most experience has been with cyclophosphamide and methotrexate. Due to RP's frequent association with vasculitis, cyclophosphamide in a daily oral dose of 1 to 2 mg/kg/day is the preferred drug for severe disease (42). To induce remission, daily oral dosing is more effective than monthly intravenous pulse therapy. Patients are started on 50 mg/day and the dose is increased by 25 mg every two weeks to a maximum of 2 mg/kg/day (usually 150 mg/day) or until the patient is brought into remission or experiences drug toxicity. The total white blood cell count should be kept above 3500 to 4000/mm^3 to help avoid infectious complications. Once remission is achieved, prednisone is tapered. After six months of remission, cyclophosphamide is tapered by 25 mg/mo to the lowest effective dose that maintains remission, as evidenced by the clinical symptoms and a normal sedimentation rate/C-reactive protein. For less severe disease in patients with normal renal function, weekly methotrexate (7.5–25 mg/wk) with folate (1 mg/day) has been an efficacious and well-tolerated, steroid-sparing medication regimen. Trentham and Le reported that 23 of 31 patients receiving methotrexate at an average weekly dose of 17.5 mg responded to therapy and were able to taper their prednisone from 19 to 5 mg/day (20). Methotrexate is started at 7.5 to 15 mg/wk and increased by 2.5 to 5.0 mg monthly to clinical response, drug toxicity, or a maximum dose at 25 mg/wk. Subcutaneous methotrexate should be used at doses higher than 20 mg/wk for better absorption. Many physicians will use cyclophosphamide initially for three to six months to bring RP under control and then switch to methotrexate to maintain remission. A combination with dapsone is also used for added therapeutic effect and for *Pneumocystis carinii* pneumonia prophylaxis. Patients who fail to initially respond or maintain their response, or who develop severe hematologic or other toxicities on cyclophosphamide or methotrexate, should be considered for cyclosporine (5 mg/kg/day) or biologic therapy (43). Due to significant potential side effects, all of these medications should be administered and monitored by a physician familiar with their use. Administration of the pneumococcal vaccine, evaluation and therapy of osteoporosis, and treatment of hyperlipidemia and hypertension to prevent accelerated atherosclerosis must be done by the treating physician.

Biologic therapies have been used successfully in RP patients who do not respond to or cannot tolerate standard therapy. The anti-TNF-α agents have been increasingly reported to be effective in such patients in isolated case reports. Infliximab, at doses of 5 mg/kg every eight weeks after loading doses, has been reported to be effective in two case reports of treatment-resistant RP, while etanercept (25 mg subcutaneously twice a week) has been used in one patient (44,45). The major concerning side effect for these agents is infection, particularly in patients with tracheobronchial disease who are prone to developing pneumonia. Finally, autologous stem cell transplant has resulted in complete remission in one patient with refractory RP (46).

Patients who develop cardiorespiratory complications despite medical therapy may require surgery. Tracheostomy or stenting may be required to alleviate localized or extensive tracheobronchial disease (47). The use of BiPAP® (Respironics, Murrysville, Pennsylvania, U.S.A.) after surgery may help keep narrowed airways from collapsing. Localized lesions in a main stem bronchus have been successfully treated with NdYAG laser ablation. Severe tracheobronchial collapse that is too severe for stenting may require tracheal reconstruction, although reported results are poor (48). Up to 33% of patients with valvular regurgitation will need valve replacement due to intractable heart failure. Frequent postoperative complications include perivalvular leak and dehiscence resulting from valvular ring dilatation and friable tissue from chronic inflammation (26). Patients with valvular disease frequently have involvement of the aortic root and ascending aorta with aneurysm formation. Complete replacement of the ascending aorta using a graft with reimplantation of the coronary arteries may be necessary. Irrespective of the type of surgery, optimum results are obtained only if the inflammation is maximally controlled with immunosuppressive medications. If possible, surgery should be delayed until this is accomplished, in order to avoid complications (49). In addition, the anesthesiologist should be alerted that tracheal intubation will be difficult in patients with laryngotracheal involvement (50).

PROGNOSIS

The prognosis of RP varies, depending upon the pattern and severity of chondral inflammation. Most patients (84%) will have intermittent flares lasting days to weeks (18). Many patients have chronic indolent symptoms between flares, and most will develop some degree of disability. A minority of patients will have a benign course free of visceral involvement or a fulminant course resulting in death. The most common complications are loss of hearing and olfaction, reduced vision (8%), phonation difficulties, and neurologic dysfunction. Potentially life-threatening complications include airway compromise from tracheal narrowing or collapse (14%), aortic or mitral valvular incompetence or rupture (8%), heart block, aortic involvement, and arterial or venous thrombosis. Earlier studies showed an overall survival rate of 74% at 5 years and 55% at 10 years (18). More recent studies show an improved survival rate of 94% at eight years, perhaps reflecting better medical and surgical therapy (20).

Pneumonia is the most common cause of death, followed by respiratory failure from airway collapse and complications of valvular heart disease and vasculitis. Poor prognostic factors predicting decreased survival include younger age (less than 50 years of age at onset), saddle nose deformity, arthritis, tracheolaryngeal involvement, renal disease, and cardiovascular inflammation including valve involvement, aortic disease, and vasculitis (18). Of note is that patients frequently have associated diseases including systemic vasculitis, various connective tissue diseases, neoplastic disease (particularly myelodys-plastic syndrome), and others that may affect the prognosis.

SUMMARY

RP is a rare disease that can affect all ages of both sexes. Diagnosis is made based on clinical signs and symptoms, since there is no single diagnostic test. Our understanding of the pathogenesis of RP has improved over the past two decades. This has led to better medical and surgical therapies with increased survival. Biologic therapies, such as anti-TNF-α agents and others, may result in better control of symptoms and prevention of disability in the future.

ACKNOWLEDGMENT

Figures are from the ACR slide collection.

REFERENCES

1. Gergely P Jr, Poor G. Relapsing polychondritis. Best Pract Res Clin Rheumatol 2004; 18(5): 723–738.
2. Knipp S, Bier H, Horneff G, et al. Relapsing polychondritis in childhood—case report and short review. Rheumatol Int 2000; 19(6):231–234.
3. Zeuner M, Straub RH, Rauh G, et al. Relapsing polychondritis: clinical and immunogenetic analysis of 62 patients. J Rheumatol 1997; 24(1):96–101.
4. Lang B, Rothenfusser A, Lanchbury JS. Susceptibility to relapsing polychondritis is associated with HLA–DR4. Arthritis Rheum 1993; 36(5):660–664.
5. Hue-Lemoine S, Caillat-Zucman S, Amoura Z, et al. HLA-DQA1 and DQB1 alleles are associated with susceptibility to relapsing polychondritis: from transgenic mice to humans. Arthritis Rheum 1999; 42:S261.
6. Serratrice J, Ene N, Granel B, et al. Severe relapsing polychondritis occurring after ear piercing. J Rheumatol 2003; 30(12):2716–2717.
7. Berger R. Polychondritis resulting from intravenous substance abuse. Am J Med 1988; 85(3): 415–417.
8. Riccieri V, Spadaro A, Taccari E, et al. A case of relapsing polychondritis: pathogenic considerations. Clin Exp Rheumatol 1988; 6(1):95–96.
9. Buckner JH, Van Landeghen M, Kwok WW, et al. Identification of type II collagen peptide 261-273-specific T cell clones in a patient with relapsing polychondritis. Arthritis Rheum 2002; 46(1):238–244.
10. Alsalameh S, Mollenhauer J, Scheuplein F, et al. Preferential cellular and humoral immune reactivities to native and denatured collagen types IX and XI in a patient with fatal relapsing polychondritis. J Rheumatol 1993; 20(8):1419–1424.
11. Buckner JH, Wu JJ, Reife RA, et al. Autoreactivity against matrillin-1 in a patient with relapsing polychondritis. Arthritis Rheum 2000; 43(4):939–943.
12. Valenzuela R, Cooperrider PA, Gogate P, et al. Relapsing polychondritis. Immunomicroscopic findings in cartilage of ear biopsy specimens. Hum Pathol 1980; 11(1):19–22.
13. Yang CL, Brinckmann J, Rui HF, et al. Autoantibodies to cartilage collagens in relapsing polychondritis. Arch Dermatol Res 1993; 285(5):245–249.
14. Hansson AS, Heinegard D, Piette JC, et al. The occurrence of autoantibodies to matrillin 1 reflects a tissue-specific response to cartilage of the respiratory tract in patients with relapsing polychondritis. Arthritis Rheum 2001; 44(10):2402–2412.
15. Hansson AS, Heinegard D, Holmdahl R. A new animal model for relapsing polychondritis, induced by cartilage matrix protein (matrillin-1). J Clin Invest 1999; 104(5):589–598.
16. Stabler T, Piette J-C, Chevalier X, et al. Serum cytokine profiles in relapsing polychondritis suggest monocyte/macrophage activation. Arthritis Rheum 2004; 50(11):3663–3667.
17. Herman JH, Greenblatt D, Khosla RC, et al. Cytokine modulation of chondrocyte proteinase release. Arthritis Rheum 1984; 27(1):79–91.
18. Michet CJ Jr, McKenna CH, Luthra HS, et al. Relapsing polychondritis. Survival and predictive role of early disease manifestations. Ann Int Med 1986; 104(1):74–78.
19. McAdam LP, O'Hanlan MA, Bluestone R, et al. Relapsing polychondritis: prospective study of 23 patients and a review of the literature. Medicine (Baltimore) 1976; 55(3):193–215.
20. Trentham DE, Le CH. Relapsing polychondritis. Ann Int Med 1998; 129(2):114–122.
21. Tillie-Leblond I, Wallaert B, Leblond D, et al. Respiratory involvement in relapsing polychondritis. Clinical, functional, endoscopic, and radiographic evaluations. Medicine (Baltimore) 1998; 77 (3):168–176.
22. Tsunezuka Y, Sato H, Shimizu H. Tracheobronchial involvement in relapsing polychondritis. Respiration 2000; 67(3):320–322.
23. Isaak BL, Liesegang TJ, Michet CJ Jr. Ocular and systemic findings in relapsing polychondritis. Ophthalmology 1986; 93(5):681–689.
24. Balsa A, Expinoza A, Cuesta M, et al. Joint symptoms in relapsing polychondritis. Clin Exp Rheumatol 1995; 13(4):425–430.
25. Buckley LM, Ades PA. Progressive aortic valve inflammation occurring despite apparent remission of relapsing polychondritis. Arthritis Rheum 1992; 35(7):812–814.
26. Lang-Lazdunski L, Hvass U, Paillole C, et al. Cardiac valve replacement in relapsing polychondritis. A review. J Heart Valve Dis 1995; 4(3):227–235.
27. Michet CJ. Vasculitis and relapsing polychondritis. Rheum Dis Clin North Am 1990; 16(2): 441–444.

28. Frances C, el Rassi R, Laporte JL, et al. Dermatologic manifestations of relapsing polychondritis. A study of 200 cases at a single center. Medicine (Baltimore) 2001; 80(3):173–179.
29. Orme RL, Nordlund JJ, Barich L, et al. The MAGIC syndrome (mouth and genital ulcers with inflamed cartilage). Arch Dermatol 1990; 126(7):940–944.
30. Letko E, Zafirakis P, Baltatzis S, et al. Relapsing polychondritis: a clinical review. Semin Arthritis Rheum 2002; 31(6):384–395.
31. Hanslik T, Wechsler B, Piette JC, et al. Central nervous system involvement in relapsing polychondritis. Clin Exp Rheumatol 1994; 12(5):539–541.
32. Damiani JM, Levine HL. Relapsing polychondritis—report of ten cases. Laryngoscope 1979; 89(6 Pt 1):929–946.
33. Foidart JM, Abe S, Martin GR, et al. Antibodies to type II collagen in relapsing polychondritis. N Engl J Med 1978; 229(22):1203–1207.
34. Kraus VB, Stabler T, Le ET, et al. Urinary type II collagen neoepitope as an outcome measure for relapsing polychondritis. Arthritis Rheum 2003; 48(10):2942–2948.
35. Krell WS, Staats BA, Hyatt RE. Pulmonary function in relapsing polychondritis. Am Rev Respir Dis 1986; 133(6):1120–1123.
36. Behar JV, Choi YW, Hartman TA, et al. Relapsing polychondritis affecting the lower respiratory tract. AJR Am J Roentgenol 2002; 178(1):173–177.
37. Miyazu Y, Miyazawa T, Kurimoto N, et al. Endobronchial ultrasonography in the diagnosis and treatment of relapsing polychondritis with tracheobronchial malacia. Chest 2003; 124(6): 2393–2395.
38. Heman-Ackah YD, Remley KB, Goding GS Jr. A new role for magnetic resonance imaging in the diagnosis of laryngeal relapsing polychondritis. Head Neck 1999; 21(5):484–489.
39. Imanishi Y, Mitogawa Y, Takizawa M, et al. Relapsing polychondritis diagnosed by Tc-99m MDP bone scintigraphy. Clin Nucl Med 1999; 24(7):511–513.
40. Mark KA, Franks AG Jr. Colchicine and indomethacin for the treatment of relapsing polychondritis. J Am Acad Dermatol 2002; 46(suppl 2 Case Reports):S22–S24.
41. Lipnick RN, Fink CW. Acute airway obstruction in relapsing polychondritis: treatment with pulse methylprednisolone. J Rheumatol 1991; 18(1):98–99.
42. Ruhlen JL, Huston KA, Wood WG. Relapsing polychondritis with glomerulonephritis: improvement with prednisone and cyclophosphamide. JAMA 1981; 245(8):847–848.
43. Ormerod AD, Clark LJ. Relapsing polychondritis—treatment with cyclosporin A. Br J Dermatol 1992; 127(3):300.
44. Mpofu S, Estrach C, Curtis J, et al. Treatment of respiratory complications in recalcitrant relapsing polychondritis with infliximab. Rheumatology (Oxford) 2003; 42(9):1117–1118.
45. Saadoun D, Deslandre CJ, Allanore Y, et al. Sustained response to infliximab in 2 patients with refractory relapsing polychondritis. J Rheumatol 2003; 30(6):1394–1395.
46. Tyndall A. Hematopoietic stem cell transplantation in rheumatic diseases other than systemic sclerosis and systemic lupus erythematosus. J Rheumatol Suppl 1997; 48:94–97.
47. Sarodia BD, Dasgupta A, Mehta AC. Management of airway complications of relapsing polychondritis: case reports and review of the literature. Chest 1999; 116(6):1669–1675.
48. Spraggs PD, Tostevin PM, Howard DJ. Management of laryngotracheobronchial sequelae and complications of relapsing polychondritis. Laryngoscope 1997; 107(7):936–941.
49. Del Rosso A, Petix NR, Pratesi M, et al. Cardiovascular involvement in relapsing polychondritis. Semin Arthritis Rheum 1997; 26(6):840–844.
50. Biro P, Rohling R, Schmid S, et al. Anesthesia in a patient with acute respiratory insufficiency due to relapsing polychondritis. J Clin Anesth 1994; 6(1):59–62.

8

Granulomatous Diseases: Wegener's Granulomatosis, Churg-Strauss Syndrome, and Nasal Natural Killer (NK)/T-Cell Lymphoma

Alexandra Villa-Forte
Vasculitis Clinic, Universidade do Estado do Rio de Janeiro, Rio de Janeiro, Brazil and Center for Vasculitis Care and Research, Cleveland Clinic Foundation, Cleveland, Ohio, U.S.A.

Anderson S. Santos
Hospital Municipal de Lagoa, Secretaria Municipal de Saúde do Rio de Janeiro, Rio de Janeiro, Brazil

Gary S. Hoffman
Lerner College of Medicine, Center for Vasculitis Care and Research, Cleveland Clinic Foundation, Cleveland, Ohio, U.S.A.

WEGENER'S GRANULOMATOSIS

INTRODUCTION

Wegener's granulomatosis (WG) is a systemic disease first described by Heinz Klinger in 1931 and later reported in greater detail by Friedrich Wegener in 1936 and 1939. The striking distinctive features noted by both physicians were an unusual pattern of both upper and lower airway involvement and glomerulonephritis (GN) that had not previously been seen in other reported forms of vasculitis. We now recognize that WG may present without all of these features being present, and, indeed, some patients may never develop disease beyond ear, nose, and throat (ENT) organs.

DEFINITION

WG is an idiopathic systemic inflammatory disease typically presenting with abnormalities affecting the upper and lower respiratory tracts and the kidneys. However, any organ system can be involved (1). WG is often referred to as an "antineutrophil cytoplasmic antibody (ANCA)-associated small-vessel vasculitis," as are microscopic polyangiitis (MPA) and Churg–Strauss syndrome (CSS) (2). In a minority of patients, however, medium- and large-sized vessels can also be affected; the presence of vasculitis is not necessary for the diagnosis; and ANCA may be lacking in a significant number of cases (3). The terminology "ANCA vasculitis" or "ANCA-associated vasculitis" remains controversial because the absence of ANCA in subsets of patients with these diseases suggests that it is not essential for pathogenesis. Nonetheless, it is possible that its presence may play a role in modifying the disease phenotype or severity.

EPIDEMIOLOGY

The prevalence of WG in the United States is about 3 per 100,000 population (4). Although more common in adults, the disease can affect all age groups. While WG is more frequent in Caucasians (>90%), it also occurs in other racial groups. There is no significant gender preference or bias.

PATHOGENESIS

The classical histopathologic features include granulomatous inflammation, necrosis, and/or vasculitis. Characteristic histologic features are more commonly seen in open lung biopsies (Fig. 1) and are seen less often (<50%) in head and neck specimens (5). The characteristic renal lesion in WG is a focal, segmental necrotizing, crescentic GN with scant or no immune-complex deposits (6).

There is evidence that both cellular and humoral components of the immune system play a role in the pathogenesis of WG. Macrophages, dendritic cells, and T-cells are necessary for granuloma formation. Antigens expressed on activated neutrophils and monocytes interact in vitro with ANCAs, resulting in enhanced neutrophil degranulation and generation of toxic oxygen radicals, which may lead to or enhance tissue injury. ANCA is present in about 55% to 75% of patients with mild disease and in more than 90% of patients with severe disease. This suggests a pathogenic role for B-cells and plasma cells. It is not yet clear how B-cells in WG may also function in their capacities as antigen-presenting and immunoregulatory cells.

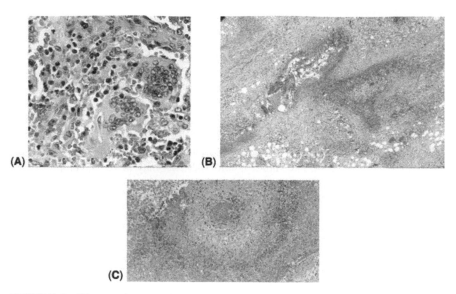

FIGURE 1 Wegener's granulomatosis: lung biopsy specimens demonstrating granuloma formation (**A**), necrosis with a geographic pattern (**B**), and vasculitis (**C**).

CLINICAL MANIFESTATIONS

WG is often described in the literature as "limited" or "generalized." Generalized disease is defined by the presence of GN, but does not necessarily indicate more severe disease. For example, patients may develop central nervous system (CNS) involvement, pulmonary hemorrhage, or gut ischemia in the absence of GN and have severe and life-threatening disease. It is therefore best to avoid terms "limited" and "generalized," and instead, note the organ systems involved and severity of illness. WG can progress over time and change from being mild to severe. Renal involvement is present in approximately 20% of patients at onset of disease and in approximately 80% later during the course of disease (Table 1) (7).

The initial symptoms typically involve the ENT region. The nose and sinuses are the most frequently affected sites in the head and neck. Symptoms of nasal mucosa inflammation include crusting, pain, epistaxis, ulceration, altered sense of smell, serosanguineous or purulent discharge, and nasal obstruction. Affected nasal mucosa results in loss of local

TABLE 1 Clinical Manifestations in Wegener's Granulomatosis

Features of disease	Prevalence at onset of disease (%)	Prevalence during course of disease (%)
Ear, nose, and throat	70	90
Lung	45	85
Glomerulonephritis	20	70–80
Eye	15	50
Skin	15	45
Musculoskeletal	30	70

Source: Adapted from Ref. 7.

lubrication and immunity. Consequently, patients frequently suffer from recurrent infections. Collapse of the nasal bridge ("saddle nose" deformity) may occur due to nasal chondritis (Fig. 2). Nasal examination typically reveals crusting, discharge, friable erythematous mucosa, and granulation tissue. Nasal septum perforation may occur. The paranasal sinuses, most commonly the maxillary and ethmoid sinuses, are affected in at least two-thirds of patients. In time, many patients develop pansinusitis. Inflammation of sinus mucosa and epithelium may result in discharge, obstruction, increased pressure, facial pain, headache, and secondary infection. Chronic inflammation usually produces sinuses lined by scar tissue and airspace obliteration. Mastoiditis may result in severe pain. Regional extension of sinus disease may lead to intracranial complications such as meningitis, epidural and subdural empyema, or cerebral abscess. Orbital complications may arise *de novo* or be a complication of disease extension from sinuses and include cellulitis, blepharitis, displacement of the globe (proptosis), extraocular muscle palsy, diplopia, visual impairment, and even blindness (8).

The middle ear is affected in at least one-third to one-half of all patients (9). Clinical features include otalgia, otitis media, and serous, purulent, or bloody discharge. Patients with chronic otitis media may present with conductive hearing loss due to thickened, scarred, or perforated tympanic membranes. Chronic otitis media can also lead to the development of a cholesteatoma (Fig. 3). Over time, the cholesteatoma increases in size and as a consequence can destroy the middle ear bones or the mastoid, or may erode into the inner ear and cause permanent hearing loss or dizziness. The facial nerve may be involved by the growth of the cholesteatoma, resulting in facial paralysis. Less often (<5% cases), hearing loss may be due to sensory neural involvement (Chapter 28). Vestibular disease may result in intermittent (~5%) or persistent (<1%) vertigo. The external ear is rarely the site of chondritis and can be associated with edema, erythema, and pain that may be identical to that of relapsing polychondritis (Chapter 7).

The oral cavity and oropharynx can develop ulcerations, edema, hyperplastic and inflamed gingiva, and sialadenitis. Rare examples of WG presenting as a parotid mass are well documented.

Subglottic stenosis (SGS) occurs in about 20% of patients. It is the result of inflammation and subsequent scar formation. Presentations include hoarseness, pain, dyspnea, cough, and stridor. Patients may have obvious wheezing, which appears to be diffuse with lung auscultation. Mistaking SGS for asthma is not unusual. If early symptoms are ignored, progression to severe stenosis may require an emergency tracheostomy.

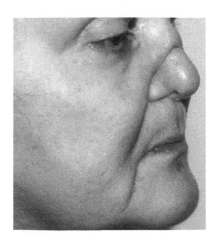

FIGURE 2 Wegener's granulomatosis: saddle nose deformity.

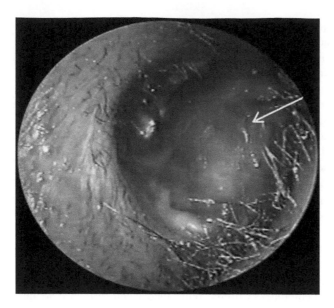

FIGURE 3 Wegener's granulomatosis: cholesteatoma.

Wheezing and dyspnea in the setting of WG and chest imaging studies that rule out active lung disease should always raise the question of SGS. The diagnosis should be pursued by nasolaryngoscopy with adequate visualization of the subglottic region (Fig. 4).

Ocular involvement may become apparent as eye or orbit pain, visual impairment, diplopia, episcleritis, scleritis, conjunctivitis, uveitis, retinitis, and dacrocystitis. Proptosis due to orbital pseudotumor is present in approximately 15% of cases and is the cause of pain, diplopia, and/or visual loss. Pseudotumor may cause vision loss in approximately 50% of patients that present with this complication (Fig. 5) (7).

Musculoskeletal disease in WG includes myalgias and migratory arthralgias. Frank arthritis can occur; but pain alone, disproportionate to findings on joint examination, is far more common. Frank myositis is rare. Constitutional symptoms, such as fever, night sweats, and weight loss, may occur with or precede characteristic organ system involvement.

Lung disease can present with focal or diffuse infiltrates, nodules that may cavitate, endobronchial stenosis, and pleuritis. Active pulmonary disease may be asymptomatic in up to one-quarter of patients. This is more common in the setting of nodules seen on chest computed tomography. Alveolar hemorrhage is almost always symptomatic and results from small-vessel vasculitis (capillaritis). It can be associated with cough, dyspnea, hemoptysis, and a rapidly falling hematocrit. Diffuse involvement may lead to ventilator dependency.

Nervous system disease in WG is less common and may result from diffuse, small-vessel involvement or mass lesions. Both may be seen in the CNS, leading to cranial neuropathies, stroke, aseptic meningitis, and intracerebral bleeds. The peripheral nervous system is most often affected by small-vessel vasculitis causing sensory neuropathies or mononeuritis multiplex (7).

Skin manifestations include palpable purpura from leukocytoclastic vasculitis, livedo reticularis, subcutaneous nodules, vesicles, papules, ulcers, small to large areas of infarction, and gangrene.

WG cardiac effects are clinically less apparent. Pericarditis is the most frequent manifestation. Myocarditis and valvular heart disease may also occur.

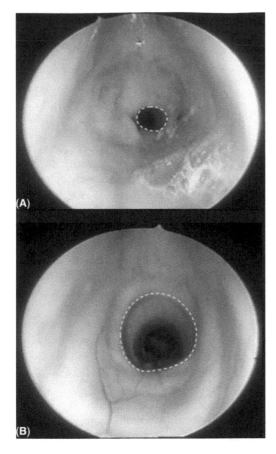

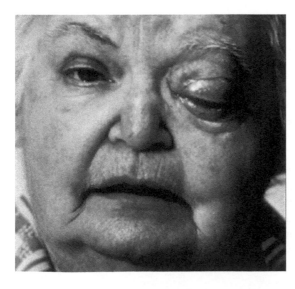

FIGURE 4 Wegener's granulomatosis: subglottic stenosis before (**A**) and after (**B**) injection of depocorticosteroids and dilatation.

FIGURE 5 Wegener's granulomatosis: orbital pseudotumor.

Other less affected sites are the pulmonary arteries, breast, and genital system. WG can affect any anatomic site, although as previously noted, it does have a unique predilection for the airways and kidneys.

DIAGNOSIS

The diagnosis is mainly based on clinical manifestations supported by laboratory abnormalities and pathology when biopsies are necessary and feasible. Anemia, leukocytosis, thrombocytosis, and high erythrocyte sedimentation rate and C-reactive protein may be present, but are neither diagnostic nor specific for WG. About 80% of all patients with WG are ANCA-positive and 80% of those patients produce ANCA with a diffuse cytoplasmic fluorescence pattern (C-ANCA) and antigen specificity for proteinase-3 (PR3-ANCA). About 10% to 20% of ANCA may have a perinuclear fluorescence pattern (P-ANCA) with specificity for myeloperoxidase (MPO-ANCA). The sensitivity of PR3-ANCA in WG is approximately 90% in patients with severe active disease and 55% to 75% in those with milder active disease (10). The combined use of indirect immunofluorescence (IIF) and antigen-specific enzyme-linked immunoassays results in diagnostic specificity of up to 98% (11). Urine sediment must be evaluated in all patients for the presence of microscopic hematuria and red blood cell casts, which are excellent surrogate markers of GN.

Differential diagnosis depends on the clinical presentation. In the setting of pulmonary–renal syndrome, WG needs to be distinguished from systemic lupus erythematosus (SLE), Goodpasture's syndrome, MPA, and CSS. MPA can closely mimic WG, except that the former lacks chronic, persistent ENT features (12). If WG presents in a classical manner and ANCA is positive, with specificity for PR3, the diagnosis is very likely. Diagnosis may be significantly delayed in patients with disease limited to the head and neck. The differential diagnosis of ENT disease includes chronic infections (e.g., tuberculous, fungal, and syphilitic), malignancy (e.g., lymphoma), sarcoidosis, CSS, and an unusual WG-mimic (13), a granulomatous syndrome that mimics WG and is associated with low surface expression of HLA class I molecules (14). Patients with class I HLA deficiency do not respond to the usual therapies for WG, which should suggest the possibility of this diagnosis. The differential diagnosis of septal perforation includes sarcoidosis, cocaine use, SLE, extranodal nasal lymphoma, lymphomatoid granulomatosis (LYG), and excessive use of intranasal corticosteroids.

TREATMENT

Systemic treatment of WG consists of a combination of glucocorticoids (GC) and a cytotoxic agent. For life- or major organ-threatening disease, daily cyclophosphamide (CYC) therapy is used (7). After three to six months, when disease remission or significant improvement is achieved, CYC is discontinued to avoid the significant morbidity associated with prolonged exposure to this agent. A less toxic agent such as methotrexate (MTX) (15) or azathioprine (AZA) (16) is used to try to sustain remission. For patients with milder forms of disease, MTX has been useful as initial and maintenance therapy (17). The optimal period of maintenance therapy has not yet been determined in randomized, controlled studies. The decision of how long to treat with cytotoxic agents must be individualized. After one month of treatment with GC (prednisone 1 mg/kg/day), the dose is slowly decreased over a period of about six months until discontinuation, if that is possible without relapse. Some patients may require low doses of GC (e.g., prednisone 5–10 mg/day) to maintain disease control.

Local treatment for disease involving the head and neck region is often necessary. Empiric experience has led to recommendations to maximize upper airway hygiene to minimize obstruction from crusts and other debris, and diminish colonization with infectious agents. For patients with chronic persistent sinus symptoms, nasal irrigation may be required up to several times a day. Water picks with nasal adaptors, or customized irrigation systems, use 200 to 1000 cc of saline or sterile water for irrigation, repeated until the return becomes clear. Since chronic nasal carriage of *Staphylococcus aureus* is associated with a higher rate of disease relapse (18), reduction of nasal colonization by irrigation, with or without nasal topical antibiotics, is advocated by most authorities. An alternative to antibiotics is to use moisturizing agents that contain lubricants such as glycerylmonoleate. Either would be applied with cotton applicators within the outer one-third of the nasal vestibule and sniffed up toward the sinuses after irrigation to help reduce symptoms from dry mucosa. For some patients with severe destruction of the nasal structures, large crusts may have to be mechanically removed. Repeated courses of oral antibiotics are occasionally necessary for patients who experience frequent or continuous ENT infections.

Surgery is usually reserved for refractory head and neck manifestations. In general, when there is a choice, it is best to consider surgery when disease is under control and GC doses are minimal. High doses of GC may pose a problem, considering the potential for this medication to impair wound healing. Unfortunately, in some patients, symptoms may be severe and surgery may be needed for prompt relief or diagnosis. Diagnosis in this case may refer to initial diagnosis of WG or to distinguishing WG from infection. Indeed, features of both can play a role in many patients.

Sinus surgery is performed to restore drainage, either through the external or intranasal approach. Both endoscopic and external approaches have been utilized. The goals include removing diseased tissue, which is the source of pain; restoring more natural drainage; and in cases with uncertainty, obtaining tissue to aid in diagnosis (8).

Repair of septal perforations is not recommended. Perforations alone are usually not the cause of significant symptoms. In addition, because it is difficult to distinguish low-grade active disease from the effects of chronic damage, there is risk that unnecessary surgery may produce an exaggerated inflammatory response, making matters worse (19).

Saddle nose deformity is a therapeutic challenge. Many patients seek reconstruction surgery, but such procedures may have significant complications. The repair may be followed by graft resorption and even worse deformity than that originally noted. This appears to be more common in patients in whom WG was not in remission and for whom medications were not minimized at the time of surgery. In a small series (13 patients, 16 surgical procedures) from the Mayo Clinic, materials for nasal reconstruction associated with failures were irradiated homografts (rib and dura mater). Autologous materials such as calvarial bone and costal cartilage provided better results. All patients were in remission at the time of surgery. Neither local nor systemic perioperative disease relapses occurred. Median follow-up was 33 months (range 10–177 months). Disease severity was evaluated as it related to the success of the procedure. Patients with only ENT disease (8/13) had a success rate of 88% (7/8 primary reconstructions). In patients with ENT and lung involvement (5/13), the success rate was 60% (3/5 primary reconstructions). None of the patients had renal disease. It was suggested that disease severity may affect the chance for a successful outcome, but because of the small number of cases, no definitive conclusions can be made (20).

Dacryocystorhinostomy for obstruction and/or recurrent infection in the lacrimal duct and sac can be performed using an external or endonasal approach. Major complications are infection and necrosis of the surgical repair area and formation of nasocutaneous fistula. As with surgery for saddle nose deformity, the likelihood of success is greater if the disease is in remission (21).

Most patients with recurrent or persistent serous otitis media resulting from Eustachian tube dysfunction can be helped by myringotomy with or without tympanostomy tube placement (Fig. 6) (22).

Mastoidectomy is indicated for selected patients with severe refractory mastoid inflammation.

Nearly all cholesteatomas require surgical excision (tympanoplasty with mastoidectomy). If left untreated, progressive destruction of the ear can occur.

Combined subglottic dilatation and intralesional injection of depo-GC has been successfully employed and has resulted in marked reduction in the need for tracheotomies for SGS (23). The stenotic lesion is injected submucosally with methylprednisolone acetate or an equivalent depo-GC preparation. If necessary, longitudinal incisions are made to release the constricting stenotic ring. Progressive serial dilatations with Maloney bougies or a Fogarty catheter balloon are then performed. Some, although not all authorities, have also recommended topical applications of mitomycin-C to inhibit fibrosis and restenosis (24); however, the value of topical mitomycin-C has not been evaluated in controlled trials. In longitudinal experiences with this technique at the National Institutes of Health (25) and Cleveland Clinic (23), none of over 40 patients required a new tracheostomy and there were only three significant complications (pneumothoraces). There were no adverse long-term sequelae (23,25).

Laser therapy for SGS should be avoided because of the high risk of producing severe laryngeal damage, more extensive scar formation, and consequent restenosis. Stents should be considered only as a last resort in WG. Metal stent placement for benign disease is frequently associated with airway complications including stent fracture, excessive granulation tissue, poor patient tolerance, inability to successfully place the prosthesis, and stent migration (26). In addition, inflammatory tissue from active WG may grow through the stent interstices, increasing the risk of restenosis (27).

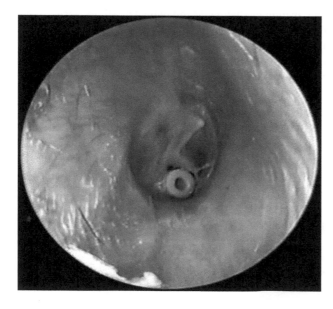

FIGURE 6 Wegener's granulomatosis: myringotomy with tympanostomy tube placement.

Tube-free tracheostomy is a relatively new procedure for patients requiring permanent tracheostomy and has the advantages of preserving the patient's voice, cough mechanism, and normal swallowing (24). Laryngotracheal reconstruction with costal cartilage graft placement has been performed in selected patients. Attempted repair with this technique has allowed successful permanent tracheostomy tube decannulation without graft failure (28).

Immunosuppressive medication is the main therapy for orbital disease.

Rarely, orbital decompression may be necessary, if proptosis is severe enough to compromise the optic nerve. Unfortunately, this procedure is usually palliative at best; it does not guarantee sight preservation or pain relief.

COMPLICATIONS AND PROGNOSIS

Prognosis has dramatically improved since the combination of CYC and GC has been utilized for severe disease presentations. Milder forms of WG, in which critical organ systems are not involved, may be effectively treated with weekly MTX or daily AZA. Recent studies have demonstrated that in severe disease, making a transition from CYC to MTX or AZA after approximately three months spares, or markedly reduces, CYC toxicities. These include cystitis, bladder cancer, lymphoma, myelodysplasia, and sterility. Almost all patients will achieve remission with these approaches to therapy. Because relapses are very common, patients should be closely monitored for early signs and symptoms of disease, so that treatment may be instituted or changed without delay.

SUMMARY

Head and neck manifestations are very common in WG and may result in significant morbidity. WG is commonly associated with PR3-ANCA and is highly responsive to treatment with GC and cytotoxic agents. Modern therapy has reduced mortality from WG, from 50% within five months to less than 20% over at least eight years of follow-up. However, disease- and treatment-related morbidity is considerable. The notion that current therapies cure WG has been abandoned for the more realistic view that therapy is life-saving and converts a usually fatal disease to a chronic one.

CHURG-STRAUSS SYNDROME

INTRODUCTION

CSS, also known as allergic granulomatosis angiitis, is an idiopathic, systemic, eosinophilic syndrome in which vasculitis may become a complication. CSS was first described as a syndrome distinct from polyarteritis nodosa (PAN) in 1951 by Jacob Churg and Lotte Strauss. Although they share many clinical and pathological features, the presence of granulomas and peripheral eosinophilia distinguishes CSS from PAN.

DEFINITION

CSS is an inflammatory condition of the upper and lower respiratory tract that is associated with asthma, hypereosinophilia, and/or vasculitis.

EPIDEMIOLOGY

CSS is rare, and the exact prevalence is not known. The annual incidence reported from Norwich County, United Kingdom was 2.4 per million (29). The disease affects all age groups (mean age 48 years). There is no significant gender predilection.

PATHOGENESIS

Although the etiology of CSS is unknown, eosinophils are thought to play a central role in tissue injury. Precipitating factors may include inhaled antigens that stimulate eosinophils. Histopathological findings are remarkable for the presence of eosinophilic infiltrates, granulomata, and, in the most typical biopsies, necrotizing vasculitis of small- to medium-sized vessels (Fig. 7) (3). There are many reports of CSS cases occurring in association with the use of leukotriene receptor antagonists and various inhaled GC, but a definite causative role for these agents in the pathogenesis of CSS has not been firmly established.

CLINICAL MANIFESTATIONS

CSS may evolve in phases. Asthma and other allergic symptoms usually precede other manifestations. In time, pulmonary infiltrates (Fig. 8) and peripheral hypereosinophilia may dominate the clinical picture, followed by the involvement of multiple organ systems. Convincing pictures of CSS may evolve several months to years after the onset of asthma. Occasionally, asthma can occur concurrently with other CSS features (30).

The most common sites of CSS involvement are the lungs, ENT organs, and nervous system (Table 2). Pulmonary manifestations include asthma, alveolar hemorrhage, infiltrates, and pleural effusions. Asthma is one of the major symptoms and is considered necessary for the diagnosis. It usually starts during adult age and may be associated with other allergic symptoms (e.g., rhinitis). The majority of patients have nervous system involvement, with peripheral neuropathy (PN) and CNS involvement occurring in 50% to 80% and 8%, respectively. Mononeuritis multiplex is the most common form of PN. CNS symptoms include stroke, meningeal symptoms, intracerebral hemorrhage, convulsions, and cognitive deficits.

Skin involvement is common, with purpura being the most frequent manifestation. Other skin lesions include papules, vesicles, ischemia, necrosis, livedo reticularis, and

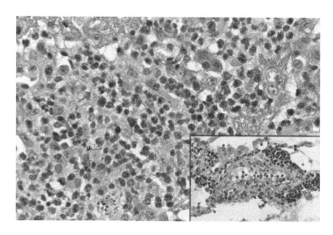

FIGURE 7 Churg-Strauss syndrome: eosinophilic pneumonia and vasculitis.

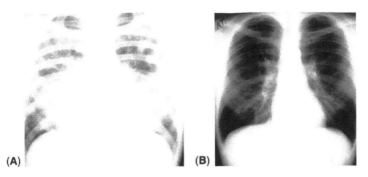

FIGURE 8 Churg-Strauss syndrome: Pulmonary infiltrates before (**A**) and after (**B**) treatment with corticosteroids and methotrexate.

Raynaud's phenomenon. Arthralgias and myalgias are frequent, but frank arthritis and myositis are uncommon. Gastrointestinal (GI) manifestations most frequently present as abdominal pain. The entire GI tract can be involved. Biopsies of affected sites may reveal vasculitis, granuloma formation, and/or inflammatory eosinophilic infiltrates. Cardiac disease may be severe and is the most frequent cause of death (30), occurring in approximately 35% (15–85%) of patients. Cardiac involvement most frequently includes heart failure, pericarditis, cardiomyopathy, and ischemic cardiomyopathy. Renal involvement is not as frequent in CSS as it is in WG and MPA. When present, renal disease is characterized by crescentic GN with scant or no immune-complex deposits.

ENT features are common in CSS. Sinusitis is one of the major manifestations and may precede the diagnosis in 60% of patients. Allergic rhinitis and nasal or sinus polyps are frequent (70%) (Fig. 9) (31). Although ENT features may be very similar to those of WG, they are usually milder and associated with less morbidity. It would be extremely unusual for CSS to cause a saddle nose deformity or SGS. Eye involvement in CSS includes episcleritis, scleritis, uveitis, retinal vasculitis, and conjunctivitis (32). Orbital pseudotumor would be very rare, and its presence should suggest WG.

Mild forms of CSS have been described, usually localized to one or few organ systems (32,33). Asthma may be absent, but allergic symptoms are frequent. Since the disease is rare, limited manifestations may not lead to suspicion of CSS.

TABLE 2 Clinical Manifestations in Churg-Strauss Syndrome

Features of disease	Prevalence at onset of disease (%)	Prevalence during course of disease (%)
Sinusitis	60	60
Lung		
Asthma	98	100
Infiltrates	37	37
Hemorrhage	3	4
Glomerulonephritis	8	8
Eye	3	3
Skin	50	50
Mononeuritis multiplex	77	78
GI	31	33
Pericardial effusion	22	23
Myocardial involvement	12	13

Abbreviation: GI, gastrointestinal.
Source: Adapted from Ref. 30.

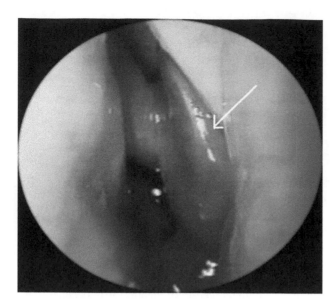

FIGURE 9 Churg-Strauss syndrome: nasal polyp.

DIAGNOSIS

The presence of a systemic disease with vasculitic manifestations preceded by asthma, allergic symptoms, and eosinophilia is suggestive of CSS. Eosinophil counts are typically greater than 1.500/mm^3. ANCAs may or may not be helpful for the diagnosis, since they are only present in 40% to 50% of patients (34). A positive ANCA is helpful, but a negative test does not rule out CSS. When present, ANCA is usually a perinuclear ("P") pattern on immunofluorescence and the antibodies are reactive to MPO. Occasionally, the antibody specificity may be to PR3, and the IIF pattern is cytoplasmic (C-ANCA). Chest imaging studies may show typical findings of bilateral patchy migratory interstitial or alveolar infiltrates. Pulmonary nodules are uncommon and cavities are very rare, the latter suggesting WG or secondary infection.

The differential diagnosis includes granulomatous diseases that may present with eosinophilia such as eosinophilic pneumonia, allergic bronchopulmonary aspergillosis, WG, parasitic and fungal infections, malignancy, and eosinophilic granuloma. When there is uncertainty about the diagnosis, pathologic confirmation should be pursued.

TREATMENT

Mild presentations may be adequately treated with corticosteroids alone. Many patients, however, cannot be tapered to low, minimally toxic doses of prednisone and require a second agent. MTX, used as has been described for milder forms of WG, may be adequate for these purposes. MTX is relatively contraindicated in patients with renal impairment. In such cases, alternative therapies that may be of value include AZA or mycophenolate mofetil. There is limited published experience regarding any of these agents in CSS. More severe cases require dual therapy with GC and CYC. Relapses requiring retreatment are common. Disease severity, as determined by organ system involvement and rate of progression, dictates choices of therapy.

COMPLICATIONS AND PROGNOSIS

Prognosis has improved dramatically with the use of GC. Remission occurs in at least 80% of patients and is associated with rapid reduction of the eosinophil count soon after onset of treatment. If treatment is delayed or inadequate, severe disease may result in death or serious morbidity from neurologic, intestinal, pulmonary, or cardiac disease.

SUMMARY

ENT and allergic symptoms are common in CSS. ENT damage is usually milder than that seen in WG. The disease is very responsive to GC, but severe manifestations require addition of a cytotoxic agent.

NASAL NATURAL KILLER (NK)/T-CELL LYMPHOMA

INTRODUCTION

Nasal natural killer (NK)/T-cell lymphoma, formerly known as "lethal midline granuloma" or "polymorphic reticulosis," is an extranodal tumor of NK-cell origin, with a predilection for the nasal cavity (35). Extranodal NK/T-cell lymphomas and LYG have been referred to as angiocentric immunoproliferative lesions, but further studies have revealed that the two diseases have different clinical features and immunophenotypes. They should therefore be considered distinct entities (Table 3). LYG is an Epstein-Barr-virus (EBV)–positive B-cell proliferative disease with a secondary T-cell response, whereas nasal NK/T-cell lymphoma is an EBV-positive NK cell or cytotoxic T-cell disorder. LYG, unlike nasal NK/T-cell lymphoma, frequently involves the lung, kidney, and CNS, and rarely the nasal area. Similarities between the two diseases include EBV positivity and histologic features (necrosis and angiocentric damage) (36). The report of the Hong Kong Workshop on Nasal and Related Extranodal Angiocentric T/NK Cell Lymphomas stated that nasal NK/T-cell lymphoma should be considered a distinct clinical-pathological entity based on its biologic behavior, characteristic immunophenotype, and strong association with EBV (37). Nasal-type NK/T-cell lymphoma is now recognized as a distinct lymphoma subtype within the

TABLE 3 EBV-Positive Extranodal Angiocentric Immunoproliferative Diseases

Disease	Sites of involvement	Phenotype	Comments
Nasal-type NK/T-cell lymphoma	Nasal cavity Paranasal sinuses Skin Subcutaneous tissue GI tract Testis	NK/T-cell	Radiation may be helpful to control localized nasal disease Poor prognosis Poor response to chemotherapy
LYG	Lung (nodules) Skin CNS Kidney GI tract Liver	B-cell	Variable clinical course: from indolent with spontaneous remission to very aggressive lymphoma

Abbreviations: CNS, central nervous system; EBV, Epstein-Barr virus; GI, gastrointestinal; LYG, lymphomatoid granulomatosis; NK, natural killer.

World Health Organization classification of lymphoid tumors and includes both nasal and extranasal tumors (38).

DEFINITION

Nasal NK/T-cell lymphoma causes destructive lesions localized exclusively or predominantly to the nasal cavity and paranasal sinuses. Extensive tissue necrosis is present. Lymphocyte proliferation has a propensity to be angiocentric and angiodestructive. The cell of origin is often an NK-cell, but some cases arise from cytolytic T-cells (NK-like T-cells that express CD56 and T-cell intracellular antigen-1 [TIA-1]), hence the term "nasal NK/T-cell lymphoma" (35).

EPIDEMIOLOGY

NK-cell neoplasms are rare. The most common and well-characterized are the nasal and nasal-type NK-cell neoplasm. Nasal NK/T-cell lymphoma is common in Asians and rare in Caucasians. The disease is also more prevalent in individuals of Native American heritage (Central and South America) (37). It occurs more commonly in males (3.3:1). The median age is approximately 50 years.

PATHOGENESIS

Molecular analyses of nasal NK/T-cell lymphomas have shown the presence of EBV in a clonal episomal form, suggesting its involvement in tumorigenesis (39). EBV is present in essentially all cases. Whether or not EBV is the ultimate cause of nasal NK/T-cell lymphomas is uncertain.

Zonal necrosis, vascular damage, prominent apoptosis, and hemophagocytosis are common features. In more than 60% of cases, the tumor cells are angiocentric and angioinvasive. The atypical cells can be a mixture of small, medium, or large cells, but most are large dysplastic cells with numerous admixed inflammatory cells (35).

In NK-cell malignancies, the cells show expression of TIA-1, granzyme B, perforin, and FAS ligand, important elements in mediating massive apoptosis and necrosis. Since angioinvasion is not seen in all cases, the cause of necrosis appears to be more complex than just physical disruption of blood vessels.

Nasal NK/T-cell tumor cells express some T-cell–associated antigens, most commonly CD2, but other T-cell markers, such as surface CD3, are usually absent. In favor of an NK-cell origin, cytoplasmic CD3, a normal marker of NK-cells, and CD56 are typically found, although CD16 and CD57 are usually negative. Molecular studies have not shown a clonal T-cell gene rearrangement in the majority of cases (40).

CLINICAL MANIFESTATIONS

Common presenting symptoms are nasal crusting, serosanguineous discharge, epistaxis, nasal swelling and obstruction, and constitutional ("B") symptoms (fever, night sweats, and weight loss). Destruction of the nasal cartilages and bone, occasionally with local infiltration into the adjacent facial areas (e.g., orbital swelling), may occur. Some cases present with a mass effect (i.e., a nasal mass or obstruction). Patients may experience long-standing symptoms before diagnosis is made. Secondary infection of necrotic tissue is not uncommon.

Localized disease may progress and involve the skin and subcutaneous tissue and less often the GI tract, testis, and upper respiratory tract.

A hemophagocytic syndrome may complicate the disease and adversely affect survival. It may occur at any time during the clinical course and is usually fatal after a period of several weeks.

DIAGNOSIS

The evaluation of patients with mid-facial destructive lesions includes imaging studies to delineate the extent of disease, as well as biopsy for immunohistochemical studies, flow cytometry, and identification of molecular studies. Extranodal tumors are difficult to diagnose and can be confused with reactive processes. There is no one specific diagnostic test; nasal NK/T-cell lymphoma diagnosis is based on a combination of clinical, histologic, immunophenotypic, and genotypic features. Clinical features that help the diagnosis include the location (nasal area), pattern of disease in extranodal sites, and rarity of nodal disease. Immunophenotyping may not be specific, but to be considered a nasal NK/T-cell tumor it must include NK-cells and/or cytotoxic T-cell–associated antigens. The most common cell phenotype is CD2+, cytoplasmic CD3+, surface CD3–, and CD56+. Absence of EBV by in situ hybridization helps to rule out nasal NK/T-cell lymphoma. Histology shows necrosis in essentially all cases, and, although common, angiocentric infiltrates are not required for the diagnosis (37).

The differential diagnosis includes LYG, an NK-cell lymphoproliferative disorder also referred to as NK-cell large granular lymphocytosis, herpes simplex infection (HIS), enteropathy-associated T-cell lymphoma (ETCL), WG, and cocaine abuse. HIS may stimulate reactive lymphoid proliferation that, in the nasal area, can mimic nasal NK/T-cell lymphoma. LYG shows many overlapping features, but is a B-cell disorder. ETCL usually involves the GI tract, and may result in extensive necrosis, but only rarely is associated with EBV (37).

TREATMENT

The optimal therapy for NK/T neoplasms is controversial due to the rarity of these diseases, their variable clinical course, and the lack of randomized clinical trials. As with other lymphomas, surgical resection of sinonasal lymphomas is not recommended. Overall complete remission with different treatment modalities is approximately 65% (39). Initial treatment with radiation therapy (RT) alone might be beneficial to patients with early stage disease, but results from small series are variable (39); the purported advantage of early RT needs to be validated in larger prospective studies. Studies in nasal-type NK/T-cell lymphoma have failed to show outcome improvement with addition of chemotherapy (CT) to RT; moreover, response to CT alone was observed to be poor, with a higher risk of local recurrence. In one study, the five-year overall survival rates for RT alone and RT plus CT were 76% and 59%, respectively (41). Investigators have suggested that CT should be reserved for the control of micrometastasis after achieving local control using RT.

COMPLICATIONS AND PROGNOSIS

Nasal NK/T-cell lymphoma is localized in its initial stages in 80% of patients; however, it can disseminate early. Prognosis is usually poor (35). The International Prognostic Index (IPI), predictive of treatment outcome in malignant lymphomas of different grades and subtypes, has been applied for this type of lymphoma. It has been suggested that patients with high IPI scores, and therefore a worse prognosis, may benefit from additional therapy to prevent relapses (39). Systemic progression is usually fatal. Life-long follow-up is recommended for all patients, in view of the possibility of delayed relapse.

SUMMARY

Nasal NK/T-cell lymphoma is an EBV-positive cytotoxic T- or NK-cell disorder that has recently been recognized as a distinct clinical entity. Prognosis is poor in most patients, regardless of therapy. The field suffers from the difficulty of conducting treatment trials for rare diseases. The state of the art has consequently been defined by empiric interventions.

REFERENCES

1. Hoffman GS, Gross WL. Wegener's granulomatosis: clinical aspects. In: Hoffman GS, Weyand CM, eds. Inflammatory Diseases of Blood Vessels. New York, NY and Basel, Switzerland: Marcel Dekker, Inc, 2002:381–397.
2. Jennette JC, Falk RJ, Andrassy K, et al. Nomenclature of systemic vasculitides. Proposal of an international consensus conference. Arthritis Rheum 1994; 37(2):187–192.
3. Hoffman GS, Langford CA. Are there different forms of life in the antineutrophil cytoplasmic antibody universe? Ann Intern Med 2005; 143(9):683–685.
4. Cotch MF, Hoffman GS, Yerg DE, et al. The epidemiology of Wegener's granulomatosis. Estimates of the five-year period prevalence, annual mortality, and geographic disease distribution from population-based data sources. Arthritis Rheum 1996; 39(1):87–92.
5. Devaney KO, Travis WD, Hoffman G, et al. Interpretation of head and neck biopsies in Wegener's granulomatosis. A pathologic study of 126 biopsies in 70 patients. Am J Surg Pathol 1990; 14 (6):555–564.
6. Weiss MA, Crissman JD. Renal biopsy findings in Wegener's granulomatosis: segmental necrotizing glomerulonephritis with glomerular thrombosis. Hum Pathol 1984; 15(10):943–956.
7. Hoffman GS, Kerr GS, Leavitt RY, et al. Wegener granulomatosis: an analysis of 158 patients. Ann Intern Med 1992; 116(6):488–498.
8. Lebovics RS. Sinonasal complications of vasculitic diseases. Cleve Clin J Med 2002; 69(suppl 2): SII152–SII154.
9. Gubbels SP, Barkhuizen A, Hwang PH. Head and neck manifestations of Wegener's granulomatosis. Otolaryngol Clin North Am 2003; 36(4):685–705.
10. Hoffman GS, Specks U. Antineutrophil cytoplasmic antibodies. Arthritis Rheum 1998; 41(9):1521–1537.
11. Vassilopoulos D, Niles JL, Villa-Forte A, et al. Prevalence of antineutrophil cytoplasmic antibodies in patients with various pulmonary diseases or multiorgan dysfunction. Arthritis Rheum 2003; 49 (2):151–155.
12. Savage CO, Winearls CG, Evans DJ, et al. Microscopic polyarteritis: presentation, pathology and prognosis. Q J Med 1985; 56(220):467–483.
13. Lamprecht P, Trabandt A, Gross WL. Clinical and Immunological Aspects of Wegener's Granulomatosis (WG) and other syndromes resembling WG. Isr Med Assoc J 2000; 2(8):621–626.
14. Moins-Teisserenc HT, Gadola SD, Cella M, et al. Association of a syndrome resembling Wegener's granulomatosis with low surface expression of HLA class-I molecules. Lancet 1999; 354(9190):1598–1603. Erratum in Lancet 2000; 356(9224):170. Baycal C [corrected to Baykal C].
15. Langford CA, Talar-Williams C, Barron KS, et al. Use of a cyclophosphamide-induction methotrexate-maintenance regimen for the treatment of Wegener's granulomatosis: extended follow-up and rate of relapse. Am J Med 2003; 114(6):463–469.
16. Jayne D, Rasmussen N, Andrassy K, et al. A randomized trial of maintenance therapy for vasculitis associated with antineutrophil cytoplasmic autoantibodies. N Engl J Med 2003; 349(1):36–44.
17. De Groot K, Rasmussen N, Bacon PA, et al. Randomized trial of cyclophosphamide versus methotrexate for induction of remission in early systemic antineutrophil cytoplasmic antibody-associated vasculitis. Arthritis Rheum 2005; 52(8):2461–2469.
18. Stegeman CA, Tervaert JW, Sluiter WJ, et al Association of chronic nasal carriage of Staphylococcus aureus and higher relapse rates in Wegener granulomatosis. Ann Intern Med 1994; 120(1):12–17.

19. Rasmussen N. Management of the ear, nose, and throat manifestations of Wegener granulomatosis: an otorhinolaryngologist's perspective. Curr Opin Rheumatol 2001; 13(1):3–11.

20. Congdon D, Sherris DA, Specks U, et al. Long-term follow-up of repair of external nasal deformities in patients with Wegener's granulomatosis. Laryngoscope 2002; 112(4):731–737.

21. Kwan AS, Rose GE. Lacrimal drainage surgery in Wegener's granulomatosis. Br J Ophthalmol 2000; 84(3):329–331.

22. Kornblut AD, Wolff SM, Fauci AS. Ear disease in patients with Wegener's granulomatosis. Laryngoscope 1982; 92(7 Pt 1):713–717.

23. Hoffman GS, Thomas-Golbanov CK, Chan J, et al. Treatment of subglottic stenosis, due to Wegener's granulomatosis, with intralesional corticosteroids and dilation. J Rheumatol 2003; 30(5):1017–1021.

24. Eliachar I, Chan J, Akst L. New approaches to the management of subglottic stenosis in Wegener's granulomatosis. Cleve Clin J Med 2002; 69(suppl 2):SII149–SII151.

25. Langford CA, Sneller MC, Hallahan CW. Clinical features and therapeutic management of subglottic stenosis in patients with Wegener's granulomatosis. Arthritis Rheum 1996; 39(10):1754–1760.

26. Zakaluzny SA, Lane JD, Mair EA. Complications of tracheobronchial airway stents. Otolaryngol Head Neck Surg 2003; 128(4):478–488.

27. Mair EA. Caution in using subglottic stents for Wegener's granulomatosis. Laryngoscope 2004; 114 (11):2060–2061.

28. Gluth MB, Shinners PA, Kasperbauer JL. Subglottic stenosis associated with Wegener's granulomatosis. Laryngoscope 2003; 113(8):1304–1307.

29. Watts RA, Carruthers DM, Scott DJ. Epidemiology of systemic vasculitis: changing incidence or definition? Semin Arthritis Rheum 1995; 25(1):28–34.

30. Guillevin L, Cohen P, Gayraud M, et al. Churg–Strauss syndrome. Clinical study and long-term follow-up of 96 patients. Medicine (Baltimore) 1999; 78(1):26–37.

31. Lanham JG, Elkon KB, Pusey CD, et al. Systemic vasculitis with asthma and eosinophilia: a clinical approach to the Churg-Strauss syndrome. Medicine (Baltimore) 1984; 63(2):65–81.

32. Nissim F, Von der Valde J, Czernobilsky B. A limited form of Churg-Strauss syndrome: ocular and cutaneous manifestations. Arch Pathol Lab Med 1982; 106(6):305–307.

33. Churg A, Brallas M, Cronin SR, et al. Formes frustes of Churg-Strauss syndrome. Chest 1995; 108 (2):320–323.

34. Sable-Fourtassou R, Cohen P, Mahr A, et al. Antineutrophil cytoplasmic antibodies and the Churg-Strauss syndrome. Ann Intern Med 2005; 143(9):632–638.

35. Greer JP, Kinney MC, Loughran TP Jr. T cell and NK cell lymphoproliferative disorders. Hematology (Am Soc Hematol Educ Program) 2001; 259–281.

36. Jaffe ES. Pathologic and clinical spectrum of post-thymic T-cell malignancies. Cancer Invest 1984; 2 (5):413–426.

37. Jaffe ES, Chan JK, Su IJ, et al. Report of the Workshop on Nasal and Related Extranodal Angiocentric T/Natural Killer Cell Lymphomas. Definitions, differential diagnosis, and epidemiology. Am J Surg Pathol 1996; 20(1):103–111.

38. Harris NL, Jaffe ES, Diebold J, et al. World Health Organization classification of neoplastic diseases of the hematopoietic and lymphoid tissues: Report of the Clinical Advisory Committee Meeting, Airlie House, Virginia, Nov, 1997. Ann Oncol 1999; 10(12):1419–1432.

39. Chim CS, Ma SY, Au WY. Primary nasal natural killer cell lymphoma: long-term treatment outcome and relationship with the International Prognostic Index. Blood 2004; 103(1):216–221.

40. Nava VE, Jaffe ES. The pathology of NK-cell lymphomas and leukemias. Adv Anat Pathol 2005; 12 (1):27–34.

41. Kim K, Chie EK, Kim CW, et al. Treatment outcome of angiocentric T-cell and NK/T-cell lymphoma, nasal type: radiotherapy versus chemoradiotherapy. Jpn J Clin Oncol 2005; 35(1):1–5.

9

Kawasaki Disease

Jane C. Burns
Department of Pediatrics, School of Medicine, University of California and Rady Children's Hospital, San Diego, California, U.S.A.

INTRODUCTION

Kawasaki disease (KD) is a systemic vasculitis of infants and children that may present initially with fever and unilateral cervical adenopathy as the only clinical features. Early diagnosis and administration of high-dose intravenous gamma-globulin (IVIG) can prevent coronary artery aneurysms, which occur in up to 25% of untreated children. The otolaryngologist may see these patients in referral and must learn to recognize the principal diagnostic criteria that constitute the clinical case definition.

DEFINITION

KD is an acute rash/fever illness of childhood that is recognized by a constellation of clinical signs and symptoms (1). The vasculitis causes damage to the coronary arteries in up to 25% of untreated children. Although an infectious trigger is suspected, the cause of KD is unknown and there is no specific laboratory-based diagnostic test. Principal clinical criteria include fever for at least four days accompanied by at least four of five clinical signs listed in Table 1. New guidelines from the American Heart Association incorporate laboratory data and echocardiographic data into the diagnostic algorithm for patients with fewer than four criteria (Table 2) (2).

EPIDEMIOLOGY

KD has been described in children of all races and ethnic backgrounds but is clearly overrepresented among Japanese and Japanese American children. In Japan and among Japanese residents of Hawaii, the annual incidence is approximately 200/100,000 children below five years of age (3). Over 185,000 children have been diagnosed with KD in Japan and more than 8000 new Japanese cases were recognized in 2001 (4). This means that approximately one in every 150 children in Japan will suffer from KD. In the continental United States, incidence estimates for KD vary from 15 to 18.8 per 100,000 children below five years of age (5,6). Using hospital discharge databases, the Centers for Disease Control and Prevention estimated that 4248 children below five years of age were diagnosed and treated in the United States in the year 2000 at a cost of $51 million (7). The variation of KD incidence among different ethnic groups is likely related to host genetic factors that influence disease susceptibility (8,9).

The etiology of KD remains unknown, although an infectious cause is suspected, based on seasonality and clustering of cases and the similarity of clinical signs to other

TABLE 1 Modified Diagnostic Criteria for KD

The diagnosis of KD is considered confirmed by the presence of fever and at least three of five clinical signs with supportive laboratory data:
1. Bilateral conjunctival injection
2. Changes of the mucous membranes of the upper respiratory tract: injected pharynx, injected, fissured lips, and strawberry tongue
3. Changes of the peripheral extremities: peripheral edema, peripheral erythema, and periungual desquamation
4. Polymorphous rash
5. Cervical adenopathy

Abbreviation: KD, Kawasaki disease.
Source: From Ref. 2.

TABLE 2 Laboratory Findings Suggestive of Kawasaki Disease

CRP $\geq$ 3.0 mg/dL
ESR $\geq$ 40 mm/hr
Albumin $\leq$ 3.0 mg/dL
Anemia for age
Elevated alanine aminotransferase and γ-glutamyl transpeptidase
Platelet count $\geq$ 450,000 after first week of fever
White blood cell count $\geq$ 15,000/μL
Urine white blood cell count $\geq$ 10 cells/hpf
CSF pleocytosis with normal CSF protein
Changes on echocardiogram including z score of LAD or RCA $\geq$ 2.5, lack of vessel tapering, perivascular brightness, decreased LV function, mitral regurgitation, and pericardial effusion

Abbreviations: CRP, C-reactive protein; CSF, cerebrospinal fluid; ESR, erythrocyte sedimentation rate; hpf, high power field; LAD, left anterior descending coronary artery; LV, left ventricle; RCA, right coronary artery.
Source: From Ref. 2.

infectious diseases. In addition, the peak incidence in infants and children less than five years of age, coupled with the rare occurrence of KD in adults and infants less than three months of age, is consistent with infection with a widely disseminated agent that causes asymptomatic infection in most hosts and the acquisition of protective immunity and passage of transplacental antibodies.

PATHOGENESIS

KD is a self-limited vasculitis that affects medium-sized, extraparenchymal muscular arteries and is now the most common cause of acquired heart disease in the pediatric age group (10,11). The systemic vasculitis is associated with elevated levels of proinflammatory cytokines including interleukin (IL)-6 and tumor necrosis factor-α and a marked acute phase response (11). Most of our knowledge of the evolution of the vasculitis in KD is derived from autopsy data (12,13). The earliest changes involve the endothelium of the musculoelastic arteries and include swelling, proliferation, enlarged nuclei, and frank degeneration with adherent platelets entrapped in fibrin (14). The endothelium of the vaso vasorum of larger arteries can be similarly involved. More advanced lesions show edema and inflammatory cell infiltrate in the subendothelial space. This progresses to destruction of the media with frank necrosis associated with infiltration of monocytes and lymphocytes of the memory T-cell (CD45RO+) and cytotoxic/suppressor (CD8+) phenotypes from both the lumen and adventitia, which results in a transmural vasculitis (15). Replacement of the intima and media with fibrous connective tissue, thinning of the media with aneurysm formation, scarring, and stenosis complete the progression of the vasculitis. The development of stenotic lesions occurs over a period of months to years, and these lesions may remain silent until the moment of acute thrombotic occlusion, often decades after the initial acute illness (16).

The finding of IgA-secreting plasma cells infiltrating into the trachea and small airways coupled with molecular evidence of an oligoclonal IgA response suggest a pathogen with a respiratory portal of entry (17,18). In addition, a synthetic antibody produced using reverse genetics and molecular methods stains intracytoplasmic inclusions in tingible macrophages, which are found infiltrating various tissues (19). Histologic examination of lymph nodes biopsied from acute KD patients and described in Kawasaki's original report revealed nonspecific changes including swelling of endothelial cells in postcapillary venules and hyperplasia of reticulum cells (20,21). Subsequent reports described focal areas of necrosis associated with microthrombi in adjacent vessels, hyperplasia of the T-cell zones of lymphoid follicles, and macrophage infiltration of B-cell zones (22,23).

CLINICAL MANIFESTATIONS

The clinical findings in acute KD evolve over the first week after onset of fever and include the features described in Table 1. The onset of fever is usually abrupt, without a prodrome, and has a spiking/remitting pattern throughout the day. More than 90% of patients develop bilateral, symmetrical dilatation of vessels in the bulbar conjunctiva with limbal sparing, which creates a "halo effect" around the iris (24). There is no exudate, and conjunctival biopsy reveals no local inflammatory response (25).

Changes of the lips and oral cavity include dryness, erythema and fissuring of the lips, diffuse erythema of the oropharynx without pharyngeal exudates or discrete intraoral lesions, and a strawberry tongue with sloughing of the filiform papillae with prominence of the fungiform and circumvallate papillae (26). Hoarseness is frequently noted and direct fiberoptic laryngoscopy has revealed marked edema and erythema of the vocal cords (Dr. Deborah Don, Rady Children's Hospital of San Diego, personal communication).

The rash is a polymorphous exanthem with nonspecific changes on biopsy (27). Target lesions, petechiae, and micropustules may be seen, but the rash is never frankly bullous, thus differentiating it from Stevens-Johnson syndrome (Chapter 22) (1,28). The rash may be dramatically accentuated in the perineum in over 50% of patients (29).

Changes in the extremities may include erythema of the palms and soles, indurative edema of the dorsa of the hands and feet, and periungual desquamation during the subacute phase (second to third week of illness). Not uncommonly, the diagnosis of KD is made retrospectively when the characteristic peeling of the fingers and toes is noted. Unfortunately, coronary artery damage from the vasculitis may already be apparent at this point in the illness.

Although unilateral or bilateral, nonsuppurative cervical lymphadenopathy with at least one node measuring at least 1.5 cm was among the original criteria described by Kawasaki, it has been noted in only 40% to 50% of patients in more recent series (1,26,30). In one series, 43 of 83 KD patients (52%) developed cervical adenopathy during their acute illness and 18 of these 43 patients (42%) were initially misdiagnosed and treated for bacterial cervical lymphadenitis (30). Patients presenting with cervical adenopathy tended to be older and have a higher erythrocyte sedimentation rate and total white blood cell count than KD patients who never developed clinically apparent cervical node enlargement. In another series of 50 KD patients from Canada, 16 of the 50 patients (32%) presented with fever and a prominent otolaryngologic condition (cervical adenitis, tonsillitis, or otitis media) that misled the treating physician and delayed the correct diagnosis of KD (31). Initial misdiagnosis is common and 60% to 90% of KD patients in various series were initially treated with antibiotics before the correct diagnosis was made (32,33). The otolaryngologist should consider the possibility of KD in any pediatric patient who is not responding to antibiotic treatment for presumed bacterial cervical lymphadenitis (33–36). Case reports have documented the association of KD with retropharyngeal soft-tissue swelling, mastoiditis, and upper airway compromise (34,37–45).

Other clinical and laboratory features that may accompany the systemic vasculitis of KD include arthralgia and arthritis, hydrops of the gallbladder with associated abdominal pain and elevated γ glutamyltranspeptidase, sterile pyuria, anterior uveitis, meningitis with cerebrospinal fluid (CSF) pleocytosis and irritability, and sensorineural hearing loss (26,46,47). Case reports from the United States and Japan have documented 20 patients with moderate-to-profound, permanent sensorineural hearing loss following the acute phase of KD (48,49). A prospective, multicenter study conducted in North America documented sensorineural hearing loss (20–35 dB) in 19 of 62 patients (30%) evaluated within 30 days after onset of fever using visual reinforcement, play audiometry, tympanometry, and brainstem auditory-evoked response testing in patients below one year of age or in patients for whom the results of behavioral audiometry were deemed unreliable (50). Persistent hearing loss was noted in 2 of 36 patients (5.5%) evaluated at least 10 days after the first evaluation. The investigators concluded that routine audiologic screening of KD patients was not warranted but that health-care providers should be aware of the possibility of profound sensorineural hearing loss as a rare complication of KD. The pathogenesis of hearing loss in this setting is unknown, although direct cytopathic effect of the causative agent in the cochlea or labyrinth, vasculitis of the vasonervorum of cranial nerve VIII, or direct immunologic attack on components of the inner ear have been proposed (50). Sensorineural hearing loss is discussed in detail in Chapter 28.

DIAGNOSIS

KD is a self-limited disease whose signs and symptoms evolve over the first 10 days of illness and then gradually resolve spontaneously in most children, even in the absence of specific therapy (26). Frequently, not all clinical criteria for KD are present on any given day. Moreover, there is no laboratory test that establishes the diagnosis, and clinicians must rely on history and physical examination to determine if patients meet clinical criteria. The development of coronary artery damage in up to 25% of untreated children is usually clinically silent and may only be recognized years later, at the time of a myocardial infarction or death (16). While the greatest concern is that KD is underdiagnosed, it is also likely that some degree of overdiagnosis occurs. Until there is a diagnostic test for KD, children will continue to be misdiagnosed and suffer preventable morbidity and mortality.

In a study from Japan, Tashiro et al. used transverse ultrasonographic evaluation of cervical lymph nodes with a 7.5- to 10-MHz transducer to distinguish between bacterial lymphadenitis, Epstein–Barr virus (EBV) infection, and KD (51). While sonograms of patients with EBV infection and KD revealed clusters of multiple, hypoechoic nodes forming a single palpable mass, sonograms of patients with documented bacterial lymphadenitis demonstrated a single, well-defined mass with a large, central hypoechoic region. Reports of computed tomography in KD patients with cervical node enlargement describe similar findings with multiple nodes forming a single, palpable mass (34,38,42).

TREATMENT

Randomized clinical trials have established that treatment within the first 10 days of onset of fever with IVIG (2 g/kg) and aspirin (80–100 mg/kg/day) reduces the risk of coronary artery damage and aneurysm formation from 20% to 25% to only 3% to 5% (52). Approximately 85% of patients will respond to a single dose of IVIG with cessation of fever and disappearance of all the clinical signs of the vasculitis. There is much speculation, but little data, on the mechanism of action of IVIG in acute KD. Possible mechanisms include cross-linking of FcγII and FcγIII receptors on macrophages, selective induction of IL-1–receptor antagonist and IL-8, or provision of specific antiagent, anti-idiotype, anticytokine, or antitoxin antibodies (53,54). Approximately 15% of KD patients will fail to respond to a single dose of IVIG and have persistent fever (55). The optimal treatment regimen for these patients has not been determined by randomized, controlled trials. These patients are at higher risk of coronary artery aneurysm formation and should receive additional immunomodulatory therapy, which may include a second dose of IVIG, high-dose pulse methylprednisolone (30 mg/kg/day × 3 days), or infliximab (5 mg/kg) (56–58).

COMPLICATIONS AND PROGNOSIS

Studies of large numbers of children have established that cardiac echocardiography is an accurate method to detect and monitor coronary artery dilatation and aneurysms in children with KD (2). Children with no coronary artery changes detectable by echocardiogram during the acute phase may have clinically silent myocardial fibrosis and impaired vasodilatory capacity of coronary and peripheral arteries (59). Thus, the long-term effects on the cardiovascular system remain uncertain for all children. For children with coronary artery aneurysms, approximately 25% will develop coronary artery stenosis (60) and may subsequently require treatment for myocardial ischemia including percutaneous transluminal angioplasty, coronary artery stenting, arterial bypass grafting, and even cardiac transplantation (2).

Sensorineural hearing loss as a complication of KD may be diagnosed, particularly in young infants, long after the resolution of acute illness. Because KD is a self-limited illness that resolves even in the absence of specific therapy, the diagnosis may be missed and the illness forgotten. Thus, a history of a rash/fever illness compatible with KD should be sought in any child undergoing evaluation of unexplained sensorineural hearing loss. Suspicion of missed KD should prompt referral to a pediatric cardiologist for echocardiography to detect possible coronary artery abnormalities.

SUMMARY

KD is an acute, self-limited vasculitis of the pediatric age group that must be diagnosed and treated in a timely manner. This presents a unique dilemma for the clinician: the disease may be difficult to recognize, there is no diagnostic laboratory test, there is an extremely effective therapy, and there is a 25% chance of serious cardiovascular damage if the therapy is not administered early in the course of the disease. Children with KD may be referred to the otolaryngologist for a variety of signs and symptoms including cervical adenitis, hoarseness, airway obstruction, torticollis, and retropharyngeal soft-tissue swelling accompanied by fever and failure to respond to appropriate antibiotic therapy. Clinical signs of KD should be sought through a careful history and physical examination in these patients, and cardiac echocardiography should be considered as an adjunct to establishing the diagnosis. Sensorineural hearing loss is a rare but potentially devastating sequela of the acute vasculitis of KD. A history of an antecedent illness compatible with KD should be sought in all pediatric patients evaluated for idiopathic sensorineural hearing loss.

REFERENCES

1. Kawasaki T, Kosaki F, Okawa S, et al. A new infantile acute febrile mucocutaneous lymph node syndrome (MLNS) prevailing in Japan. Pediatrics 1974; 54(3):271–276.
2. Newburger JW, Takahashi M, Gerber MA, et al. Diagnosis, treatment, and long-term management of Kawasaki disease: a statement for health professionals from the Committee on Rheumatic Fever, Endocarditis and Kawasaki Disease, Council on Cardiovascular Disease in the Young, American Heart Association. Circulation 2004; 110(17):2747–2771.
3. Holman RC, Curns AT, Belay ED, et al. Kawasaki syndrome in Hawaii. Pediatr Infect Dis J 2005; 24 (5):429–433.

4. Burns JC, Cayan DR, Tong G, et al. Seasonality and temporal clustering of Kawasaki syndrome. Epidemiology 2005; 16(2):220–225.
5. Bronstein DE, Dille AN, Austin JP, et al. Relationship of climate, ethnicity and socioeconomic status to Kawasaki disease in San Diego County, 1994 through 1998. Pediatr Infect Dis J 2000; 19 (11):1087–1091.
6. Holman RC, Shahriari A, Effler PV, et al. Kawasaki syndrome hospitalizations among children in Hawaii and Connecticut. Arch Pediatr Adolesc Med 2000; 154(8):804–808.
7. Holman RC, Curns AT, Belay ED, et al. Kawasaki syndrome hospitalizations in the United States, 1997 and 2000. Pediatrics 2003; 112(3):495–501.
8. Burns JC, Shimizu C, Shike H, et al. Family-based association analysis implicates IL-4 in susceptibility to Kawasaki disease. Genes Immun 2005; 6(5):438–444.
9. Burns JC, Shimizu C, Gonzalez E, et al. Genetic variations in the receptor-ligand pair CCR5 and CCL3L1 are important determinants of susceptibility to Kawasaki disease. J Infect Dis 2005; 192 (2):344–349.
10. Taubert KA, Rowley AH, Shulman ST. Nationwide survey of Kawasaki disease and acute rheumatic fever. J Pediatr 1991; 119(2):279–282.
11. Burns JC, Glode MP. Kawasaki syndrome. Lancet 2004; 364(9433):533–544.
12. Burns JC, Felsburg PJ, Wilson H, et al. Canine pain syndrome is a model for the study of Kawasaki disease. Perspect Biol Med 1991; 35(1):68–73.
13. Naoe S, Takahashi K, Masuda H, et al. Kawasaki disease. With particular emphasis on arterial lesions. Acta Pathol Jpn 1991; 41(11):785–797.
14. Amano S, Hazama F, Hamashima Y. Pathology of Kawasaki disease: I. pathology and morphogenesis of the vascular changes. Jpn Circ J 1979; 43(7):633–643.
15. Brown TJ, Crawford SE, Cornwall ML, et al. CD8 T lymphocytes and macrophages infiltrate coronary artery aneurysms in acute Kawasaki disease. J Infect Dis 2001; 184(7):940–943.
16. Burns JC, Shike H, Gordon JB, et al. Sequelae of Kawasaki disease in adolescents and young adults. J Am Coll Cardiol 1996; 28(1):253–257.
17. Rowley AH, Shulman ST, Spike BT, et al. Oligoclonal IgA response in the vascular wall in acute Kawasaki disease. J Immunol 2001; 166(2):1334–1343.
18. Rowley AH, Shulman ST, Mask CA, et al. IgA plasma cell infiltration of proximal respiratory tract, pancreas, kidney, and coronary artery in acute Kawasaki disease. J Infect Dis 2000; 182(4): 1183–1191.
19. Rowley AH, Baker SC, Shulman ST, et al. Detection of antigen in bronchial epithelium and macrophages in acute Kawasaki disease by use of synthetic antibody. J Infect Dis 2004; 190(4): 856–865.
20. Kawasaki T. Acute febrile mucocutaneous syndrome with lymphoid involvement with specific desquamation of the fingers and toes in children. Arerugi 1967; 16(3):178–222.
21. Shike H, Burns JC, Shimizu C. Translation of Dr. Tomisaku Kawasaki's original report of fifty patients in 1967. Pediatr Infect Dis J 2002; 21(11):online, http//www.pidj.com.
22. Corbeel L, Delmotte B, Standaert L, et al. Kawasaki disease in Europe. Lancet 1977; 1(8015): 797–798.
23. Giesker DW, Pastuszak WT, Forouhar FA, et al. Lymph node biopsy for early diagnosis in Kawasaki disease. Am J Surg Pathol 1982; 6(6):493–501.
24. Smith LB, Newburger JW, Burns JC. Kawasaki syndrome and the eye. Pediatr Infect Dis J 1989; 8 (2):116–118.
25. Burns JC, Wright JD, Newburger JW, et al. Conjunctival biopsy in patients with Kawasaki disease. Pediatr Pathol Lab Med 1995; 15(4):547–553.
26. Burns JC, Mason WH, Glode MP, et al. Clinical and epidemiologic characteristics of patients referred for evaluation of possible Kawasaki disease. United States Multicenter Kawasaki Disease Study Group. J Pediatr 1991; 118(5):680–686.
27. Sato N, Sagawa K, Sasaguri Y, et al. Immunopathology and cytokine detection in the skin lesions of patients with Kawasaki disease. J Pediatr 1993; 122(2):198–203.
28. Kimura T, Miyazawa H, Watanabe K, et al. Small pustules in Kawasaki disease. A clinicopathological study of four patients. Am J Dermatopathol 1988; 10(3):218–223.
29. Friter BS, Lucky AW. The perineal eruption of Kawasaki syndrome. Arch Dermatol 1988; 124(12):1805–1810.
30. April MM, Burns JC, Newburger JW, et al. Kawasaki disease and cervical adenopathy. Arch Otolaryngol Head Neck Surg 1989; 115(4):512–514.
31. Park AH, Batchra N, Rowley A, et al. Patterns of Kawasaki syndrome presentation. Int J Pediatr Otorhinolaryngol 1997; 40(1):41–50.

32. Kryzer TC, Derkay CS. Kawasaki disease: five-year experience at Children's National Medical Center. Int J Pediatr Otorhinolaryngol 1992; 23(3):211–220.
33. Seicshnaydre MA, Frable MA. Kawasaki disease: early presentation to the otolaryngologist. Otolaryngol Head Neck Surg 1993; 108(4):344–347.
34. Murrant NJ, Cook JA, Murch SH. Acute ENT admission in Kawasaki disease. J Laryngol Otol 1990; 104(7):581–584.
35. Kao HT, Huang YC, Lin TY. Kawasaki disease presenting as cervical lymphadenitis or deep neck infection. Otolaryngol Head Neck Surg 2001; 124(4):468–470.
36. Waggoner-Fountain LA, Hayden GF, Hendley JO. Kawasaki syndrome masquerading as bacterial lymphadenitis. Clin Pediatr (Phila) 1995; 34(4):185–189.
37. Puczynski MS, Stankiewicz JA, Ow PE. Mucocutaneous lymph node syndrome mimicking acute coalescent mastoiditis. Am J Otol 1986; 7(1):71–73.
38. McLaughlin RB Jr, Keller JL, Wetmore RF, et al. Kawasaki disease: a diagnostic dilemma. Am J Otolaryngol 1998; 19(4):274–277.
39. Shetty AK, Homsi O, Ward K, et al. Massive lymphadenopathy and airway obstruction in a child with Kawasaki disease: success with pulse steroid therapy. J Rheumatol 1998; 25(6):1215–1217.
40. Rothfield RE, Arriaga MA, Felder H. Peritonsillar abscess in Kawasaki disease. Int J Pediatr Otorhinolaryngol 1990; 20(1):73–79.
41. Hester TO, Harris JP, Kenny JF, et al. Retropharyngeal cellulitis: a manifestation of Kawasaki disease in children. Otolaryngol Head Neck Surg 1993; 109(6):1030–1033.
42. Burgner D, Festa M, Isaacs D. Delayed diagnosis of Kawasaki disease presenting with massive lymphadenopathy and airway obstruction. Br Med J 1996; 312(7044):1471–1472.
43. Homicz MR, Carvalho D, Kearns DB, et al. An atypical presentation of Kawasaki disease resembling a retropharyngeal abscess. Int J Pediatr Otorhinolaryngol 2000; 54(1):45–49.
44. Bradley MK, Crowder TH. Retropharyngeal mass in a child with mucocutaneous lymph node syndrome. Clin Pediatr (Phila) 1983; 22(6):444–445.
45. Korkis JA, Stillwater LB. An unusual otolaryngological problem—mucocutaneous lymph node syndrome (Kawasaki's syndrome) case report. J Otolaryngol 1985; 14(4):257–260.
46. Dengler LD, Capparelli EV, Bastian JF, et al. Cerebrospinal fluid profile in patients with acute Kawasaki disease. Pediatr Infect Dis J 1998; 17(6):478–481.
47. Ting EC, Capparelli EV, Billman GF, et al. Elevated gamma-glutamyltransferase concentrations in patients with acute Kawasaki disease. Pediatr Infect Dis J 1998; 17(5):431–432.
48. Sundel RP, Newburger JW, McGill T, et al. Sensorineural hearing loss associated with Kawasaki disease. J Pediatr 1990; 117(3):371–377.
49. Sundel RP, Cleveland SS, Beiser AS, et al. Audiologic profiles of children with Kawasaki disease. Am J Otol 1992; 13(6):512–515.
50. Knott PD, Orloff LA, Harris JP. Sensorineural hearing loss and Kawasaki disease: a prospective study. Am J Otolaryngol 2001; 22(5):343–348.
51. Tashiro N, Matsubara T, Uchida M, et al. Ultrasonographic evaluation of cervical lymph nodes in Kawasaki disease. Pediatrics 2002; 109(5):E77.
52. Newburger JW, Takahashi M, Beiser AS, et al. A single intravenous infusion of gamma globulin as compared with four infusions in the treatment of acute Kawasaki syndrome. N Engl J Med 1991; 324 (23):1633–1639.
53. Ravetch JV, Lanier LL. Immune inhibitory receptors. Science 2000; 290(5489):84–89.
54. Ruiz de Souza V, Carreno MP, Kaveri SV, et al. Selective induction of interleukin-1 receptor antagonist and interleukin-8 in human monocytes by normal polyspecific IgG (intravenous immunoglobulin). Eur J Immunol 1995; 25(5):1267–1273.
55. Burns JC, Capparelli EV, Brown JA, et al. Intravenous gamma-globulin treatment and retreatment in Kawasaki disease. US/Canadian Kawasaki Syndrome Study Group. Pediatr Infect Dis J 1998; 17 (12):1144–1148.
56. Sundel RP, Burns JC, Baker A, et al. Gamma globulin re-treatment in Kawasaki disease. J Pediatr 1993; 123(4):657–659.
57. Wright DA, Newburger JW, Baker A, et al. Treatment of immune globulin-resistant Kawasaki disease with pulsed doses of corticosteroids. J Pediatr 1996; 128(1):146–149.
58. Burns JC, Mason WH, Hauger SB, et al. Infliximab treatment for refractory Kawasaki syndrome. J Pediatr 2005; 146(5):662–667.
59. Newburger JW, Burns JC. Kawasaki disease. Vasc Med 1999; 4(3):187–202.
60. Kato H, Sugimura T, Akagi T, et al. Long-term consequences of Kawasaki disease. A 10- to 21-year follow-up study of 594 patients. Circulation 1996; 94(6):1379–1385.

10

Epstein-Barr, Herpes Simplex, and Herpes Zoster Infections

Kedar K. Adour
Department of Head and Neck Surgery, Kaiser Permanente Medical Center, Oakland, California, U.S.A.

INTRODUCTION

The three most common types of herpes viruses that infect humans are the Epstein-Barr virus (EBV), herpes simplex virus types 1 (HSV-1) and 2 (HSV-2), and herpes zoster virus (HZV), more properly called the varicella zoster virus (VZV). All three have a DNA genomic core encased in a nucleocapsid surrounded by the viral envelope, but each produces different clinical manifestations. A common feature shared by all three viruses is the ability either to persist in a nonreplicating state in specific cells or to replicate, thereby producing secondary disease or asymptomatic viral shedding.

EPSTEIN-BARR VIRUS

DEFINITION

In 1968, researchers determined that EBV causes heterophile-positive infectious mononucleosis (1). The clinical presentation of mononucleosis includes fever, sore throat, headache, white patches in the oropharynx, swollen neck glands, and lethargy.

EPIDEMIOLOGY

EBV is a member of the herpesvirus family and is one of the most common human viruses. It occurs worldwide and is estimated to have infected as many as 95% of adults in the United States. After birth, infants become susceptible when maternal EBV antibody protection disappears. In children, EBV infection is usually mild and indistinguishable from other mild childhood illnesses. EBV infection causes infectious mononucleosis in 35% to 50% of infected adolescents. Mononucleosis is not easily spread and is found in saliva and mucus passed from person to person through intimate contact, the reason for the lay terminology, "kissing disease." Clinical symptoms of infectious mononucleosis generally develop four to seven weeks after exposure. The condition occurs most commonly in persons between the ages of 15 years and 35 years and rarely recurs (2).

PATHOGENESIS

Like other members of the herpesvirus family, the EBV DNA viral genome is encased in a nucleocapsid surrounded by the viral envelope. EBV initially infects oropharyngeal epithelial cells; there, the virus replicates and then primarily infects B lymphocytes (B + EBV) and is disassembled. The genome is thus transported to the nucleus in a state of viral latency. Nearly all seropositive persons actively shed virus in the saliva. During primary viral infection, the EBV-infected B cells rapidly proliferate. The infection is usually brought under control by cytotoxic T cells, and this process often results in infectious mononucleosis. After the acute infection resolves, the virus persists in the peripheral B cells without causing disease; however, in males with X-linked lymphoproliferative disorder, the initial B + EBV proliferation is not contained and may result in fatal mononucleosis (1).

CLINICAL MANIFESTATIONS

Classic symptoms of infectious mononucleosis are the triad of fever, pharyngitis, and cervical lymphadenopathy. In addition to fever, systemic symptoms include fatigue and generalized lymphadenopathy. Oral hairy leukoplakia, a collection of hairy or corrugated white lesions located on the lateral surface of the tongue, is common. Sometimes splenomegaly or mild hepatitis may develop. Uncommon manifestations include heart problems, jaundice, pneumonitis, blood dyscrasia, and cerebritis (2). In patients with HIV infection, infection of epithelial cells by EBV is often represented by oral hairy leukoplakia.

DIAGNOSIS

The diagnosis is suggested by the clinical features. The most frequently used serologic test is the EBV-specific heterophile antibody test (the "monospot test," "mononucleosis spot test," or Paul–Bunnell test), which gives a positive result (2). Other abnormal laboratory findings include elevated white blood cell (WBC) count ranging from 1.0×10^9/L to 1.5×10^9/L; of these WBCs, 50% or more are "atypical" lymphocytes with oval, kidney-shaped nuclei and vacuolated cytoplasm. Thrombocytopenia is common, and levels of hepatic enzymes may be elevated.

Cytomegalovirus (CMV) can produce symptoms that mimic those of infectious mononucleosis, but give a negative result when subjected to the heterophile antibody test. The diagnosis must be made by isolating the CMV virus. CMV-type mononucleosis usually has both slower onset and slower resolution. Most infected patients recover without sequelae.

TREATMENT

No specific therapy is available to treat infectious mononucleosis. Most practitioners advise bed rest, increased fluid intake, and use of pain relievers such as acetaminophen or ibuprofen. Aspirin should not be given to children younger than 16 years, because doing so may trigger the rare but potentially fatal disorder known as Reye's syndrome (2). Antibiotic drugs are not given for viral disease but should be given to treat any superimposed streptococcal or sinus infection. Treatment with piperacillin/tazobactam is probably the causative agent in systemic rash. Early reports individually implicated corticosteroid or ampicillin treatment as causing peritonsillar abscess formation, but have since been disproved (3).

Many practitioners believe that for most patients with infectious mononucleosis, no specific therapy is indicated. Because corticosteroid drugs shorten the duration of fever and oropharyngeal symptoms, allowing patients the benefit of such treatment seems prudent. Corticosteroid therapy is used for patients with severe complications such as impending upper-airway obstruction, acute hemolytic anemia, severe cardiac involvement, or neurologic disease.

Acyclovir, which inhibits EBV replication and reduces viral shedding, is effective in treating oral hairy leukoplakia; however, because the immune response prevents acyclovir from having any clinically significant effect on the symptoms of mononucleosis, acyclovir is not recommended for treating this condition (2).

COMPLICATIONS AND PROGNOSIS

Most patients with infectious mononucleosis have the triad of fever, lymphadenopathy, and pharyngitis. The most common complication is swollen tonsils with obstructed

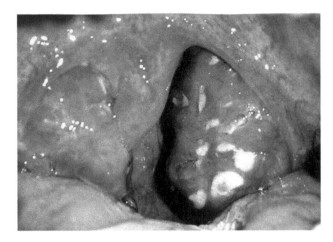

FIGURE 1 Photograph of a patient with mononucleosis shows obstructive tonsillitis.

breathing (Fig. 1) (3). Splenomegaly, palatal petechiae, and hepatomegaly develop in another 10% of infected patients. The main serious complication is enlarged spleen and its possible rupture. Less common complications include hemolytic anemia, thrombocytopenia, aplastic anemia, myocarditis, hepatitis, rash, and neurologic complications, such as Guillain–Barré syndrome, encephalitis, and meningitis.

Symptoms such as fever and sore throat usually lessen within two to three weeks. Fatigue, enlarged lymph nodes, and swollen spleen may last weeks longer. Most signs and symptoms ease within a few weeks, although two to three months may elapse before patients feel completely normal (4).

SUMMARY

Infectious mononucleosis is caused by the ubiquitous EBV virus, which is estimated to infect 80% to 95% of the U.S. population. In infants, the disease is unremarkable and mimics the usual benign diseases of childhood. In adolescents and in young adults under the age of 35 years, primary infection with EBV can cause lymphadenopathy, fever, and pharyngitis, a symptom triad often called "mono," "glandular fever," or the "kissing disease." Treatment for symptoms consists of bed rest, increased fluid intake, and use of anti-inflammatory pain relievers. The disease is inflammatory and immune-related, and clinical experience suggests that corticosteroid drugs should be used because they dramatically relieve the symptoms and shorten the duration of fatigue. Corticosteroid drugs should be used also to treat the most common complications of mononucleosis, i.e., respiratory obstruction (from enlarged tonsils) and splenomegaly.

*H*ERPES SIMPLEX VIRUS TYPE 1

INTRODUCTION

All herpes viruses can establish a persistent state after primary infection.

Persons who become infected with a herpesvirus are susceptible to periodic viral reactivation releasing transmissible virus. The latent sites determine clinical manifestations and are variable. HSV-1, HSV-2, and VZV have structure and propensity similar to all members of the herpesvirus family. The double-stranded DNA genome is surrounded by a nucleocapsid and becomes dormant and persistent in the nucleus of sensory cells. Although circulating antibodies are present in both diseases, HSV antibodies are not protective: Reactivation is common, and recurrence is not accompanied by increase in the quantity of circulating antibodies. HSV reactivation with replication produces secondary neurocutaneous disease or may manifest as asymptomatic viral shedding (5,6).

In VZV infection, the antibodies remain protective until later in life, when antibody protection is lost and recurrence manifests as segmental neurocutaneous disease ("shingles") with a concomitant rise in antibodies. VZV rarely recurs a second time. Another factor common to HSV and VZV is that both viruses are responsible for syndromes affecting multiple nerves and dermatomes.

DEFINITION

HSV-1 and HSV-2 are almost identical in structure; however, whereas HSV-1 has been associated with head and neck disease, HSV-2 primarily causes genital infection. As a result of oral–genital sexual encounters, both types of viruses can be isolated from the oral or genital area. The two viruses can cause identical lesions; however, herpetic encephalitis is usually caused by HSV-1 infection, whereas meningitis is usually caused by HSV-2 infection (7). (Discussion of genital herpes is beyond the scope of this chapter.)

EPIDEMIOLOGY

HSV-1 is ubiquitous, and HSV-1 infection is often acquired in the first decade of life by contact with oral secretions. Presence of antibodies to HSV-1 in a general population increases with age and correlates with socioeconomic status (7). By adulthood, 50% of people in the highest social strata are infected, as are 85% of people in lower social strata. Of those who are infected, more than 25% have recurrent episodes, which usually manifest as mucocutaneous herpes labialis. Between symptomatic episodes, HSV-1 can be shed in as many as 10% of healthy persons with a history of cold sores. This shedding spreads the infection. HSV-1 is transmitted chiefly by contact with infected saliva. The mode of transmission is by close personal contact. Aerosol spreading rarely occurs, because the virus is inactivated readily at room temperature and by drying (6).

PATHOGENESIS

With the exception of the optic and olfactory nerves, the HSV-1 genome has been detected in all sensory cranial ganglia (Fig. 2) and from cervical ganglia 2 and 3. When HSV-1 is injected into the cornea of experimental animals, the virus proceeds to the otic ganglion, then to the trigeminal ganglion, the glossopharyngeal and vagal ganglia, and finally down to the level of the second and third cervical ganglia. The virus also crosses the midline to infect contralateral ganglia.

HSV-1 infection occurs in three stages: the primary disease stage, the dormant (latent) stage, and the recurrent disease stage.

In the primary disease stage, infection is initiated by contact with infected oral secretions or lesions. The virus enters through mucocutaneous membranes or through a break in the skin. In the latent stage, the virus travels up the sensory nerves that reside in the nucleus of the cranial and spinal ganglia, where the virus is protected from circulating

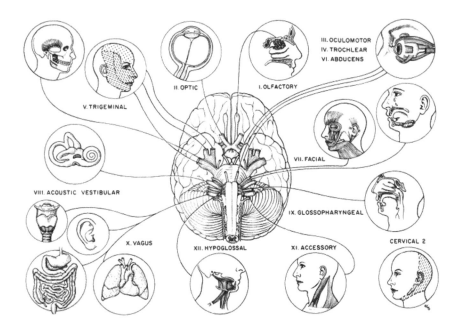

FIGURE 2 Schematic drawing of the cranial and cervical 2–3 nerves shows multiple areas of potential signs and symptoms of HSV-1 reactivation. *Abbreviation*: HSV-1, herpes simplex virus type 1.

antibodies but can be reactivated. Disease recurrence is triggered by multiple factors, including fever, trauma, emotional stress, sunlight, menstruation, and ovulation (5).

Because every replication begins in ganglion cells, every case of recurrent HSV infection starts as ganglionitis (8). When the virus is episodically reactivated in multiple ganglia, it does so as polyganglionitis episodica (PGE). The virus only then passes down the axons to induce radiculitis and finally mucocutaneous disease. The virus also travels up the axon to the brain stem to form a localized arachnoiditis, but usually does not cause generalized encephalitis.

When the virus genome leaves the nucleus, it acquires a nuclear protein coat from the nucleus and thus forms a nucleocapsid. This nucleocapsid acquires an envelope of lipoprotein from the plasma membrane of the infected cell (Fig. 3). This alteration in the host cell membrane and deposition of neural protein in perineural areas leads to processes— T lymphocyte sensitization and virally induced immune response—that cause demyelinization. The mucocutaneous vesicles caused by the virus invading epithelial cells merely represent the visible perimeter of the infected area. These virally mediated cranial neurologic syndromes include many sensory symptoms as well as motor paralysis (9).

CLINICAL MANIFESTATIONS

The primary episode of HSV-1 infection manifests after the patient is exposed to secretions containing viable HSV-1, which then incubate for three to six days. Mucocutaneous lesions, which can be painful, develop into vesicles that erupt for one to two weeks (Fig. 4). In many cases, areas of gingivostomatitis and surrounding skin lesions are prominent and

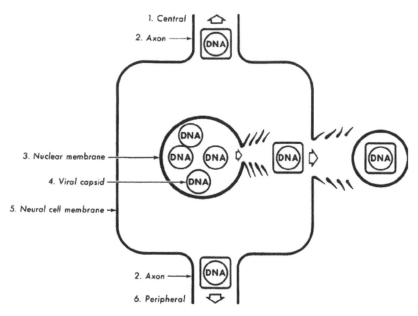

1. Central
2. Axon
3. Nuclear membrane
4. Viral capsid
5. Neural cell membrane
2. Axon
6. Peripheral

FIGURE 3 Schematic representation of HSV replication within sensory ganglion cells shows centripetal and centrifugal migration and envelopment with portions of neural cell lipoproteins. *Abbreviation*: HSV, herpes simplex virus. *Source*: From Ref. 8.

are associated with lymphadenopathy. Systemic symptoms include fever, malaise, myalgia, anorexia, and dysphagia. Painful, shallow ulcers are formed by breakdown of individual vesicles. Skin vesicles persist longer and develop into crusted ulcers that heal in five to seven days (6).

Recurrent infection can be either subclinical (characterized by viral excretion without formation of lesions) or overt (characterized by formation of mucocutaneous lesions). Many affected patients have prodromal dysesthesia, paresthesia, and a burning sensation at the site of impending vesicular lesions. Typical lesions are small, painful, fluid-filled vesicles that form crusts and shallow ulcers within three to five days. Localized lymphadenopathy can

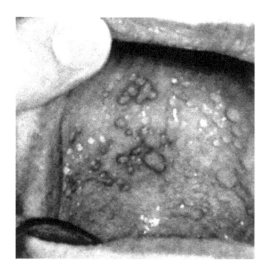

FIGURE 4 Photograph shows recurrent oral herpes simplex ulceration of the palate.

occur; unlike primary infection, however, constitutional symptoms are minimal. Recurrent episodes last three to seven days and can be frequent or occur once or twice in a lifetime. Over time, the number of annually recurrent episodes tends to decrease. The neurologic manifestation of recurrent infection depends on the neural ganglia specifically involved in the reactivation: Whereas the sensory component of the peripheral neurologic system is separated from the motor system, motor fibers in the cranial nerves traverse the ganglion in direct contact with sensory ganglion cells. This intimate contact is postulated to lead to virally induced demyelinization of motor fibers and subsequent paralysis or palsy (8).

Every sensory system has an inhibitory system, and in the cranial nerves, the inhibitory fibers traverse the ganglion. Decreased function of the ganglion cells cause hypofunction, whereas loss of inhibition creates a hyperactive state such as intolerance to light, sound, and touch. Photophobia results from reduction in the number of inhibitory impulses reaching the optic nerve; phonophobia results from reduction in the number of such impulses reaching the auditory nerve. To emphasize the similarity of symptoms associated with loss of inhibition at different nerve sites, this discussion will refer to phonophobia in place of hyperacusis and will refer to somatophobia in place of hyperesthesia (8).

Reactivation can occur in one ganglion or in multiple ganglia. When occurring in multiple ganglia, reactivation represents polyganglionitis. Table 1 lists the signs and symptoms associated with cranial and cervical ganglia function, decreased function, and loss of inhibition, as well as the clinical syndromes that these processes are postulated to cause (Fig. 5).

The most visible clinical manifestation of herpetic polyganglionitis is Bell's palsy, a condition which commonly affects the trigeminal, glossopharyngeal, vagal, vestibular-cochlear, and cervical nerves (9). Otherwise-healthy patients affected with this condition present with a one-sided facial droop (Fig. 6) and complain of pain behind the ear as well as facial numbness on the affected side. Other symptoms may include dysgeusia and phonophobia (hyperacusis) resulting from loss of inhibitory impulses to the cochlea, probably originating from the olivocochlear bundle of cranial nerve VIII. Results of physical examination confirm numbness of the face (trigeminal nerve) and postauricular area (second and third cervical nerves) (Fig. 7). All patients with Bell's palsy have unilateral inflammation of the fungiform papillae of the tongue (Fig. 8). Some patients with Bell's palsy have unilateral inflammation of the circumvallate papillae (Fig. 9), which are supplied by the glossopharyngeal nerve (8). Other patients may have partial motor paresis of the palate (Fig. 10), which is supplied by vagus nerve.

The features of migraine headache are not clearly differentiated from those of severe tension headache caused by muscle contraction. Both types of headache are usually unilateral, have a female-to-male predominance of 3:1, are activated by stress and menstruation, and are associated with varying neurologic signs and symptoms. The unilateral nature of the headache is not fully explained by describing the pathophysiology causing both types of headache.

Most clinicians agree that a vascular effect is inherent in migraine headache. In addition, the HSV-1 genome has been shown in temporal artery biopsy specimens (12). A common finding in patients with migraine headache is a unilateral increase in somatic sensitivity (somatophobia) of the postauricular and occipital area when the hair is combed, yet astute testing shows numbness (hypesthesia) of that area. This finding is typical of both HSV and herpes zoster. Recurrent herpes simplex PGE explains the prodrome, unilaterality, chronicity, familial incidence, female predominance, age distribution, findings of sterile inflammation, and neurologic dysfunction characteristic of migraine headache.

Temporomandibular joint dysfunction syndrome (formerly called Costen's syndrome) is a prime example of polyganglionitis (11). Manifestations include occipital

(*Text continues on page 137*)

TABLE 1 Clinical Signs and Symptoms of Polyganglionitis Episodica (HSV-1 Reactivation) Associated with Each Cranial Nerve

Cranial nerve	Decreased function	Questionable symptoms	Decreased inhibition	Associated diagnosis
Optic	Scotomata		Photophobia	Migraine
Trigeminal (motor)	Paresis of muscles of mastication	Bruxism	Late-onset contracture pain (somatophobia)	Temporomandibular joint syndrome
Trigeminal (sensory)	Hypesthesia; dysesthesia			Atypical facial pain; tic douloureux
Facial (motor)	Paralysis		Late-onset contracture with synkinesis	Bell's palsy
Facial (visceral sensory)	Dysgeusia			
Facial (autonomic)	Decreased salivary flow			
Auditory	Hearing loss	Tinnitus	Phonophobia	Sudden hearing loss; cochlear Ménière's disease
Vestibular	Decreased caloric response; decreased gag reflex	Positional nystagmus	Spontaneous nystagmus	Vestibular vertigo; hearing loss + vertigo = Ménière's disease
Glossopharyngeal (somatic sensory)	Ageusia/hypogeusia	Dysgeusia	Somatophobia	Globus; pharyngeal pain neuralgia (Sluder's syndrome)
Glossopharyngeal (visceral sensory)				Part of Bell's palsy
Glossopharyngeal (autonomic)	Decreased parotid salivation			Sjögren's syndrome
Vagal (motor)	Paresis of palate, vocalis, cricothyroid, esophageal muscles	Heart block	Dysphagia; late-onset spastic dysphonia	Paralytic or spastic dysphonia, cricopharyngeal spasm, idiopathic blocked ear
Vagal (somatic sensory)	Hypesthesia; decreased cough reflex		Somatophobia	Choking or coughing spells; carotidynia
Vagal (autonomic)	Bradycardia, hyposecretion of glandular elements	Paroxysmal tachycardia; hypersecretion of glandular elements		Cardiac arrhythmia; sudden death syndrome; esophageal and gastric dysfunction
Cervical 2 and 3	Hypesthesia		Somatophobia	Occipital headache; part of Bell's palsy

Abbreviation: HSV-1, Herpes simplex virus type 1.

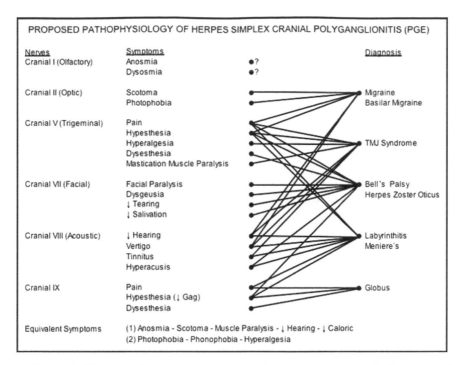

FIGURE 5 Diagram describes signs, symptoms, and proposed diagnosis of herpes simplex-1 polyganglionitis.

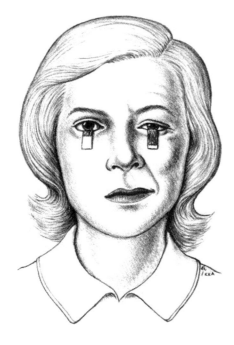

FIGURE 6 Illustration shows a woman with right-sided facial droop as well as decreased lacrimation indicated by Shirmer tear test. *Source*: From Ref. 10.

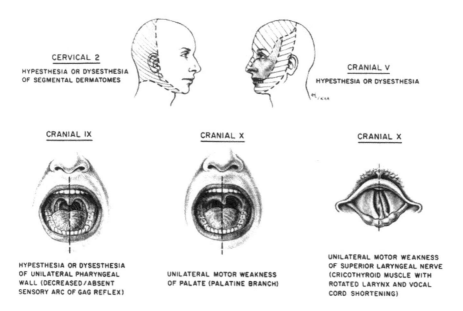

CERVICAL 2
HYPESTHESIA OR DYSESTHESIA
OF SEGMENTAL DERMATOMES

CRANIAL V
HYPESTHESIA OR DYSESTHESIA

CRANIAL IX

CRANIAL X

CRANIAL X

HYPESTHESIA OR DYSESTHESIA
OF UNILATERAL PHARYNGEAL
WALL (DECREASED/ABSENT
SENSORY ARC OF GAG REFLEX)

UNILATERAL MOTOR WEAKNESS
OF PALATE (PALATINE BRANCH)

UNILATERAL MOTOR WEAKNESS
OF SUPERIOR LARYNGEAL NERVE
(CRICOTHYROID MUSCLE WITH
ROTATED LARYNX AND VOCAL
CORD SHORTENING)

FIGURE 7 Illustration of cranial and cervical nerves often affected in Bell's palsy and in HZV facial paralysis. *Source*: From Ref. 10.

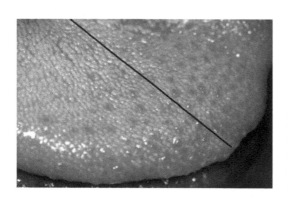

FIGURE 8 Photograph of tongue of patient with left-sided Bell's palsy shows unilateral inflammation of fungiform papillae on the left with minor extension across the midline. This condition occurs in 100% of patients with Bell's palsy.

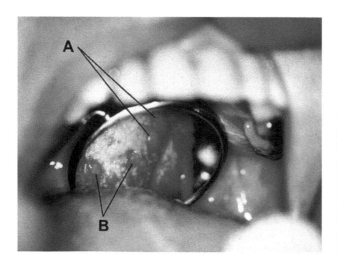

FIGURE 9 Photograph (*mirror view*) shows unilateral inflammation of circumvallate papillae in a patient with left-sided Bell's palsy and dysgeusia. (A) Inflamed circumvallate papillae on the left side. (B) Normal circumvallate papillae on the right side. *Source*: From Ref. 9.

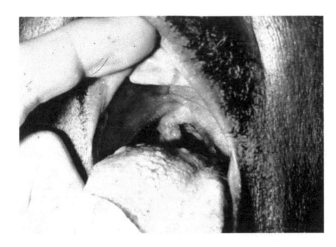

FIGURE 10 Photograph of a patient with right-sided Bell's palsy shows how unilateral palatal weakness becomes more apparent when the tongue is used to stretch palatal folds. *Source*: From Ref. 11.

headache (cervical nerves 2 and 3), stuffy sensation in the ears (cranial nerve X), tinnitus with hearing loss (cranial nerve VIII, the auditory nerve), earache (cranial nerve V), dizziness with nystagmus (cranial nerve VIII, the vestibular nerve), burning throat (cranial nerve IX), and masseter muscle weakness (cranial nerve V).

Clinical manifestations related to the auditory-vestibular system (cranial nerve VIII) can be traced to either branch of the nerve. *Vestibular neuritis* or *neuronitis* describes the vertigo associated with viral reactivation within the vestibular ganglion alone. *Acute sudden hearing loss* or *cochlear Ménière's disease* describes the hearing loss, tinnitus, and phonophobia associated with viral replication in the cochlear division. Involvement of both nerves suggests a clinical diagnosis of classical Ménière's disease. Many patients with this diagnosis complain of pharyngeal pain (cranial nerve IX) and facial hypesthesia (cranial nerve V), symptoms which further document involvement of multiple nerves (13).

DIAGNOSIS

The diagnosis of HSV-1 infection is best confirmed by isolating the virus in tissue culture. Results of tissue culture are often positive within 48 hours after inoculation, and immunofluorescent staining of the tissue culture cells can enable quick identification of HSV and distinction between HSV types 1 and 2 (7).

Because innumerable cases of recurrent HSV-1 infections occur daily, this method of diagnosis is neither practical nor necessary. Histologic diagnosis using scrapings from a mucocutaneous lesion shows multinucleated giant cells as well as epithelial cells that contain eosinophilic inclusion bodies (visible on Tzank smears). Polymerase chain reaction (PCR) techniques can rapidly detect HSV DNA in clinical specimens: Whereas confirmation of HSV encephalitis previously required brain biopsy, PCR study of cerebral spinal fluid is a noninvasive technique as sensitive as brain biopsy (6).

Antibody testing can document seroconversion in patients with primary HSV-1 but has no value for confirming recurrent infection.

TREATMENT

Treatment of primary HSV-1 infection is well established; however, treatment of mucocutaneous, recurrent HSV-1 infection is less well defined, and treatment of polyganglionitis is controversial (8). Symptomatic and asymptomatic recurrent disease accompanied by viral shedding is self-limited; therefore, therapy is designed to reduce severity, duration, and frequency of symptoms. In general, early treatment achieves the best therapeutic response.

Acyclovir binds viral DNA and ends viral replication by acting as a chain terminator. Although acyclovir is safe and extremely well tolerated, its oral availability is only about 15%, and its half-life is only about 2.5 hours. The drug penetrates most body tissues, including the brain, and crosses the placenta. Intravenous administration of acyclovir increases its concentration by tenfold. Because the drug is excreted through the kidneys, adjustment must be made for patients with renal impairment.

Because of the poor bioavailability and short half-life of acyclovir, oral treatment regimens of the drug require that it be administered five times per day. Valacyclovir and famciclovir are newer drugs with longer half-lives and better intestinal absorption. Valacyclovir, the prodrug of acyclovir, produces higher peak levels and has 55% bio-availability. Famciclovir, the prodrug of penciclovir, has a half-life 10 times longer than acyclovir and 77% bioavailability. Contraindications include hypersensitivity. Concurrent administration of probenecid or cimetidine may increase toxicity of either valacyclovir or famciclovir.

To treat the primary infection, patients receive a 7- to 10-day regimen of 200 mg acyclovir orally five times daily (or 400 mg orally three times daily) (14); valacyclovir 1000 mg orally twice daily (15); or famciclovir 250 mg orally three times daily (16). Patients who are immunocompromised or have disseminated disease should receive acyclovir intravenously every eight hours for 5 to 10 days with appropriate adjustment made for the patient's weight and the severity of disease.

Recurrent mucocutaneous disease is best treated in the prodromal stage or within 48 hours after formation of vesicles. Treatment should consist of 200 mg acyclovir given orally five times per day or 500 mg valacyclovir given orally twice per day or 125 mg famciclovir given orally three times per day for five days. In patients with intact immune systems, adding a regimen of steroid drugs lessens the severity of disease and dries the vesicles but does not shorten the course of the disease. Use of steroid agents in patients with HIV can cause fulminant oral candidiasis.

Patients with HSV-1 ocular infection should receive a double dose of acyclovir. Topical steroid agents are contraindicated for these patients, who should receive referral to an ophthalmologist.

For long-term suppression of recurrent episodes, patients should receive 100 mg acyclovir twice daily (14), 500 mg valacyclovir daily (15), or a 125- to 250-mg dose of famciclovir twice daily (16).

Unfortunately, treatment of neurologic symptoms associated with polyganglionitis is determined on the basis of each treating physician's own philosophy. Because the disease is both inflammatory and a virally induced immune complex, use of steroid drugs is the most effective method of reducing the severity and duration of sensory symptoms (17). Methylprednisolone can reduce symptoms of acute vestibular vertigo (neuritis, neuronitis, and labyrinthitis) within hours after treatment (18). For affected patients who have associated nausea and vomiting, intravenous administration of a single 100-mg bolus of methylprednisolone relieves the vertigo within hours. Adults receive follow-up treatment consisting of 40 to 60 mg generic prednisone given orally for five days. For adults with unilateral parietal–occipital headache and evidence of other cranial nerve involvement, 40 mg prednisone given twice daily for three to four days has proved highly effective.

Now that Bell's palsy has been recognized as a form of polyganglionitis, treatment with steroid agents and acyclovir has become an accepted form of therapy (19). As with any herpetic disease, the most effective treatment is given early, i.e., within three days after the onset of the palsy. Patients diagnosed with Bell's palsy should receive 500 mg valacyclovir twice daily, 250 mg famciclovir three times daily, or 200 mg acyclovir five times daily. For these patients, prednisone treatment begins with at a dosage of 60 mg twice daily and is then tapered downward in increments of 5 mg per dose for the next seven days. The role of surgical decompression remains controversial; this treatment should be undertaken only under strict guidelines (which are beyond the scope of this chapter).

COMPLICATIONS AND PROGNOSIS

Ocular infection resulting from autoinoculation during acute herpetic gingivostomatosis or asymptomatic oropharyngeal infection is not an uncommon complication of HSV-l infection in children. The condition manifests as unilateral follicular conjunctivitis or as an acute herpetic keratoconjunctivitis with dendritic corneal ulcers, and can recur in as many as 25% of patients. HSV-1 infection can be associated with progressive scarring of the cornea and has been a leading infectious cause of blindness (20).

Types of skin infection complicating HSV-1 infection include eczema herpeticum, herpetic whitlow, and herpes gladiatorum. Eczema herpeticum occurs in patients with underlying dermatitis, skin breakdown (such as occurs with burns), and pemphigus. Herpetic whitlow is an infection of the fingers at or near the cuticle or at a break in the skin. The condition is associated with exposure to saliva and is observed most commonly in health-care workers and in children. Herpes gladiatorum manifests as scattered skin lesions and is most often observed in wrestlers exposed to infectious saliva.

Visceral infection resulting from viremia with and without skin lesions can infect many organs to cause esophagitis, adrenal necrosis, interstitial pneumonitis, cystitis, arthritis, and hepatitis. Hepatitis is often associated with blood dyscrasia that produces intravascular coagulation.

Herpes simplex encephalitis accounts for 10% to 20% of all cases of acute necrotizing encephalitis in the United States. The condition most often occurs after primary infection and, as has been suggested, by reinfection with a different strain of HSV-1. Herpes simplex encephalitis produces nonspecific findings: headache, meningeal irritation, altered mental status, and seizures. In affected patients, magnetic resonance imaging (MRI) often shows focal necrosis of the temporal and orbital frontal region. This necrosis causes symptoms of anosmia, memory loss, and olfactory hallucinations. PCR imaging is the most sensitive noninvasive method of showing HSV-1 DNA. Untreated patients have an estimated mortality rate of 70%. Even with treatment, patients with herpes simplex encephalitis have a high incidence of neurological sequelae (6).

Complications associated with cranial polyganglionitis vary widely according to the nerve or nerves affected. Corneal ulceration is not uncommon in patients with Bell's palsy. Late complications of Bell's palsy include mid-face contracture with synkinesis and begin at three to four months after the facial nerve has degenerated and begun to regenerate (9).

HERPES ZOSTER VIRUS

INTRODUCTION

Herpes zoster virus is more properly called VZV because it produces contagious varicella (chickenpox), usually in childhood, and then resides latently in cranial nerve and dorsal root ganglia. Reactivation in adults usually occurs in those aged 50 years and older and manifests either as segmental herpes zoster (shingles) or as a central nervous system disease syndrome (21). In many affected patients, reactivation causes postherpetic neuralgia.

EPIDEMIOLOGY

In children, epidemic primary infection with VZV manifests as chickenpox. One suggestion is that every person who has had chickenpox harbors latent virus; molecular analyses of DNA have shown that VZV infection in adults represents reappearance of the childhood virus infection. Of all people who live to be 85 years of age, about half will have an attack of zoster, and about 10% of this affected population will have at least two attacks. One study found 100 cases per 100,000 person-years among people aged between 15 years and 35 years, with an increase in each decade to 450 cases per 100,000 by age 75 years. The proportion of Americans older than 65 years is increasing, so rates of VZV infection and its associated complications will also increase (22). The lifetime risk of VZV infection is estimated at between 10% and 20%. Compared with persons who are seronegative for HIV, persons who are seropositive for HIV have a higher frequency of VZV infection. This higher frequency of VZV infection can be expected for any population with immunodeficiency.

PATHOGENESIS

Like HSV-1, VZV is a double-stranded DNA virus which, in humans, has a propensity to reside in a latent, noninfective state in sensory neural ganglia; unlike HSV-1, however, VZV cannot be cultured from human ganglia cells. Unlike herpes simplex reactivation, VZV reactivation causes serum antibody levels to rise during virus reactivation. Neurologic damage begins before the characteristic rash appears. Studies using PCR analysis have found the genome in blood vessels and in other types of tissue. The mechanisms causing reactivation of VZV to an active infective state have not been identified (23).

CLINICAL MANIFESTATIONS

Because VZV becomes latent in cranial nerve, dorsal root, and autonomic ganglia along the entire neuroaxis, the virus can manifest anywhere on the body. Typically, the activated virus causes a prodrome consisting of skin sensitivity and mild-to-severe radicular pain, and after five days, a rash appears. The pain is associated with itching and dysesthesia. As with HSV-1, VZV infection decreases sensation in the affected dermatome, yet the affected skin is exquisitely sensitive to touch. The rash may continue to produce pustules that lead to crusting and ulceration. In many affected patients, healing is delayed beyond two weeks and is accompanied by increased skin pigmentation and scarring. Lesions can erupt outside the affected dermatome but rarely cross the midline and are not clinically significant. Distribution of 10 or more lesions outside a single dermatome suggests early evidence of viral dissemination. The term "zoster sine herpete" is used to describe VZV that is reactivated without the typical pattern of skin eruption.

Of the facial nerves, the ophthalmic division of the trigeminal nerve is most frequently affected in herpes zoster (Fig. 11), and this event can cause optic keratitis, a potential cause of blindness. The most visible sign of motor nerve involvement is facial paralysis as seen in Ramsay Hunt syndrome, a condition which is more properly described as *herpes zoster cephalicus* (Fig. 7). Patients affected with this condition also have palatal and laryngeal paralysis and hearing loss. Acute facial paralysis with pain and hearing loss is pathognomonic of herpes zoster infection. The diverse manifestations of VZV activation

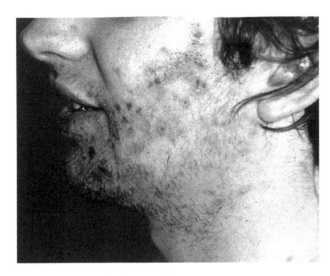

FIGURE 11 Photograph shows varicella zoster virus affecting the third division of the trigeminal nerve and minor vesicles apparent in the first division.

are exemplified in Figure 12, which illustrates VZV affecting a left thoracic dermatome concomitantly with left-sided facial palsy. A diagnosis of zoster sine herpete should be considered for patients who have acute facial paralysis accompanied by moderate-to-severe pain and no vesicle formation (23).

DIAGNOSIS

The diagnosis of VZV is generally not difficult if the characteristic dermatomal rash and pain are present. Diagnosis is most difficult during the prodromal phase, when patients have pain but no visible lesions.

In patients who have the characteristic rash, a Tzanck preparation shows presence of multinucleated giant cells and thus provides strong supportive evidence of zoster infection. The Tzanck preparation and immunofluorescence have proved superior to viral isolation for diagnosing early lesions. Samples obtained from patients during the acute stage of

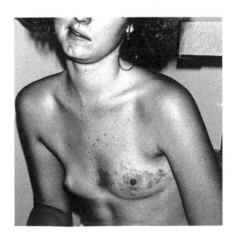

FIGURE 12 Photograph shows patient with varicella zoster virus of the thoracic dermatome and concomitant right facial palsy.

disease show a fourfold higher level of VZV antibody titer compared with serum samples obtained from convalescent patients, but this observation comes too late to have value for determining treatment (23).

TREATMENT

Treatment of VZV has no universally accepted protocol. The goal of treatment should be to inactivate the virus, control pain, reduce severity of the vesicular eruption, and reduce complications (including postherpetic neuralgia). Oral treatment with antiviral agents [acyclovir (14), valacyclovir (15), or famciclovir (16)] should be continued for 7 to 10 days. Patients should receive 800 mg acyclovir orally five times a day, 500 mg famciclovir orally three times a day, or 1 g valacyclovir orally three times a day. Although antiviral drugs reduce duration of pain and development of vesicles, addition of oral 40 to 60 mg prednisone orally twice per day further reduces the inflammatory reaction, further controls pain, and reduces both the severity and the duration of vesicular eruption. We have only anecdotal evidence that treatment with corticosteroid agents may reduce incidence of postherpetic neuralgia, but these drugs do reduce pain, promote healing of the vesicular eruptions, and are an appropriate adjuvant to treatment. Many treatments have been suggested for postherpetic neuralgia, but proof of their effectiveness is lacking. The U.S. Food and Drug Administration (FDA) has approved a topical lidocaine patch for treating postherpetic neuralgia, but a recent study questions its effectiveness.

A recent (2005) prospective multicenter study (24) tested the hypothesis that vaccination against VZV would decrease the incidence, severity, or both of herpes zoster and postherpetic neuralgia among older adults. They found that the zoster vaccine markedly reduced morbidity from herpes zoster and postherpetic neuralgia among older adults. On May 25, 2006, the Food and Drug Administration (FDA) licensed Zostavax, a new vaccine to reduce the risk of shingles (herpes zoster) for use in people 60 years of age and older.[a]

COMPLICATIONS

About one in eight patients with herpes zoster infection has at least one complication of this condition. Major complications include postherpetic neuralgia, uveitis, motor deficits, skin infection, and systemic involvement (with manifestations such as meningoencephalitis, pneumonia, deafness, or dissemination). Postherpetic neuralgia occurs most frequently in patients older than 50 years of age and can be prolonged and intractable despite early antiviral therapy. The pain is often excruciating and does not respond well to conventional methods of pain control. Granulomatous vasculitis has recently been added to the list of complications (25).

SUMMARY

Because herpes zoster virus (VZV) is identical to the varicella virus the VZV abbreviation is preferable. After an episode of chickenpox (varicella) resolves, the virus subsides to a latent, noninfective state in the nucleus of sensory ganglia. Later in life, when antibody immunity is reduced, VZV is reactivated and manifests as radicular disease, commonly known as "shingles." The virus is latent in multiple ganglia, and reactivation in specific nerves causes a variety of neurologic syndromes, the most visible of which affect the head and neck as

---

[a]Zostavax is manufactured by Merck & Co., Inc., of Whitehouse Station, New Jersey.

herpes zoster cephalicus (described also as Ramsay Hunt syndrome) or as Costen's syndrome. In 10% to 20% of affected patients, symptoms include hearing loss, vertigo, and muscle paralysis. Treatment usually consists of antiviral agents and corticosteroid drugs, but this approach is not universally accepted. Despite early and adequate treatment, postherpetic neuralgia develops and persists in many patients as a complication that defies treatment.

Acknowledgments

Editorial assistance was provided by the medical editing service of the Permanente Medical Group Physician Education and Development Department.

References

1. Cohen JI. Epstein-Barr virus infection. N Engl J Med 2000; 343(7):481–492.
2. Ebell MH. Epstein-Barr virus infectious mononucleosis. Am Fam Physician 2004; 70(7):1279–1287.
3. Johnsen T, Katholm M, Stangerup SE. Otolaryngological complications in infectious mononucleosis. J Laryngol Otol 1984; 98(10):999–1001.
4. Straus SE. The chronic mononucleosis syndrome. J Infect Dis 1988; 157(3):405–412.
5. Corey L, Spear PG. Infections with herpes simplex viruses (1). N Engl J Med 1986; 314(11):686–691.
6. Corey L, Spear PG. Infections with herpes simplex viruses (2). N Engl J Med 1986; 314(12):749–757.
7. Langenberg AG, Corey L, Ashley RL, et al. A prospective study of new infections with herpes simplex virus type 1 and type 2. Chiron HSV Vaccine Study Group N Engl J Med 1999; 341(19):1432–1438.
8. Adour KK, Hilsinger RL Jr, Byl FM. Herpes simplex polyganglionitis. Otolaryngol Head Neck Surg 1980; 88(3):270–274.
9. Adour KK, Byl FM, Hilsinger RL Jr, et al. The true nature of Bell's palsy: analysis of 1,000 consecutive patients. Laryngoscope 1978; 88(5):787–801.
10. Adour KK. Facial nerve testing and evaluation. In: House JW, O'Connor AF, eds. Handbook of Neurological Diagnosis. New York, New York: Marcel Dekker, 1987.
11. Adour KK. Acute temporomandibular joint pain-dysfunction syndrome: neuro-otologic and electromyographic study. Am J Otolaryngol 1981; 2(2):114–122.
12. Powers JF, Bedri S, Hussein S, et al. High prevalence of herpes simplex virus DNA in temporal arteritis biopsy specimens. Am J Clin Pathol 2005; 123(2):261–264.
13. Adour KK, Byl FM, Hilsinger RL Jr, et al. Meniere's disease as a form of cranial polyganglionitis. Laryngoscope 1980; 90(3):392–398.
14. Mattison HR, Reichman RC, Benedetti J, et al. Double-blind, placebo-controlled trial comparing long-term suppressive with short-term oral acyclovir therapy for management of recurrent genital herpes. Am J Med. 1988; 85(2A):20–25.
15. Reitano M, Tyring S, Lang W, et al. Valacyclovir for the suppression of recurrent genital herpes simplex virus infection: a large-scale dose range-finding study. J Infect Dis 1998; 178:603–610.
16. Mertz GJ, Loveless MO, Levin MJ, et al. Oral famciclovir for suppression of recurrent genital herpes simplex virus infection in women. A multicenter, double-blind, placebo-controlled trial. Collaborative Famciclovir Genital Herpes Research Group. Arch Intern Med 1997; 157:343–349.
17. Strupp M, Zingler VC, Arbusow V, et al. Methylprednisolone, valacyclovir, or the combination for vestibular neuritis. N Engl J Med 2004; 351(4):354–361.
18. Ariyasu L, Byl FM, Sprague MS, et al. The beneficial effect of methylprednisolone in acute vestibular vertigo. Arch. Otolaryngol Head Neck Surg 1990; 116(6):700–703.
19. Adour KK, Ruboyianes JM, Von Doersten PG, et al. Bell's palsy treatment with acyclovir and prednisone compared with prednisone alone: a double-blind, randomized, controlled trial. Ann Otol Rhinol Laryngol 1996; 105(5):371–378.
20. Wilhelmus KR, Beck RW, Moke PS, et al. Acyclovir for the prevention of recurrent herpes simplex virus eye disease. Herpetic Eye Disease Study Group. N Engl J Med 1998; 339(5):300–306.
21. Weller TH. Varicella and herpes zoster. Changing concepts of the natural history, control, and importance of a not-so-benign virus. N Engl J Med 1983; 309(23):1434–1440.
22. Arvin A. Aging, immunity, and the varicella-zoster virus. N Engl J Med 2005; 352(2):2266–2267.
23. Gnann JW Jr, Whitley RJ. Clinical practice. Herpes zoster. N Engl J Med 2002; 347(5):340–346.

24. Oxman MN, Levin MJ, Johnson GR, et al. A vaccine to prevent herpes zoster and postherpetic neuralgia in older adults. N Engl J Med 2005; 352:2271–2284.
25. Gilden DH, Kleinschmidt-DeMasters BK, LaGuardia JJ, et al. Neurologic complications of the reactivation of varicella-zoster virus. N Engl J Med 2000; 342(9):635–645. Erratum in N Engl J Med 2000; 342(14):1063.

11

Bacterial Diseases: Diphtheria, Cat-Scratch Disease, Gonorrhea, and Necrotizing Fasciitis

Andrew K. Patel
Department of Surgery, Division of Otolaryngology-Head and Neck Surgery, University of California, San Diego, California, U.S.A.

Terence M. Davidson
Department of Surgery, Division of Otolaryngology-Head and Neck Surgery, University of California and VA San Diego Healthcare System, San Diego, California, U.S.A.

DIPHTHERIA

INTRODUCTION

Once known as the "strangling angel of children," diphtheria is a preventable, acute, toxin-mediated disease caused by *Corynebacterium diphtheriae* (Table 1). In the fifth century BCE, Hippocrates described a disease characterized by sore throat, membrane formation, and death through suffocation. In 1826, the French physician Bretonneau named the condition "diphtherite," from the Greek word for leather, because the characteristic membrane resembled leather (1). The bacterium was identified by Klebs in 1884 and first cultivated by Loeffler one year later. Subsequently, Roux and Yersin purified the toxin in 1889, and an antitoxin was invented shortly thereafter, with development of the toxoid in the 1920s (2).

The bacterial exotoxin causes many of the severe manifestations of diphtheria. Clinically, the disease is characterized by pharyngitis and a membrane that may cover the tonsils, pharynx, and larynx. Although diphtheria was one of the most common causes of death of children in the prevaccine era, today diphtheria is rare and seldom considered within the differential diagnosis in developed areas of the world. Sporadic cases do occur, however, and epidemic diphtheria spread through the Soviet Union as recently as the 1990s. Furthermore, the disease is prevalent in many developing countries, and the importation of cases into the United States or other developed countries may occur. The majority of nasopharyngeal *C. diphtheriae* infections results in asymptomatic carriers, and approximately one in seven individuals develops clinical disease.

EPIDEMIOLOGY

In the prevaccine era, diphtheria was a feared, highly endemic childhood disease found in temperate climates. Despite a gradual decline in deaths in the developed parts of the world, attributed to improved living standards, diphtheria remained a leading cause of death of children until widespread vaccination was implemented. Despite the decrease in reported cases in the United States, a recent re-emergence in the former Soviet Union in 1994 caused 50,000 cases and roughly 1800 deaths (3). Epidemic diphtheria primarily affected children younger than age 15, but recently has shifted to affect adults who lack natural exposure to toxigenic *C. diphtheria* in the vaccine era and did not receive booster vaccinations. The factors governing the periodicity of diphtheria outbreaks are not understood. No gender difference has been described in terms of acute infection, although lack of immunity has been noted in elderly women compared to men.

PATHOLOGY/PATHOPHYSIOLOGY

C. diphtheria is a member of a group of irregular, non–spore-forming, aerobic Gram-positive bacilli characterized by growth in facultative anaerobic conditions and catalase- and oxidase-positivity. Although other coryneform bacteria are ubiquitous in nature, *C. diphtheria* exclusively exists on human mucous membranes and skin. Transmission is via infected respiratory droplets or skin wound for two to four weeks in untreated infected individuals, although antibiotic treatment greatly reduces the risk of transmission after 48 hours, and asymptomatic respiratory carriers factor greatly in disease transmission (4). Diphtheria immunization protects against disease but does not prevent carriage.

TABLE 1 Diphtheria: Key Points

Overview
  Preventable, acute toxin-mediated disease caused by *Corynebacterium diphtheriae*
  Currently rare in most developed nations after the implementation of vaccination
Pathophysiology of C. diphtheria
  Aerobic and facultative anaerobic Gram-positive bacilli
  Exists exclusively on human mucous membranes and skin
  Potent exotoxin is synthesized by some strains after 2–4 days of incubation, taken up by cells
    and inhibiting protein synthesis, causing necrosis with formation of a tough
    pseudomembrane of leukocytes, dead host cells, fibrin, and erythrocytes, which may
    precipitate airway obstruction
Symptomatology (by location of infection)
  Nasal—typically infants, serosanguinous and mucopurulent rhinitis, excoriation of the nares
    and upper lip, and a white septal pseudomembrane may be seen
  Pharynx—pharyngitis, tonsillitis, low-grade temperature, and a white-to-gray
    pseudomembrane extending from the tonsils to the posterior pharyngeal pillars and
    nasopharynx. The most common site for clinical diphtheria. Hoarseness and a barking
    cough accompany the progression of disease
  Larynx—worsening hoarseness, dyspnea and inspiratory stridor, and later a tracheobronchitis
  Malignant or "bull-neck" diphtheria—extensive pseudomembrane formation, halitosis, massive
    swelling of the tonsils and uvula, thick speech, cervical lymphadenopathy, striking
    edematous swelling of the submandibular region and anterior neck, and severe toxicity
  Toxin production accompanied by profound malaise, weakness, cervical lymphadenitis,
    cervical soft tissue swelling causing a "bull neck," and occasionally palatine paralysis and
    upper respiratory obstruction with inspiratory stridor
  Cutaneous—associated with tropics, prevalent in Southeast Asia. The characteristic, deep,
    rounded, crater-like lesions are covered with an eschar and take months or even years to heal
  Diphtherial neuropathy usually involves the cranial nerves, causing diplopia, slurred speech,
    and dysphagia
Diagnosis
  Isolation on specialized growth media including potassium tellurite (Tinsdale agar) to inhibit
    other oral flora
  Treatment is reserved for patients carrying toxigenic strains, identified by streaking of the
    organism and controls on toxin-antibody impregnated paper and observing for
    immunoprecipitation lines
  PCR may also be used to detect toxin genes
Treatment
  Removal of membrane by direct laryngoscopy or bronchoscopy may be necessary to prevent
    or alleviate airway obstruction
  Diphtheria antitoxin must be delivered promptly to prevent myocarditis, neuritis, or death, after
    administration of intradermal skin test for horse serum sensitivity
  Penicillin G or erythromycin antibiotic course, with repeated nasopharyngeal cultures to
    confirm eradication of carrier state
  Bed rest for 12 days to prevent sudden cardiac death from myocarditis
  Strict isolation
Prognosis
  Mortality rate reported from most series varies from 5% to 10%
  Vaccinated patients experience a mild illness

Abbreviation: PCR, polymerase chain reaction.

The diphtheria organisms remain in the superficial layers of the respiratory mucosa and induce a local inflammatory reaction. The potent exotoxin released by the organism is taken up by cells and inhibits protein synthesis, causing necrosis. Initially, a gray exudate of dead host cells and white blood cells forms, which is easily removed. After the addition of fibrin and red blood cells, the tough gray-brown pseudomembrane is produced; this is difficult to remove, and bleeds after such attempts. Subsequently, bacterial superinfection may occur with *Staphylococcus aureus* and *Streptococcus pyogenes*.

PATHOGENESIS

Diphtheria toxin (DT) is one of the most extensively studied bacterial toxins, due to the fact that the causative organism was one of the first bacteria isolated and grown in pure culture, and the toxin among the first toxins discovered (3). Diphtheria exotoxin is a 62 kDa polypeptide composed of a B subunit which binds to cell receptors at clathrin-coated pit sites of endosome, followed by release of the active A subunit. The A subunit is released by proteolytic cleavage of a peptide bond with reduction of a disulfide bridge, followed by a conformational change in the B subunit in the acidic pH of the endosome, allowing release of the A subunit into the cytoplasm. The A subunit inactivates elongation factor-2 (EF-2) via ADP-ribosylation, thus acting as a polypeptide chain terminator of host cell protein synthesis. The cell is then unable to repair its own membranes, and cytotoxicity results. The toxin is very potent: a single molecule is enough to inactivate all of the EF-2 in a cell and halt protein synthesis within a few hours. The estimated human lethal dose of DT is 0.1 mg/kg.

CLINICAL MANIFESTATIONS

After an incubation of two to four days, colonizing toxigenic diphtheria strains produce toxin locally with initiation of the signs and symptoms of disease (5). In nasal disease, typically seen in infants, the illness appears similar to the common cold but then progresses to a serosanguinous and mucopurulent rhinitis. Excoriation of the nares and upper lip and a white septal pseudomembrane may be seen. Spread of the disease to the pharynx occurs next, causing a sore throat, tonsillitis, low-grade temperature and a white to gray pseudo-membrane extending from the tonsils to the posterior pharyngeal pillars and nasopharynx, the most common site for clinical diphtheria. Hoarseness and a barking cough accompany the progression of disease. Laryngeal diphtheria most often develops as an extension of pharyngeal involvement, although occasionally it may be an isolated manifestation of diphtheria. As toxin production continues, there is profound malaise, weakness, cervical lymphadenitis, soft tissue swelling of the neck causing a "bull neck," and occasionally palatine paralysis and upper respiratory obstruction with inspiratory stridor. A small percentage of patients present with malignant or "bull-neck" diphtheria, with extensive pseudomembrane formation, foul breath, massive swelling of the tonsils and uvula, thick speech, cervical lymphadenopathy, striking edematous swelling of the submandibular region and anterior neck, and severe toxicity. Further spread of the disease downward to the larynx, causing worsening hoarseness, dyspnea and inspiratory stridor, and later a tracheo-bronchitis with edema and membrane formation extending along the entire tracheobronchial tree, will often precede respiratory failure.

In mild cases, or those modified by anti-toxin treatment, the membrane is coughed up between the 6th and 10th days, although a sudden and acute airway obstruction may occur from a partially detached piece of membrane. In severe cases, this obstruction is manifested by progressive hypoxia, restlessness, cyanosis, severe prostration, coma, and death. Of note, systemic signs of diphtheria are minimal in laryngeal involvement, due to the poor absorption of the toxin from the laryngeal mucous membrane. In general, however, the laryngeal involvement is associated with tonsillar and pharyngeal diphtheria, resulting in both obstruction and severe toxemia.

In addition to the classic respiratory form of diphtheria, a cutaneous form exists which is associated with the tropics and is prevalent in Southeast Asia. The characteristic, deep, rounded, crater-like lesions are covered with an eschar and take months or years to heal. The lesion acts as a potential reservoir for transmission and spread of the pharyngeal form of the disease. On rare occasions, clinical infection with *C. diphtheriae* can be seen in other sites such as the ear, conjunctivae, or vagina.

DIAGNOSIS

The differential diagnosis includes infectious mononucleosis, adenovirus or herpes simplex infection, Vincent's angina, pharyngitis due to *Arcanobacterium haemolyticum*, candidiasis, streptococcal tonsillitis, and acute epiglottitis. The tonsillar exudate of infectious mononucleosis is creamy in color, does not extend beyond the tonsil, and does not produce bleeding if removed. Streptococcal pharyngotonsillitis is associated with more severe local symptoms and a higher fever. Epiglottitis is acute in onset and is not associated with a local membrane. In the head and neck, diphtherial neuropathy usually involves the cranial nerves, causing diplopia, slurred speech, and dysphagia.

C. diphtheria colonizes the human respiratory tract alone. Isolation of the organism occurs on specialized growth media including potassium tellurite (Tinsdale agar) to inhibit other oral flora. Treatment is reserved for patients carrying toxigenic strains, identified by streaking of the organism and controls on toxin-antibody impregnated paper and observing for immunoprecipitation lines. Polymerase chain reaction (PCR) may also be used to detect toxin genes.

TREATMENT

Removal of membrane by direct laryngoscopy or bronchoscopy may be necessary to prevent or alleviate airway obstruction. Diphtheria antitoxin must be delivered promptly to prevent myocarditis, neuritis, or death. DT is present in infected individuals in a circulating, or unbound form, a form bound to the surface of cells, and also internalized into the cytoplasm. The antitoxin is able to neutralize circulating toxin and may affect the bound form to some degree, but has no effect on the internalized fraction of toxin. Due to the delay in bacteriologic confirmation of diphtheria, the decision to treat with antitoxin is determined by clinical and epidemiological evidence and must be considered whenever there is a membrane present in the throat or nares. The antitoxin is of equine origin, and an intradermal skin test can be performed to evaluate the possibility of horse serum sensitivity. If this test is negative, the total dose of antitoxin should be administered. This total dose varies, depending on the site of diphtheria involvement, ranging from 10,000 to 20,000 units for anterior nasal diphtheria to increasing doses for tonsillar, pharyngeal, laryngeal, or nasopharyngeal diphtheria, up to 80,000 to 120,000 units for patients with brawny cervical edema (4). The antitoxin is available via the Centers for Disease Control and Prevention (CDC) as an investigational agent at this time in the United States.

Penicillin and erythromycin are effective agents for treatment of diphtheria, with penicillin being the preferred agent, for a duration of 14 days. Antibacterial therapy is not a substitute for antitoxin treatment. Bed rest should be enforced for 12 days due to the risk for myocarditis (5). Sudden death can be caused by myocardial failure from excessive activity. Palatal and pharyngeal paralysis from neuritis may cause aspiration, requiring gastric or duodenal feedings, and diaphragmatic paralysis may require mechanical ventilation. For patients with laryngeal diphtheria, treatment with intubation or tracheostomy also may be required. In addition to administration of antitoxin and antibiotics, strict isolation procedures are required to limit propagation of the disease.

Treatment of the carrier state of diphtheria may include a single dose of intramuscular penicillin G or a 7- to 10-day course of oral erythromycin, followed by nasopharyngeal cultures at 14 days to confirm eradication of the carrier state. Persistence of the carrier state after the initial course of antibiotics is followed by an additional 10-day course of erythromycin and repeated cultures, in addition to evaluation for a nasal foreign body.

Immunization with diphtheria toxoid is the only effective means of primary prevention. The primary series is four doses of diphtheria toxoid (given with tetanus toxoid and pertussis vaccine) at 2, 4, 6, and 15 to 18 months; a preschool booster dose is given at ages 4 to 6 years. Thereafter, tetanus and diphtheria toxoid for adults (Td) boosters should be given as part of the adolescent immunization visit (i.e., between 11 and 13 years of age), followed by doses administered every 10 years.

PROGNOSIS

Before the turn of the century, the mortality from diphtheria was estimated at 30% to 50% (1). The initiation of diphtheria antitoxin use in 1894, followed by the use of large-scale vaccination practices in 1922, resulted in the dramatic fall in the mortality rate to 10% (2). Despite the refinement in the care of critically ill patients since that time, the mortality rate reported from most series varies from 5% to 10% (5). Notable risk factors for death due to diphtheria include extensive, virulent disease and delays in receiving diphtheria antitoxin, seeking medical attention, or diagnosis. Mortality rates are lower for those patients who receive antitoxin within the first two days of the illness. Vaccinated patients typically experience a mild illness. Sudden death may be caused by rapid airway obstruction due to membrane detachment, myocarditis resulting in heart failure, or respiratory paralysis from phrenic nerve involvement. Although patients who develop myocarditis or neuritis generally recover completely, some patients may sustain permanent heart damage.

SUMMARY

Despite a greatly reduced incidence over the past 50 years, diphtheria remains endemic in many developing nations. Though immunization has had a dramatic effect on the incidence of diphtheria, a decline in incidence began well before the onset of widespread immunization. The major virulence of *C. diphtheria* is a result of its toxin production. Within a few days of respiratory infection, the toxin produces a local adherent pseudomembrane composed of dead host epithelial cells, leukocytes, fibrin, and red blood cells. This gray-green or black membrane can be local, or can extend widely to cover the entire pharyngeal or tracheobronchial mucosa. There is a marked underlying soft tissue edema and regional lymphadenitis producing the bull neck appearance. Palatal paralysis is an early local effect of the toxin. Myocarditis, renal tubular necrosis and demyelination, and axon degeneration within cranial or peripheral nerves are prominent features of the more severe infections with *C. diphtheriae*. Diphtheria can be prevented by active immunization with formalin-detoxified DT (toxoid). Diphtheria, at the end of the twentieth century, remains a serious disease, associated with a high case–fatality rate.

CAT-SCRATCH DISEASE

INTRODUCTION

Cat-scratch disease (CSD), also known as cat-scratch fever or benign lymphoreticulitis, is an uncommon disease found worldwide (Table 2). The search for the etiologic agent of CSD has spanned several decades and taken unexpected turns. Interest in the topic has been high enough to generate over 900 publications since the first accurate clinical description in 1950 (6). During this time, the clinical description of CSD has remained remarkably stable.

EPIDEMIOLOGY

In the United States, roughly 22,000 cases of CSD are diagnosed annually, with 2000 resulting in hospital admissions. Over 90% of individuals with the illness report some form of contact with cats, often kittens. The male:female ratio is 3:2. In 80% to 90% of cases, patients are younger than 21 years (7).

TABLE 2   Cat-Scratch Disease: Key Points

> *Overview*
> Benign and self-limited infection with a course lasting 6–12 wk
> *Bartonella henselae* usually introduced into host via scratch from the claw or tooth of a kitten
>   younger than 6 mo of age
>
> *Pathophysiology of CSD*
> Gram-negative bacteria found in cat saliva for several months after cat infection, though
>   generally the cat reservoir is asymptomatic
> Fleas act as the vector of transmission between cats
> Human-to-human transmission does not occur
>
> *Symptomatology*
> After an incubation of 7–12 days after a cat scratch or bite, skin lesions develop followed by
>   tender regional lymphadenopathy
> Half of patients report low-grade fevers and malaise
> In most patients, the lymphadenopathy ranges from 1–5 cm; while the majority of lesions
>   regress over 2–6 mo, they may last for as long as 2 yr. Suppuration is seen in approximately
>   10% of cases.
> In the head and neck, atypical manifestations of CSD appear in up to 14% of patients,
>   specifically Parinaud's oculoglandular syndrome (6%), encephalopathy (2%), and
>   osteomyelitis (0.3%).
>
> *Diagnosis*
> Current diagnostic options include the *Bartonella* serology, the *B. henselae* IFA test utilizing
>   fluid aspirate or tissue from an affected lymph node, a lymph node biopsy, or a CSD skin
>   test
>
> *Treatment*
> In the immunocompetent host, CSD is not a serious illness and does not require treatment
>   beyond reassurance
>
> *Prognosis*
> After an episode of CSD, healthy individuals usually develop lifelong immunity preventing
>   reinfection
> In children with normal immune systems, spontaneous healing with full recovery is the norm,
>   usually with complete resolution of lymphadenopathy after 2–6 mo

Abbreviations: CSD, cat-scratch disease; IFA, indirect fluorescence antibody.

Untreated, CSD is a benign and self-limited infection with a course lasting 6 to 12 weeks (7). The principal clinical feature of CSD is tender regional lymphadenopathy, typically in the head and neck, as well as axillary and inguinal regions. Affected lymph nodes may be suppurative (7,8). A primary cutaneous lesion (typically a 0.5–1 mm papule or pustule) at the site of cat bite or scratch is reported from 25% to 60% of cases (8). Approximately 75% of patients report a bite or scratch to the head, neck, or upper limb. After an incubation period of 3 to 30 days (usually 7–12 days) after the injury, the skin lesions develop and precede lymphadenopathy by one to two weeks. Low grade fevers and malaise accompany lymphadenopathy in up to half of patients with CSD (9). Other studies have reported nausea and vomiting, sore throat, anorexia, headache, and splenomegaly, while brief nonspecific maculopapular eruptions, erythema nodosum, figurate erythemas, and thrombocytopenic purpura have also been described.

PATHOLOGY/PATHOPHYSIOLOGY

Most CSD begins with a scratch from the claw or tooth of a kitten younger than six months of age. It can also be inflicted by an adult cat, or from contact of the animal's saliva with broken skin or the eye. Previous investigations into the responsible organism identified a family of α-proteobacteria based on 16S ribosomal RNA gene sequences (6). Currently it is believed that *Bartonella henselae,* a Gram-negative bacterium, is the causative organism in CSD. In California, about 40% of cats carry Bartonella (9). Fleas are the vector transmitting the infection between cats, with bacteria subsequently found in the animal's saliva. In cats, the carrier state is generally asymptomatic (although experimental inoculations have produced a mild illness with fever, anemia, and transient neurological dysfunction) and an animal may carry the bacteria for months. The disease seems to rarely occur following a dog scratch or even from porcupine quills, cactus spines, or rosebush thorns. Most cases of CSD occur in children between the ages of 2 and 14, and in veterinarians. For reasons yet to be determined, most cases occur in the fall or winter months (75% of cases occur between September and March). CSD is not transmitted between human hosts.

CLINICAL MANIFESTATIONS

In the head and neck, atypical manifestations of CSD appear in up to 14% of patients, specifically Parinaud's oculoglandular syndrome (6%), encephalopathy (2%), and osteomyelitis (0.3%); other atypical manifestations are hepatic granulomas (0.3%) and pulmonary disease (0.2%) (7). In general, these complications resolve without sequelae. Parinaud's oculoglandular syndrome is manifested by conjunctival granuloma, periauricular lymphadenopathy, and nonsuppurative conjunctivitis. Encephalopathy, manifested as fever and coma that progress to convulsions, may last for days to weeks; cerebrospinal fluid is unremarkable. Other atypical presentations may commence with arthritis, synovitis, thrombocytopenic purpura, or erythema nodosum. Optic neuritis with transient blindness may also occur. Specifically, neuroretinitis manifests as fairly sudden loss of visual acuity, usually unilaterally, sometimes preceded by an influenza-like syndrome or development of unilateral lymphadenopathy. The most striking, if not most common, retinal manifestation is papilledema associated with macular exudates in a star formation, although this is not pathognomonic and usually follows a favorable spontaneous course.

Among patients with this disease, 50% have involvement of a single node, 20% have involvement of several nodes in the same region, and 30% have involvement of nodes in

TABLE 3   Typical and Atypical Features of Cat-Scratch Disease

Typical features of CSD	Chronic tender lymphadenopathy (49%) Fever (38–41°C) lasting 1–7 days (32%) Malaise or fatigue (30%) Anorexia, emesis, weight loss (15%) Headache (14%) Splenomegaly (11%) Pharyngitis (8%) Transient truncal maculopapular rash (5%)

Atypical features (16%) of CSD	Conjunctival granuloma with conjunctivitis and
	   preauricular adenopathy (6%)
	CNS, including encephalopathy/encephalitis with seizures,
	   combative behavior, extreme lethargy, or coma (2%)
	Cranial/peripheral nerve involvement, including facial nerve paresis,
	   myelitis, neuroretinitis, polyneuritis, radiculitis, optic neuritis with
	   transient blindness
	Thrombocytopenic purpura
	Osteitis/osteomyelitis (0.3%)
	Hepatomegaly/hepatosplenomegaly with hepatic granulomata (0.3%)
	Skin symptoms, including erythema nodosum, erythema marginatum,
	   erythema multiforme
	Pulmonary disease (0.2%)

Abbreviations: CSD, cat-scratch disease; CNS, central nervous system.

multiple sites (7). In 80% of cases, the lymphadenopathy ranges from 1 to 5 cm. While the majority of lesions regress over two to six months, they may last for as long as two years. Suppuration is seen in about 10% of cases. Cellulitis is rare (Table 3).

DIAGNOSIS

The differential diagnosis of CSD can include virtually all known causes of lymphadenopathy. As a general rule the diagnosis is favored by chronicity, unilateral occurrence, tenderness, and characteristic sites of involvement, such as the axillary, epitrochlear and preauricular nodes. Cervical, femoral, inguinal, and generalized lymph node involvement is less specific for CSD and necessitates more care in differential diagnosis. The most common diagnoses in a series of patients with adenopathy and negative CSD skin test were pyogenic lymphadenitis or abscess, lymphogranuloma venereum, benign or malignant neoplasms, and cervical adenitis caused by typical or atypical mycobacteria. Tularemia, toxoplasmosis, plague, and Kawasaki disease must be considered because of the need for specific therapy. In addition, brucellosis, syphilis, sporotrichosis, histoplasmosis, toxoplasmosis, infectious mononucleosis syndromes, lymphoma, and other neoplasms must also be included in the differential diagnosis.

    The clinical diagnosis of CSD depended for many years on a patient meeting three of the following four criteria: (*i*) history of traumatic cat contact; (*ii*) positive skin-test response to CSD skin-test antigen; (*iii*) characteristic lymph node lesions; and (*iv*) negative laboratory investigation for unexplained lymphadenopathy (7). Biopsy is rarely required, due to the development of reliable serologic testing. A pathologic feature of CSD-affected tissues has been the formation of granulomas, ringed by lymphocytic infiltrates and multinucleated giant cells in affected lymph nodes. In the primary inoculation site, the tissue demonstrates small areas of frank necrosis surrounded by concentric layers of histiocytes and lymphocytes with nucleated giant cells.

Current diagnostic options include the Bartonella serology, the *B. henselae* indirect fluorescence antibody test utilizing fluid aspirated or tissue from an affected lymph node, a lymph node biopsy, or a CSD skin test. Current tests under investigation are DNA amplification (highly selective) and PCR (highly specific).

TREATMENT

In the immunocompetent host, CSD is not a serious illness and does not require treatment beyond reassurance. However, in severe cases, treatment with antibiotics may have utility. Furthermore, in the immunodeficient patient, antibiotic therapy is recommended.

PROGNOSIS

After an episode of CSD, healthy individuals usually develop lifelong immunity, preventing reinfection. In children with normal immune systems, spontaneous healing with full recovery is the norm, usually with complete resolution of lymphadenopathy after two to six months. In immunocompromised people, treatment with antibiotics generally leads to recovery, with the order of preferred antibiotic agent as follows: rifampin, ciprofloxacin, gentamicin, and trimethoprim-sulfamethoxazole (9). Azithromycin may shorten the duration of lymphadenopathy, as was demonstrated in a small, prospective, comparative study. Complications of CSD include Parinaud's syndrome, encephalopathy, neuroretinitis, and osteomyelitis.

SUMMARY

Traumatic cat contact results in either bacillary angiomatosis in the immunocompromised patient or CSD in the immunocompetent patient. It appears that CSD is not easily acquired. In the immunocompetent host, CSD is not a serious illness and does not require treatment, with healthy individuals usually developing lifelong immunity, preventing reinfection. The final identification of *B. henselae* represents the convergence of fascinating data from eclectic fields of study, including AIDS-related opportunistic infections, epidemiology, pathology, molecular biology, microbiology, and veterinary medicine. The diagnosis of CSD can be overlooked easily if the clinician fails to obtain an adequate history, especially in the case of the atypical syndromes, and not uncommonly in the case of adults with the typical syndrome whose clinicians are inexperienced with CSD. With domestic cats representing the single largest category of companion animals in the United States, the importance of accurate history regarding animal exposure cannot be emphasized enough when evaluating a patient with findings consistent with CSD. Fortunately, in most cases, whether typical or atypical, spontaneous resolution occurs.

*G*ONORRHEA

INTRODUCTION

Gonorrhea is one of the oldest known human illnesses, and references to sexually acquired urethritis can be found in ancient Chinese writings, the biblical Old Testament (Leviticus), and other works of antiquity (Table 4). Galen (AD 130) introduced the term "gonorrhea" ("flow of seed"), implying interpretation of urethral exudate as semen. The causative organism was described by Neisser in 1879 and was first cultivated in 1882 by Leistikow and Löffler (10). Untreated infections were understood to resolve spontaneously over several

TABLE 4   Gonorrhea: Key Points

Overview
   The most common reportable infectious disease, causing symptomatic or asymptomatic
      localized infections including urethritis, cervicitis, proctitis, pharyngitis, and conjunctivitis
      after an incubation period of 2–8 days
   Disseminated infections occur either by extension to adjacent organs (pelvic inflammatory
      disease, epididymitis) or by bacteremic spread (skin lesions, tenosynovitis, septic arthritis,
      endocarditis, and meningitis)

Pathophysiology of gonorrhea
   Neisseria gonorrhoeae are Gram-negative cocci, usually seen in pairs with the adjacent sides
      flattened
   Gonorrhea is usually acquired by sexual contact. Gonococci adhere to columnar epithelial
      cells, penetrate them, and multiply on the basement membrane
   Transmission from the pharynx to sexual contacts is rare
   Adherence is facilitated through pili and opa proteins. Gonococcal lipopolysaccharide
      stimulates the production of tumor necrosis factor, which causes cell damage
   Gonococci may disseminate via the bloodstream. Strains that cause disseminated infections
      are usually resistant to serum and complement
   In the head and neck, pharyngeal gonococcal infection is significant, because it is the principal
      origin of gonococcemia

Symptomatology (by location of infection)
   Pharyngeal gonococcal infection is most often asymptomatic

Diagnosis
   Gonorrhea cannot be diagnosed solely on clinical grounds
   Pharyngeal culture on selective medium is often required to differentiate *N. gonorrhoeae* from
      other *Neisseria* species and evaluate antimicrobial resistance
   A nonamplified DNA probe test is available but is not as sensitive as culture
   Serologic tests are not recommended for uncomplicated infections

Treatment
   Recommended treatment for uncomplicated infections is a third-generation cephalosporin or a
      fluoroquinolone plus an antibiotic (e.g., doxycycline) effective against possible coinfection
      with *Chlamydia trachomatis*
   Sex partner(s) should be referred and treated
   No effective vaccine yet exists
   Condoms are effective in preventing gonorrhea

Prognosis
   Isolated pharyngeal infection is rare, complications occur infrequently if ever, and most cases
      resolve spontaneously within a few weeks or in response to therapy for genital or rectal
      infection

weeks or months, but reinfection was recognized to occur. Many therapies were tried, but truly effective treatment did not become available until the advent of the sulfonamides in the 1930s and penicillin in 1943. Growth of fundamental knowledge about the organism and the host response to infection was slow for 80 years, but a remarkable surge of new information began in the 1970s, and, currently, as much is known of the molecular biology of the gonococcus and the pathogenesis of gonorrhea as that of any bacterial pathogen. Public health control efforts have met with variable success, and gonorrhea remains a prime example of the influence that social, behavioral, and demographic factors can have on the epidemiology of an infectious disease despite highly effective, readily available antimicrobial therapy. Although the most common portal of entry is the genitourinary tract, head and neck manifestations of infection include gonococcal pharyngitis, gingivitis, stomatitis, and glossitis. Gonococcal pharyngitis is an uncommon but well-described manifestation. Gonorrhea remains a major public health problem worldwide, is a significant cause of morbidity in developing countries, and may play a role in enhancing transmission of HIV.

EPIDEMIOLOGY

Since 1995, gonorrhea has become the second most frequently reported infectious disease, after chlamydial infection, in the United States (11). The World Health Organization estimates that there are approximately 100 million gonorrheal infections each year throughout the world. The reported number of cases of gonorrhea in the United States in 2002 was roughly 362,000, although the true incidence is estimated to be twice that number. This number had been decreasing yearly after a peak of 1 million cases in 1978, until 1997 through 1998, when the rates increased over 10% in women and 7.4% in men, according to the Centers for Disease Control and Prevention.

The highest incidences occur in young (ages 15–30 years), single persons of low socioeconomic and educational attainment, in inner-city residents, and in some rural settings, especially in the Southeast. The incidence of reported gonorrhea is 30-fold higher in African Americans than in whites or persons of Asian or Pacific-Island ancestry; the rates in those of Hispanic or Native American ethnicity are three-fold and four-fold higher than in whites, respectively (12). The differences between racial and ethnic groups are reflections of differing sex-partner-network structures, socioeconomic attainment, education, and access to health care. Persons of lower socioeconomic status selectively attend public clinics, where reporting is more complete than in the private sector, but this bias accounts for only a small part of the observed differences between racial and ethnic groups. The incidence of gonorrhea is several times higher in men who have sex with men (MSM) than in heterosexuals. Rates of gonorrhea and other sexually transmitted diseases (STDs) rose dramatically among MSM in the United States and other industrialized countries from 1997 to 2002, in association with improved therapy and survival of persons with HIV infection. The risk of contracting gonorrhea via conventional intercourse is 50% for women and about 20% for men following a single exposure (12). Urethral-to-pharyngeal transmission by fellatio also occurs frequently, and pharyngeal gonococcal infection is especially common among MSM. Conflicting data exist on the efficiency of transmission of pharyngeal infection to the urethra by fellatio. Both transmission and acquisition of gonorrhea by cunnilingus appear to be very rare. Transmission by kissing is rare to nonexistent. Pharyngeal gonococcal infection is found in about 5% of heterosexual men, 5% to 10% of heterosexual women, and 10% to 20% of MSM with gonorrhea (11). Pharyngeal gonococcal infection, most often asymptomatic, may be more common in pregnant women because of altered sexual practices. Gonococci die rapidly on drying, so that transmission by fomites is rare. Perinatal transmission, with neonatal ophthalmitis or pharyngeal infection, is now rare. Gonorrhea in prepubertal children older than one year almost always results from sexual abuse.

PATHOLOGY/PATHOPHYSIOLOGY

Neisseria gonorrhoeae is a nonmotile, non–spore-forming, Gram-negative coccus that characteristically grows in pairs (diplococci), with flattened adjacent sides in the configuration of "coffee beans." All *Neisseria* species, including *Neisseria meningitidis*, rapidly oxidize dimethyl- or tetramethyl-paraphenylene diamine, the basis of the diagnostic oxidase test. The cell envelope of *N. gonorrhoeae* is similar to that of other Gram-negative bacteria. Specific surface components of the envelope have been related to adherence, tissue and cellular penetration, cytotoxicity, and evasion of host defenses, both systemically and at the mucosal level.

Stratified squamous epithelium can resist invasion by the gonococcus, whereas columnar epithelium is susceptible to it. Gonorrhea can occur in the genitalia of males or females without signs or symptoms. The primary infection can also occur in the rectal or pharyngeal mucosa of either sex. Gonococci attach to the mucosal epithelium and then penetrate between and through the epithelial cells to reach the subepithelial connective tissue by the third or fourth day of infection. An inflammatory exudate quickly forms beneath the epithelium. In the acute phase of infection, numerous leukocytes accumulate (many with phagocytosed gonococci), causing a characteristic profuse yellow-white discharge in males. In the absence of specific treatment, the inflammatory exudate in the subepithelial connective tissue is replaced by macrophages and lymphocytes. Direct extension of the infection occurs through the lymphatic vessels and less often through the blood vessels. Acute urethritis is the most common manifestation in males, and the infection can then spread to the posterior urethra, Cowper's glands, seminal vesicles, prostate, and epididymis, which leads to perineal, perianal, ischiorectal, or periprostatic abscesses.

Conjunctivitis beyond the newborn period follows direct spread of the gonococcus, usually via fingers contaminated with genital secretions. It rarely results from gonococcemia. Conjunctivitis is often severe, with profuse purulent discharge, chemosis, eyelid edema, and ulcerative keratitis, and presentations may mimic orbital cellulitides.

PATHOGENESIS

Pili are filamentous projections that traverse the outer membrane of the organism and are composed of repeating protein subunits (pilin) that help gonococci attach to mucosal surfaces by binding to the host cell receptor CD46 (13). Attachment is also mediated by a family of outer membrane proteins, designated opacity proteins, which bind to either CD66 or heparin-like molecules on host cells. Attachment and invasion of host epithelium are influenced by antigenic variations of pili and opacity proteins and by variations in the core sugars of lipooligosaccharide (LOS) components of the organism's outer membrane. These variations also help the organism evade the immune response.

When *N. gonorrhoeae* is grown on translucent agar, various colonial morphologies can be seen. Fresh clinical isolates initially form colony types P+ and P++ (formerly called T1 and T2). These organisms have numerous pili extending from the cell surface. After 20 to 24 hours, P− (formerly T3 and T4) colonies—in which the cells are nonpiliated—predominate. These nonpiliated organisms are not virulent. The shift between P+ or P++ and P− colony types is termed "phase variation" and is mediated by chromosomal rearrangement. The protein that constitutes pili (pilin) has regions of considerable antigenic variability between strains of *N. gonorrhoeae*. Single strains of *N. gonorrhoeae* also can produce pili of different antigenic composition (antigenic variation), which has made the possibility of a pilus-based vaccine against *N. gonorrhoeae* less feasible. Piliated gonococci are better able to attach to human mucosal surfaces than nonpiliated organisms. Pili also contribute to killing by neutrophils.

Typical urethral infections result in moderately severe inflammation, probably due to the release of toxic lipopolysaccharide and peptidoglycan fragments and to chemotactic factors that attract neutrophilic leukocytes. The reasons that some gonococcal strains selectively cause asymptomatic genital infection are poorly understood, but this propensity may be related to differences in the ability of the organism to bind complement-regulatory proteins that downregulate the production of chemotactic peptides.

The gonococcus has a cell envelope like other Gram-negative bacteria; it consists of three layers: an inner cytoplasmic membrane, a middle peptidoglycan cell wall, and an outer membrane. The outer membrane contains LOS, phospholipid, and a variety of proteins. One of them is protein I, which functions as a porin and is believed to play an important role in pathogenesis. Preliminary data suggest that it may facilitate endocytosis of the organism or otherwise trigger invasion. Protein I is also the basis of the most commonly used gonococcal serotyping system because there is consistent antigenic variation between different strains. Certain *N. gonorrhoeae* protein I serovars are associated with resistance of the organism to the bactericidal effect of normal nonimmune serum and an increased propensity to cause bacteremia. Gonococcal LOS is an endotoxin that differs from the polysaccharides of most Gram-negative bacteria in that it lacks O-antigenic side chains. Some components of LOS are also related to resistance of *N. gonorrhoeae* to serum bactericidal activity. LOS also demonstrates interstrain antigenic variations, which are the basis of another serotyping system.

CLINICAL MANIFESTATIONS

In the head and neck, pharyngeal gonococcal infection is asymptomatic as a rule, although rare cases present with exudative pharyngitis and cervical lymphadenopathy. Symptomatic patients usually present with findings suggestive of tonsillitis. The tonsils are enlarged with a white-yellow exudate arising from the crypts. Patients may show evidence of oropharyngeal trauma, particularly on the soft palate or uvula. Fever (8%) and lymphadeno-pathy (9%) are uncommon findings (11). Organisms are found within the cellular debris at the base of crypts. Isolated pharyngeal infection is rare; complications occur infrequently, if ever, and most cases resolve spontaneously within a few weeks or in response to therapy for genital or rectal infection. In addition, transmission of pharyngeal infection to other sites is inefficient. Gonococcal oropharyngitis is common among homosexuals and among children who are victims of sexual abuse. Infection follows orogenital contact. For asymptomatic patients, evidence suggests that the presence of *N. gonorrhoeae* in the oropharynx may be self-limited. This does not justify withholding treatment, however, because dissemination from the pharynx can still occur. Dissemination occurs in roughly 1% to 3% of cases, typically in patients asymptomatic relative to the pharyngeal or urogenital infection (10). Manifestations of dissemination can include low grade fever, migratory polyarthralgias involving the large joints, septic arthritis, or dermatitis.

Bacterial conjunctivitis may affect one or both eyes. Presenting symptoms may include red, injected (hyperemic) conjunctiva; discharge may be watery or purulent. Matted eyelids are common. Pseudomembranes may be present; they do not cause bleeding when removed. True membranes occur, as well; these are fibrin coagulated exudates attached to inflamed conjunctiva, which cause bleeding if removed. This differentiation between pseudomembranes and true membranes is not as important as once thought, because both have similar etiologies (i.e., infection with β-hemolytic *Streptococcus*, *Gonococcus*, *C. diphtheriae*). *N. gonorrhoeae* is commonly considered first for neonatal conjunctivitities, that is, those occurring within the first month of life. When conjunctivitis occurs within the first two to five days of life, *Neisseria* must be considered. If infection with this organism is suspected, early treatment is imperative to prevent rapid corneal ulceration and penetration. Gonococcal conjunctivitis is a sight-threatening infection when it occurs in the neonatal period, because the Gram-negative intracellular diplococci can easily penetrate the cornea. Corneal ulceration may occur within hours. Signs of *Neisseria* conjunctivitis include a hyperacute, purulent, yellow-green discharge. Conjunctivitis beyond the newborn period follows direct spread of the gonococcus, usually via fingers contaminated with genital secretions. It rarely results from gonococcemia. Conjunctivitis is often severe with chemosis, eyelid edema, and ulcerative keratitis; and presentations may mimic orbital cellulites.

DIAGNOSIS

Due to the asymptomatic nature of pharyngeal gonococcal infection, testing persons at risk for pharyngeal gonococcal infection is optional, although most providers routinely test MSM. Culture is the only approved test. Pharyngeal cultures are positive in 15% to 54% of children with genital gonococcal infections (12). Because organisms are found in the base of tonsillar crypts, it is recommended to obtain Gram stain and culture specimens from deep within the crypts. Pharyngeal infection almost always coexists with genital infection, and genital cultures should also be obtained. A typical Gram stain reveals intracellular Gram-negative diplococci. This finding should be confirmed on culture on modified Thayer-Martin medium because the pharynx can be colonized by other *Neisseria* species. Acute HIV infection should also be considered in the differential diagnosis of pharyngitis in persons with appropriate risk factors.

The Gram stain for diagnosis of gonorrhea is considered to be positive if typical Gram-negative diplococci are seen in association with polymorphonuclear leucocytes. A positive Gram stain from a male urethral specimen is highly sensitive and specific for gonococcal infection; however, in females, the adult cervix and the vagina of prepubertal children may be colonized with other *Neisseria* species, rendering the Gram stain less reliable. Similarly, Gram-stained smears of rectal and pharyngeal specimens are not useful to determine infection at these sites.

Diagnostic specimens of the pharynx, rectum, and vagina or urethra should be taken and immediately plated onto selective media appropriate for isolation of *N. gonorrhoeae* (e.g., Thayer-Martin media) and then placed in an atmosphere enriched with carbon dioxide, which is done most easily using an extinction candle jar. Isolation of gonococci from sites containing many saprophytic organisms (vagina, cervix, pharynx, and rectum) is enhanced if selective media containing antibiotics (e.g., Thayer-Martin media) are used; these media inhibit most of the normal flora and permit only the growth of gonococci and meningococci. Specimens from other usually sterile sites (blood, synovial fluid, or cerebrospinal fluid) should be inoculated only onto nonselective (antibiotic free) media such as enriched chocolate agar. *N. gonorrhoeae* organisms are Gram-negative, oxidase-positive diplococci, and their presence should be confirmed with additional tests, including rapid carbohydrate tests, enzyme-substrate tests, and rapid serologic tests. Failure to perform appropriate confirmatory tests may lead to misidentification of other organisms as *N. gonorrhoeae*.

Although culture of *N. gonorrhoeae* is well standardized and widely available, there have always been concerns about the loss of viability during transport to the laboratory. Enzyme immunoassays for detection of *N. gonorrhoeae* were introduced in the 1980s but were not satisfactory in terms of sensitivity or specificity. In the late 1980s, a nonamplified DNA probe was introduced (PACE 2, GenProbe, San Diego, California, U.S.A.). The overall sensitivity of the DNA probe compared with that of culture of endocervical specimens from women has been on the order of 95%. Data are similar for male urethral specimens, with sensitivities of 98.8% to 100% and specificities >99% compared with culture. There are now four nucleic acid amplification tests (NAATs) approved by the U.S. Food and Drug Administration (FDA) for the detection of *N. gonorrhoeae* in clinical specimens: PCR (Amplicor, Roche Molecular Diagnostics, Pleasanton, California, U.S.A.); transcription-mediated amplification (TMA) (GenProbe, San Diego, California, U.S.A.); and strand displacement amplification (SDA) (ProbeTec, Becton Dickson, Franklin Lakes, New Jersey, U.S.A.). PCR and SDA are DNA amplification tests; TMA is an RNA ampli-fication assay. A fourth NAAT, ligase chain reaction (LCX assay, Abbott Diagnostics, Abbott Park, Illinois, U.S.A.) was withdrawn from the market by the manufacturer in 2002 because of poor quality control.

TREATMENT

In the preantibiotic era, gonorrhea usually persisted for two to three months before host defenses finally eradicated the infection. These defenses include serum opsonic and bactericidal antibodies, as well as mucosal antibodies of the IgG and IgA classes. All gonococci produce IgA1 protease, an enzyme that inactivates the major class of secretory IgA, perhaps contributing to persistence of mucosal infection.

Most cases of pharyngeal gonococcal infection resolve spontaneously, and transmission from the pharynx to sexual contacts is rare.

During the 20 years before 1976, all *N. gonorrhoeae* strains were sensitive to penicillin, but a gradual increase had been noted in the mean MIC (13). The first reports of penicillinase-producing *N. gonorrhoeae* (PPNG) arising in the Far East occurred in the 1970s. PPNG strains have accounted for more than 30% of isolates of *N. gonorrhoeae* in the United States. There has also been a similar increase in tetracycline-resistant *N. gonorrhoeae*. These resistant strains cause the same disease spectrum as penicillin-sensitive organisms. In 1983 an outbreak of chromosomally mediated penicillin-resistant gonococci was reported from North Carolina; subsequently, it has occurred in other areas of the country. Although strains of *N. gonorrhoeae* with decreased susceptibility to ceftriaxone do occur, no documented clinical treatment failures have been observed related to decreased gonococcal susceptibility to ceftriaxone in the United States.

Routine preventive prophylaxis of gonococcal ophthalmia includes (*i*) 1% silver nitrate (with no irrigation with saline solution, which might reduce efficacy) and (*ii*) ophthalmic ointments containing tetracycline (1%) or erythromycin (0.5%), per the 2002 CDC guidelines. Use of bacitracin ointment (not effective) and penicillin drops (sensitizing) is not recommended. Data on use of povidone-iodine are limited; initial studies suggested less efficacy. Silver nitrate is no longer manufactured in the United States. Systemic therapy is imperative. Patients are hospitalized and given hourly eyewashes with normal saline until discharge is eliminated. This reduces the bacterial load and forces hourly monitoring of the cornea.

The infant born to a mother with untreated gonorrhea should have orogastric and rectal cultures taken routinely and blood cultures taken if the infant is symptomatic. A full-term infant should receive a single injection of ceftriaxone [50 mg/kg intravenously (IV) or intramuscularly (IM), not to exceed 125 mg]. Although ceftriaxone is not usually given to newborn infants, it is indicated in this specific setting.

The first-line regimen for treatment of uncomplicated gonococcal infection in adults recommended by the CDC 2002 guidelines is cefixime (400 mg orally, single dose); ciprofloxacin (500 mg orally, single dose); single-dose ceftriaxone (125 mg IM); or a single-dose oral quinolone (ciprofloxacin, 500 mg, ofloxacin, 400 mg, levofloxacin, 250 mg, or gatifloxacin, 400 mg). However, cefixime is no longer available, as the manufacturer ceased production in 2002. Spectinomycin is not as effective in treating pharyngeal gonorrhea. Each regimen should also include a regimen effective against possible coinfection with *Chlamydia trachomatis* such as azithromycin (1 g orally in a single dose) or doxycycline (100 mg orally, two times a day for seven days). Recent data from the CDC's Gonococcal Isolate Surveillance Project from several sites in California are also demonstrating an increased prevalence of quinolone resistance in the state and further suggest that use of quinolones in California is probably not advisable.

PROGNOSIS

The most common complication is acute salpingitis, or pelvic inflammatory disease, leading in turn to infertility and ectopic pregnancy. Other complications are epididymitis, posterior urethritis, urethral stricture, Bartholin gland abscess, and perihepatitis. Bacteremia may occur, with production of characteristic cutaneous lesions, arthritis, and rarely endocarditis or meningitis.

SUMMARY

Gonorrhea, an STD involving infection of columnar and transitional epithelium by *N. gonorrhoeae,* continues to be a significant sexually transmitted infection causing a generally asymptomatic pharyngeal infection that may later become disseminated. In some cases of *N. gonorrhoeae,* erythema, edema, vesicles, ulcers, and pain may be present in the oral cavity. These patients are more likely to develop systemic gonorrhea. Major virulence mechanisms include production of pili and IgAase. Gonococci are very fragile and fastidious organisms, resulting in a lack of transmission by fomites, the need for calcium alginate swabs to collect specimens, and nutrient media such as Thayer-Martin media required to culture the organism. In the head and neck, pharyngeal gonococcal infection is significant, because it is the principal origin of gonococcemia. Treatment of uncomplicated gonococcal infections currently is a single dose of cefixime, ceftriaxone, or ciprofloxacin if chlamydial infection has been ruled out. Disseminated infections (bacteremias, meningitis, endocarditis, septic arthritis) require parenteral antibiotic (ceftriaxone, cefotaxime or ceftizoxime). Previous investigations into gonococcal vaccines, most of which are composed of gonococcal pili, found that they were not protective. Control rests on better education, proper reporting, follow-up of patients and their contacts, use of condoms, and chemoprophylaxis to prevent neonatal gonoccocal conjunctivitis.

*N*ECROTIZING FASCIITIS

INTRODUCTION

Necrotizing fasciitis (NF), a fulminant soft-tissue infection that causes necrosis of fascia and subcutaneous tissue while sparing skin and muscle initially, was first described by Wilson in the 1950s (Table 5) (14,15). The disease is known by several eponyms, including hospital gangrene, Meleney's synergist gangrene, hemolytic streptococcal gangrene, and synergistic necrotizing cellulites, among others. It is most commonly seen in adults, involving the perineum, extremities, and abdominal wall, though it may affect any part of the body. Immunocompromised patients are at increased risk of developing this infection. These infections require early diagnosis, aggressive surgical debridement, and appropriate antibiotic therapy. Failure to do so results in an extremely high mortality rate, ranging from 80% to 100%, and even with rapid intervention and treatment, mortality remains approximately 30% to 50%. NF of the head and neck is rare, most commonly reported due to odontogenic infections.

EPIDEMIOLOGY

Risk factors for infection include an immunocompromised or elderly state, diabetes mellitus, alcoholism, chronic renal failure, peripheral vascular disease, injection drug use,

TABLE 5 Necrotizing Fasciitis: Key Points

Overview
  NF is a rare, life-threatening, soft-tissue infection characterized by rapidly spreading
    inflammation and necrosis of the skin, subcutaneous fat, and fascia
  After an incubation period of 1–4 days, an acute onset of symptoms with moderate to marked
    toxemia, a putrid discharge, and pain out of proportion to the physical examination findings

Pathophysiology of NF
  Clinical manifestations include extensive dissection and necrosis of the superficial and often
    the deep fascia. The infection undermines adjacent tissue and leads to marked systemic
    toxicity
  Thrombosis of subcutaneous blood vessels leads to necrosis of the overlying skin
  Most cases of fasciitis follow surgery or minor trauma. The highest incidence is seen in
    patients with small vessel diseases such as diabetes mellitus
  When careful bacteriologic techniques are used, anaerobes, particularly *Peptostreptococcus*,
    Bacteroides, and *Fusobacterium* species, are found in 50–60% of cases. Aerobic
    organisms, especially *Streptococcus pyogenes*, *Staphylococcus aureus*, and members of
    the Enterobacteriaceae have also been isolated
  Most infections are mixed aerobic–anaerobic infections, but a type of NF caused solely by
    S. pyogenes has been reported and is referred to by the lay press as "flesh eating bacteria"

Symptomatology (by location of infection)
  Initial local pain is replaced by numbness or analgesia as the infection involves the cutaneous
    nerves
  Clinically, the hallmarks of mixed aerobic–anaerobic soft tissue infections are tissue necrosis,
    a putrid discharge, gas production, the tendency to burrow through soft tissue and fascial
    planes, and the absence of classic signs of tissue inflammation

Diagnosis
  A Gram stain of tissue fluid and blood cultures should be obtained to assist in guiding antibiotic
    therapy
  Radiologic testing may detect air within the tissue, highly suggestive of NF

Treatment
  Treatment includes broad-spectrum antibiotic coverage, nutritional supplements,
    hemodynamic support, wound care, and prompt surgical debridement

Prognosis
  Untreated, NF has been noted to have an extremely high mortality rate, ranging from 80–100%,
    and even with rapid intervention and treatment, mortality remains approximately 30–50%

Abbreviation: NF, necrotizing fasciitis.

postpartum patients, or a combination of these factors (16). The unifying thread among these risk factors appears to be a compromised fascial blood supply coupled with the introduction of exogenous microbes. However, various studies have reported that 13% to 31% of patients were previously healthy individuals with no identifiable risk factors (15). The incidence of NF in adults has been reported to be 0.40 cases per 100,000 population, while the incidence in children is 0.08 cases per 100,000 population (16).

PATHOLOGY/PATHOPHYSIOLOGY

NF usually originates in traumatic musculoskeletal wounds or operative sites, or follows other types of injuries such as minor cuts, scrapes, and insect bites. In the head and neck, the most common source of infection is odontogenic, with one series describing mandibular molar abscesses as the most common site of origin (17). In the head and neck region, bacterial penetration into the fascial compartments can result in a related syndrome known as Ludwig's angina, or it may develop into NF (18). NF is caused by aerobic and anaerobic microorganisms causing massive tissue destruction and toxic shock syndrome. These infections are characterized by the absence of clear local boundaries or palpable limits, which contributes to the frequent delay in diagnosis and subsequent surgical debridement. The infections may be clostridial or nonclostridial in origin. The causative agent may be a single organism, most commonly Group A β-hemolytic streptococcal infection or *S. aureus*, or may be polymicrobial (19). The polymicrobial infections are caused by mixed aerobic and anaerobic pathogens. Many pathogens have been described, including β-hemolytic streptococci, staphylococci, coliforms, enterococci, pseudomonads, *Bacteroides*, and *Vibrio vulnificus*. The clinical features of NF caused by *V. vulnificus* are different from those of NF caused by classic pathogens: when caused by *V. vulnificus*, especially in the warmer half of the year, the predominant skin lesions are edema and subcutaneous bleeding, and there is no superficial necrosis.

Histology reveals obliterative endarteritis and thrombosis of the subcutaneous vessels. Other changes are necrotic superficial fascial and microbial colonization of the skin and fascia. Myonecrosis is rarely seen, except in clostridial infections. The presence of vesiculation, ecchymosis, crepitus, anesthesia, and necrosis is indicative of advanced disease. As the infection moves along the deep fascial plane, the speed of spread is directly proportional to the thickness of the subcutaneous layer.

Staphylococci and streptococci produce extracellular enzymes that damage connective tissue. Bacterial metabolism may produce insoluble hydrogen, nitrogen, nitrous oxide, and hydrogen sulfide gases that result in subcutaneous emphysema. Though classically associated with clostridial infections, organisms such as *Escherichia coli*, *Klebsiella*, *Peptostreptococcus*, and *Bacteroides* may also produce subcutaneous emphysema. The more common anaerobic organisms seen in NF of the head and neck include *Peptostreptococcus*, *B. melaninogenicus*, and *Fusobacterium*.

PATHOGENESIS

The exact mechanism of this rapidly spreading gangrenous infection has not been established. The release of enzymes such as hyaluronidase and proteolytic portions of cell membranes have been shown to be contributing factors to the necrosis.

CLINICAL MANIFESTATIONS

Cervical NF (CNF) initially involves the superficial musculoaponeurotic system and superficial fascial planes of the head and neck, or it may result from a deep soft-tissue infection, such as pharyngitis or dental infection, which spreads along the deep fascial planes. These virulent bacteria, alone or in synergistic combination, produce a severe necrotizing infection of the fascia and soft tissues of the head, neck, and scalp. If the disease is not recognized in time, the infection can rapidly involve the great vessels or mediastinum, producing life-threatening systemic toxicity and sepsis. The affected skin is red, hot, smooth, shiny, tense, and tender. At the time of presentation, most patients are toxic with high fever and a rapidly progressive nonfluctuant swelling of the face and neck. Lymphadenopathy and lymphangitis are not usually found.

Initially, there is cellulitis which leads to invasion of the deeper tissues. Clinically, at this stage, skin changes of erythema and edema are seen. Redness, pain, and edema progress to central patches or dusky blue discoloration within 24 to 48 hours, and these areas become gangrenous by the fourth or fifth day. Anesthesia of the involved skin is very characteristic. Progressive tissue necrosis causes an invasion by the normal flora. Continuous bacterial overgrowth and synergy causes a decrease in oxygen tension and development of local ischemia, with proliferation of anaerobic organisms. After 8 to 10 days, necrotic tissue separates from the underlying ischemic but viable tissue.

NF can be divided into five types (20).

1. NF type I—polymicrobial
2. NF type II—Grp A streptococcal
3. Clostridial myonecrosis—gas gangrene
4. Fournier's gangrene
5. Lemierre's syndrome

NF type I is caused by non-Grp-A streptococci and anaerobes and/or facultative anaerobes. It is usually seen after trauma or surgery with involvement of subcutaneous fat and fascia. Surrounding muscles are typically not involved. Gas formation is common.

NF type II is caused by *S. pyogenes* alone or with *Staphylococcus*. It is usually associated with streptococcal toxic shock syndrome. Predisposing factors are trauma, surgery, and varicella infections.

Clostridial myonecrosis is characterized by its fulminant onset. The predominant features are muscle necrosis and gas production. The commonest causative organism is *Clostridium perfringens*.

Fournier's gangrene (J. A. Fournier, 1883) is NF of the scrotum. Lemierre's syndrome (A. Lemierre, 1936) is an oropharyngeal infection with secondary thrombophlebitis of the internal jugular vein and frequent metastatic infections, caused by *Fusobacterium necrophorium*.

DIAGNOSIS

The diagnosis of NF is initially based solely on clinical findings, which vary significantly between patients. The differential diagnosis includes cellulitis of dental origin, erysipelas, deep neck-space infections, and gangrenous necrosis due to *Clostridium*.

Pain out of proportion to other clinical findings is an important clue to the diagnosis of this condition. A careful examination should be undertaken for evidence of an entry site such as a small break or sinus in the skin, from which a grayish, turbid semipurulent material may be expressed ("dishwater pus"), as well as for the presence of skin changes (brawny hue or brawny induration). Due to the presence of gas-producing organisms, detection of subcutaneous air is a classic finding in NF, although this finding is not always detectable on x-ray imaging. Although radiologic evaluation is controversial and recommended only for patients in whom the disease is not seriously considered, due to the delay in surgical intervention, computed tomography of the head and neck is the imaging study of choice to confirm the presence of gas and provide detailed anatomical information (18). A critical element of diagnosis is a high clinical index of suspicion for the infection, given that subcutaneous or radiologic changes may not readily be apparent early in the disease and may delay the required early, aggressive surgical intervention. During the procedure, a confirmatory Gram stain should be performed on tissue fluid.

TREATMENT

Treatment involves wide local surgical debridement supported by intravenous antibiotics and other supportive treatment. It is essential that all areas of necrotic tissue be debrided, including direct visualization of infected tissue and radical resection of affected areas.

Debridement is performed not only to control the primary infectious process but also to remove the necrotic tissue, which is the source of secondary infection as well as of toxin production. Fasciotomy incisions need to be planned according to the area involved; however, they should be parallel to the major blood vessels, thus maintaining the blood supply to the surrounding tissue. All involved fascial planes and head and neck spaces must be debrided and drained. Extension of the CNF after peritonsillar abscess or odontogenic infection to the layers of the deep cervical fascia can lead to involvement of the carotid sheath, cervical viscera, and deep neck musculature, with further extension to the mediastinum and anterior thoracic wall (17). The infection spreads along the middle layer of deep cervical fascia. Characteristic of NF is the ability to dissect between fascia with little resistance. A finding during surgery suggests that gas and purulent fluid dissect into fascial compartments far away from sites of skin duskiness, crepitus, and fluctuance.

Excision to the point of bleeding tissue is a useful guide for debridement. Although extirpation of the infected tissue may result in significant deformity, incomplete procedures are associated with higher rates of persistence, reoperation, morbidity, and mortality. Antimicrobial therapy directed against Gram-negative and Gram-positive aerobes and anaerobes (such as vancomycin and a carbapenem), in addition to high-dose penicillin G for treatment of clostridial pathogens, should be administered (18). Most patients should be returned to the operating room on a scheduled basis to determine if disease progression has occurred, so that serial debridement may be required. There are some centers which advocate the use of hyperbaric oxygen for treating this condition.

PROGNOSIS

Mortality is higher in patients over 50 years of age, those with associated systemic illnesses such as diabetes mellitus or peripheral vascular diseases, and when there is a delay in diagnosis. These infections require a rapid diagnosis, because mortality rates up to 76% have been reported without early intervention (15). Even in the setting of optimal management, the mortality due to NF ranges from 30% to 50%. In the small number of cases described in the literature, patients with a peritonsillar abscess demonstrated a mortality rate of 33%, in comparison with 25% for patients with a predominantly odontogenic cause of CNF (17). The mortality rate for CNF is higher than that of the upper face infection, presumably because of the tendency for it to spread to the mediastinum, chest, and carotid sheath. CNF associated with a peritonsillar abscess is an extremely rare condition. The general condition of patients with CNF deteriorates more rapidly than for other regions, resulting in a higher mortality rate than in patients with upper face and scalp infections. The death rate is associated with comorbidity, but also with depth of infection and complications such as mediastinitis and fatal vascular complications. Involvement of the neck carries a death rate of 32%, attributed to the spread of the necrotizing process to the adjoining cervical viscera and thoracic cavity (17). In comparison, NF of the scalp and upper face has been reported to have a better prognosis, with a mortality rate of 12.5%.

SUMMARY

NF is a serious soft-tissue infection that is characterized by rapidly progressive necrosis of the subcutaneous tissue and superficial fascia. It is often associated with systemic toxicity, and, in a significant number of cases, is fatal. The pathogenic organisms implicated in the disease include *Streptococcus*, *Staphylococcus*, *Pseudomonas*, *Enterobacteria*, and a variety of anaerobes. Treatment involves wide local surgical debridement supported by intravenous antibiotics and other supportive treatment. The mortality rate in the setting of optimal treatment is 30% to 50%, and ranges from 80% to 100% for infections which were untreated or did not receive early intervention. Though NF in the head and neck is rare, patients may present with symptoms of odontogenic infections, and vigilance must be maintained to ensure that prompt and aggressive treatment is initiated.

R*EFERENCES*

1. Kleinman LC. To end an epidemic. Lessons from the history of diphtheria. N Engl J Med 1992; 326:773–777.
2. Pappenheimer AM Jr, Murphy JR. Studies on the molecular epidemiology of diphtheria. Lancet 1983; 2(8356):923–926.
3. Collier RJ. Understanding the mode of diphtheria toxin: a perspective on progress during the 20th century. Toxicon 2001; 39(11):1793–1803.
4. Bortolussi R, Mailman T. Aerobic Gram-positive Bacilli. In: Cohen J, Powderly W, eds. Infectious Diseases. Vol. 2. 2nd ed. NY: Mosby, 2004:2162–2166.
5. Wharton M. Diphtheria. In: Gershon AA, Hotez PJ, Katz SL, eds. Krugman's Infectious Diseases of Children, 11th ed. Philadelphia, PA: Mosby, 2004:85–95.
6. Emmons RW, Riggs JL, Schachter J. Continuing the search for the etiology of cat scratch disease. J Clin Microbiol 1976; 4(1):112–114.
7. Carithers HA. Cat scratch disease: an overview based on a study of 1,200 patients. Am J Dis Child 1985; 139(11):1124–1133.
8. Margileth AM. Cat scratch disease. Adv Pediatr Infect Dis 1993; 8:1–21.
9. Adal KA, Cockerell CJ, Petri WA Jr. Cat scratch disease, bacillary angiomatosis, and other infections due to *Rochalimaea*. N Engl J Med 1994; 330(21):1509–1515.
10. Wiesner PJ, Tronca E, Bonin P, et al. Clinical spectrum of pharyngeal gonococcal infection. N Engl J Med 1973; 288(4):181–185.
11. Lewis LS, Glauser TA, Joffe MD. Gonococcal conjunctivitis in prepubertal children. Am J Dis Child 1990; 144(5):546–548.
12. McClure EM, Stack MR, Tanner T, et al. Pharyngeal culturing and reporting of pediatric gonorrhea in Connecticut. Pediatrics 1986; 78(3):509–510.
13. Johnson SR, Morse SA. Antibiotic resistance in *Neisseria gonorrhoeae*: genetics and mechanisms of resistance. Sex Transm Dis 1988; 15(4):217–224.
14. Meleney FL. Hemolytic streptococcus gangrene. Arch Surg 1924; 9:317–364.
15. Rea WJ, Wyrick WJ Jr. Necrotizing fasciitis. Ann Surg 1970; 172(6):957–964.
16. Pai NB, Gerst PH, Yousuf AM, et al. Necrotizing fasciitis in immunocompromised patients. Contemp Surg 1996; 4:12.
17. Skitarelic N, Mladina M, Morovic M, et al. Cervical necrotizing fasciitis: sources and outcomes. Infection 2003; 31(1):39–44.
18. Mathieu D, Neviere R, Teillon C, et al. Cervical necrotizing fasciitis: clinical manifestations and management. Clin Infect Dis 1995; 21(1):51–56.
19. Giuliano A, Lewis F, Hadley K, et al. Bacteriology of necrotizing fasciitis. Am J Surg 1977; 134(1):52–57.
20. Bisno AL, Stevens DL. Streptococcal infections of skin and soft tissues. N Engl J Med 1996; 334(4):240–245.

12

Tuberculosis and Atypical Mycobacteria

Theodoros F. Katsivas
*Owen Clinic and Department of Medicine, Division of Infectious Diseases,
University of California, San Diego, California, U.S.A.*

TUBERCULOSIS

INTRODUCTION

Despite global efforts to control it, tuberculosis (TB) remains an urgent issue in all areas of the world, including the most developed nations. The emergence of the HIV epidemic and its impact on TB epidemiology, multidrug-resistant strains, malnutrition, poverty, and growing concentration of populations in urban centers, are all factors that make TB difficult to control. Worldwide, TB is second only to HIV as a cause of death resulting from a single infectious agent. Prior to the era of effective chemotherapy, treatment for TB was confined to isolation, sanatorium regimens, and surgical intervention for cavity closure and resection of the affected lung lobe. Isoniazid (INH) appeared in 1952 and rifampicin or rifampin (RMP) in 1970; however, TB is far from controlled at the time of this writing.

DEFINITION

TB is a chronic granulomatous disease with worldwide prevalence caused by *M. tuberculosis* (1) and less often by *M. bovis* (both referred to as the tubercle bacilli). Historically present since the early evolutionary stages of our species, mycobacteria have evolved to effectively infect and establish latency in almost all mammalian and other species. *M. tuberculosis* is an aerobic, non–spore-forming, slow-growing bacillus with a lipid-laden thick cell wall that tends to grow in parallel groups, exhibiting serpentine cording morphology. *M. tuberculosis* complex (MTB complex) refers to a group of genetically related mycobacteria and includes *M. tuberculosis*, *M. bovis*, *M. microti*, *M. canetti*, and *M. africanum*. Mycobacteria appear faintly positive or colorless on Gram stain. The term "acid-fast bacilli" (AFB) is almost synonymous with mycobacteria, although Nocardia species and other organisms can also be variably acid fast. The classic Ziehl–Neelsen stain, the modified Kinyoun stain and the auramine-rhodamine fluorochrome stains are commonly used for AFB. Multidrug-resistant tuberculosis (MDR-TB) is defined as being resistant to INH and rifamycin (RMP or rifabutin).

EPIDEMIOLOGY

Approximately one-third of the global human population is infected with *M. tuberculosis* (or *M. bovis*), with 8 million new cases of TB and 2 million deaths annually. The World Health Organization declared TB a global public health emergency in 1993, focusing on implementation of directly observed therapy (DOT) in most cases.

In the United States, a continuous decline in TB incidence rates was observed until 1985, when rates began to increase again, due to factors including illicit drug use, homelessness, HIV infection, irregular adherence to drug therapy, and evolution and spread of drug-resistant strains. Since 1992, TB rates in the United States have declined and in 2004, with effective TB-control programs, reached the lowest in recorded history (mean 4.9 cases per 100,000 population) (2). Most of the TB cases in the United States occur in foreign-born immigrants, ethnic minorities, and medically underserved populations. Rates of MDR-TB are variable, with a global median of 1% of all active TB cases, but rates can be as high as 10% to 15% in certain areas of the world. The goal of the National TB Control Program is to achieve less than one case per 100,000 by the year 2010.

PATHOGENESIS

Humans are the only reservoir for *M. tuberculosis*. Other than rare cases of ingestion, sexual transmission, or direct cutaneous inoculation, the vast majority of TB transmission occurs by inhalation of infectious respiratory droplet nuclei. Prolonged contact in a relatively contained area is necessary for transmission, and transmission in the outdoors or via fomites is rare.

The risk of infection from close contact with smear-positive sputum varies from 30% to 80% (3,4). The risk is less if the sputum is smear negative and culture positive; nonetheless, one study reported a rate of 17% for this risk (5). HIV coinfected patients can easily transmit the disease, even with negative chest X rays. In patients who are smear positive, infectiousness readily diminishes after initiation of appropriate chemotherapy. In 2005, the Centers for Disease Control and Prevention issued revised criteria for removal of patients from respiratory isolation (2) that were in line with prior stringent criteria from 1990 (6) and 1994 (7,8). According to those criteria, after initiation (2) of anti-TB therapy, three consecutive negative sputum smears (8 to 24 hours apart, with at least one an early-morning specimen) are required for the safe removal of the patient from isolation.

Within 2 to 12 weeks after inoculation of the lungs, the immune response controls the local infection, immunity develops, and the skin test becomes positive. Latency is established [latent TB infection (LTBI)] and the patient is asymptomatic and noninfectious. Local infection and infection to the draining lymphatics can be seen on chest X ray; this is known as the Ranke complex or primary complex (Ghon focus and draining lymphatics and hilar lymph nodes). Hematogenous dissemination is rare during primary infection.

Only 3% to 4% of persons will develop the disease during the first year after the infection. Infants and older persons are at greatest risk. In non–HIV-infected individuals, the risk of reactivation is 5% to 15% overall. In HIV-infected patients, the risk is dramatically higher by 7% to 10% per year.

CLINICAL MANIFESTATIONS

In the majority of TB cases, the lungs are the site most commonly involved. Primary TB or TB of childhood refers to the primary infection usually affecting the mid-lung fields. Adult or postprimary disease is characterized by caseation, cavity formation, and fibrosis. TB can affect many extrapulmonary sites, including the gastrointestinal tract, liver, lymph nodes and reticuloendothelial system, central nervous system, pericardium, pleura and peritoneum, bone and joint structures, and kidneys and genital tract. It can also disseminate hematogenously as miliary TB. The discussion of clinical manifestations will focus on the head and neck organs, relevant to the otorhinolaryngologist (9–12).

Head and Neck Manifestations
Tuberculous Lymphadenitis (Scrofula). This represents the most common form of extrapulmonary TB (13), and in 80% to 90% of cases, it is the only site of infection. In HIV-negative patients, it is usually bilateral and posterior cervical in location, presenting as an erythematous, painless mass along the anterior border of the sternocleidomastoid, typically without systemic symptoms (11). The tuberculin skin test (TST) is positive in more than 75% of patients. In HIV-positive patients, multiple sites may be involved, often with mediastinal and intra-abdominal lymphadenopathy, pulmonary or other organ involvement, and systemic symptoms. The TST is often negative in these patients. Of the patients, 10%

present with a fluctuant mass and 5% with sinus tract draining serosanguinous discharge. Chest radiographs are indicative of past or active infection in less than 20%.

Fine needle aspiration (FNA) may reveal granulomas, but the cultures and smears are rarely positive in HIV-negative patients. The opposite occurs in HIV-infected patients, where cytohistologic findings are not often typical, but the FNA yield of acid-fast smears and cultures is higher. Excisional biopsy is required for definitive diagnosis if the FNA is inconclusive, basically to exclude lymphoma or other infectious agents (atypical mycobacteria or fungi). Drains are not required to avoid fistula formation.

Complications of cervical lymph node involvement are node enlargement with pain, suppuration, sinus formation, and appearance of new nodes. These occur in 25% to 30% of patients, even during or postchemotherapy, and do not necessarily indicate failure of drug treatment. While some do not recommend surgical excision of scrofulous nodes, there are many who do, justifying it with the 25% to 30% drug-failure rate.

Pregnant patients with TB lymphadenitis are managed with topical care and aspiration of fluctuant collections until after delivery, due to concerns of teratogenicity. Antibacterial treatment can be initiated postpartum.

Ocular TB.   TB produces various ocular syndromes, including choroidal tubercles, uveitis (Chapter 6), iritis, and episcleritis. In suspected cases, a prompt referral to an ophthalmologist should be made.

Tuberculous Otitis.   Tuberculous otitis media is rare and usually represents hematogenous spread. Roughly one-half of the cases have no other evidence of present or past TB. The classic clinical picture is painless otorrhea with multiple tympanic perforations, exuberant granulation tissue, early severe hearing loss, and mastoid bone necrosis (see Chapter 25 for further discussion of otorrhea). The finding of multiple tympanic membrane perforations is most likely TB, possibly pathognomonic. Nonetheless, the diagnosis is difficult, even when tissue is available. Tuberculous otitis may be complicated by facial nerve paralysis, which is discussed in detail in Chapter 29. Response to drug therapy is excellent, and surgery usually is not required.

Nasal TB.   Tuberculomas with destructive characteristics in the nasal cavity can be seen and are part of the differential for nasal destructive lesions, companions to Wegener's granulomatosis and lymphoma (these are discussed in Chapters 8 and 17, respectively). Polyps can also be seen in the inferior turbinate. A positive AFB smear from the nasal cavity needs to be followed with culture to rule out infection from *M. leprae*, since nasal infection is common in lepromatous leprosy.

Pharyngeal TB.   The most common sites are the adenoids, posterior pharynx and the tonsils. Most of those infections are primary infections. They were more common in the past, associated with ingestion of nonpasteurized milk that was infected with *M. bovis*. No specific characteristics are present and in many cases, biopsies are performed to rule out cancer; however, response to anti-TB therapy is prompt, and resolution is the rule.

Tuberculous Sialadenitis.   The parotid and submandibular glands are most commonly infected and can be the sole site of disease. Minor salivary glands have also been involved (15). In most cases, computed tomography (CT) imaging, FNA, and culture have not been helpful. Surgical excision is recommended if medical treatment fails and/or diagnostic confirmation is required. Pathology will show granulomatous inflammation and nucleic acid amplification testing (NAAT) by polymerase chain reaction (PCR) will be positive. Postoperatively, nine months of anti-TB therapy is recommended.

Tuberculous Laryngitis.   The pathogenesis of TB laryngitis has changed with the implementation of active chemotherapy. In the preantibiotic era, TB laryngitis was often encountered in advanced disease, along with oral and epiglottic lesions, tonsillar ulcers, otitis media, and bronchogenic spread. Once diagnosed with laryngeal TB, patients respond promptly to antibacterial therapy; the prevalence of laryngeal TB has decreased dramatically since the introduction of this therapy; and most of the laryngeal cases now seen are due to hematogenous dissemination (9,11).

TB laryngitis is highly contagious, due to the effective aerosolization of bacilli-laden secretions during speaking, sneezing, or coughing. Lesions vary from erythema to ulceration and exophytic masses resembling carcinoma. The most common initial symptom is hoarseness. Systemic symptoms of weight loss, fever, night sweats, and fatigue are often present; cough, wheezing, hemoptysis, dysphagia, odynophagia, and otalgia are the dominant local symptoms. Stridor may develop secondary to subglottic fibrosis and narrowing, local tumor mass, or vocal cord paralysis.

Sputa samples reveal AFB in up to 30% of cases. If biopsy is performed to rule out carcinoma, the tissue should be sent for AFB culture. Histology will reveal granulomatous inflammation. Appropriate respiratory precautions should be taken to avoid aerosol formation and occupational exposure of health-care personnel.

Oral and Esophageal TB. Nonhealing ulcers of the tongue or oropharynx and nonhealing sockets after tooth extraction may be due to TB. The esophagus can be eroded by an adjacent caseous node, which leads to stricture with obstruction or tracheoesophageal fistula formation, and rarely, fatal hematemesis from an aortoesophageal fistula.

Systemic Manifestations

Cutaneous TB. Facial lesions due to conditions associated with TB have been described; these include erythema induratum of Bazin, papulonecrotic tuberculids, and others. *M. tuberculosis* DNA has been detected in erythema induratum skin lesions by PCR, and erythema nodosum has been attributed to primary TB. Skin involvement may result from exogenous inoculation, spread from an adjacent focus to the overlying skin, or hematogenous spread, often seen in patients with AIDS and tuberculous bacteremia. Any unexplained skin lesion, particularly one with nodular or ulcerative components, may be due to TB, especially in AIDS patients; and biopsy and cultures are warranted.

Skeletal TB. More than 30% of skeletal TB cases involve the spine (tuberculous spondylitis or Pott's disease). The most commonly affected area is the lower thoracic spine, followed by the lumbar, cervical, and sacral areas. The mode of spread to the spine is usually hematogenous, but it also can result from contiguous disease or lymphatic spread from TB pleuritis. In contrast to common bacterial causes of spinal osteomyelitis that initially present as discitis with adjacent vertebral body involvement, TB spondylitis typically begins within the anterior vertebral body. With time, spread to the adjacent disc and vertebra occurs, and vertebral body wedging develops.

Pott's disease is a disease of older age in developed countries and presents with local symptoms of pain and stiffness without systemic manifestations such as fever or weight loss. Initial roentgenograms can be negative. Thus, the diagnosis can be difficult to make, and late complications often appear. These can include paraspinal abscess and sinus tract formation as well as neurological symptoms from spinal instability and cord compression. Paraspinal cold abscesses develop in 50% of patients and can extend along tissue planes and present as masses in remote areas such as the supraclavicular, inguinal, popliteal, or posterior iliac regions.

Bone biopsy rarely yields bacilli but can reveal bone marrow granulomas in about 75% of cases.

The most serious complication is lower extremity paralysis (Pott's paraplegia) from spinal instability and cord compression, inflammatory arachnoiditis, or vasculitis.

A 12-month course of treatment is recommended for Pott's spondylitis. In a review of uncomplicated cases, response rates to systemic chemotherapy and bed rest until pain resolved exceeded 90% (16). Laminectomy does not appear to be dramatically helpful for neurologic complications unless there are advancing defects and severe instability of the spine. In a series of complicated patients, needle aspiration of the paraspinal abscesses along with steroids seemed to be beneficial to successful management (16).

DIAGNOSIS

LTBI is diagnosed by a purified protein-derivative skin test or TST after excluding active TB disease. The typical cutoff point is 10 mm induration, but for HIV-positive patients, 5 mm induration is considered a positive reaction.

Newer Food and Drug Administration (FDA)–approved in vitro cytokine-based immunoassays for the detection of TB infection are being introduced (QuantiFERON®). This test does not cross-react with the bacille CalmetteGuérin (BCG) vaccine strain (an attenuated strain of *M. bovis*) or with other nontuberculous mycobacteria (NTM).

Appropriate clinical specimens for diagnostic testing include sputum, bronchial washings, blood, morning-voided urine, and gastric secretions. The gold standard test to assess the presence of mycobacteria in a clinical specimen is culture on solid media, although this takes three to eight weeks to complete. Correct species identification and drug susceptibility testing then are conducted on the isolated organisms. Acid-fast staining of the clinical specimen is fast but less sensitive than culture and does not distinguish between different mycobacterial species.

NAAT based on PCR has intermediate sensitivity and identifies bacteria as members of the MTB complex but cannot distinguish between dead and living organisms; and drug susceptibility testing is not possible. The sensitivity and specificity of nucleic acid amplification is over 95% for AFB-smear–positive samples, but for smear-negative cases, sensitivity ranges from 40% to 77%. Specificity remains over 95%.

TREATMENT

Treatment for TB has significantly reduced the mortality of the disease, which, in the preantibiotic era, was estimated at 50% within two years of diagnosis (3). Failures occur due to primary drug resistance or inappropriate drug regimen, but most commonly because of nonadherence to the long-term therapeutic regimen, because as patients feel better, their motivation to complete the long-term treatment course declines. Therefore, the responsibility of adherence has been transferred to the health system, and global efforts are under way to establish DOT as a means of monitoring a successful regimen.

The treatment strategies for TB are focused on the use of three or more active drugs; of these, INH and RMP are the most important; also included in the armamentarium are ethambutol, pyrazinamide, streptomycin, quinolones, and second-line agents. Selection of a drug regimen, monitoring and length of treatment, resistance testing, and other treatment issues should be addressed after consulting with a specialist and local public health authorities.

COMPLICATIONS AND PROGNOSIS

Local complications are described in detail with each site of infection. As a rule, a high degree of suspicion and early diagnosis can lead to timely diagnostic workup and avoidance of most late complications.

TB has a good prognosis if treated aggressively and early. Most failures occur because of poor followup or antibacterial resistance. Involvement of infectious disease specialty services and Public Health authorities is imperative.

SUMMARY

TB remains a highly prevalent infection with serious morbidity and mortality today. Manifestations in the head and neck area are frequently difficult to diagnose, and often, initiation of anti-TB treatment is based on clinical suspicion alone. Clinical specimens should be sent for AFB smears, NAAT, and culture when a high degree of suspicion is present. The association of TB with HIV makes those patients specifically prone to extensive disease and serious complications.

*A*TYPICAL MYCOBACTERIA

INTRODUCTION

Atypical mycobacteria, also known as mycobacteria other than tuberculosis (MOTT) or non-NTM, are any mycobacterial species other than the MTB complex and *M. leprae*. This group includes about 100 organisms, of which 60 are identified as causes of clinical disease.

DEFINITION

The atypical mycobacteria organisms are categorized by their growth rate on culture media and the presence of pigment. The most commonly encountered is the *M. avium* complex (MAC), which includes two organisms, *M. avium* and *M. intracellulare*. Table 1 lists the most commonly encountered organisms in the head and neck area. Atypical mycobacteria can cause pulmonary disease, disseminated infection in advanced immunosuppression or HIV infection, bone involvement, and lymphadenitis. The mode of transmission is usually via ingestion of contaminated water or food by fomites or rarely by direct inoculation.

TABLE 1 Nontuberculous Mycobacterial Head and Neck Pathogens

Mycobacterium avium	*Mycobacterium tusciae*
Mycobacterium intracellulare	*Mycobacterium palustre*
Mycobacterium bohemicum	*Mycobacterium interjectum*
Mycobacterium kansasii	*Mycobacterium elephantis*
Mycobacterium chelonei	*Mycobacterium heidelbergense*
Mycobacterium malmoense	*Mycobacterium porcinum*
Mycobacterium fortuitum	*Mycobacterium smegmatis*
Mycobacterium marinum	*Mycobacterium genavense*
Mycobacterium genovense	*Mycobacterium lacus*
Mycobacterium scrofulaceum	*Mycobacterium novocastrense*
Mycobacterium haemophilum	*Mycobacterium houstonense*
Mycobacterium simiae	*Mycobacterium goodie*
Mycobacterium abscessus	*Mycobacterium immunogenum*
Mycobacterium lentiflavum	*Mycobacterium mageritense*

CLINICAL MANIFESTATIONS

Cervical Lymphadenitis

Lymphadenitis is a common manifestation of MAC and atypical mycobacteria in children aged one to five years (17). MAC appears to have replaced *M. scrofulaceum* as the most common etiologic agent for scrofula in young children (18). In individuals aged 12 years and older, *M. tuberculosis* remains the most common etiologic agent, and a suspicion for more disseminated disease and immunosuppression should arise in these patients (19). Other atypical mycobacteria seen are *M. scrofulaceum*, *M. malmoense* (in northern Europe), *M. abscessus*, *M. fortuitum*, *M. lentiflavum*, *M. tusciae*, *M. palustre*, *M. interjectum*, *M. elephantis*, and *M. heidelbergense*. Infection usually presents as a firm, painless, erythematous mass without fluctuance or systemic symptoms, which is bilateral in 10% of cases. Sinus tracts and fistulas can form as the condition becomes chronic.

Diagnosis is difficult, and the differential should include bacterial infections, cancer, lymphomas, TB, and bartonellosis. Chest radiographs are typically normal and the TST is negative unless the patient has been previously vaccinated with BCG.

FNA can be used for diagnosis, but the yield of positive AFB smears is low (around 30–50%). Excisional biopsy provides more tissue for diagnosis and is also curative. AFB cultures are important to isolate the infectious agent and for reliable antibacterial susceptibility testing.

Otitis Media and Mastoiditis

Usually affecting older children and adolescents, otitis from atypical mycobacteria presents as a chronic otitis not responding to common antibacterial therapy. The middle-ear space and mastoid may be filled completely with inflammatory granulation tissue that later extends to the external auditory canal. Biopsy is necessary to rule out a malignancy and to obtain tissue for culture, including AFB and fungal examinations.

Cutaneous Disease

Mycobacteria can be directly inoculated to the skin of the head and neck area or disseminated hematogenously in immunosuppressed patients. Plaques, papules, ulcers, or nodules are the common presentations. The most common agents are the *M. fortuitum* group, *Mycobacteria chelonae*, *M. abscessus*, *Mycobacteria marinum* ("fish tank granuloma" or "swimming pool granuloma"), *Mycobacteria ulcerans* ("Buruli ulcer," found in Australia and tropical countries) *M. kansasii*, *M. haemophilum*, *M. porcinum*, *M. smegmatis*, *M. genavense*, *M. lacus*, *M. novocastrense*, *M. houstonense*, *M. goodii*, *M. immunogenum*, and *M. mageritense*.

Other Head and Neck NTM Infections

Chronic sinusitis has been associated with NTM, and MAC has been reported as a cause of chronic mastoiditis (20) in an infant and of aphthous oral ulcers in HIV patients.

DIAGNOSIS

Isolation of the organism from an infected tissue specimen is required to confirm the diagnosis. As with TB, excisional biopsy yields adequate tissue and is preferred to FNA, especially in HIV-negative patients, to avoid fistulization; however, culture yield is quite low as the condition becomes chronic. Positive AFB smears with negative nucleic acid amplification test for MTB complex is suggestive; often, response to presumptive therapy is used as a criterion for diagnosis.

TREATMENT

Treatment of choice for atypical mycobacterial lymphadenitis is complete excision of the affected node, without need for antimicrobial chemotherapy, depending on the site and if rupture has not occurred. If surgery is not an option, in cases of cutaneous disease or if the condition is chronic, combination treatment with a macrolide and/or quinolone-containing regimen can be used, with varying degrees of success. Antimicrobial resistance is often a problem with the atypical mycobacteria group.

COMPLICATIONS AND PROGNOSIS

Overall, NTM infections of the head and neck carry a good prognosis and complications are rare. However, diagnosis requires a high degree of suspicion and is often delayed due to the low incidence of the disease and the poor yield of the smears and cultures. In cases of immunocompromised hosts, the possibility of disseminated disease needs to be considered and the prognosis is guarded.

SUMMARY

NTM infections of the head and neck are rare in the immunocompetent host. Usually representing a disease of children, they can be effectively treated by surgical excision and/or combination antibacterial therapy. In the immunocompromised host, those infections are often seen as part of disseminated disease and are better managed via a multidisciplinary approach.

REFERENCES

1. Fitzgerald D, Haas DW. *M. tuberculosis*. In: Mandell GL, Bennett JE, Dolin R, eds. Principles and Practice of Infectious Diseases. Vol. 2. 6th ed. New York, NY: Elsevier/Churchill Livingstone, 2005:2852–2886.
2. Jensen PA, Lambert LA, Iademarco MF, et al. CDC. Guidelines for preventing the transmission of *M. tuberculosis* in health-care settings, 2005. MMWR Recomm Rep 2005; 54(17):1–141.
3. Styblo K. Recent advances in epidemiological research in tuberculosis. Adv Tuberc Res 1980; 20:1–63.
4. Stead WW. Tuberculosis among elderly persons: an outbreak in a nursing home. Ann Intern Med 1981; 94(5):606–610.
5. Behr MA, Warren SA, Salamon H, et al. Transmission of *M. tuberculosis* from patients smear-negative for acid-fast bacilli. Lancet 1999; 353(9151):444–449. Erratum in Lancet 1999; 353 (9165):1714.
6. Dooley SW Jr, Castro KG, Hutton MD, et al. Guidelines for preventing the transmission of tuberculosis in health-care settings, with special focus on HIV-related issues. MMWR Recomm Rep 1990; 39(RR-17):1–29.
7. Guidelines for preventing the transmission of *M. tuberculosis* in health-care facilities, 1994. Centers for Disease Control and Prevention. MMWR Recomm Rep 1994; 43(RR-13):1–132.
8. Guidelines for preventing the transmission of *M. tuberculosis* in health-care facilities, 1994—CDC. Notice of final revisions to the "Guidelines for Preventing the Transmission of *M. Tuberculosis* in health-care facilities, 1994." Fed Regist 1994; 59(208):54242–54303.
9. Manolidis S, Frenkiel S, Yoskovitch A, et al. Mycobacterial infections of the head and neck. Otolaryngol Head Neck Surg 1993; 109(3 Pt 1):427–433.

10. Lee KC, Schecter G. Tuberculous infections of the head and neck. Ear Nose Throat J 1995; 74(6):395–399.
11. Munck K, Mandpe AH. Mycobacterial infections of the head and neck. Otolaryngol Clin North Am 2003; 36(4):569–576.
12. Cleary KR, Batsakis JG. Mycobacterial disease of the head and neck: current perspective. Ann Otol Rhinol Laryngol 1995; 104(10 Pt 1):830–833.
13. Bayazit YA, Bayazit N, Namiduru M. Mycobacterial cervical lymphadenitis. ORL J Otorhinolaryngol Relat Spec 2004; 66(5):275–280.
14. Kim YH, Jeong WJ, Jung KY, et al. Diagnosis of major salivary gland tuberculosis: experience of eight cases and review of the literature. Acta Otolaryngol 2005; 125(12):1318–1322.
15. Bradley PJ. Benign salivary gland disease. Hosp Med 2001; 62(7):392–395.
16. Janssens JP, Haller R. Spinal tuberculosis in a developed country. A review of 26 cases with special emphasis on abscesses and neurologic complications. Clin Orthop Relat Res 1990; (257):67–75.
17. Schaad UB, Votteler TP, McCracken GH Jr, et al. Management of atypical mycobacterial lymphadenitis in childhood: a review based on 380 cases. J Pediatr 1979; 95(3):356–360.
18. Wolinsky E. Mycobacterial lymphadenitis in children: a prospective study of 105 nontuberculous cases with long-term follow-up. Clin Infect Dis 1995; 20(4):954–963.
19. Inderlied CB. Mycobacteria. In: Cohen J, Powderly W, eds. Infectious Diseases. Vol. 2. Mosby: St. Louis, MO, 2004:2285–2308.
20. Stewart MG, Troendle-Atkins J, Starke JR, et al. Nontuberculous mycobacterial mastoiditis. Arch Otolaryngol Head Neck Surg 1995; 121(2):225–228.

13

Fungal Rhinosinusitis

Gregory C. Barkdull
Department of Surgery, Division of Otolaryngology-Head and Neck Surgery, University of California, San Diego, California, U.S.A.

Terence M. Davidson
Department of Surgery, Division of Otolaryngology-Head and Neck Surgery, University of California and VA San Diego Healthcare System, San Diego, California, U.S.A.

INTRODUCTION

Rhinosinusitis is one of the most common reasons for physician visits in the United States. Disease impact studies have revealed a significant reduction in quality of life and high socioeconomic cost measured in lost schooldays and workdays. Current estimates indicate chronic rhinosinusitis (CRS) afflicts 37 million people annually in the United States.

Acute rhinosinusitis is thought to be caused by an inflammatory reaction of the paranasal mucous membranes in response to a viral or bacterial infection. The pathophysiology of CRS is less clear. The traditional hypothesis has been that repeated acute inflammatory episodes, with or without an underlying anatomic predisposition, lead to obstruction of sinus ostia with resulting impairment of the mucociliary transport system. The diseased sinuses fail to ventilate and drain. Some patients go on to develop nasal polyposis in response to the chronic inflammation. Histopathologic studies of nasal mucosa obtained during sinus surgery have revealed the presence of an eosinophilic infiltrate. Several systemic diseases, including cystic fibrosis, immune deficiency, or primary ciliary dyskinesia, may predispose patients to development of sinusitis. It remains unclear why in some patients recurrent acute rhinosinusitis develops into CRS. Investigators are working on understanding the relationship between infection, allergy, and nasal polyposis. Recently, it has been proposed that fungus may be the inciting environmental factor that initiates the chain of events culminating in the condition known as CRS (1).

In 1999, investigators at the Mayo Clinic raised the possibility that a previously unrecognized nonallergic fungal inflammatory process is responsible for the majority of cases of CRS. Using an extremely sensitive culture technique, they demonstrated positive fungal cultures in 97 of 101 consecutive patients who underwent endoscopic sinus surgery for CRS (1). This observation was tempered by the finding that 14 of 14 healthy controls also demonstrated positive fungal cultures from nasal mucus. Despite this observation, an important difference remained between the two patient populations. Histologic examination of the resected mucosa from patients with CRS revealed heterogenous tissue eosinophilia. The eosinophils appeared to be migrating through the epithelium into the mucus of the nasal and sinus lumen. Furthermore, these eosinophils appeared to cluster around fungal elements within the mucus. They hypothesized that the targeting of fungi trapped within the nasal mucus by an eosinophilic reaction could produce the inflammation seen in patients with CRS. This hypothesis does not explain why some patients appear to mount a vigorous inflammatory response to the environmentally ubiquitous fungi, while others do not (2). Perhaps, the presence of incidental fungal elements in both diseased and healthy individuals merely reflects the natural function of the nasal mucus as a particle-trapping filter.

Further research will determine whether fungi truly have a role in the pathogenesis of all cases of CRS. There are, however, several well-described manifestations of fungal sinusitis. These include the noninvasive forms of fungal infection [allergic fungal sinusitis (AFS), saprophytic infections, and fungus balls] as well as the invasive forms (acute invasive fungal sinusitis and chronic invasive fungal sinusitis). This chapter will review their presentation, pathophysiology, diagnosis, and management.

DEFINITIONS

Fungal sinusitis, when used loosely, can be a misleading term. It actually refers to a spectrum of fungal-associated diseases of the nose and paranasal sinuses, each with a unique presentation and management implications (Table 1). When communicating with

TABLE 1 Fungal-Associated Diseases of the Nose and Paranasal Sinuses (? is used to indicate controversy)

Classification	Immunologic status	Prognosis	Treatment
Noninvasive forms			
Allergic fungal sinusitis	Atopic	Good	Surgery, oral and topical steroids, immunotherapy, nasal irrigation, ? antifungals
Eosinophilic fungal rhinosinusitis/CRS	? Normal	Good	Surgery, nasal irrigation, topical nasal steroids, ? antifungals
Fungus ball	Normal	Excellent	Surgical removal
Saprophytic	Normal	Excellent	Office removal, nasal irrigation
Invasive forms			
Acute	Compromised	Guarded	Reversal of immunocompromise, surgery, antifungals
Chronic	Normal	Fair	Surgery, antifungals

Abbreviation: CRS, chronic rhinosinusitis.

members of the health-care team, it is important to characterize the specific manifestation of fungal sinusitis (3).

AFS is characterized by paranasal sinus inflammation, evidence of fungal-specific allergy, and the presence of allergic mucin. Histopathologic examination of allergic mucin reveals necrotic inflammatory cells and eosinophils containing Charcot–Leyden crystals along with various fungal elements. A variety of fungal species have been implicated, including *Alternaria*, *Bipolaris*, *Aspergillus*, and *Curvalaria*. Patients usually are atopic, have elevated total IgE, and demonstrate allergic responses to fungal antigen testing. A combination of endoscopic sinus surgery, systemic and topical steroids, and adjunctive immunotherapy usually results in significant relief of symptoms and can induce disease remission.

The definition of CRS set forth by the U.S. Food and Drug Administration is 12 weeks of persistent inflammation of the paranasal sinuses. As discussed in the introduction, investigators have proposed that eosinophilic fungal rhinosinusitis may account for the majority of cases of CRS. This is based on their finding of fungal elements in nearly all cases of CRS. While their hypothesis is currently being investigated, no one has conclusively demonstrated that fungi, and the immune system's response to them, are the underlying etiology of CRS.

Fungus balls are common and grow in the wet moist cavities of the paranasal sinuses irrespective of the immunologic status of the host. Some cases are asymptomatic while others mimic chronic sinusitis. They can occasionally become a source for invasive infection if the host develops an immunocompromised state. Fungus balls are usually located in the maxillary antrum. They are composed of mucin, hemorrhagic blood, and *Aspergillus*, *Alternaria*, or *Mucor*. Treatment consists of surgical removal and drainage.

Saprophytic fungal infections occur when fungal spores land and germinate on mucus crusts. This is commonly seen after sinonasal surgery. Treatment is simply removal of the crusts on which the fungal spores are growing.

Acute invasive fungal sinusitis occurs in patients with impaired host defenses, including patients with uncontrolled diabetes, primary or acquired immunodeficiency, or leukemia, or those on immunosuppressive therapy in the transplant setting. Histopatho-logic examination reveals fungal elements invading tissue. The typical pathogens are members of the order *Mucorales*. Without reversal of the immunocompromised state and prompt medical and surgical therapy, this condition is generally fatal (3).

Chronic invasive fungal sinusitis is seen in the immunocompetent patient. It is rare and usually not lethal. *Aspergillus flavus* accounts for many of the indolent, chronic cases of invasive fungal disease seen in Sudan. Other species include *Aspergillus fumigatus*, *Alternaria*, *Pseudallescheria boydii*, *Sporothrix schenckii*, and *Bipolaris* species. Histology reveals a granuloma composed of giant cells containing hyphae. In some patients, surgical exenteration is curative, while in others, the disease is persistent despite medical and surgical treatment (3).

*A*LLERGIC FUNGAL SINUSITIS

INTRODUCTION

AFS appears to be an allergic reaction to aerosolized, environmental fungi that occurs in immunologically normal hosts. The immune response is believed to be an IgE-mediated type-I hypersensitivity reaction. The ensuing inflammation manifests as noninvasive fungal rhinosinusitis. It was first described in 1981 by Millar and Lamb. Katzenstein further detailed the histopathologic findings in 1983, describing allergic mucin characterized by necrotic inflammatory cells, eosinophils, and Charcot–Leyden crystals.

EPIDEMIOLOGY

AFS is estimated to account for 5% to 10% of cases of CRS. It typically affects young, immunocompetent patients. They frequently have a history of asthma or atopy (56% and 77%, respectively) (4). There appears to be geographic variation, with a higher incidence in the southern United States.

PATHOPHYSIOLOGY

Fungi implicated in the development of AFS are predominantly of the dematiaceous family, and include *Alternaria*, *Curvularia*, *Bipolaris specifera*, and *Exserohilum* species. *Aspergillus* was originally implicated but is now understood to account for only 10% to 20% of cases (4). The presence of these fungi is insufficient to cause disease, as these same fungi are cultured from the nasal mucus of healthy patients as well. It has been suggested that the pathology seen in susceptible individuals is the result of an allergic response to the fungal antigens. In support of this hypothesis, fungal-specific immediate-hypersensitivity skin testing is frequently positive. These patients have an elevated serum total IgE and fungal-specific IgG. Histologic analysis of allergic mucin shows a characteristic eosinophilic infiltrate, fungal hyphae, and Charcot-Leyden crystals within the eosinophils. The immune response results in local mucosal edema that causes obstruction of the involved sinus ostia, perpetuating the process.

Molecular investigations have uncovered further evidence in support of this model. Extracellular major basic protein (MBP) and neutrophil elastase have been detected within the allergic mucin. The presence of these proteins in high quantities is indicative of eosinophil and neutrophil activation (5). Local fungal-specific IgE and IgG can be demonstrated in the mucin of two-thirds of AFS cases, suggesting a role for locally produced IgE (6). In AFS, it is likely that germinating hyphae contained within the allergic mucin provide persistent IgE-mediated antigenic stimulation that drives the paranasal inflammation (3).

CLINICAL MANIFESTATIONS

The clinical presentation of AFS can be similar to CRS. Patients often report chronic nasal congestion and nasal obstruction that has failed to respond to antibiotic therapy. Examination of the nasal cavity may reveal nasal polyps within the olfactory cleft, middle meatus, and sphenoethmoid recess. Occasionally, locally destructive changes from long-standing polyposis lead to proptosis and malar flattening (7). AFS is unilateral in more than 50% of patients but may involve several sinuses bilaterally, and bone erosion and extrasinus extension have been reported. The allergic mucin characteristic of this condition is thick and glue-like, with a heterogeneous brown appearance that has been compared to peanut butter.

DIAGNOSIS

Computed tomography (CT) of the paranasal sinuses may show hyperdensities with small calcifications that represent allergic mucin concretions. There may be adjacent hypodense opacification of the involved sinus with air-fluid levels representing retained mucus. More advanced disease can lead to loss of adjacent bony sinus margins and even erosion of the anterior skull base due to expansile pressure. There may be extensive polyps that accompany mucosal thickening. Magnetic resonance imaging (MRI) reveals low signal intensity on T1-weighted images and areas of signal void on T2-weighted images, possibly due to the presence of paramagnetic metals within the allergic mucin concretions (3).

While AFS may be suspected based on the clinical signs and symptoms, and positive allergy testing, definitive diagnosis requires histopathologic confirmation. The identification of allergic mucin at the time of surgery with the absence of histologic evidence of fungal invasion confirms the diagnosis. The presence of mucosal necrosis, granulomas, or giant cells is indicative of a more serious, chronic invasive fungal sinusitis and must be distinguished from AFS (8). Fungal stains of the allergic mucin reveal hyphae of a variety of fungal species. *Bipolaris* is most common, but *Alternaria*, *Exserohilum*, *Curvularia*, and *Aspergillus* have been identified. Patients have elevated specific and total IgE levels and positive skin testing. Total IgE levels are often high at the time of presentation, but decrease as therapy is instituted (8).

As AFS is an immune-mediated condition, an alternative diagnosis must be sought in patients who are immunocompromised. They should undergo biopsy of diseased mucosa and bone to rule out invasive fungal infection. It is also important to consider a broad differential diagnosis in patients with extensive nasal polyps. The presence of asthma and aspirin sensitivity should alert the clinician to Samter's syndrome. Other causes of CRS and nasal polyps include Churg–Strauss syndrome, inhalant allergies, and cystic fibrosis.

Ancillary studies that can assist with treatment planning and counseling include smell testing, acoustic rhinometry, skin testing for inhalant allergies, and endoscopically guided biopsy and/or cultures from the middle meatus (5).

TREATMENT

Successful control of AFS involves complementary medical and surgical approaches. Unfortunately, recurrence rates are high; therefore, the goal is to extend the disease-free interval between revision surgeries.

Oral corticosteroids have an important role in the management of this disease. They are often started preoperatively, at a dose of 60 mg of prednisone for three days, followed by a two-to-four-week taper. This regimen can improve surgical visibility and reduce intraoperative bleeding by shrinking the polyps. Some surgeons, on the other hand, prefer to wait for several weeks after surgery to administer steroids, to avoid interference with postoperative healing. The use of perioperative oral steroids appears to increase the disease-free interval and time to recurrence (9).

Surgical treatment involves conservative endoscopic removal of nasal polyps and inspissated allergic mucin. This procedure requires a sinus CT scan to inform the surgeon about anatomic variations. Many centers now use image guidance systems that allow real-time three-dimensional intraoperative localization. This is particularly useful for nasal polyps and even more so for revision polypectomy where normal sinus landmarks may be absent due to previous procedures. Microdebriders are very efficient for resection of nasal polyps but because of their potential to damage surrounding structures, they are used with image guidance. The mucin of AFS can be difficult to remove. Simple lavage is usually insufficient and microdebriders facilitate removal.

After surgical opening of the sinus cavities, patients continue twice-daily nasal irrigation and topical nasal steroids. Doses up to three to four times the usual for allergic rhinitis have been used. Office endoscopy with debridement of allergic mucin can prolong remission. Monitoring of total serum IgE can be helpful in the followup of these patients. Increasing total serum IgE often precedes the need for a return to the operating room.

Long-term oral corticosteroid therapy can effectively suppress this disease; however, it is fraught with side effects. Patients need to be monitored for diabetes, osteoporosis, and cataracts. The oral steroid protocol used by Schubert and Goetz is detailed in Table 2.

Immunotherapy may have a role in AFS. Immunotherapy works by inducing specific IgG "blocking antibody." Patients with AFS, however, already have elevated IgG and IgE; therefore, immunotherapy was initially thought to be contraindicated. Mabry demonstrated an absence of ill effects and possible improvement in patients receiving immunotherapy with fungal antigens, and it is now considered accepted practice to offer patients this treatment (Table 3). After formal testing for common allergens and all available fungal antigens, definitive immunotherapy is initiated. This can be continued for a three-to-five-year period. Furthermore, patients also are instructed on environmental modification and mold avoidance. This approach reduces the need for maintenance systemic steroids and revision surgery (2).

Antifungal therapy has been proposed, and oral itraconazole and voriconazole have good in vitro activity against dematiaceous fungi, but they have not been shown to be useful and are generally not recommended.

TABLE 2 Oral Corticosteroid Protocol for AFS

1. Prednisone 0.5 mg/kg postoperatively and then daily for 2 wk
2. The same dose is given every other day for weeks 3 through 6
3. The dose is then tapered down to 5 mg every other day by week 12
4. Maintenance dosing of 5 mg every other day is maintained for 1 yr or longer
5. Acute episodes of rhinosinusitis are treated with a short burst of prednisone

Abbreviation: AFS, allergic fungal sinusitis.
Source: From Ref. 8.

TABLE 3   Immunotherapy Protocol for AFS

1. Surgical exenteration of disease from the sinuses and pathologic confirmation of the diagnosis.
2. Allergy evaluation and testing (RAST or quantitative skin test) for typical nonfungal antigens and all molds and fungi available.
3. Instruct patient in avoidance measures for molds.
4. Prepare a vial of all positive nonfungal antigens and a second vial of all positive fungal antigens. Perform a skin test with each.
5. Administer immunotherapy weekly, with dose advancement as tolerated, placing one injection from each vial in a different arm.
6. Observe the patient at regularly scheduled intervals, adjusting dosage as necessary if local reactions or changes in nasal symptoms occur. Patients should also undergo regular endoscopic examination to monitor for reaccumulation of allergic mucin or reformation of polyps and for cleaning and adjustment of medical management.
7. Once dosage advancement is completed, the antigens may be combined into one vial and treatment continued for a 3–5 yr regimen.

Abbreviation: AFS, allergic fungal sinusitis; RAST, radioallergosorbent test.
Source: From Ref. 2

COMPLICATIONS AND PROGNOSIS

If allowed to progress unabated, AFS can be locally destructive due to the pressure placed on adjacent bone and tissues. Complications include permanent deformity of the nasal bones, exophthalmos, and even blindness as a result of optic nerve compression.

When patients receive comprehensive medical and surgical treatment and complementary immunotherapy, the prognosis for this group of patients is excellent.

SUMMARY

Management of patients with AFS is challenging and there are high rates of recurrence. However, with close followup and appropriate medical and surgical intervention, these patients can enjoy dramatic improvements in the quality of their lives. Hopefully, in the years to come, we will develop treatments that can offer the benefit of oral steroids without the systemic side effects.

EOSINOPHILIC FUNGAL SINUSITIS

INTRODUCTION

Recently, Ponikau and colleagues have reported that fungi are present in over 90% of patients with CRS as well as 100% of healthy controls when very sensitive culture techniques are used. The discovery of fungi with an associated eosinophilic infiltrate in nearly all patients with CRS has led Ponikau to coin the term "eosinophilic fungal sinusitis." Furthermore, he has proposed that the host response to fungi is the underlying mechanism behind CRS.

EPIDEMIOLOGY

Rhinosinusitis holds the distinction as being the most frequent cause of physician visits in the United States. Up to 14% of the U.S. population reports symptoms of CRS (2). If the hypothesis put forth by Ponikau is shown to be valid, then eosinophilic fungal sinusitis is one of the most prevalent conditions seen today.

PATHOPHYSIOLOGY

The etiology and pathogenesis of CRS currently is unknown; however, there are several new insights into the potential mechanisms of CRS.

The hypothesis proposed by Ponikau involves fungus-dependent activation of the immune system with subsequent recruitment of eosinophils to the nasal mucus. This is supported by histopathologic studies of nasal mucus that demonstrate fungal elements surrounded by clusters of eosinophils (10). It has been hypothesized that eosinophils play a defensive role against fungal hyphae trapped in the mucus. Eosinophils release granule-associated cationic proteins, MBP, eosinophilic peroxidase, and eosinophil-derived neurotoxin, which are toxic to both fungi, and unfortunately, nasal mucosal epithelium. The weakened nasal and sinus epithelium may then be susceptible to bacterial invasion, infection, and additional tissue inflammation. Cytokines and growth factors released by the inflamed mucosa can promote the formation of nasal polyps (1). Over time, infection can involve the underlying bone with resulting low-grade osteomyelitis. The chronic inflammation and scarring contributes to permanent obstruction of the natural sinus ostia. Critics of this model point out there is inconclusive evidence that the fungi cultured in these patients are pathogenic or even colonizers of the nasal mucosa. They argue that the fungal elements seen on histopathologic analysis and the organisms cultured from the nasal mucus merely represent airborne contamination. Proponents of this model, however, have gone on to use highly sensitive polymerase chain reaction (PCR) assays on mucosal tissue removed from patients with CRS and demonstrated the presence of fungal DNA (11). They speculate this may represent true mucosal disease or even endocytosis and antigen presentation of fungal elements.

Efforts to identify the strains of fungi in patients with CRS have demonstrated a remarkable diversity. Stammberger's group reported fungal cultures on 233 subjects, in which 619 fungal strains were cultured and 81 species identified. There were up to nine separate species isolated per patient. The most prevalent isolates were *Penicillium*, *Aspergillus* species, *Cladosporium*, *Alternaria*, and *Aurobasidium* (12). Interestingly, Gosepath reported on 27 of 27 surgical specimens from patients with CRS and found all positive for fungal DNA. His controls, consisting of 15 patients with healthy ethmoid mucosa, however, tested positive when using pan-fungal PCR primers. Species-specific analysis revealed that many of the patients with CRS were positive for *Alternaria*, while none of the healthy controls were, possibly implicating *Alternaria* as an important pathogen (11). In an effort to establish the early and ubiquitous nature of fungal presence in nasal mucus, Lackner examined neonates. His group demonstrated that by four months of life, 17 of 18 healthy neonates had positive fungal cultures and concluded that fungi must be considered a normal content of nasal mucus. Fungi that were cultured included *Alternaria alternate*, *A. fumigatus*, *Penicillium commune*, *Acremonium polychromum*, and *Cladosporium cladosporioides* (13).

Immunologic studies suggest that these patients have an abnormal systemic response to fungi. Interleukin-5 (IL-5) and interleukin-13 (IL-13) are known to be key cytokines for eosinophilic reactions and play a role in eosinophil chemotaxis. In 2004, Shin obtained peripheral blood lymphocytes from patients with CRS and exposed them to fungal antigens from *Alternaria*, *Aspergillus*, *Cladosporium*, and *Penicillium* species. He demonstrated that over 90% of these patients exhibited a peripheral blood lymphocyte response by producing IL-5 and IL-13. Control lymphocytes from healthy patients, however, did not produce IL-5 and IL-13 (14). Interestingly, less than 30% of the patients in the CRS group had specific IgE antibodies to the fungi tested. These observations suggest that there is a systemic immune response to fungal antigens in patients with CRS, and it may not require the presence of IgE-specific antibodies.

If CRS is the result of chronic bacterial infection, a neutrophilic infiltrate would be expected. Histomorphologic analysis of mucosal tissue from patients with CRS, however, reveals an eosinophilic infiltrate. Eosinophils are known to be involved in host defenses against fungi and parasites but are not part of the defense against bacteria (15). This also correlates with the contention that the immune response to fungi plays a role in CRS.

CLINICAL MANIFESTATIONS

Symptoms of eosinophilic fungal sinusitis, by definition, are those of CRS. These include facial pain and pressure, congestion, fullness, nasal obstruction, nasal discharge, and hyposmia. Associated symptoms can include headache, fever, halitosis, dental pain, and cough.

DIAGNOSIS

Patients must meet the accepted criteria for CRS, which includes 12 weeks of paranasal inflammation. This diagnosis is strengthened by abnormal radiographic findings. The study of choice is a limited sinus CT scan with coronal cuts, which may demonstrate mucosal thickening and air-fluid levels. Greater than 8 mm of mucoperiosteal thickening is considered abnormal. In contrast to AFS, these patients do not necessarily have elevated fungal-specific IgE or positive skin testing for fungal antigens.

Successful fungal cultures have been greatly enhanced by new techniques that first release fungal hyphae from nasal mucin. Pretreatment with dithiothreitol frees the organisms by breaking sulfur hydrogen bonds. Specific histologic stains, including Gomori methenamine silver stain and fluorescein-labeled chitinase stain, have enabled selective visualization of fungal organisms (11). Using these techniques, Ponikau has identified fungus in nearly all of his patients with CRS (1).

TREATMENT

Antifungal therapy for eosinophilic fungal rhinosinusitis is still under investigation. Several preliminary trials have reported improvement in objective and subjective findings in patients with CRS, who were treated with nasal irrigation using amphotericin B (16,17). These patients were irrigated with 20 mL of amphotericin B (100 μg/mL) twice daily for up to 12 months. The authors report complete disappearance of nasal polyps in 35% to 39% of patients. These studies, however, lack control groups, randomization, and blinding. It is unclear whether the improvement is due to the antifungal agent or simply a nonspecific benefit associated with nasal irrigation. Significant benefit has been reported with the use of hypertonic saline alone. A prospective, double-blind, placebo-controlled investigation published by Weschta in 2004 failed to show benefit from amphotericin washes. In this trial, patients used 200 μL of amphotericin B in each nostril, at a concentration of 3 mg/mL, four times a day for eight weeks. A response was noted in only 2 of 28 patients, which was not significantly different from the control group (18). Another important observation from studies of ciliary beat frequency has shown that several antifungals, including amphotericin, clotrimazole, and itraconazole, have the potential for dose-dependent ciliotoxicity. Higher concentrations of amphotericin resulted in ciliary stasis within two hours of administration. This suggests that there may be undesirable repercussions of amphotericin irrigation (11). Oral antifungal therapy has also been studied. Kennedy conducted a multicenter trial of oral terbinafine for six weeks in patients with CRS. This prospective study was well done, adequately blinded, and randomized. It failed to show any benefit when compared to placebo even in patients with positive fungal cultures (19).

Eosinophil production, chemotaxis, and degranulation are inhibited by steroids. Therefore, topical steroids are attractive in that they may exert a local benefit without systemic side effects. Multiple studies have shown a modest decrease in polyp size and improvement in nasal airflow. The molecular effects of topical nasal steroids in patients with CRS and nasal polyposis have been evaluated by Burgel. He found that eight weeks of intranasal steroids improved nasal airflow and decreased polyp size, with a corresponding decrease in intraepithelial eosinophils. Mucin production, IL-8, and tumor necrosis factor-α levels, however, were unchanged (20).

Nasal irrigation with saline solution is a mainstay of treatment and should be performed in conjunction with topical nasal steroids. Irrigation is thought to reduce antigen load by removing airborne fungal elements deposited on the nasal mucus film. The current recommendations from the UCSD Nasal Dysfunction Clinic are twice daily, hypertonic, pulsatile irrigation. This is best delivered with a WaterPik®-type device. The Grossan Hydropulse is a commercially available device that performs well.

Endoscopic sinus surgery is an option for patients with CRS, who fail to respond to nasal irrigation, nasal steroids, and long-term antibiotic therapy. Patients with extensive nasal polyposis tend to have a more dramatic improvement in their symptoms. Surgery typically involves polypectomy with anterior ethmoidectomy and maxillary antrostomy. Patients with more extensive disease may require frontal sinus, posterior ethmoid, and sphenoid procedures. Postoperatively, patients are instructed to perform twice-daily nasal irrigation and use topical intranasal steroids. To reduce polyp recurrence, this regimen is continued indefinitely. If specific allergens are identified, environmental modifications and immunotherapy are recommended as appropriate.

COMPLICATIONS AND PROGNOSIS

Complications of eosinophilic fungal rhinosinusitis or CRS are uncommon because most acute exacerbations are bacterial and are successfully treated with antibiotics. Rarely, patients can progress to frontal bone osteomyelitis. Extensive polyps can thin out and erode bone, altering facial structure and resulting in orbital and anterior cranial fossa dehiscence. Orbital complications, including preseptal and orbital cellulitis and subperiosteal abscess, still occur. These patients must be started on intravenous antibiotics and evaluated for surgical intervention. More serious complications include cavernous sinus thrombophlebitis, meningitis, epidural abscess, and brain abscess (5).

The prognosis for this group of patients is optimistic. Those patients with a propensity to develop polyps will require revision surgery in the future, because polyp recurrence is generally the rule; however, their quality of life can be dramatically improved with appropriate medical and surgical intervention.

SUMMARY

The role of fungus in CRS remains to be fully elucidated. The hypothesis has been put forth that an inappropriate host response to fungal organisms may be the underlying pathogenic factor in CRS and nasal polyposis. It is clear that fungal hyphae are present in nasal mucin in both patients with CRS and healthy controls; however, the significance of this finding remains controversial. Future studies will need to identify why certain individuals mount a vigorous immunologic response to ubiquitous environmental fungi, with resulting sinonasal inflammation and the development of CRS, while others do not. Finally, there is hope that better treatments will be developed as our understanding of the pathophysiology of CRS improves.

FUNGUS BALL

Fungal colonization of the maxillary sinus occasionally manifests as a fungus ball. This clinical entity is, on occasion, referred to as mycetoma; however, this is an inappropriate term, because mycetoma refers to a locally destructive subcutaneous fungal infection that can involve muscle and bone. A maxillary sinus fungal ball, on the other hand, is not invasive. It is typically unilateral, may or may not be symptomatic, and occurs in an immunocompetent host. MR imaging may demonstrate heterogenous opacification with hypointense signal on T2-weighted images. CT imaging may reveal calcification centers within the fungal concretion (Fig. 1). Surgical exploration of the involved sinus reveals thick, mucinous, or clay-like concretions. This form of fungal infection usually has a benign course, and endoscopic sinus surgery is the treatment of choice. It is important to recognize that patients who become immunosuppressed are at risk for progression to invasive disease; therefore, expedient removal is recommended (3). Steroids are not necessary and there is no role for antifungal therapy.

SAPROPHYTIC FUNGAL DISEASE

Saprophytic fungal disease is a superficial growth of fungus on mucopurulent crusts within the sinonasal cavity. This is occasionally seen on the crusts that form after sinus surgery. The hyphae are not found invading the nasal mucosa or deeper tissues. Treatment involves simple removal of the crusts along with the resident hyphae. The prognosis is excellent and residual crusts can be loosened and washed free with the addition of nasal irrigation. There is no role for steroids or antifungal therapy.

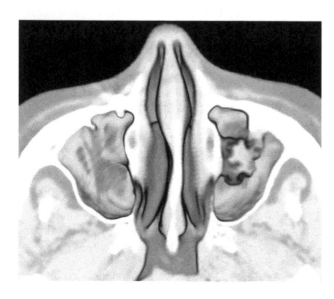

FIGURE 1 Axial image of a three-dimensional reconstructed maxillofacial CT scan in a patient confirmed at the time of surgery to have a left maxillary sinus fungus ball. *Abbreviation*: CT, computed tomography.

Acute Invasive Fungal Sinusitis

INTRODUCTION

Acute invasive fungal sinusitis must be suspected when an immunocompromised patient develops fever and signs of inflammation of the paranasal sinuses. Prompt recognition is critical because the infection can evolve over hours. In the current era of transplant immunosuppression, chemotherapy, and advanced HIV, clinicians must be able to make the diagnosis and institute prompt therapy. Unfortunately, the causative zygomycetous fungi are ubiquitous in nature. As a consequence, immunosuppressed patients are exposed to these fungi during day-to-day activities.

EPIDEMIOLOGY

Acute invasive fungal sinusitis occurs almost exclusively in poorly controlled diabetics and immunosuppressed patients. Diabetics account for 50% to 70% of cases. The remainder are associated with solid-organ and bone-marrow transplant, hematologic malignancy, chemotherapy-induced neutropenia, advanced HIV infection, and dialysis patients. Rare cases have been reported in patients with hemochromatosis and protein-calorie malnutrition.

PATHOPHYSIOLOGY

Mucormycosis is the most common form of acute invasive fungal infection and is caused by pathogens within the order *Mucorales. Rizopus oryzae* is the most virulent and common species within the order. Other members, in decreasing frequency, include *Absidia, Cunninghamella, Rhizomucor, Syncephalastrum, Saksenaea, Apophysomyces*, and *Mucor*. Mucormycosis is discussed in detail in Chapter 14.

Rhinocerebral infection is the most common manifestation of mucormycosis. Infection begins with inhalation of spores that usually land on the nasal turbinates. Fungal hyphae grow and invade the mucosa of the paranasal sinuses. As the infection continues, hyphae grow along and into blood vessels, resulting in vascular infarction. Invasion progresses through soft tissue, muscle, cartilage, and bone. The infection spreads to the hard palate and nose where it can result in septal and palatal necrosis. These areas of infarction appear black on gross inspection and are surrounded by a rim of yellow, dying tissue. If allowed to continue, it can breach the orbits and cribriform plate. Death occurs following direct infection of the brain or by invasion of the carotid vessels, with resulting cerebral infarction (Fig. 2).

R. oryzae has an enzyme, ketone reductase, which promotes survival in high glucose, acidic conditions. It is no surprise that patients with diabetic ketoacidosis are especially vulnerable to infection. Iron overload and deferoxamine also increase the risk of mucormycosis. Increased iron uptake by the fungus seems to stimulate growth.

Aspergillus infection can also become invasive in immunocompromised hosts, with extension into the mucosa and bone. This fulminant necrotizing form is seen in AIDS patients with CD4 counts below 50 and in the setting of persistent neutropenia. *A. fumigatus* is the most common pathogen, and the infection can be fatal within days, due to hematogenous dissemination (5).

CLINICAL MANIFESTATIONS

Initial clinical manifestations of rhinocerebral mucormycosis mimic those of acute bacterial sinusitis. Therefore, the clinician needs a high index of suspicion when evaluating

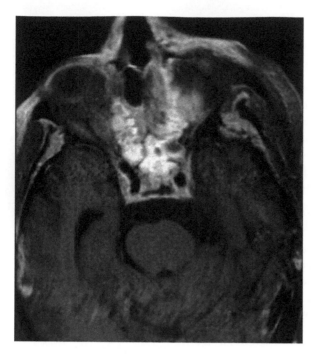

FIGURE 2 1.5 Tesla multiplanar MR with axial T1-weighted post-gadolinium imaging in a patient with biopsy-proven mucormycosis. There is near complete opacification of ethmoid sinuses. Ill-defined peripheral enhancement extends into the right medial rectus and left orbital apex. Abnormal signal surrounds both carotid arteries within their course through the cavernous sinus. *Abbreviation*: MR, magnetic resonance.

an immunosuppressed patient. Fever, headache, and cough may be the only symptoms. The presence of epistaxis, sinonasal ulceration or eschar, palatal eschar, proptosis, decreased vision, or facial swelling is alarming and suggestive of invasive disease (21). Rapid disease progression follows. Patients may initially report facial pain that progresses to facial anesthesia as trigeminal nerve invasion occurs. Once infection reaches the frontal lobes, mental status changes and obtundation ensues. Spread from the sphenoid sinus to the adjacent cavernous sinus is heralded by cranial nerve palsy or visual loss.

Mucormycosis is not limited to the head and neck region. Pulmonary mucormycosis is rapidly progressive and often fatal. Patients present with fever and hemoptysis. Transmission is by inhalation of spores with subsequent development of a necrotizing pneumonia that can spread to the mediastinum and heart. Gastrointestinal, cutaneous, and renal involvement have also been reported.

DIAGNOSIS

Physical examination should be complemented by full nasal endoscopy. Necrotic areas or sites of mucosal ulceration should be biopsied for immediate frozen section analysis (22). The presence of characteristic fungal hyphae invading the tissue confirms the diagnosis. The hyphae of zygomycetous fungi are broad and irregularly branched and have rare septations. This is in contrast to the hyphae of *Aspergillus*, which are narrow and have regular branching and septations. Special stains and fungal cultures can identify the species; however, these studies take too long to be of use in the initial management. Furthermore, these pathogens are notoriously difficult to culture.

TREATMENT

Once invasive fungal elements are confirmed on frozen section, antifungal therapy and surgical debridement should be initiated without delay. Efforts should also be directed toward restoration of immune function, by withdrawing immunosuppressive medications or addressing the predisposing illness.

Amphotericin B continues to be the drug of choice, at doses of 0.8 to 1.5 mg/kg/day. Nephrotoxicity is the dose-limiting factor, but amphotericin B lipid complex can minimize the renal side effects and allow dose escalation up to 5 to 7 mg/kg/day in patients with kidney disease. An alternative agent for zygomycetes is the second-generation triazole posaconazole (23). Itraconazole, voriconazole, and Casopofungin should not be used for rhinocerebral mucormycosis but can be considered for invasive *Aspergillus*.

Medical therapy alone rarely contains infection, especially in the setting of neutropenia or severe immunosuppression. As a rule, involved tissue should be surgically resected as soon as possible. Transnasal endoscopic surgery, external ethmoidectomy, or a Caldwell–Luc procedure are performed for limited disease; more extensive disease requires radical surgical resection, including medial maxillectomy, total maxillectomy with orbital exoneration, or even more extensive craniofacial resection. In a retrospective analysis performed by Gillespie in 1998, 9 of 10 survivors underwent complete surgical resection. Obvious disease was left behind in nine of nine patients who died of the disease (24). This supports the principle that complete surgical resection is required to obtain a cure.

Systemic antifungal therapy should be continued even if all necrotic tissue is fully debrided, given the high likelihood of unapparent local and disseminated disease (7). In general, therapy should be continued until there is a clear clinical remission and as many immunocompromising conditions as possible are reversed.

Once in remission, patients may be transitioned to oral itraconzole or voriconazole as chronic suppressive therapy. Empiric coverage with amphotericin B should be resumed during subsequent periods of immunocompromise.

Hyperbaric oxygen has been used in some patients with mucormycosis, but no benefit has been demonstrated (25).

COMPLICATIONS AND PROGNOSIS

Invasive fungal sinusitis is devastating. Many patients will not survive, and those who do often are left with permanent disfigurement. The overall mortality ranges from 25% to 75%. The most important predictor of survival is successful correction of the predisposing condition. This includes control of ketoacidosis in diabetics and reversal of the underlying immunocompromised state. Risk factors associated with death include delayed diagnosis, presence of hemiparesis, bilateral sinus involvement, leukemia, renal disease, and treatment with deferoxamine.

SUMMARY

Acute invasive fungal sinusitis is a devastating infection that requires prompt diagnosis and initiation of comprehensive medical and surgical therapy to avoid patient demise. Unfortunately, the incidence of these cases seems to be on the rise as more patients are undergoing bone marrow and organ transplant. An estimated 4% of bone marrow transplant recipients will develop an invasive fungal infection during their lifetime.

CHRONIC INVASIVE FUNGAL SINUSITIS

INTRODUCTION

In contrast to acute invasive fungal sinusitis, chronic invasive fungal sinusitis can occur in immunocompetent hosts. The disease is endemic to Sudan and is primary caused by *A. flavus* (5).

EPIDEMIOLOGY

This manifestation of fungal sinusitis is rare in the United States. It seems to be more prevalent in areas with high levels of environmental spores, such as Sudan, Saudi Arabia, and other warm, tropical, and desert climates. It is occasionally seen in patients with diabetes.

PATHOPHYSIOLOGY

Chronic invasive fungal sinusitis progresses over months to years. It may initially involve only the turbinates or ethmoid sinuses but can breach the orbit and subsequently the skull base if allowed to progress. Ultimately, intracranial extension results in the demise of the patient, unless appropriate treatment is undertaken (3). Histopathology shows fungal invasion into the mucosa with chronic inflammatory infiltrate of lymphocytes, giant cells, and necrotizing granulomas (8).

CLINICAL MANIFESTATIONS

Patients with chronic invasive fungal sinusitis, who present early, have the typical symptoms of CRS. If they endure the symptoms for months, the disease can progress with resulting visual changes from orbital invasion. Eventually, mental status changes occur due to brain involvement. Examination may reveal tenderness and erythema over the maxillary or frontal sinuses. Proptosis or fixation of the globe suggests more advanced disease.

DIAGNOSIS

Radiologic examination with CT imaging frequently shows involvement of a single paranasal sinus with a mass lesion and thickening of the adjacent mucoperiosteum. Bone destruction and orbital involvement can be seen in advanced cases. Early endoscopic evaluation should be followed by biopsy of diseased mucosa and bone. Frozen section analysis revealing evidence of hyphae penetrating into the submucosa, vessels, or bone confirms the diagnosis. Aspiration of sinus contents and middle meatus cultures should be sent to microbiology for specific fungal stains and PCR analysis in an effort to identify the causative pathogen.

TREATMENT

As in cases of acute invasive fungal sinusitis, surgical debridement and antifungal therapy are the mainstays of treatment. Steroids should be avoided. These patients require close followup for many years, because relapses can occur.

COMPLICATIONS AND PROGNOSIS

Chronic invasive fungal sinusitis has a better overall prognosis than the acute form and can frequently be controlled with surgery and antifungal agents. Unfortunately, though, some patients have multiple relapses and eventually develop orbital and cerebral complications.

SUMMARY

Chronic invasive fungal sinusitis is rare in the United States. The prognosis is better than for the acute invasive form, in part, due to the fact that the patients afflicted have normal immune systems. The clinician must distinguish chronic invasive fungal sinusitis from AFS, because invasive fungal infections should never be treated with systemic steroids.

REFERENCES

1. Ponikau JU, Sherris DA, Kern EB, et al. The diagnosis and incidence of allergic fungal sinusitis. Mayo Clin Proc 1999; 74(9):877–884.
2. Branovan DI. Pathophysiology of rhinosinusitis. In: Rice DH, Schaefer SD, eds. Endoscopic Paranasal Sinus Surgery. 3rd ed. Philadelphia, PA: Lippincott Williams & Wilkins, 2004:53–68.
3. Furguson BJ, Johnson JT. Infectious causes of rhinosinusitis. In: Cummings CW, Flint PW, Haughey BH, eds. Cummings Otolaryngology-Head and Neck Surgery. Vol. 2. 4th ed. Philadelphia, PA: Mosby, 2005:1188–1192.
4. deShazo RD, Swain RE. Diagnostic criteria for allergic fungal sinusitis. J Allergy Clin Immunol 1995; 96(1):24–35.
5. Bachert C, van Cauwenberge P. Nasal polyps and sinusitis. In: Adkinson NF Jr, Yunginger JW, Busse WW, et al., eds. Middleton's Allergy: Principles and Practice. 6th ed. Philadelphia, PA: Mosby, Section E, 2003:1421–1436.
6. Collins M, Nair S, Smith W, et al. Role of local immunoglobulin E production in the pathophysiology of noninvasive fungal sinusitis. Laryngoscope 2004; 114(7):1242–1246.
7. Pelton S. Otitis, sinusitis and related conditions. In: Cohen J, Powderly WG, eds. Infectious Diseases. 2nd ed. Philadelphia, PA: Mosby, 2004:352–356.
8. Schubert MS. Allergic fungal sinusitis. Otolaryngol Clin North Am 2004; 37(2):301–326.
9. Sohail MA, Al Khabori MJ, Hyder J, et al. Allergic fungal sinusitis: can we predict the recurrence? Otolaryngol Head Neck Surg 2004; 131(5):704–710.
10. Eliashar R, Levi-Shaffer F. The role of the eosinophil in nasal diseases. Curr Opin Otolaryngol Head Neck Surg 2005; 13:171–175.
11. Gosepath J, Brieger J, Vlachtsis K, et al. Fungal DNA is present in tissue specimens of patients with chronic rhinosinusitis. Am J Rhinol 2004; 18(1):9–13.
12. Buzina W, Braun H, Freudenschuss K, et al. Fungal biodiversity—as found in nasal mucus. Med Mycol 2003; 41(2):149–161.
13. Lackner A, Stammberger H, Buzina W, et al. Fungi: a normal content of human nasal mucus. Am J Rhinol 2005; 19(2):125–129.
14. Shin SH, Ponikau JU, Sherris DA, et al. Chronic rhinosinusitis: an enhanced immune response to ubiquitous airborne fungi. J Allergy Clin Immunol 2004; 114(6):1369–1375.
15. Braun H, Buzina W, Freudenschuss K, et al. 'Eosinophilic fungal rhinosinusitis': a common disorder in Europe? Laryngoscope 2003; 113(2):264–269.
16. Ponikau JU, Sherris DA, Kita H, et al. Intranasal antifungal treatment in 51 patients with chronic rhinosinusitis. J Allergy Clin Immunol 2002; 110(6):862–866.
17. Ricchetti A, Landis BN, Maffioli A, et al. Effect of anti-fungal nasal lavage with amphotericin B on nasal polyposis. J Laryngol Otol 2002; 116(4):261–263.
18. Weschta M, Rimek D, Formanek M, et al. Topical antifungal treatment of chronic rhinosinusitis with nasal polyps: a randomized, double-blind clinical trial. J Allergy Clin Immunol 2004;113(6):1122–1128.
19. Kennedy DW, Kuhn FA, Hamilos DL, et al. Treatment of chronic rhinosinusitis with high-dose oral terbinafine: a double blind, placebo-controlled study. Laryngoscope 2005; 115(10):1793–1799.

20. Burgel PR, Cardell LO, Ueki IF, et al. Intranasal steroids decrease eosinophils but not mucin expression in nasal polyps. Eur Respir J 2004; 24(4):594–600.
21. Bhansali A, Bhadada S, Sharma A, et al. Presentation and outcome of rhino-orbital-cerebral mucormycosis in patients with diabetes. Postgrad Med J 2004; 80(949):670–674.
22. Hofman V, Castillo L, Betis F, et al. Usefulness of frozen section in rhinocerebral mucormycosis diagnosis and management. Pathology 2003; 35(3):212–216.
23. Tobon AM, Arango M, Fernandez D, et al. Mucormycosis (zygomycosis) in a heart-kidney transplant recipient: recovery after posaconazole therapy. Clin Infect Dis 2003; 36(11):1488–1491.
24. Gillespie MB, O'Malley BW Jr, Francis HW. An approach to fulminant invasive fungal rhinosinusitis in the immunocompromised host. Arch Otolaryngol Head Neck Surg 1998; 124(5):520–526.
25. Ferguson BJ, Mitchell TG, Moon R, et al. Adjunctive hyperbaric oxygen for treatment of rhinocerebral mucormycosis. Rev Infect Dis 1988; 10(3):551–559.

14

Mucormycosis

Andrew K. Patel
*Department of Surgery, Division of Otolaryngology-Head and Neck Surgery,
University of California, San Diego, California, U.S.A.*

Terence M. Davidson
*Department of Surgery, Division of Otolaryngology-Head and Neck Surgery,
University of California and VA San Diego Healthcare System, San Diego, California,
U.S.A.*

Case Example

A 51-year-old woman was transferred from a small community emergency department for subspecialty evaluation. The patient had presented to that facility the previous night complaining of headache and fever for three days with a sudden loss of vision in her left eye. During our evaluation, the patient reported that one week earlier, she fell, striking the left side of her face and sustaining several small abrasions. She denied other facial trauma. Further history revealed a general malaise and gradual weight loss for about one month's duration. She also admitted to falling occasionally in the past. Her past medical history included non-insulin-dependent diabetes mellitus for "several years." She was non-compliant with her oral hypoglycemic medication. She denied other past medical history.

The patient was noted to have a blood pressure of 164/86 mmHg, a pulse rate of 82 beats/min, a respiratory rate of 18 breaths/min, and a rectal temperature of 99.6°F. Fingerstick glucose was 284 mg/dL. The patient was alert and oriented, although somewhat apprehensive. Her left eye was proptotic; her sclera were muddy bilaterally. Marked chemosis was noted on the left. The left periorbital area was swollen and erythematous with abrasions sustained with her recent fall. The left eye had no light perception, with the pupil midpoint and fixed. The left-sided extraocular muscles were paralyzed. The right eye exam and extraocular muscles were normal. There was a 4 cm black necrotic area on the left hard palate. The neck exam was normal. Examination of the chest was without abnormalities. The abdomen was benign. The extremities were normal except for dry, flaking skin.

Screening serum chemistries showed a sodium level of 132 mEq/L, potassium of 3.1 mEq/L, chloride of 95 mEq/L, and bicarbonate of 18 mmol/L, resulting in an anion gap of 21 mmol/L. Serum glucose was 272 mg/dL and liver function panel was normal except for a lactate dehydrogenase of 307 U/L. Screening coagulation studies were normal. Serum acetone was markedly positive. Complete blood count (CBC) revealed a white cell count of 12,800/mm^3 with a leftward shift. The rest of the CBC findings were within normal range. The electrocardiogram and chest X ray were normal.

In consideration of the patient's history of diabetes, the positive serum acetone, the low serum bicarbonate, and the high anion gap, the diagnosis of diabetic ketoacidosis (DKA) was made. Therefore, the patient was treated with intravenous insulin and normal saline. It was believed that she also had an infection of the soft tissues of the left orbit; infection and paralysis of the third nerve by a retro-orbital abscess could explain the unilateral blindness and proptosis.

This was confirmed by contrast-enhanced computed tomography (CT) of the head, orbits, and paranasal sinuses. The CT showed no intracranial abnormalities. No midline shift was present. There were no signs of intracranial abscess or infection. There was an air fluid level present in the left maxillary sinus, without evidence of bone destruction. Fluid and mucosal thickening were noted in the left ethmoid and frontal sinuses with no evidence of bone destruction. An air fluid level was present in the left sphenoid sinus. The CT scan further revealed left periorbital soft-tissue swelling. The left retrobulbar fat appeared infiltrated and "dirty." The left extraocular muscles were swollen. These changes suggested orbital cellulitis. No discrete abscess collection was seen. The left eye was proptotic. On one CT image, the left superior ophthalmic vein was prominent, suggesting thrombosis. The cavernous sinus appeared normal and there was a loss of fat planes in the left masticator space, suggesting infection.

Because of her immunocompromised state, her presentation with DKA, the CT findings of retrobulbar infiltration, and the necrotic areas in the mouth, the diagnosis of mucormycosis with possible retrobulbar abscess was suspected. Urgent otolaryngology and ophthalmology consultations were obtained. A biopsy of the left palate lesion was obtained (Fig. 1).

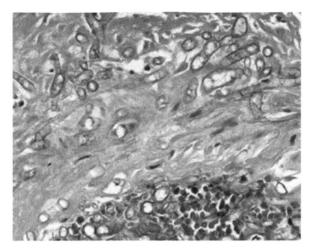

FIGURE 1 Mucormycosis fungal elements with broad and branching nonseptated hyphae. The consulting services concurred with the diagnosis, and the patient urgently went for surgical debridement. Surgical specimens of the left sinus system and the hard palate lesion tested positive for mucormycosis. The patient later underwent serial debridements, enucleation of the left eye, drainage of the retrobulbar abscess, and aggressive intravenous antifungal treatment. The patient did well after her debridements and antifungal treatment and survived to discharge one month later. *Source.* (Photo) Courtesy of Dr. Marco A. Ayala, LT and Dr. Gretchen S. Folk, LCDR, DC, USNR, Naval Medical Center San Diego, CA, U.S.A.

INTRODUCTION

Mucormycosis (zygomycosis and phycomycosis) is one of the most acute, fulminant fungal infections known. Invasive fungal infections are major medical complications in immunocompromised patients (Table 1). The recent rise in the incidence of cancer and the increased use of newer medical treatment modalities, including organ transplantations, have resulted in growing numbers of highly immunosuppressed individuals. Although aspergillosis and candidiasis are among the most common invasive mycoses in such patients, there is evidence that the incidence of infectious diseases caused by *Zygomycetes* has risen significantly over the past decade. Species of the genera *Rhizopus* and *Mucor* are the common pathogens of this group. Other genera, including *Absidia*, *Cunninghamella*, *Rhizomucor*, and *Apophysomyces*, have also been reported to cause disease. Patients with diabetes, malignancies, neutropenia, solid organ or bone marrow transplants, or iron overload and those suffering from severe malnutrition or receiving immunosuppressive agents, deferoxamine therapy, or broad-spectrum antimicrobial drugs are at highest risk for zygomycosis. Also at risk are individuals with primary breakdown in the integrity of the cutaneous barrier due to trauma, surgical wounds, needle sticks, or burns. Less than 5% of cases involve normal adult hosts. The clinical spectrum of zygomycosis is now broader, and it can be difficult to distinguish between mucormycosis and entomophthoramycosis, both of which can manifest as disease ranging from a superficial infection to an angioinvasive infection with high mortality. Treatment of zygomycosis requires several simultaneous approaches: surgical intervention, antifungal therapy, and medical management or correction of the underlying condition that is predisposing the patient to the disease. Lipid formulations of amphotericin B are the antifungal agents of choice for treatment of

TABLE 1   Mucormycosis: Key Points

Overview

Mucormycosis is an acute and rapidly developing fungal infection caused by fungi of the class *Zygomycetes* and the third most common invasive fungal infection in immunocompromised patients.

The *Mucorales* organisms are ubiquitous thermotolerant saprophytic fungi, abundant in nature and found in bread, fruits/vegetables, soil, and manure, as well as in the mouth, nose, stool, and sputum of healthy individuals. Unlike most pathogenic fungi, these can grow anaerobically.

Pathophysiology of mucormycosis

Acquisition primarily via inhalation of spores without human-to-human transmission.

Principal site of disease: rhinocerebral, pulmonary, cutaneous, GI, disseminated, central nervous system. Opportunistic infections primarily pulmonary and rhinocerebral.

Diabetic patients appear to be more frequently colonized, and serum from diabetics with ketoacidosis fails to provide normal inhibition of fungal growth.

Other risk factors include severe burns, hemodialysis with deferoxamine, immunosuppression, severe malnutrition, and neutropenia.

Invasion, thrombosis, and necrosis are the characteristic findings in this disease. After the fungal spores have germinated at the site of infection, the hyphal elements are very aggressive and tend to invade blood vessels, nerves, lymphatics, and tissues. The infarction leads to further tissue hypoxia and acidosis, resulting in a vicious cycle that enhances rapid growth and infection. The paucity of a granulomatous reaction is quite characteristic. The fungal hyphae sometimes have little or no inflammation around them.

Symptomatology (by location of infection)

Rhinocerebral—75% of reported cases, often in poorly controlled diabetics with DKA, neutropenic or immunosuppressed patients, or in azotemic patients. Left undiagnosed, may be rapidly fatal. Hyphae invade the paranasal sinuses and palate from the ironical cavity. From the sinuses, especially the ethmoid sinus, the infection spreads to involve the retro-orbital region or the CNS. Epistaxis, severe unilateral headache, alteration in mental status, and eye symptoms such as lacrimation, irritation, or periorbital anesthesia are common symptoms. Examination of the nose may reveal the classic black necrotic turbinates (too often mistaken for dried blood) or nasal septum perforation; however, at the early stage of infection, the nasal mucosa may appear only inflamed and friable. Facial cellulitis and palatal necrosis may be seen. The early eye findings include mild proptosis, periorbital edema, decreased visual acuity, or lid swelling. In more advanced orbital involvement, exophthalmos, complete ophthalmoplegia, conjunctival hemorrhage, blindness, fixed and dilated pupil, and corneal anesthesia may be found. These conditions result from fungal invasion of the roof of the orbit, affecting the nerves (i.e., the third, fourth, and sixth cranial nerves and the ophthalmic branch of the fifth cranial nerve), muscles, and orbital vessels, a condition also known as the "orbital apex syndrome." The infection can spread through the superior orbital fissure or the cribriform plate to involve the brain. Cavernous sinus thrombosis is a frequent complication, usually resulting from hematogenous spread from the ophthalmic veins. This spread results in additional cranial nerve involvement outside the orbital apex, specifically the trigeminal nerve ganglion and the root of the facial nerve, leading to ipsilateral paresthesia of the face or peripheral facial palsy. Internal carotid artery thrombosis, resulting from retrograde spread from the ophthalmic artery or invasion from the cavernous sinus, is another late complication, leading to cerebral infarction. The middle ear may be involved by means of the blood, CSF, or Eustachian tube. CT or MRI is useful in better defining the bone destruction and soft-tissue involvement, which may be important in guiding subsequent surgical intervention.

Pulmonary mucormycosis usually occurs in patients with hematologic malignancies or diabetes. The presentation usually is acute, and patients are often profoundly ill, with variable complaints of cough and fever. No pathognomonic clinical or radiographic findings exist. Sputum culture usually is negative.

Cutaneous mucormycosis is rare and is primarily a nosocomial infection in burn and blunt trauma victims. Local infection has resulted from using contaminated elastic bandages. The involved area is erythematous and painful, with various degrees of central necrosis that can progress to gangrenous cellulitis.

(Continued)

TABLE 1 Mucormycosis: Key Points *(Continued)*

GI mucormycosis is the least common form of infection. It is seen primarily in patients suffering from intrinsic abnormalities of the GI tract or severe malnutrition. The infection is thought to arise from fungi entering the body with food. Any part of the GI tract is susceptible to infection, with the stomach, terminal ileum, and colon being the most common sites. Wall invasion, ischemic infarction, and ulceration are characteristic. The diagnosis is frequently made at autopsy.

Disseminated mucormycosis is defined as an infection occurring in two or more noncontiguous organ systems. The distant sites are infected by bloodstream invasion from a local site. Although any organ can be affected, the lungs and CNS are the two common sites. The outcome of this infection is almost invariably fatal.

Isolated CNS mucormycosis results from hematogenous spread and is seen primarily in intravenous drug addicts.

Diagnosis

The diagnosis of any form of mucormycosis depends on direct and histologic examinations of scrapings and biopsies of necrotic material. In contrast to most fungi, these organisms are readily seen in H&E-stained tissue. The Gomori methenamine silver stain usually is adequate.

Swabs of discharge or abnormal tissue are not adequate and can give erroneous information. Fungal cultures are occasionally positive, but a negative culture result does not exclude the diagnosis or make it less likely.

No skin tests or serologic methods are adequate for diagnosing mucormycosis, and blood cultures are not helpful.

Treatment

Successful outcome in treating this aggressive infection relies on early diagnosis by invasive procedures, immediate correction of the underlying predisposing condition, urgent surgical debridement, and early systemic amphotericin therapy.

Endoscopic surgery has a role in early rhinocerebral cases.

Amphotericin B is the only drug with proven clinical efficacy, and a high therapeutic dosage (e.g., 1.0–1.5 mg/kg/day, if tolerated) should be achieved as soon as possible. This may be reduced to alternate-day dosing after the patient is stabilized. Typically, a cumulative dose of 2–5 g may be needed to achieve cure. Lipid-complexed amphotericin could enable continued aggressive therapy in the nephrotoxic patient.

Colony-stimulating factors may accelerate neutrophil return in neutropenic patients.

Prognosis

Mucormycosis remains a disease with guarded prognosis.

Rhinocerebral mucormycosis is the most common form of infection and is thought to have an overall mortality rate of about 50%.

Patients who develop hemiplegia or nasal deformity have higher mortality rates.

Deeper cutaneous infections of the extremities usually require amputation, and when the head or trunk is involved, the condition is commonly fatal.

The most aggressive approach we can take toward this lethal disease is rapid diagnosis and immediate institution of surgical debridement plus systemic and local chemotherapy.

Abbreviations: CNS, central nervous system; CSF, cerebrospinal fluid; CT, computed tomography; GI, gastrointestinal; H&E, hematoxylin and eosin; MRI, magnetic resonance imaging.

zygomycosis. A novel antifungal triazole, posaconazole, has been developed and may become approved for treatment of zygomycosis. The clinical experience with adjunctive treatments such as colony-stimulating factors, interferon-γ, and hyperbaric oxygen therapy is still limited.

DEFINITION

Mucormycosis is the common name given to several different diseases caused by fungi of the class *Zygomycetes*, order *Mucorales*. Organisms of the class *Zygomycetes* were first noted to cause disease in humans in publications from the 1800s. Platauf is credited with the first description of zygomycosis in the human nasopharynx in his 1885 paper entitled "Mycosis Mucorina" (1). His descriptions, in German, are detailed enough to suggest that this first case of disseminated disease in a cancer patient was caused by *Absidia corymbifera*. It was over 65 years later that Harris reported the first case of successful cure in a young girl who improved after correction of her DKA (2). She was the only known survivor until 1961, when Gass reported the successful management of a patient with amphotericin B, which became available in the 1950s (3).

The information that emerged over the next several decades was based predominantly on tissue morphology and rarely confirmed by culture. As a result, many of the early cases, and some of the cases still reported today, relied on the morphologic tissue findings of coenocytic, angioinvasive hyphae suggesting infection with one of the *Mucorales*. The majority of cases reported had no culture identification; instead, the infection was identified as a "mucormycosis" or *Mucor* infection, despite this lack of culture confirmation. Even with the poor showing with culture results, it soon became obvious that *Rhizopus* species, and not *Mucor* species, were the predominant organisms causing disease. Other important information was also being collected by astute clinicians and researchers regarding the association of zygomycosis with cancer, antibiotic or prednisone use, diabetes, deferoxamine and desferrioxamine therapy, transplantation, and the associated forms of immunosuppressive therapies.

With the development of diagnostic tools that allowed earlier diagnosis, with better surgical and antifungal interventions, and with more sophisticated laboratory methods for identifying these agents, more patients are surviving these previously fatal infections. The variety of organisms causing disease has also expanded. In addition to *Rhizopus*, *Mucor*, and *Absidia*, human diseases due to *Rhizomucor*, *Apophysomyces*, *Saksenaea*, *Cunninghamella*, *Cokeromyces*, and *Syncephalastrum* species have all been confirmed. The manifestations of disease have also evolved from primarily rhinocerebral, pulmonary, and disseminated disease to include gastrointestinal (GI), cutaneous/subcutaneous, allergic disease, and even asymptomatic colonization.

EPIDEMIOLOGY

Mucormycosis is extremely rare, making it difficult to calculate incidence accurately. In a population-based epidemiological assessment, the cumulative incidence of invasive mycotic infections was 178.3 cases per million per year, with zygomycosis comprising 1.7 infections per million per year based on data from the San Francisco Bay Area (4). A recent review of mucormycosis cases at one U.S. cancer center showed that it was present in 0.7% of patients at autopsy and in 20 patients per 100,000 admissions (5). Less than 5% of cases involve normal adult hosts. Researchers estimate that the incidence in hematologic malignancy is approximately 1%. The incidence of *mucor* in allogeneic bone marrow transplants is 1.9%; however, most cases do not involve the central nervous system (CNS). No racial factors predisposing people to mucormycosis are known; reviews of cases from single institutions show an equal sex distribution; and mucormycosis is found in patients of a wide age range.

The major mode of disease transmission for the *Zygomycetes* is presumed to be via inhalation of spores from environmental sources. No reports of confirmed human-to-human transmission exist in the literature. The presence of neutropenia with an absolute neutrophil count of less than 1000/μL for one week or more poses the major risk for these patients. For patients in whom myelosuppressive therapies have been administered, and neutropenia and fever have persisted for longer than 7 to 10 days despite antibiotic therapy, a diagnosis of a fungal infection, including zygomycosis, should be suspected (Table 2).

TABLE 2 Diseases Associated with Mucormycosis ($n = 145$)

Disease state	n	Frequency (%)
Diabetes mellitus	87	60
Renal disease	11	7
Renal transplant	10	7
Deferoxamine toxicity	9	6.2
Leukemia	8	5.5
Steroid therapy	6	4.2
Hematologic disorder	5	3.4
No underlying disease	3	2
Others (nine disorders)	11	7

Note: HIV is not an independent risk factor for mucormycosis.
Source: Adapted from Ref. 6.

PATHOGENESIS

The *Zygomycetes* represent relatively uncommon isolates in the clinical laboratory, reflecting either environmental contaminants, or, less commonly, a clinical disease called *Zygomycosis*. There are two orders of *Zygomycetes*-containing organisms that cause human disease, the *Entomophthorales* and the *Mucorales*.

The *Entomophthorales* derive their name from the Greek word "entomon," meaning insect, reflecting their original identification as pathogens or parasites infecting insects. The *Entomophthorales* cause distinctive clinical syndromes, which are usually clearly separable from those produced by the agents causing mucormycosis. Entomophthoromycosis is the currently accepted general term used to describe the disease caused by these fungi. Extremely rare in North America, they are usually found in Africa, Southeast Asia, Indonesia, and South America (7). Entomophthoramycosis is a tropical infection of the subcutaneous tissue or paranasal sinuses, caused by species of *Basidiobolus* and *Conidiobolus*, respectively.

The majority of human illness is caused by the *Mucorales*. These organisms are ubiquitous saprophytic fungi and are abundant in nature. They have been recovered from bread, fruits, vegetables, soil, and manure. The spores from these molds are transmitted by inhalation, via a variety of percutaneous routes, or by ingestion of spores. Human zygomycosis caused by the *Mucorales* generally occurs in immunocompromised hosts as opportunistic infections. Zygomycosis occurs only rarely in immunocompetent hosts. The disease manifestations reflect the mode of transmission, with rhinocerebral and pulmonary diseases being the most common manifestations. Cutaneous, GI, and allergic diseases are also seen. The *Mucorales* are associated with angioinvasive disease, often leading to thrombosis, infarction of involved tissues, and tissue destruction mediated by a number of fungal proteases, lipases, and mycotoxins (7).

Traditionally, the *Mucorales* are divided into six families of significance in causing human or animal disease: *Mucoraceae*, *Cunninghamellaceae*, *Saksenaea*, *Thamnidiaceae*, *Syncephalastraceae*, and *Mortierellaceae* (8). Under this classification system, the vast majority of human zygomycotic disease is caused by the members of the family *Mucoraceae*. The taxonomy of these fungi is based on a morphologic analysis of the fungus, in addition to carbohydrate assimilation and maximal temperature compatible with growth. These organisms typically grow in two to five days on most media. However, cycloheximide inhibits the growth of these fungi, and media that contain this compound, such as mycosel and mycobiotic agar, should not be used.

Routine stains, such as potassium hydroxide and hematoxylin and eosin (H&E), help visualize mucor hyphae, while Grocott methenamine stains (GMS) and periodic acid-Schiff stains help demarcate fungal elements in tissue (8). The *Rhizopus* species are mucoraceous *Zygomycetes*, which produce wide ribbon-like aseptate hyphae in tissues stained with GMS. Another useful stain is Cresyl violet, which stains *Mucor* fungi walls brick red, while other fungi are stained purple or blue. There is a great deal of variation of hyphal width, ranging from 6 to 50 μm (typically 6–15 μm) (7). Branching occurs at wide angles nearing 90°. The organisms are inexplicably difficult to grow from infected tissue. When growth does take place, it is rapid and profuse on most media at room temperature. Identification is based on the gross and microscopic appearance of the mold.

Fungal Infections in the Immunocompromised Host

For the most part, the *Mucorales* are considered to be opportunistic pathogens. They require a breakdown in the immune defenses, particularly disease processes that lead to neutropenia or neutrophil dysfunction. Although neutrophil dysfunction induced by ketoacidosis underlies the majority of cases of human zygomycosis, neutropenia induced by bone marrow suppression during chemotherapy or immunosuppression induced following transplantation is causing a growing proportion of cases. Specifically, the growing numbers of immunocompromised patients receiving organ transplants or cytotoxic therapies are changing the epidemiology of rhinocerebral mucormycosis (RCM). While diabetes mellitus accounts for 70% to 90% of RCM in earlier literature reviews, more recent studies have reported underlying diabetes in only 27% to 60% of patients with this disease (9). Currently, most patients with RCM have underlying hematologic disorders or are immunosuppressed recipients of organ transplants.

The mechanism responsible for increased susceptibility in various patient groups to mucormycosis is not clear. The reactive oxygen species generated by the phagocyte respiratory burst (including superoxide, hydrogen peroxide, and hypochlorous acid) have been demonstrated to be fungicidal against *Rhizopus* hyphae. The manner in which diabetes and steroid therapy interfere with the ability of the fungus to elicit these toxic phagocyte products is not known. Some researchers have postulated that once infection is established, neutrophils have a pivotal role in killing hyphae. This is presumed because hyphae are too large to be ingested, so the killing is an extracellular process. In the setting of DKA, each of four phases of neutrophil activation is impaired, essentially inducing functional neutropenia. Defensins, cationic proteins obtained from mammalian phagocytic cells, also have significant ability to kill *Rhizopus oryzae* spores and hyphae (7). The relative importance of oxidative and nonoxidative fungicidal mechanisms in the normal state and in situations of immunosuppression or diabetes remains a mystery.

At this time, it is still not possible to develop a unifying concept of the pathogenesis of mucormycosis. It is clear, however, that undefined defects of macrophages and neutrophils, present in diabetic and steroid-treated animals, are important in allowing the replication of the *Mucorales*. Moreover, immunologically healthy people can suppress the growth of the *Mucorales* and clear them from the lung with great efficiency. Finally, the relative paucity of cases of mucormycosis in patients with the acquired immunodeficiency syndrome (AIDS) attests to the importance of the neutrophil in inhibiting fungal spore development. However, cases of mucormycosis in AIDS patients do occur and may be secondary to quantitative and qualitative defects in neutrophils.

In the late 1980s, physicians began to notice the occurrence of a fulminant form of zygomycosis in patients on hemodialysis who were receiving deferoxamine/desferrioxamine for iron or aluminum overload (5). The more liberally the iron chelator was used, the more likely zygomycosis was to develop. A large body of evidence supports the theory that the *Zygomycetes* are able to utilize iron bound to iron chelators to enhance their growth, in which the drug acts as an iron siderophore to *Mucorales* species, even in the absence of iron overload. The presence of acidosis together with deferoxamine therapy may also be a fatal combination. By inhibiting the binding and sequestration of iron by transferrin, acidosis also serves to keep the concentrations of iron in the plasma high, allowing its use as a growth factor by the *Zygomycetes*. It has also been demonstrated that iron overload states, such as hemochromatosis, even in the absence of chelator usage, may pose a slightly increased risk for the development of zygomycosis in humans.

Most of the current understanding of the pathogenesis of mucormycosis is derived from the mouse and rabbit models of infection. In addition, *Mucorales* contains a ketone reductase system that lets it thrive in a glucose-rich, acidotic, and ketotic environment. *Mucorales* hyphae have a predilection for growth into arteries, lymphatics, and nerves. Vascular invasion of the hyphae produces a fibrin reaction and the development of *Mucor thrombi,* which occlude vessels, producing ischemia and infarction. This infarction produces the black, necrotic eschars in the nasal and oral cavities and on the face that are characteristic of mucormycosis. Vascular occlusion also produces an acidotic tissue that is ideal for fungal growth and is protected from intravenously administered antifungal agents.

Mucormycosis in Children

In addition to cases involving immunosuppressed children, mucormycosis also has been observed in neonates (especially very-low-birth-weight premature infants weighing less than 1000 g), burn patients, and children with a history of incidental trauma. As with adult patients, the occurrence of mucormycosis depends on host immunity, but the mechanisms of increased susceptibility in certain hosts remain perplexing. In a pooled review by Kline of 41 cases of RCM in children aged 2 months to 18 years, 49% of cases were found in children with diabetes mellitus and 15% of cases were found in children with leukemia (10). In 10% of cases in these children, no predisposing conditions were present. In neonates, these invasive fungal infections have been observed to be rapidly fatal; the time from clinical symptoms to death ranges from 6 to 42 days.

CLINICAL MANIFESTATIONS

The dramatic invasive infections caused by the *Zygomycetes* are well known to clinicians. The main categories of human disease with the *Mucorales* are sinusitis/rhinocerebral, pulmonary, cutaneous/subcutaneous, GI, and disseminated zygomycosis. Other disease states occur with a much lower frequency and include cystitis, vaginal or GI colonization, external otitis, and allergic disease. Mucormycosis has a rapid onset, which has been estimated at one to seven days after inoculation.

Rhinocerebral Mucormycosis

RCM represents one-third to one-half of all cases of *Zygomycosis*. The process originates in the nose and paranasal sinuses following inspiration of fungal spores. It is estimated that 70% of the cases of rhinocerebral zygomycosis occur in the setting of DKA (7). Disease starts with symptoms consistent with sinusitis. Low-grade fever, dull sinus pain, drainage, and soft-tissue swelling are initially seen, followed in a few days by double vision, increasing fever, and obtundation. Examination reveals a unilateral generalized reduction of ocular motion, chemosis, and proptosis. Facial skin adjacent to paranasal sinuses may be invaded by direct extension, turning progressively red, purple, and black. Fever, decreased vision, and facial swelling are the most common complaints in the first 72 hours of the disease (6). Other common complaints include facial pain and nasal congestion or discharge. Headache was found early in the disease in only 25% of patients in one large study but may be a common late finding.

Schwartz noted that these nerve abnormalities are often consistent with orbital apex syndrome (unilateral ptosis, proptosis, visual loss, complete ophthalmoplegia, and ophthalmic and maxillary nerve anesthesia and anhidrosis) (11). Most cases of orbital apex syndrome are due to mucormycosis or *Aspergillus*, and visual loss is usually irreversible. In contrast with typical bacterial orbital cellulitis, patients with RCM may have minimal preseptal lid erythema, more pain in the forehead or temple than in the eye, and early onset of decreased sensation in the first and second divisions of cranial nerve V. The facial edema associated with RCM may be confused with periorbital cellulitis. The periorbital edema described for RCM is soft, cool, and nontender, differentiating it from the warm, tender, taut edema of cellulitis (9). Mucormycosis can be further distinguished from cellulitis by examining the character of the ptosis, if present; RCM produces a paralytic ptosis in which the eyelid can be raised easily by the examiner, whereas the edematous ptosis of cellulitis is resistant to opening. Altered mental status may be the only finding in some patients, and this disorder should be considered particularly in diabetic patients with altered mental states, who do not improve after 24 to 48 hours with correction of electrolyte abnormalities. Abramson et al. specifically noted a "characteristic" presentation that combines some of the most common findings: a dark, necrotic epistaxis ipsilateral to facial pain and soft periorbital swelling (9).

The disease may become rapidly progressive, extending into neighboring tissues. Involved tissues become red, then violaceous, and finally black as vessels are thrombosed and the tissues undergo necrosis. Extension into the periorbital region of the face and ultimately into the orbit is often found, even at presentation. Periorbital edema, proptosis, and tearing are early signs of orbital involvement. Ocular or optic nerve involvement is first suggested by pain, blurring, or loss of vision in the infected eye. Cranial nerve palsies may also be seen. Extension from the sinuses into the mouth often occurs, producing painful, black, necrotic ulcerations into the hard palate, which are sharply delineated and respect the midline. A bloody nasal discharge is generally the first sign of that the disease has invaded through the nose and sinuses and into the brain. Patients may demonstrate an altered mental state due either to ketoacidosis or to CNS invasion. Specifically, coma may be due to direct invasion of the frontal lobe.

Once the eye is infected, fungal disease can readily progress up the optic nerve, again gaining access to the CNS. Fungal invasion of the globe or ophthalmic artery leads to blindness. Angioinvasion is often seen and may result in systemically disseminated disease. Decidedly uncommon forms of rhinofacial disease published in the literature include isolated sinusitis and calcified fungal ball of the sinus. Early cases with rhinocerebral zygomycosis were almost uniformly fatal. There is still a high mortality rate with rhinocerebral disease, but curative interventions have been made with early diagnosis and aggressive surgical and antifungal treatment. The nature of the underlying disease is the most important determinant of survival, with up to 75% of immunocompetent individuals surviving in some series, compared to 60% of diabetics or 20% of individuals with other systemic disease achieving cure (6).

Pulmonary Mucormycosis

Pulmonary mucormycosis manifests as progressive severe pneumonia accompanied by high fever and toxicity. A pleuritic rub and ronchi may be evident over the affected area. The necrotic center of large infiltrates may cavitate. Fatal hemoptysis may occur from cavities formed near the hilum. Hematogenous spread to other areas of the lung, as well as to the brain and other organs, is common. Survival beyond two weeks is unusual.

Gastrointestinal Mucormycosis

GI invasion presents as one or more ulcers that tend to perforate, generally in patients who are severely malnourished, and may occur throughout the GI tract. The presentation is nonspecific with abdominal pain, distension, nausea, and vomiting. Hematogenous dissemination can originate from the GI tract, lung, or paranasal sinuses. Sometimes no portal of entry can be found. Due to the rapid course and delay in diagnosis, this disease is seldom diagnosed in life.

Primary Cutaneous Mucormycosis

Primary cutaneous inoculation is uncommon but occurs in burn eschars, underneath occlusive dressings, and at sites of minor trauma in immunocompromised adults and low-birth-weight neonates. In burn patients, *Mucor* generally involves the skin and only rarely causes the rhinocerebral form. In the cutaneous form of mucormycosis, presentation occurs with minimal pain, variable systemic toxicity, rapid progression with low-grade fever, and anesthesia of the lesion. The lesion appears as a central black, necrotic area with a purple raised margin or may appear as a black ulcer. Multiple reports in the literature document inoculation of *Rhizopus* and other spores from nonsterile elastic bandages or from the use of nonsterile tongue depressors. Use of properly sterilized bandages, dressings, and other supplies should eliminate this transmission of mucormycosis. Treatment is more successful in cutaneous mucormycosis than in other forms, though curative surgical intervention may be quite disfiguring or may require amputation of the affected limb (Table 3).

TABLE 3 Signs and Symptoms of Mucormycosis at Presentation ($n = 114$)

Sign/symptom	n	Frequency (%)
Fever	50	44
Nasal necrosis/ulceration	43	38
Facial/periorbital swelling	39	34
Decreased vision	34	30
Ophthalmoplegia	33	29
Sinusitis	30	26
Headache	29	25
Facial pain	25	22
Altered mental status	25	22
Leukocytosis	22	19
Nasal discharge	20	18
Nasal stuffiness	19	17
Corneal anesthesia	19	17
Palatal/gingival necrosis	16	14
Afferent papillary defect	15	13
CN VII palsy	13	11
Periorbital pain	13	11

Source: Adapted from Ref. 6.

DIAGNOSIS

Imaging Studies in Mucormycosis

Maxillofacial CT scan is used for initial investigation in rhinocerebral infection. The CT scan may demonstrate ethmoid and sphenoid mucosal thickening or sinusitis as well as orbital or intracranial extension and is valuable in planning surgical debridement.

Magnetic resonance imaging (MRI) with enhancement may be helpful in assessing patients with allergic fungal sinusitis and in patients in whom invasive fungal sinusitis is suspected. MRI is helpful in evaluating CNS spread in invasive fungal sinusitis and may be superior to CT in assessing the need for further surgical intervention. MRI additionally helps to define early vascular intracranial invasion before clinical signs develop.

Chest CT and chest X rays may be useful in the setting of pulmonary infection to evaluate consolidation, cavitation, nodular lesions, or effusions. A predilection for upper lobe involvement is common in pulmonary infection.

Abdominal CT in the setting of GI mucormycosis may demonstrate a mass associated with the GI tract in addition to splenic or renal involvement.

Cytologic Testing

Demonstration of fungal elements from cytologic preparations (i.e., sputa, inflammatory fluid aspirates from abscesses or sinusitis infection, and genitourinary and gynecologic specimens) may be difficult, due to the difficulty in extracting fungal elements from invaded tissues (8). Cultures of blood and cerebrospinal fluid (CSF) are negative. CSF, if inadvertently examined, may show an increased opening pressure, modest neutrophilic pleocytosis, normal or slightly elevated protein levels, or low glucose. In most cases, CSF study findings are normal. Smear and culture of sputum may be positive during cavitation of a lung lesion. Fine needle aspiration can yield a diagnosis, but should not preclude definitive therapy.

Evaluation of Tissue Specimens

The diagnosis of zygomycosis is easily made on tissue section from the margin of a necrotic lesion. Involved tissue demonstrates focal areas of infection and may appear nodular or may produce extensive areas of necrosis with accompanying hemorrhage into the tissue. Specifically, histology demonstrates invasion along the elastic lamina of blood vessels, with hyphae of the fungus extending into and occluding the lumens of the blood vessels they have invaded, followed by thrombosis and tissue necrosis (7). Abscess formation with central tissue necrosis, acute inflammatory exudate, and peripheral tissue invasion by hyphal elements is quite common. An acute inflammatory exudate often accompanies these infections in non-neutropenic patients.

Demonstration of the fungal elements with fungal specific stains such as Calcofluor white stain or Grocott-Gomori methenamine silver stain is recommended. The specimen should not be crushed or ground, because the nonseptate hyphae are prone to damage. The key feature associated with the *Zygomycetes* on direct examination of cytologic specimens is the presence of wide, ribbon-like, aseptate, hyaline hyphal elements, often in the setting of extensive necrotic debris. The width of the hyphal element varies substantially. Branching of the hyphae is seen, with wide-angle (generally around 90°) bifurcations noted.

Invasion of the blood vessels (angioinvasion) by hyphal elements is generally seen in infections with the *Mucorales* but usually not with the *Entomophthorales*. The hallmark of a zygomycosis includes the demonstration of wide, ribbon-like, hyaline, predominantly aseptate hyphae with wide-angle (45–90°) branching. The hyphae often are not preserved well and may become crinkled or gnarled in the tissue sections. This is often referred to as a "crinkled cellophane" appearance of the hyphal elements. To the inexperienced observer, these artifactual folds in the hyphae may be confused with septations. Cross sections of hyphal elements often give tissues a vacuolated appearance. These cross sections vary in diameter and may be confused with yeast cells. In H&E-stained tissue section, the *Entomophthorales* demonstrate hyphal encasement by eosinophilic material.

Fungal Culture

The *Mucorales* grow well on both nonselective and fungal-selective media. The growth of the *Mucorales* tends to be rapid, with mycelial elements expanding to cover the entire plate in only a few (1–7) days. Organisms of the order *Mucorales* are characterized by an erect aerial mycelium that is described as fibrous or "cotton candy-like." The mycelium tends to be quite high, with some isolates reaching the lid of the petri dish at mature growth. It is this vigorous growth characteristic that is responsible for the group being designated as "lid lifters."

Laboratory Studies

Urea and electrolytes are used to monitor disturbances of homeostasis and direct correction of acidosis. Blood glucose monitoring should be rapidly instituted for the treatment of unstable diabetes. Arterial blood gases assist in determining the degree of acidosis and direct corrective treatments. A full blood examination is indicated, including assessment of neutrophil count, monitoring of recovery after withdrawal of cytotoxic therapies, and institution of colony-stimulating factor treatment. Iron studies permit assessment of the presence of iron overload as shown by high ferritin levels and a low total iron-binding capacity. At this time, molecular techniques for detection of *Zygomycetes* by polymerase chain reaction or other methods such as enzyme-linked immunosorbent assays are not widely available and are reserved primarily for research purposes. Further development and validation will be required before their inclusion in clinical practice becomes routine.

TREATMENT

The role of surgery in the treatment of mucormycosis cannot be overemphasized. Because of their propensity for invading blood vessels, the *Mucorales* cause extensive tissue infarction, thereby impairing the delivery of antifungal agents to the site of infection. This often leaves surgery as the only modality that may effectively eliminate the invading microorganisms. In one small study of 10 patients with RCM, all patients were noted to have involvement of the pterygopalatine fossa, and it was noted that facial soft tissues, palate, and infratemporal fossa were potentially infected via connecting pathways from the pterygopalatine fossa (12). The study concluded that debridement of the pterygopalatine fossa seems to be a definitive method of managing RCM, based on this limited cohort. In addition, Mohs micrographic surgery has been reported as a tissue-sparing technique in the management of the cutaneous form of mucormycosis. It is important to understand the urgency of surgical resection. This is a true surgical emergency and is an operation that requires immediate attention. A case diagnosed in the late afternoon cannot be scheduled for the following day; rather, it must be operated that evening, even if late at night.

Amphotericin B is the first-line drug of choice for most cases of zygomycosis caused by the *Mucorales*. Amphotericin mediates its antifungal action by modifying fungal cell walls. This drug binds to ergosterol and causes increased cell wall permeability. With permeabilization, ions leak from the cell and the membrane depolarizes. The maximal tolerated doses are given until progression is halted. Endoscopic examination of paranasal sinuses can help assess progression. With the deoxycholate formulation, a dosage of 1 to 1.5 mg/kg daily is indicated. Amphotericin B lipid complex or liposomal amphotericin B, each at 5 mg/kg daily, appear to be as effective as and less toxic than conventional amphotericin B. Therapy is continued for a total of 10 to 12 weeks. Amphotericin B has also been applied topically in the orbital cavities in patients with RCM, although it is not clear whether this is beneficial.

Amphotericin B is not effective in all cases, particularly if the patient presents late in the disease course and has inoperable or disseminated disease. *Mucor* reacts variably to amphotericin. Sensitivity testing is not standardized and does not necessarily correlate with disease. The therapeutic activity of amphotericin B is also limited by its potentially severe side effects. Impaired renal function often leads to cessation of therapy. The liposomal preparation of amphotericin B may help to alleviate this problem and allow for higher doses of medication to be administered. Although synergism of amphotericin B and rifampin in treating zygomycosis has been suggested by some authors, this has not been demonstrated conclusively in clinical trials.

None of the currently available azoles (ketoconazole, itraconazole, fluconazole, or voriconazole) or echinocandins has a role in the treatment of mucormycosis. *Mucor* is highly resistant to itraconazole in vitro. A new, broad-spectrum triazole, posaconazole (not yet clinically available), has been shown to be active in a murine model of mucormycosis, although no parenteral form is available.

Currently, the role of colony-stimulating factors as adjuncts to surgical and antifungal therapy still remains unclear, beyond that of increasing the neutrophil count in patients with neutropenia.

Some case reports have suggested benefit from adding hyperbaric oxygen to standard therapy (13). Proponents suggest that oxygen-based free radicals are believed to be responsible for the fungistatic and fungicidal effects of hyperbaric oxygen, which may potentiate the antifungal effect of amphotericin B by reversing tissue hypoxia, which protects fungal protoplasts from lysis. Because of the uncontrolled nature of the observations and the absence of a rationale for treating an aerobic fungus with oxygen, this form of therapy cannot be routinely recommended at present.

COMPLICATIONS, PROGNOSIS, AND PREVENTION

Mucor is a disease with protean findings and diverse outcomes. These infections are often fatal, although patients with limited sinonasal disease may have a better prognosis, especially with early diagnosis, aggressive surgical resection, and aggressive antifungal therapy. There is a markedly poorer prognosis for those patients with hemiplegia, facial necrosis, and nasal deformity (12). Among patients with RCM, 70% of survivors are left with residual defects (14). In a meta-analysis by Yohai et al, it was believed that the survival rate declines when interval from diagnosis to treatment is longer than six days (6).

Once the patient is stable, amphotericin should be continued in the outpatient setting, administered either as a home infusion or in an ambulatory infusion center. At this point, the frequency of amphotericin infusion is often reduced to every other day or more, depending on renal function. Follow-up MRI or CT scans at the end of therapy should demonstrate significant improvement and lack of inflammation (15). Physicians have observed chronic presentations and late sequelae after successful therapy; therefore, patients require long-term monitoring to detect recurrence or signs of indolent residual infection (16).

Measures to decrease the incidence of zygomycosis in patients at risk are difficult, at best. There is no routine antifungal prophylaxis available, and with the low prevalence of zygomycosis, there is no real indication to provide it. With rare exception, mycoses are not transmissible from patient to patient. Gown, glove, or mask isolation of hospitalized patients with mycoses is not indicated. The most common preventive interventions attempted consist of modifications and controls in the environment that reduce the risk of exposure to airborne spores. Most of these control measures are focused on easily identified patients at risk, i.e., those expected to be profoundly neutropenic for prolonged periods. The most effective, and expensive, method of protection is to confine the patient to a hospital room supplied with sterile laminar airflow. Although this measure reduces the risk of disease to an insignificant level, infection can still develop if patients are moved from the protected environment to other areas of the hospital for performance of essential procedures. Transplantation and chemotherapeutic wards are often isolated with Hepafilter treatment of the air supply and positive pressure to exclude the recruitment of dust into the ward, which provides significant protection. Dust should be kept to a minimum in the environment that houses these neutropenic patients. Additionally, flower arrangements and live plants are often excluded from such wards since they may harbor a variety of fungal agents. Patients, when neutropenic below 1000/mL, are asked to wear masks when leaving the cancer or transplant wards, particularly when going outside. The monitoring of air quality, particularly during times of building renovation and excavation in the vicinity of transplant centers, is also an important infection-control measure.

Preventive measures for patients other than the transplant and chemotherapy population require addressing the underlying risk factors for developing zygomycosis. Adequate control of diabetes, the use of iron chelators other than deferoxamine (such as substitution of hydroxypyridinone chelators for deferoxamine in patients who require such therapy), limitation of the use of aluminum-containing buffers in dialysis, and aggressive direct and culture-based detection of zygomycosis are among the best preventive measures. Keeping a high level of suspicion for zygomycosis in patients at risk can aid in early diagnosis and implementation of appropriate therapy.

SUMMARY

With the increasing prevalence of diabetes and immunosuppressive conditions, zygomycosis has emerged as an important fungal infection. The increasing number of organ transplantations and new immunosuppressant therapies also may be changing the demographics of this disease. In the setting of diabetes mellitus, hematological or solid-organ malignancies, transplantation, neutropenia, steroid therapy, and other immunocompromising conditions, the *Mucorales* tend to produce angioinvasive disease. Approximately 12% of fungal infections in patients with hematologic diseases have been found to be caused by the order *Mucorales*, the best-known pathogens being of the family *Mucoraceae,* including the genera *Rhizopus*, *Absidia*, *Mucor*, and *Rhizomucor*. The disease manifestation differs tremendously, depending upon the organism causing the disease and upon the underlying risk factor for acquiring the disease. The full spectrum of disease seen with these agents includes rhinocerebral, pulmonary, cutaneous, abdominal-pelvic and gastric, and disseminated presentations. Diagnosis of mucormycosis remains a major problem. Even in the presence of hematogenous dissemination of fungi, blood cultures are negative, and the detection of specific antibodies in patients with mucormycosis has revealed poor sensitivity and specificity. Therefore, tissue biopsy and histologic identification of fungi remain the gold standard of diagnosis. Because the diagnosis is often made after death, the real incidence of mucormycosis may be underestimated. A high degree of suspicion, careful clinical examination, precise radiologic localization, and early aggressive treatment of mucormycosis are essential for the outcome of patients with an otherwise very poor prognosis. Therapy should begin immediately upon suspicion of diagnosis. Optimal treatment of mucormycosis involves both aggressive surgical debridement and appropriate systemic antifungal therapy. In particular, early surgical intervention has been associated with improved prognosis and survival rate. Overall, disease with the *Mucorales* tends to be fulminant and is fatal in all cases if not aggressively treated.

REFERENCES

1. Platauf AP. Mycosis mucorina. Virchows Arch 1885; 102:543–564.
2. Harris JS. Mucormycosis; report of a case. Pediatrics 1955; 16(6):857–867.
3. Gass JD. Acute orbital mucormycosis. Report of two cases. Arch Ophthalmol 1961; 65:214–220.
4. Rees JR, Pinner RW, Hajjeh RA, et al. The epidemiological features of invasive mycotic infections in the San Francisco Bay area, 1992–1993: results of population-based laboratory active surveillance. Clin Infect Dis 1998; 27(5):1138–1147.
5. Kontoyiannis DP, Wessel VC, Bodey GP, et al. Zygomycosis in the 1990s in a tertiary-care cancer center. Clin Infect Dis 2000; 30(6):851–856.
6. Yohai RA, Bullock JD, Aziz AA, et al. Survival factors in rhino–orbital–cerebral mucormycosis. Surv Ophthalmol 1994; 39(1):3–22.
7. Segal BH, Walsh TJ. Opportunistic fungal infections. In: Cohen J, Powderly W, eds. Infectious Diseases. Vol. 1, 2nd ed. New York: Mosby, 2004:1161–1162.
8. Hostetter MK. Fungal infections in childhood. In: Gershon AA, Hoetz PJ, Katz SL, eds. Krugman's Infectious Diseases of Children. Vol. 1, 11th ed. Philadelphia, PA: Mosby, 2004:187–201.
9. Abramson E, Wilson D, Arky RA. Rhinocerebral phycomycosis in association with diabetic ketoacidosis. Report of two cases and a review of clinical and experimental experience with amphotericin B therapy. Ann Intern Med 1967; 66(4):735–742.
10. Kline MW. Mucormycosis in children: review of the literature and report of cases. Pediatr Infect Dis 1985; 4(6):672–676.
11. Schwartz JC. Rhinocerebral mucormycosis: three case reports and subject review. J Emerg Med 1985; 3(1):11–19.
12. Blitzer A. Patient survival factors in paranasal sinus mucormycosis. Laryngoscope 1980; 90 (4):635–648.
13. Giiter MF, Henderson LT, Afsari KK. Adjunctive hyperbaric oxygen therapy in the treatment of rhinocerebral mucormycosis. Infect Med 1996; 13:130–136.
14. Warwar RE, Bullock JD. Rhino-orbital-cerebral mucormycosis: a review. Orbit 1998; 17(4):237–245.
15. Peterson KL, Wang M, Canalis RF, et al. Rhinocerebral mucormycosis: evolution of the disease and treatment options. Laryngoscope 1997; 107(7):855–862.
16. Sugar AM. Mucormycosis. Clin Infect Dis 1992; 14(suppl 1):S126–S129.

15

Syphilis

Jacob Husseman
*Department of Surgery, Division of Otolaryngology-Head and Neck Surgery,
University of California, San Diego, California, U.S.A.*

Terence M. Davidson
*Department of Surgery, Division of Otolaryngology-Head and Neck Surgery,
University of California and VA San Diego Healthcare System, San Diego, California,
U.S.A.*

INTRODUCTION

Syphilis, "The Great Imitator," with its myriad manifestations, is a disease with a rich background, colorful history, and never-ending speculation. The very origin remains controversial. The Columbian theory proposes that syphilis is a disease of the New World that was carried back to the European continent by Columbus and his sailors. Chronologically, this is supported by an outbreak of the disease in Naples in 1494 with documentary evidence linking Columbus's crew to the event. Additionally, syphilitic lesions have been noted in discovered remains of precontact Native Americans. The alternative suggests that the disease was present, at least in some form, pre-Columbus and spread through Europe with developing urbanization. Proponents refer to sporadic documentation of syphilitic symptoms throughout Europe prior to Columbus's era and note descriptions of similar symptoms described by Hippocrates and possibly dating back to biblical passages. Furthermore, it has been suggested that systemic syphilis evolved from a microbiological cousin, *Treponema pertenue*, a subspecies of *Treponema pallidum*. This organism certainly existed in the early European era and was the source of yaws, a localized soft-tissue infection primarily afflicting children. It has also been proposed that both theories have some truth to them, and in fact, the Old World and New World strains of *T. pallidum* merged, resulting in the entity later known as syphilis.

Regardless of the origin, the first major outbreak of what is believed to be modern-day syphilis spread through the late fifteenth and into the sixteenth century. This was dubbed the Great Pox and produced significant morbidity and mortality with the spread of armies and population throughout Europe. It was first named *morbus gallicus*, or the "French disease," due to an outbreak in the French army; however, finger-pointing was prevalent, with Italians and Dutch also calling it the "Spanish disease," Germans and Russians calling it the "Polish disease," French naming it the "English disease" and "Italian disease," and the Arab population referring to the "Disease of the Christians."

While the lack of microbiology in that era precludes the confirmation of *T. pallidum* as the source of the outbreak, the disease process, including its sexual transmission, was well documented in the sixteenth century. In 1530, it received its current moniker, syphilis, at the hand of the Italian physician and scientist Girolamo Fracastoro. In his poem entitled "Syphilis, sive Morbus Gallicus," or "Syphilis, or the French Disease," he describes a shepherd by the name of Syphilis who is afflicted with the disease after disobeying the commands of Apollo.

From its original outbreak, which has been described as having an impact similar to the twentieth-century development of AIDS, syphilis continued with epidemic waves. However, while the original affliction was much more virulent, with rapid progression and more severe symptoms, further epidemics resembled the more indolent disease process with which we are now familiar. These were particularly pronounced during the Napoleonic wars, nineteenth-century industrialization, and World Wars I and II. Over the years, many notable figures are alleged or speculated to have been afflicted with syphilis, including Franz Schubert, Friedrich Nietzsche, Paul Gauguin, Vincent van Gogh, Oscar Wilde, Joseph Stalin, James Joyce, Al Capone, and Howard Hughes. While not often considered a disease of the modern era, it remained the leading cause of neurological and cardiovascular disease of middle-aged individuals as late as the early 1900s (1). At the turn of the twentieth century, syphilis picked up the nickname "lues" from the Latin phrase "*lues venereum*," which translates as "disease" or "pestilence." The term was applied generally to sexually transmitted diseases but then was used primarily as a substitute for syphilis, although the phrase is found infrequently in modern literature.

During the twentieth century, our understanding of syphilis rapidly progressed with a few key events. Fritz Schaudinn and Erich Hoffmann identified the spirochete *T. pallidum* from serum in 1905. One year later, August von Wassermann developed a complement fixation test to detect antibodies against the bacteria, allowing identification of millions of previously undiagnosed individuals. Paul Ehrlich then began his work with arsenic derivatives and in 1910 patented arsphenamine, which was found to be a significant improvement in treatment, though plagued by recurrences. The discovery of penicillin by Alexander Fleming in 1928 led to John Mahoney's breakthrough demonstration of this antibiotic's utility in treating syphilis in 1943. Penicillin was widely available by the post–World-War-II era, and in combination with public health measures, it facilitated the near-eradication of this historical plague. However, this effective treatment has left most current health-care providers relatively unfamiliar with the disease, with many never having seen a case of syphilis. Recent epidemiological data demonstrate an increasing incidence, particularly among the population of men who have sex with men. As such, a review of syphilis including its head and neck manifestations is of timely benefit.

DEFINITION

Syphilis is caused by the gram-negative spirochete *T. pallidum*. As referred to in the introduction, there are several subspecies of *T. pallidum*. Although there is striking antigenic and genetic overlap within the species, the other subspecies including *endemicum*, *pertenue*, and *carateum* are generally of little virulence and produce nonvenereal disease. The name *T. pallidum* is commonly used to refer to subspecies *pallidum*, the etiology of syphilis. These spiral-shaped bacteria are approximately 5 to 15 μm long and roughly 0.2 μm in width (Fig. 1). The bacterium is surrounded by an outer membrane rich in phospholipids but relatively free of exposed surface proteins. It demonstrates corkscrew motility by way of endoflagella, which attach to either end of the organism and wrap around the body between the cytoplasmic membrane and the outer membrane. Darkfield microscopy is utilized for visualization of the bacteria, and the characteristic movement patterns of *T. pallidum* allow visual differentiation from other nonpathogenic treponemes (2).

T. pallidum has one of the smallest genomes among known bacteria and lacks many genes required for the synthesis of necessary compounds. It achieves glycolysis but scavenges many of its metabolic requirements from the host. The organism is actually quite fragile and does not live outside of a mammalian host; humans are the only known natural vectors. It cannot be cultured on artificial media, though there has been some success with growth in tissue culture, typically using rabbit testis. The difficulty with growing *T. pallidum* in the laboratory has translated to a relative paucity of information regarding its pathogenic features. There are no known virulence factors to distinguish *T. pallidum* from other nonpathogenic treponeme species. It is known to be capable of invasion and survival

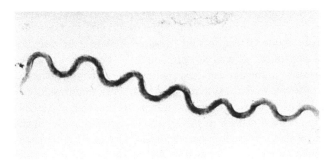

FIGURE 1 This photomicrograph shows the unique spiral morphology of *Treponema pallidum*. *Source:* Courtesy of the CDC Public Health Image Library; special thanks to Bill Schwartz.

in a wide variety of tissues and organs, based on its various clinical manifestations as well as findings in animal models. Nonetheless, the nature of this invasion is not yet understood. It may be related to the organism's ability to attach to a large diversity of cell types including epithelial, fibroblastic, and endothelial by way of adhesion molecules. Nonpathologic treponemal species do not adhere to cultured cells (3).

EPIDEMIOLOGY

Though more likely to affect individuals who belong to lower socioeconomic groups, lack access to healthcare, or have multiple sexual partners, syphilis is a venereal disease found worldwide. The World Health Organization estimated that 12 million new cases of syphilis occurred in 1999, largely in developing countries, where it remains a leading cause of perinatal and neonatal deaths (4).

As noted earlier, after the first outbreak of syphilis in the 15th century, the disease remained quite common throughout Europe with periodic epidemic flares. It spread throughout the United States with similar numbers. The U.S. Surgeon General of 1937, Thomas Parran, considered it the greatest health problem in the United States and estimated that 10% of Americans would be infected with syphilis at some point (1). The reporting of syphilis and recording of statistical data began in 1941, when there were over 100,000 primary and secondary cases in the United States. Public health measures and early use of penicillin dropped the incidence to 66.4 cases per 100,000 in 1947, and widespread use of penicillin nearly eradicated the disease by 1956, with only 3.9 cases per 100,000. Over the following decades, the incidence waxed and waned, with a few minor epidemics. By the 1970s, syphilis in the United States was found primarily among the homosexual male population. With the outbreak of HIV, the 1980s brought a new epidemic, and increased numbers of heterosexual and congenital syphilis were noted. A peak of 20 cases per 100,000 developed in 1990. Further public health measures and a Centers for Disease Control and Prevention (CDC)-sponsored plan to eradicate the disease facilitated gradual decline to a nadir of 2.1 cases per 100,000 in 2000 (5,6).

The latest data available from the CDC indicate that after a 13-year decline, the incidence of primary and secondary syphilis again increased in the United States, with a rate of 2.7 cases per 100,000 in 2004. This increase was attributed largely to an outbreak among men who have sex with men, with an estimated 64% of all reported cases from this population. Racial disparities continue to persist, with the rate among African Americans about six times higher than that among Caucasians (6). The distribution throughout the United States is highly skewed to the southeastern states, where syphilis remains an epidemic for unclear reasons. The disease is prevalent during the years of peak sexual activity, with most new cases affecting those 15 to 30 years old.

PATHOGENESIS

Direct sexual contact is the primary mode of acquisition, though syphilis can also be passed by close contact with an active lesion, as well as congenitally. The risk of disease spread with sexual intercourse is greatest in the early stages, particularly when the primary lesion, or chancre, is present. Risk of sexual transmission remains high when manifestations of secondary syphilis are present, but as it progresses to latent syphilis, the risk of sexual transmission is thought to be nearly resolved as long as the host is immunologically intact (7). While transmission to the anogenital region is most common, any contact with an active lesion, especially with a primary chancre, can transmit the organism through small breaches in the epithelial surface. Oropharyngeal mucosa involvement is therefore noted with some frequency. Congenital syphilis is typically seen with fetal infection in utero upon *T. pallidum* crossing the placental barrier. However, infection can also occur during passage through the birth canal. Transmission is most likely when the mother is in early stages of syphilis; nonetheless, there remains potential for fetal infection even in latent syphilis. Blood-borne transmission via transfusion or needle-stick is theoretically possible, though exceptionally rare.

CLINICAL MANIFESTATIONS

William Osler was quoted as stating, "He who knows syphilis, knows medicine." Its multiple organ system involvement and diverse presentations have earned syphilis the title of the great imitator. Certainly, one could rarely be faulted for including the disease in a differential diagnosis. The manifestations of syphilis are largely dependent on the stage of the disease. We will review these in order, with a focus on the pathology found in the head and neck.

Primary Syphilis

Primary syphilis is defined by the presence of a chancre that develops at the site of inoculation. The initial lesion usually appears approximately three weeks after infection, although the incubation period can range from 10 to 90 days. The primary chancre appears as a single painless papule, and can often go unnoticed by the patient. After a short time, the lesion will become indurated, and then erode and ulcerate. The lesion generally remains clean and dry unless secondary infection occurs. Regional lymphadenopathy commonly presents within one week of the chancre's appearance. The lesion will spontaneously resolve in a period of three to six weeks, although adenopathy may persist slightly longer. Darkfield examination of exudate from a lesion will demonstrate numerous motile spirochetes and is the gold standard for diagnosis.

Although the site of inoculation usually involves the anogenital region, with the external genitalia being the most common location for a primary chancre, syphilis also presents with head and neck manifestations. After the external genitalia, the lips are the next most common site of chancre formation (Fig. 2). Inoculation can occur throughout the oral cavity, with the tongue and tonsil most likely to be involved. Lesions of the oral cavity are more likely to become superinfected. Though much more rare, chancres involving the

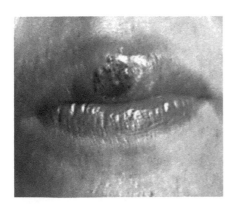

FIGURE 2 A chancre is the defining lesion of primary syphilis. This image demonstrates a chancre of the lip, the most common site of presentation after the external genitalia. *Source:* Courtesy of the CDC Public Health Image Library.

larynx and the nose have also been reported. Cervical adenopathy is frequently associated with such primary infections of the head and neck region.

Secondary Syphilis

Approximately eight weeks after the initial presentation of a chancre, a generalized infection ensues. This is a result of proliferation and systemic dissemination of *T. pallidum* and persists until a sufficient immune response develops. Constitutional symptoms including fever, headache, arthralgias, malaise, pharyngitis, and generalized lymphadeno-pathy are common. The dominant feature of secondary syphilis is a mucocutaneous rash, which appears in 90% of patients. While there is significant variation, the characteristic rash begins as small pink to red macules symmetrically distributed on the trunk and extremities, also involving mucous membranes. This will progress to a papular rash and spread to the distal extremities to involve the palms and soles. Eventually the rash will develop a coppery color and become papulosquamous. It will often have the appearance of pityriasis rosea and follow skin cleavage lines, although distinguishable by its involvement with the palms and soles. The timeframe for resolution of this rash is quite variable, ranging from a few days to several months. Sometimes the papules coalesce into moist, broad plaques, called condyloma lata, that are typically gray-white in appearance. These plaques are highly infectious and tend to form in moist skin folds.

With the hematogenous spread of the bacteria, nearly any organ system can be involved in secondary syphilis. The kidneys may demonstrate acute nephrotic syndrome and glomerulonephritis secondary to immune-complex injury. Direct liver invasion will lead to syphilitic hepatitis. The intestine may be involved, showing wall thickening or ulceration, which sometimes can be confused with malignancy. Synovitis and periosteitis have also been described, and uveitis is not uncommon.

One of the areas in which head and neck manifestations become apparent is with central nervous system (CNS) involvement, which may occur in up to 40% of secondary syphilis. This most commonly presents with headache and meningismus; acute aseptic meningitis will be apparent in 1% to 2% of patients (7). Symptoms of visual disturbance, hearing loss, tinnitus, dizziness, and facial weakness may appear with cranial nerve or temporal bone involvement. Nerves II through VIII are affected most frequently. Labyrinthine involvement in secondary syphilis is more likely to produce abrupt, bilateral, rapidly progressive hearing loss, with vestibular symptoms less frequent. CNS involvement may also produce various distal neurologic deficits. The likelihood of progressing to late neurosyphilis is increased with CNS involvement during secondary syphilis; approximately 8% to 10% of untreated patients will do so (7).

Other head and neck manifestations of secondary syphilis are related to the initial mucocutaneous rash (Fig. 3). Facial lesions will follow the hairline of the temporal and frontal scalp and also present with cracking papules at the corners of the lips. Involvement of hair follicles can lead to temporary alopecia in the scalp, beard, eyebrows, and eyelashes. There may be superficial scaling of the skin, including the face and neck, termed "papulosquamous syphilids." Hypopigmented lesions called collaris veneris may appear on the lateral neck. Similar to the condylomata lata that develop in moist skin folds, the mucous membrane lesions of the rash may coalesce into lesions known as mucous patches (Fig. 4). They may present throughout the upper aerodigestive tract. Mucous patches are usually asymptomatic and appear as a slightly elevated flat plaque covered by a silvery gray membrane with a mildly erythematous periphery. As with the condylomata lata, these lesions are teeming with spirochetes and are highly infectious. They may become painful with secondary infection. Laryngeal involvement may produce laryngitis and hoarseness,

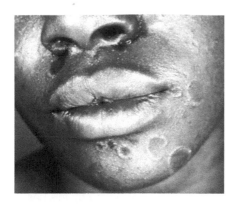

FIGURE 3 The rash of secondary syphilis can involve the face, as seen in this image illustrating the annular papulosquamous lesions. *Source:* Courtesy of the CDC Public Health Image Library; special thanks to Susan Lindsley.

while nasal involvement tends to present as acute rhinitis with scant thick discharge and mucosal inflammation.

Secondary syphilis symptoms persist for a variable time frame, but generally will resolve within one year. Once the lesions of secondary syphilis have resolved, an individual is considered to be in the latent phase. The first year of this period is considered the early latent phase, during which infected individuals maintain a higher potential for disease transmission. Relapses of secondary syphilis do occur and tend to do so in the early latent phase. Immunocompromised patients are at greater risk for recurrence, which tends to be milder than the initial symptoms. If an individual had not been diagnosed in the primary stage, consistent clinical symptoms and positive serologic testing will confirm syphilis in the secondary stage.

Tertiary Syphilis
Latent syphilis is defined as the period of persistent positive testing with a specific treponemal antibody assay in the absence of disease manifestations. Prospective data regarding untreated syphilis indicate that one-third of patients will clear the disease, one-third will persist with latent syphilis, and one-third will progress to late or tertiary syphilis (8). With the advent of penicillin treatment, late syphilis is rarely seen today. When the disease does advance to the tertiary stage, it involves a slowly progressive inflammatory process. Latent syphilis can persist for years to decades before the manifestations of late syphilis present. As with secondary syphilis, tertiary syphilis can involve nearly any organ

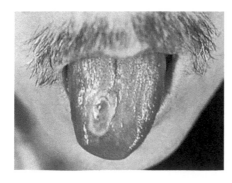

FIGURE 4 A mucous patch characteristic of secondary syphilis. These lesions affecting the mucosal surfaces of the oral cavity and oropharynx are teeming with *Treponema pallidum* and are highly infectious. *Source:* Courtesy of the CDC Public Health Image Library; special thanks to Susan Lindsley.

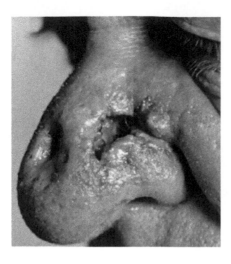

FIGURE 5 When syphilis goes untreated, gummas may develop nearly anywhere during the tertiary stage. Though benign, these lesions are locally destructive as demonstrated by this nasal gumma. *Source:* Courtesy of the CDC Public Health Image Library; special thanks to Susan Lindsley.

system; however, the hallmark findings include gummatous syphilis, neurosyphilis, and cardiovascular syphilis.

The gumma is a granulomatous lesion that can appear in any organ but typically affects the mucocutaneous surfaces and skeletal system. While considered benign, they can be locally destructive, and symptoms, if any, are related to the organ system involved. They vary in size from microscopic nodules to large masses. They begin as irregularly shaped nodules or plaques with a tendency toward central necrosis and ulceration (Fig. 5). When skin lesions ulcerate, they tend to heal with thin, atrophic scars and leave punched-out lesions. Though gummas can develop anywhere, there is a predilection for the arms, back, and face, and may be triggered by minor trauma. Complications within the head and neck can include palatal perforation, saddle-nose deformity secondary to destruction of nasal cartilage, and glossitis. Gummatous involvement of the larynx can produce hoarseness or late complications of subglottic stenosis, vocal cord adhesions, or arytenoid fixation. Gummas can also be seen in the middle ear with resulting tympanic membrane perforation or erosion of the ossicles. Biopsy of a lesion often fails to demonstrate spirochetes and it is thought that gummas represent an intense inflammatory response to a few bacteria. The lesions tend to respond well to antibiotic therapy.

While infrequently seen now, neurosyphilis had significant impact in the past. It is estimated to have caused 5% to 10% of first-time admissions to U.S. mental health hospitals prior to World War II and widespread availability of penicillin (9). As discussed previously, hematogenous dissemination and direct invasion can produce acute neurosyphilis during the secondary stage; however, the CNS can also be involved in tertiary neurosyphilis. Most commonly, this infection is asymptomatic and picked up with an abnormal finding on cerebrospinal fluid (CSF) analysis. This may occur in up to 40% of untreated syphilitics (7). As this asymptomatic infection is curable with antibiotic therapy, lumbar puncture should be performed if the adequacy of prior treatment is in question.

The pathology of symptomatic tertiary neurosyphilis is divided among parenchymatous and meningovascular neurosyphilis, although a combination of the two is nearly always present. The former is an insidious process involving direct destruction of neurons and has a peak incidence of 10 to 20 years after infection. Cerebral cortex destruction can cause general paresis while involvement of the spinal cord may lead to a clinical entity known as tabes dorsalis. This results from demyelinization of the posterior column as well as dorsal roots and ganglia. The manifestations include hypotonia, areflexia, a wide-based ataxic gait, paresthesias, sudden paroxysms of lower limb pains known as lightning pains, bowel and bladder dysfunction, and loss of positional, vibratory, and temperature sensation. Optic involvement is also common, with most cases demonstrating the classic Argyll-Robertson pupil that is unreactive to light but will accommodate to near vision. Gun barrel sight also develops with progressive degeneration of the optic nerve working inward from the periphery, leaving the patient with intact vision but a narrowed visual field. Though rarely seen any longer, tabes dorsalis was the most common presentation of late syphilis prior to penicillin treatment. Parenchymatous disease also produces cognitive decline and psychiatric symptoms with hallucinations and slowly progressive dementia.

Meningovascular neurosyphilis presents slightly earlier, usually 5 to 10 years after infection. As opposed to the destructive nature of parenchymatous disease, this is an inflammatory process and is characterized by endarteritis obliterans involving the small vessels of the meninges, brain, and spinal cord. The symptoms typically begin abruptly relating to multiple small areas of infarction, most commonly in the distribution of the middle cerebral artery. The clinical outcome entails a wide spectrum but can include hemiparesis, aphasia, and seizures.

The aspect of neurosyphilis most relevant to the otolaryngologist is the phenomenon of otosyphilis, historically known as luetic otitis or labyrinthitis. While otic involvement can develop at any stage of the disease, it is typically seen as a late manifestation of tertiary neurosyphilis. The pathology and symptoms seen in late otosyphilis are distinct from what is seen in early disease. While otic involvement in early syphilis is related to treponeme-induced labyrinthitis and direct neuritis of cranial nerve VIII, late otosyphilis demonstrates the obliterative endarteritis characteristic of tertiary neurosyphilis. This produces a periostitis of the otic capsule, particularly the semicircular canals. Gummatous involvement may enhance the osteitis and periostitis. Eventually, the membranous labyrinth undergoes atrophy and fibrosis. The endolymphatic sac and duct become narrowed. Middle-ear involvement can produce fibrosis of the ossicles with a resulting conductive hearing loss (10). The hearing loss of late otosyphilis begins at high frequencies but may progress to complete loss if untreated. While early syphilis usually entails abrupt, bilateral loss, tertiary disease tends to have an indolent nature and often begins quite asymmetrically, so as to seem only a unilateral loss. Vestibular symptoms are much more prevalent in tertiary otosyphilis and often are associated with the tinnitus and fluctuating hearing of Ménière's disease. Tertiary otosyphilis classically presents between 5 and 15 years after infection but may develop as late as 50 years later. Coinfection with HIV tends to accelerate and intensify the process, with symptoms often appearing within the first five years and progressing more rapidly (11).

The final area of particular interest in tertiary syphilis is cardiovascular involvement. Similar to the meningovascular pathology of neurosyphilis, the cardiovascular system is also affected by endarteritis obliterans. It affects the vaso vasorum, predominantly of the ascending aorta, and appears 10 to 30 years after the initial infection. The result is necrosis of the elastic tissue of the medial aortic wall, leading to saccular aneurysms. Affected individuals are often asymptomatic, with aneurysms detected on chest radiography performed for other reasons. Proximal disease may lead to stretching of the aortic valve and insufficiency, which in turn may lead to left ventricular failure. The aneurysms rarely dissect due to extensive scarring but can potentially rupture. Symptomatic disease presents in approximately 10% of untreated syphilitics, but pathologic lesions have been found at autopsy in up to 83% of those with untreated neurosyphilis (12). With regard to otolaryngologic manifestations, these aneurysms are of interest due to potential compression against the recurrent laryngeal nerve and resulting dysphonia.

Congenital Syphilis

Fetal infection with syphilis is highly dependent on the mother's stage of disease. Mothers with untreated primary or secondary disease are extremely likely to pass the infection, while those with latent disease have rates of transmission as low as 2%. Appropriate treatment of the mother during pregnancy generally prevents fetal infection. When infection does occur, the outcome can range from spontaneous abortion to a healthy-appearing child at birth with only latent infection.

Similar to acquired syphilis, congenital infection is divided into early and late stages. There are often no abnormalities noted at birth, but exam or diagnostic findings are nearly always present by three months of age. However, the severity of early disease can range from asymptomatic imaging findings to severe, life-threatening multiorgan/system disease. Early congenital syphilis characteristically first presents with a serosanguinous nasal discharge and rhinitis known as snuffles. The rash of early syphilis is a diffuse maculopapular rash that develops into epithelial sloughing. Vesicles or bullae may also be present and the fluid within is highly infectious. Oral mucous patches are often seen. Facial lesions on the lips and nose, as well as anal lesions, may heal with radiating scars known as rhagades. Visceral involvement is relatively frequent, with the liver often heavily infected, leading to jaundice, splenomegaly, anemia, and thrombocytopenia. Bony abnormalities related to osteochondritis and periostitis are prevalent and are particularly noted in the long bones on imaging. CNS involvement is common in early congenital syphilis.

Children who survive the early disease manifestations will then enter a latent phase. Late symptoms may present years to decades later. Skeletal defects from the osteochondritis and periostitis are quite notable, with characteristic facies consisting of a high arched palate, protruding mandible, frontal bossing, and saddle-nose deformity. Other structural defects include palatal and nasal septum perforations, anterior bowing of the lower extremities known as saber shins, and bilateral knee effusions termed Clutton's joints. Hutchinson's triad consists of eighth nerve deafness, interstitial keratitis, and peg-shaped, centrally notched, widely spaced central incisors known as Hutchinson's teeth. Congenital otosyphilis is usually more severe than that seen with acquired syphilis. It typically presents with sudden onset, profound, bilateral hearing loss with rare vestibular symptoms. Untreated, congenital syphilis frequently progresses to neurosyphilis with sequelae similar to the acquired form of disease.

DIAGNOSIS

There are four general modalities used in diagnostic testing for syphilis: histopathology, darkfield microscopy, serology, and CSF examination. Histopathology employing Warthin–Starry staining or with specific immunofluorescent antibody preparations is sometimes used on biopsy tissue of late syphilitic lesions if darkfield examination is unavailable. Otherwise, histopathology is largely reserved for autopsy material. Darkfield microscopy is considered the gold standard and quickest method of diagnosis with primary, secondary, and early congenital syphilis. Transudate from a moist primary chancre, condyloma latum, or mucous patch is examined under darkfield for the characteristic corkscrew appearance and spiraling motion. Aspirates from lymph nodes may also be useful, particularly in secondary syphilis. Oral lesions should not be used, as *T. pallidum* can be confused with nonpathogenic treponemes normally found in the oral cavity.

There are two types of serologic testing for syphilis: standard nontreponemal and specific treponemal antibody tests. Nontreponemal tests are quick and inexpensive, making them ideal for screening. The specific treponemal antibody tests are more specific for either current or past infection. Generally, a nontreponemal test is first used for screening and then infection is confirmed with a specific antibody test.

Four types of nontreponemal tests exist. These are all based on an antigen developed from the Venereal Disease Research Laboratory (VDRL), which consists of cardiolipin, cholesterol, and lecithin. They screen for IgG and IgM antibodies directed against this antigen, which is produced when host cells interact with *T. pallidum*. The antigen was originally generated from extracts of beef livers and hearts and was found to cross-react with antibodies produced with syphilis infection, albeit with many false-positives. The antigen has since been purified and is now more specific; however, false-positives may still be seen in association with pregnancy, other spirochete infections, multiple viral or bacterial infections, and various autoimmune diseases. Nonetheless, the tests remain 97% to 98% specific (2). In addition to the VDRL test, the other nontreponemal tests include the rapid plasma reagin (RPR), unheated serum reagin (USR), and toluidine red unheated serum test (TRUST). The nontreponemal tests do not turn positive until one to four weeks after development of a primary chancre. All of the tests are quantitative with the highest titers in secondary syphilis. In fact, particularly high antibody titers seen in secondary disease and pregnancy can produce a prozone phenomenon with false-negative testing. This can be corrected with serum dilution. Given the quantitative nature, the nontreponemal tests are quite useful in assessing response to treatment. After successful treatment, a nontreponemal assay should become nonreactive within one year in a case of primary syphilis or within two years when treating secondary disease. Tertiary syphilis may take up to five years before testing turns negative after adequate treatment (7).

In addition to the nontreponemal tests, there are several assays, which measure antibodies specific for *T. pallidum*. The two primary tests are the fluorescent treponemal antibody absorption (FTA-abs) and the microhemagglutination assay for antibodies to *T. pallidum* (MHA-TP). The MHA-TP is somewhat easier to use than the FTA-abs, but slightly less sensitive in early disease. There is no strong persuasion to use one test over the other, and both continue to be used throughout laboratories worldwide. These specific antibody tests are significantly more expensive than the nontreponemal tests and thus are generally only used for confirmation of the diagnosis. Once positive, the tests usually remain positive for life, and repeat testing is not indicated. However, about 10% of patients may revert to a nonreactive result after treatment.

If neurosyphilis is suspected, CSF examination can be used to confirm the diagnosis. CSF testing is not necessarily indicated for routine primary and secondary syphilis, although certain conditions may prompt it. These include treatment failure, evidence of tertiary disease including gumma or aortitis, HIV infection, or known neurologic, ophthalmic, or auditory symptoms. The most commonly employed test is the CSF-VDRL, which is highly specific though insensitive. A moderate mononuclear pleocytosis and elevated protein level in the CSF are also suggestive of neurosyphilis in the correct clinical setting. The FTA-abs test should not be used with CSF, as traces of blood may produce a false-positive result.

Diagnosis of otosyphilis remains somewhat problematic, especially in those patients with no known history of congenital or acquired syphilis. It is a diagnosis of exclusion, and has been defined as a positive serologic test for syphilis with otherwise unexplained hearing loss or vestibular disturbance (10). Confirmation as well as evaluation for active neuro-syphilis can be achieved by CSF analysis including CSF-VDRL. The benefit of routine syphilis screening in patients with idiopathic sensorineural hearing loss is called into question by an investigation showing a positive result in only 1 of 182 patients (13). Other studies, however, have suggested otosyphilis to be the cause of 6.5% of previously unexplained sensorineural hearing loss and 7% of Ménière's disease (14,15). As syphilitic cochleovestibular dysfunction may be treatable, especially if early in the process, these statistics suggest screening may be worthwhile, especially in those patients with risk factors.

TREATMENT

Parenteral penicillin G is the standard therapy for syphilis. While this treatment has been used for over 50 years and its efficacy is well established, the recommendation is based on clinical studies and expert opinion rather than randomized clinical trials (16). It has been found that adequate treatment requires serum concentrations to be maintained above a threshold of 0.03 units/mL for 10 days (17). A single intramuscular dose of 2.4 million units of penicillin G will maintain a supratherapeutic level for two weeks. The CDC provides treatment recommendations based on the stage of disease, as well as associated comorbidities and other special circumstances (Table 1).

While a single dose of intramuscular penicillin G has been found to be highly effective in the early stages of syphilis, other situations may require more extensive treatment. Gummatous and cardiovascular tertiary syphilis should be treated with weekly doses of penicillin G given for three weeks. With one-third of latent syphilis cases advancing to the tertiary stage, those in the late or unknown stages of latency should also receive this regimen. Although not officially recommended by the CDC, many practitioners favor the extended three-week treatment for patients coinfected with HIV, even if only in the early stages of syphilis. All of these individuals should also undergo CSF examination prior to therapy to assess for possible CNS involvement. Neurosyphilis requires special care, as adequate bactericidal levels of antibiotic are not found in the CSF after a single dose of penicillin G (18). It is therefore recommended that neurosyphilis patients be treated with a 10- to-14-day course of intravenous penicillin and followed closely with serial testing of the CSF to ensure eradication. Pregnant women should receive treatment appropriate to the stage of their disease. As no other antibiotic has been shown to effectively treat the fetus, penicillin-allergic patients should undergo desensitization. If congenital infection does occur, the CDC recommends at least a 10-day course of intravenous aqueous penicillin G.

Data regarding the management of otosyphilis are lacking and there are no prospective clinical trials to support any given regimen. General consensus from a prior review of the literature suggests that an extended treatment with penicillin in combination with steroids is indicated (19). This literature review revealed practices ranging from weekly intramuscular injections to multiple intravenous infusions daily, with length of treatment anywhere from 15 days to 1 year. The CDC currently recommends that auditory syphilitic disease be treated the same as neurosyphilis: aqueous penicillin G given as three to four million units intravenously every four hours for 10 to 14 days. For those with questionable follow-up, an alternative is a one-time intramuscular dose of 2.4 million units of penicillin G followed by probenecid 500 mg orally, four times daily for 10 to 14 days. Data regarding corticosteroid usage are also lacking, and the above-referenced review by Darmstadt and Harris revealed a wide discrepancy in treatment regimens, but a tendency for better outcomes with combined antibiotic and steroid therapy. Their recommendation entails 40 to 60 mg of prednisone daily for a minimum of two weeks. If improvement occurs, the steroid can be slowly tapered until recurrence of symptoms. Long-term maintenance, if needed, should consist of alternate-day dosing.

Recommended follow-up is dependent on the stage at the time of treatment and should include serial serologic testing. Those with early syphilis should be assessed at 3, 6, and 12 months with expected seronegativity by one year. Patients with late latent or gummatous disease should have follow-up extended to two years to ensure seronegative

TABLE 1 CDC Recommended Syphilis Treatment Regimens

Stage/comorbidity	Primary recommendation	Alternative therapy
Primary, secondary, or early latent disease in adults	Benzathine penicillin G 2.4 million units i.m. in a single dose	Data for alternative treatments are lacking. These regimens have been used in nonpregnant, penicillin-allergic patients: doxycycline (100 mg orally twice daily for 14 days) or tetracycline (500 mg 4 times daily for 14 days)
Primary, secondary, or early latent disease in children	Benzathine penicillin G 50,000 units/kg i.m., up to the adult dose of 2.4 million units in a single dose	
Late latent syphilis or latent syphilis of unknown duration in adults	Benzathine penicillin G 7.2 million units total, administered as 3 doses of 2.4 million units i.m. each at 1 wk intervals	
Late latent syphilis or latent syphilis of unknown duration in children	Benzathine penicillin G 50,000 units/kg i.m., up to the adult dose of 2.4 million units, administered as 3 doses at 1 wk intervals (total 150,000 units/kg up to the adult total dose of 7.2 million units)	
Tertiary syphilis (gummatous or cardiovascular involvement; *not* neurosyphilis)	Benzathine penicillin G 7.2 million units total, administered as 3 doses of 2.4 million units i.m. each at 1 wk intervals	
Neurosyphilis (including otologic involvement)	Aqueous crystalline penicillin G 18–24 million units per day, administered as 3–4 million units i.v. every 4 hr or continuous infusion, for 10–14 days	If compliance is questioned: Procaine penicillin 2.4 million units i.m. once daily plus Probenecid 500 mg orally 4 times a day, both for 10–14 days
Primary and secondary syphilis among HIV-infected persons	Benzathine penicillin G, 2.4 million units i.m. in a single dose	
Latent syphilis among HIV-infected persons	Benzathine penicillin G, at weekly doses of 2.4 million units for 3 wk	
Syphilis during pregnancy	Treatment during pregnancy should consist of the penicillin regimen appropriate for the stage of syphilis	No alternatives to penicillin have been proven effective for treatment of syphilis during pregnancy. Pregnant women who have a history of penicillin allergy should be desensitized and treated with penicillin
Congenital syphilis	Aqueous crystalline penicillin G, 100–150,000 units/kg i.v. daily in 2 or 3 divided doses for a minimum of 10 days or procaine penicillin G, 50,000 U/kg i.m. daily for a minimum of 10 days	

Abbreviations: CDC, Centers for Disease Control and Prevention; i.m., intramuscular; i.v., intravenous.

results by the end of the second year. A fourfold increase in titers or lack of fourfold decrease in titers by 12 to 24 months suggests treatment failure (2). CSF examination and repeat treatment are then indicated. Cardiovascular involvement or neurosyphilis prompts the need for lifelong follow-up. Neurosyphilis should be followed with serologic and CSF examinations every three to six months until all antibody testing is negative.

COMPLICATIONS AND PROGNOSIS

A phenomenon known as the Jarisch–Herxheimer reaction is a known complication resulting from antibiotic treatment of syphilis, and patients should be informed before initiating therapy. This typically develops within the first few hours of treatment and presents with fever, tachycardia, mild hypotension, headache, myalgias, arthralgias, exacerbation of skin lesions, and sometimes obtundation. The reaction is self-limited, but tends to last 12 to 24 hours. It is more likely to occur in patients with secondary syphilis. The reaction may be more serious in pregnant women, who can enter early labor or develop fetal distress. Patients with neurosyphilis or cardiovascular syphilis may also experience more serious and sometimes life-threatening manifestations. The reaction is well managed with non-steroidal anti-inflammatory medications as well as prednisone.

It is also worthwhile to discuss the interaction between syphilis and HIV disease. Given that both are sexually transmitted and associated with at-risk sexual behaviors, coinfection is common. The two may interact and enhance transmission of each other. With concomitant HIV infection, syphilis tends to present more aggressively. There is a tendency for involvement of more organ systems, atypical rashes, and greater constitutional symptoms, as well as increased rate of progression to neurosyphilis. Treatment failure is also more frequent, likely relating to the underlying immunocompromised state. Serologic responses are often altered with HIV-coinfected patients, showing high antibody titers sometimes leading to false-positive surveillance testing after adequate treatment (7). Frequent, extended follow-up is critical in such coinfected patients.

When syphilis is treated early, the prognosis is excellent. Primary and secondary disease treated appropriately with penicillin G has shown an 89% to 95% cure rate with initial therapy (20). Of those who fail to improve, most will respond to a second treatment. Late syphilis typically can be halted from further progression, although existing neurologic and cardiovascular injury cannot be reversed. Scarring from prior destructive mucocutaneous lesions will also remain, to varying degrees. Due to T. pallidum's ability to access tissues that are less immune-accessible, such as the eye, ear, and CNS, infection may remain in these sites even after adequate treatment. However, this persistent, sequestered infection usually produces no manifestations unless the host is immunocompromised. Data regarding the otologic response to treatment are mixed, but the trend across studies suggests that approximately 15% to 35% will gain at least some improvement with a combination of antibiotic and steroid therapy (21). Some factors associated with better response to intervention include fluctuating hearing loss, symptoms less than five years in duration, and age less than 60 (22). Isolated vertigo or tinnitus also tends to respond well, although if secondary to endolymphatic hydrops, the outcome is less promising. If left untreated, otosyphilis tends to take a progressive course, generally resulting in complete hearing loss and persistent vestibular symptoms.

SUMMARY

A disease of great historical significance, though rarely seen today, syphilis is truly protean in its manifestations. *T. pallidum* demonstrates the ability to invade nearly any tissue or organ system with resulting diverse pathology. It is unusual for an otolaryngologist to make the diagnosis of syphilis, given the initial symptoms of genital lesions and truncal rash. Nonetheless, with the recent trend of increasing incidence and the diffuse head and neck manifestations, it is certainly an entity to keep within the differential diagnosis when evaluating lesions of the head and neck. Otologic symptoms may be of particular interest, as these may sometimes manifest in a patient who is unaware of prior infection and is otherwise in asymptomatic, latent disease.

REFERENCES

1. Parran T. Shadow on the Land: Syphilis. New York: Reynal & Hitchcock, 1937.
2. Kinghorn GR. Syphilis. In: Cohen J, Powderly W, eds. Infectious Diseases. Vol. 1. 2nd ed. Edinburgh, NY: Mosby, 2004:807–816.
3. Lafond RE, Lukehart SA. Biological basis for syphilis. Clin Microbiol Rev 2006; 19(1):29–49.
4. World Health Organization. Global prevalence and incidence of selected curable sexually transmitted infections: overview and estimates. Geneva: WHO, WHO/HIV AIDS/2001.02.
5. Singh AE, Romanowski B. Syphilis: review with emphasis on clinical, epidemiologic, and some biologic features. Clin Microbiol Rev 1999; 12(2):187–209.
6. Centers for Disease Control and Prevention. Sexually Transmitted Disease Surveillance, 2004. U.S. Department of Health and Human Services Centers for Disease Control and Prevention, National Center for HIV, STD, and TB Prevention, Division of STD Prevention: Atlanta, GA, September 2005.
7. Tramont EC. *Treponema pallidum* (Syphilis). In: Mandell GL, Bennett JE, Dolin R, eds. Mandell, Douglas, and Bennett's Principles and Practice of Infectious Diseases. 6th ed. New York, NY: Elsevier/Churchill Livingstone, 2005:2768–2783.
8. Gjestland T. The Oslo study of untreated syphilis; an epidemiologic investigation of the natural course of the syphilitic infection based upon a re-study of the Boeck-Bruusgaard material. Acta Derm Venereol 1955; 35(suppl 34):3–368.
9. Catterall RD. Neurosyphilis. Br J Hosp Med 1977; 17(6):585–604.
10. Becker G. Late syphilitic hearing loss: a diagnostic and therapeutic dilemma. Laryngoscope 1979; 89 (8):1273–1288.
11. Johns DR, Tierney M, Felsenstein D. Alteration in the natural history of neurosyphilis by concurrent infection with the human immunodeficiency virus. N Engl J Med 1987; 316(25):1569–1572.
12. Rosahn PD. Autopsy studies in syphilis. J Vener Dis Infect 1947; 649(suppl 21):1–67.
13. Gagnebin J, Maire R. Infection screening in sudden and progressive idiopathic sensorineural hearing loss: a retrospective study of 182 cases. Otol Neurotol 2002; 23(2):160–162.
14. Zoller M, Wilson WR, Nadol JB Jr, et al. Detection of syphilitic hearing loss. Arch Otolaryngol 1978; 104(2):63–65.
15. Pulec JL. Ménière's disease: results of a two and one-half-year study of etiology, natural history and results of treatment. Laryngoscope 1972; 82(9):1703–1715.
16. Rolfs RT. Treatment of syphilis, 1993. Clin Infect Dis 1995; 20(suppl 1):S23–S38.
17. 1998 Guidelines for treatment of sexually transmitted diseases. Centers for Disease Control and Prevention. MMWR Recomm Rep 1998; 47(RR-1):1–111.
18. Mohr JA, Griffiths W, Jackson R, et al. Neurosyphilis and penicillin levels in cerebrospinal fluid. JAMA 1976; 236(19):2208–2209.
19. Darmstadt GL, Harris JP. Luetic hearing loss: clinical presentation, diagnosis, and treatment. Am J Otolaryngol 1989; 10(6):410–421.
20. Schroeter AL, Lucas JB, Price EV, et al. Treatment for early syphilis and reactivity of serologic tests. JAMA 1972; 221(5):471–476.
21. Pletcher SD, Cheung SW. Syphilis and otolaryngology. Otolaryngol Clin North Am 2003; 36(4):595–605, vi.
22. Gleich LL, Linstrom CJ, Kimmelman CP. Otosyphilis: a diagnostic and therapeutic dilemma. Laryngoscope 1992; 102(11):1255–1259.

16

Human Immunodeficiency Virus and Acquired Immune Deficiency Syndrome

Theodoros F. Katsivas
Owen Clinic and Department of Medicine, Division of Infectious Diseases,
University of California, San Diego, California, U.S.A.

INTRODUCTION

The head and neck complications of the human immunodeficiency virus (HIV) disease/ acquired immune deficiency syndrome (AIDS) described in this chapter may also be encountered in non–HIV-infected persons; however, widespread involvement, atypical features, and poor clinical response to treatment are often seen in the context of HIV infection (1) trend that has not significantly changed after the widespread use of highly active antiretroviral therapy (HAART) (2–4). Therefore, the threshold for testing for the presence of HIV infection should be low in cases where clinical suspicion arises; this scenario can present itself in the emergency department, the outpatient setting, or the hospital. Given that about 50% of patients will develop some head and neck symptoms during the course of the disease (5,6), the otorhinolaryngologist can be called to assist with diagnosis and management of HIV-related complications (6). In this chapter, we will list entities which are frequently or specifically seen in HIV infection. As the field is undergoing rapid evolution, some of these entities may become obsolete in the near future, while novel ones may emerge.

DEFINITION

HIV infection is prevalent worldwide and is universally fatal if left untreated, leading to and being the etiologic agent of AIDS. Initial reports in 1981 of cases of men who have sex with men in major U.S. cities, presenting with a combination of malignancies and infections usually encountered in severe immunosuppression, were quickly followed by the definition of what we know today as AIDS. The Centers for Disease Control (CDC) published the current case definition criteria in 1993 (7), which include a set of clinical parameters in three different categories and also three categories of quantification of the primary cellular immunologic marker of the infection, the CD4+ T-lymphocyte count (CD4 cell) (Table 1).

EPIDEMIOLOGY

HIV is estimated to have caused 65 million human infections worldwide with 25 million deaths since the beginning of the epidemic (8), according to the World Health Organization and the Joint AIDS United Nations program data as of the end of 2005. The epidemic has different characteristics in different geographic areas, but overall remains the fourth leading cause of death, with a staggering 95% of those occurring in young adults in the developing world, mostly in sub-Saharan Africa. The epidemic continues to intensify in Africa and there are alarming signs that prevalence rates will take off in areas of Asia and Eastern Europe.

In the United States, there were an estimated 1.2 million people living with HIV/AIDS (8,9). The majority of people with HIV in the United States are men who have sex with men, and sex between men remains the dominant mode of transmission. One of the striking facets of the epidemic in the United States is the concentration of HIV infections among African-Americans. Despite constituting only 12.5% of the country's population, African-Americans accounted for 48% of new HIV cases in 2003. AIDS has become one of the top three causes of death for African-American men aged 25 to 54; it is the number one cause of death for African-American women aged 25 to 34 years, in most of these cases acquired via heterosexual transmission (9).

TABLE 1 Centers for Disease Control Definition of CD4 Lymphocyte Count and Clinical Categories of HIV Infection[a]

Categories of CD4 cell counts
Category 1: ≥500 cells/mL
Category 2: 200–499 cells/mL
Category 3: ≤200 cells/mL
Clinical categories
   Category A
      Asymptomatic HIV infection
      Persistent generalized lymphadenopathy
      Acute (primary) HIV infection
   Category B
      Bacillary angiomatosis
      Candidiasis, oropharyngeal (thrush)
      Candidiasis, vulvovaginal; persistent, frequent, or poorly responsive to therapy
      Cervical dysplasia (moderate or severe)/cervical carcinoma in situ
      Constitutional symptoms such as fever (38.5°C) or diarrhea lasting greater than 1 mo
      Hairy leukoplakia, oral
      Herpes zoster (shingles), involving at least 2 distinct episodes or more than 1 dermatome
      Idiopathic thrombocytopenic purpura
      Listeriosis
      Pelvic inflammatory disease, particularly if complicated by tubo-ovarian abscess
      Peripheral neuropathy
   Category C
      Candidiasis of bronchi, trachea, or lungs
      Candidiasis, esophageal
      Cervical cancer, invasive
      Coccidioidomycosis, disseminated or extrapulmonary
      Cryptococcosis, extrapulmonary
      Cryptosporidiosis, chronic intestinal (>1 mo duration)
      Cytomegalovirus disease (other than liver, spleen, or nodes)
      Cytomegalovirus retinitis (with loss of vision)
      Encephalopathy, HIV-related
      Herpes simplex: chronic ulcer(s) (>1 mo duration); or bronchitis, pneumonitis, or
        esophagitis
      Histoplasmosis, disseminated or extrapulmonary
      Isosporiasis, chronic intestinal (>1 mo duration)
      Kaposi's sarcoma
      Lymphoma, Burkitt's (or equivalent term)
      Lymphoma, immunoblastic (or equivalent term)
      Lymphoma, primary, of brain
      Mycobacterium avium complex or *Mycobacterium kansasii*, disseminated or
        extrapulmonary
      Mycobacterium tuberculosis, any site (pulmonary or extrapulmonary)
      Mycobacterium, other species or unidentified species, disseminated or extrapulmonary
        Pneumocystis jirovecii (*carinii*) pneumonia
      Pneumonia, recurrent
      Progressive multifocal leukoencephalopathy
      Salmonella septicemia, recurrent
      Toxoplasmosis of brain
      Wasting syndrome due to HIV

[a]Categories A3, B3, C1, C2, and C3 meet the case definition for AIDS.
Source: From Refs. 7, 31.

PATHOGENESIS

HIV is one of the human retroviruses of the family Lentivirus; there are solid data that humans have acquired HIV from other primates via cross species transmission. After exposure to HIV, a symptomatic illness termed primary HIV infection (PHI) occurs in one to four weeks in more than half the patients; however, clinical immunodeficiency or AIDS develops after a long period of clinical latency that follows PHI. Clinical latency is a dynamic period where active viral replication occurs and immunologic abnormalities begin to emerge, most notable of which are quantitative and qualitative defects in the CD4+ T-lymphocyte pool. The average length of the latency period in adults is estimated to be about 10 years. Opportunistic infections (OIs) are the hallmarks of progression to AIDS and usually occur with CD4 counts of less than 200 cells/mm^3.

CLINICAL MANIFESTATIONS—SYSTEMIC

An extensive discussion of the systemic manifestations of HIV/AIDS would be quite lengthy and beyond the scope of this chapter. Note will be made of the PHI, which presents with fever, myalgias, pharyngitis, arthralgias, headache, and malaise. Nonpruritic maculo-papular rash of the face and trunk is reported in 30% to 70% of cases (10) Generalized lymphadenopathy, nausea, vomiting, neurological complications, oral ulceration, and candidiasis might be observed. Since PHI can present before antibody test seroconversion, diagnostic testing should utilize measurement of specific viral antigens or viral load for detection of HIV infection.

CLINICAL MANIFESTATIONS—HEAD AND NECK

Infectious Complications of HIV/AIDS

Bacterial Infections

Linear gingival erythema.   Also known as HIV gingivitis, a fiery red linear discoloration of the gingival margin can be seen in HIV disease, even without significant plaque formation (Fig. 1). Patients complain of spontaneous bleeding or are asymptomatic. Referral to an HIV dental specialist is recommended and usually involves debridement, local care, and systemic antibiotics.

   Necrotizing ulcerative periodontitis and stomatitis.   Rarely encountered in the asymptomatic HIV-infected individual, this form of periodontal disease occurs in up to 50% of AIDS patients (11). Halitosis is a common complaint, along with severe pain and bleeding. On exam, gingival necrosis of the tips of the interdental papillae with formation of ulcers is found (Fig. 2).

   Rapid progression can lead to loss of periodontal tissue and also bone with loosening and loss of teeth. Lesions can resemble the rapidly destructive lesions of noma, as are seen

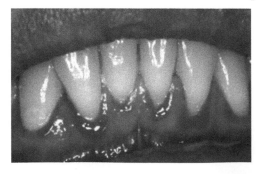

FIGURE 1 Linear gingival erythema. *Source*: Courtesy of the International AIDS Society-U.S.A. From Refs. 3, 4, 11.

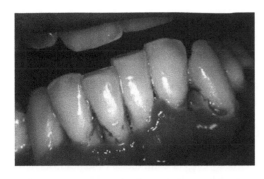

FIGURE 2   Necrotizing ulcerative periodontitis. *Source*: Courtesy of the International
AIDS Society-U.S.A. From Refs. 3, 4, 11.

with severe malnutrition and coexisting chronic infections in developing countries.
Anaerobic indigenous flora seems to play a role in maintaining the destructive character of
the lesion, but the pathogenesis is unclear.

Treatment is best left to an HIV dental specialist and includes debridement of
necrotic tissue, aggressive local care with antiseptics and chlorhexidine mouthwashes, and
systemic antibiotics with some degree of anaerobic coverage, such as doxycycline,
amoxicillin/clavulanate, metronidazole, or clindamycin.

Other Bacterial Causes of Stomatitis.   Cases of *Klebsiella, Enterobacter cloacae*,
and *Mycobacterium avium* complex stomatitis with oral nodules, masses, or oral ulcers
have been reported in HIV-infected persons. These responded to etiologic treatment with
systemic antibiotics.

Bacillary Angiomatosis—Bartonellosis.   Caused by the species *Bartonella quin-
tana* and *Bartonella henselae,* bacillary angiomatosis has been reported to present with oral
papules that resemble Kaposi's sarcoma (KS), and biopsy, special stains (Warthin–Starry
stain), and culture may be required for definite diagnosis. Serology for specific antibodies
is available. The infection responds well to macrolides and doxycycline.

Syphilis.   Infection with *Treponema pallidum* can present with head and neck
symptoms. Primary syphilitic chancre can occur in the oral or nasal mucosa or the perioral
skin at the site of inoculation. This usually has the appearance of an indurated, relatively
painless ulcer. Mucous patches of secondary syphilis and the rash associated with it can be
found in the head and neck area. Syphilis is discussed in detail in Chapter 15.

Mycobacterial Infections

Tuberculosis.   Tuberculosis (TB, from *Mycobacterium tuberculosis* and/or *Mycobacterium
bovis*) is a major cause of morbidity and mortality in HIV disease. It usually presents as
reactivation of a pulmonary primary focus, with a risk of 7% to 10% per year for HIV-infected
persons regardless of CD4 lymphocyte count, versus 10% per lifetime for HIV-negative
persons. There can be involvement of the lungs, central nervous system (CNS), or other
organs, with rhinosinusitis, diffuse or localized (scrofula) lymphadenopathy, skin and mucosal
ulcers, chronic otitis, and laryngeal involvement. Fever, chills, night sweats, and weight loss
may be the presenting symptoms of any form of tuberculosis. Hemoptysis may be a symptom
of laryngeal, tracheobronchial, or pulmonary disease. The clinical presentation becomes more
atypical as the immunosuppression worsens; pulmonary TB presenting with essentially
normal chest X ray is not uncommon in CD4 counts of less than 50 cells/mm^3. TB can also
coexist with other OIs in the same host. For the reasons above, all HIV patients with any
symptoms that could be associated with TB need to undergo clinical screening with skin
testing, chest X rays, and appropriate samples submitted for acid-fast smears and cultures. A
more detailed discussion of TB appears in Chapter 12.

Mycobacterium Avium Complex and Atypical Mycobacteria. *M. avium* complex can be a cause of significant morbidity and mortality for AIDS patients, usually becoming a problem with CD4 counts of less than 50 cells/mm^3. Other atypical mycobacteria (*Mycobacterium kansasii*, *Mycobacterium fortuitum*, *Mycobacterium gordonae*, and *Mycobacterium hominis*) sometimes can be isolated from clinical samples, but their role as pathogens and their management are controversial. Further discussion of atypical mycobacteria can be found in Chapter 12.

Fungal Infections

Oroesophageal Candidiasis or Candidosis. Oroesophageal candidiasis or candidosis is a superficial infection of the oral, pharyngeal, and esophageal mucosa caused by the fungus *Candida*. It represents the most common fungal OI among HIV-infected individuals; about 90% of all patients will develop it during the course of the disease. Normally present in the oral cavity in healthy persons, *Candida* can overgrow and through upregulation of genes or via infection with more virulent strains can cause infection. In 75% of cases, the oral infection is associated with concurrent involvement of the esophagus or the larynx and tracheobronchial tree, especially in deep immunosuppression. Typically seen in the pre-HIV era as a complication of antibiotic treatment, it has been one of the cardinal presentations of advanced HIV infection with CD4 counts of less than 200 cells/mm^3, but can be seen during acute HIV infection or in the asymptomatic stage. Presence of oral candidiasis or oral hairy leukoplakia (OHL) predicts the development of AIDS in HIV-infected persons, independent of CD4 counts (12). Despite the reduction of incidence in the HAART era, it remains a significant cause of morbidity and malaise in persons with severe immunodeficiency. Other well-known coexisting predisposing factors are steroid use, antibiotics, diabetes, anemia, xerostomia, radiation therapy, use of dentures, and dehydration (13).

Most of the cases are actually asymptomatic and the person is often unaware of the presence of the infection; with time, soreness, dysgeusia, hoarseness, aspiration with laryngeal involvement and burning, dysphagia to solids and liquids, and odynophagia develop when the esophagus is involved.

The most commonly encountered species (in 77% or more) involved in this infection is *Candida albicans*, but frequently other species, including *Candida tropicalis*, *Candida guilliermondii*, *Candida dubliniensis*, *Candida glabrata*, *Candida krusei*, and *Candida parapsilosis*, are present, some of which might be inherently resistant to fluconazole.

The oral lesions assume a characteristic appearance in different forms:

1. Pseudomembranous or common thrush (Figs. 3 and 7)
2. Erythematous candidiasis (Figs. 4 and 6)
3. Angular cheilitis (perleche) (Fig. 7) and
4. Atypical; including exfoliative cheilitis and palatal papillary hyperplasia.

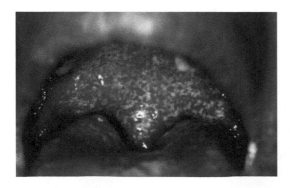

FIGURE 3 Pseudomembranous form of oral candidiasis of the buccal mucosa. *Source*: Courtesy of the International AIDS Society-U.S.A. From Refs. 3, 4, 11.

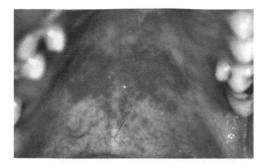

FIGURE 4 Erythematous form of oral candidiasis of the palate. *Source*: Courtesy of the International AIDS Society-U.S.A. From Refs. 3, 4, 11.

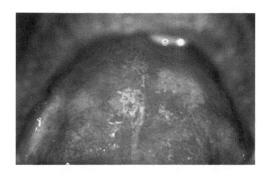

FIGURE 5 Pseudomembranous candidiasis of the soft palate. *Source*: Courtesy of the International AIDS Society-U.S.A. From Refs. 3, 4, 11.

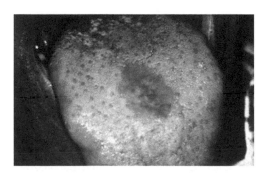

FIGURE 6 Erythematous candidiasis on the dorsal tongue surface. *Source*: Courtesy of the International AIDS Society-U.S.A. From Refs. 3, 4, 11.

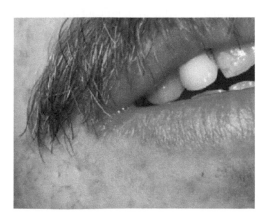

FIGURE 7 Angular cheilitis. *Source*: From Ref. 21.

Pseudomembranous candidiasis is the most common form, accounting for 70% to 80% of all cases. The lesions appear as soft, white, curdled papules, which increase in size and can coalesce, forming large whitish or creamy plaques, which typically are easily dislodged when scraped by a tongue blade, revealing an erythematous base. They can form in any area of the oropharynx and often at multiple sites in the esophagus.

Erythematous candidiasis may coexist with plaques or present by itself, usually as red macular coalescing lesions on the dorsal tongue (median rhomboid glossitis) or forming a mucous surface eruption (enanthem) over the hard and soft palate.

Angular cheilitis is a commonly overlooked manifestation of oral candidiasis, manifesting with ulceration and erythema over the oral commissures.

The diagnosis is usually made clinically from the history and physical examination with the characteristic lesions; a swab smear submitted to the lab for a rapid potassium oxide (KOH) preparation in the pseudomembranous form, or biopsy for more specialized periodic acid-Schiff (PAS) or Giemsa stains in other forms can readily demonstrate an abundance of spores and hyphae (Fig. 8), strongly supporting the diagnosis.

Culture is not useful in establishing the diagnosis, since the fungus will be present as normal flora in samples of healthy volunteers, but it can assist in identifying the causative species for sensitivity testing in cases of treatment failure.

When atypical or mixed lesions are simultaneously present in the oral cavity (for example, erythematous plaques and ulcers), empiric treatment for candidiasis is warranted. In cases of azole treatment failure or if there is clinical presentation consistent with concurrent esophagitis, a barium swallow may reveal a cobblestone appearance and upper endoscopy may reveal whitish ulcerative plaques; biopsies should be performed for culture and to rule out other pathogens including herpes simplex or cytomegalovirus (CMV), or lesions such as lymphoma or KS (6).

Topical treatment can be with nystatin either as tablets or as troches (100,000 or 200,000 units) dissolved slowly in the mouth four times daily between meals for two weeks, or with clotrimazole 10 mg troches dissolved in the mouth slowly four to six times daily for two weeks.

Extensive disease, persistent and advanced immunosuppression, poor patient compliance, poor palatability, and recurrence are factors that favor systemic treatment. Many clinicians prefer to treat systemically with azoles: ketoconazole 200 mg daily; itraconazole 200 mg twice daily, or fluconazole 100 to 200 mg daily, each for two weeks. In recurrent disease, longer duration treatment is optional. Ketoconazole and itraconazole capsules require significant stomach acidity for absorption, while itraconazole suspension and fluconazole have more favorable bioavailability. All azoles exhibit extensive drug interactions with many drug classes and are pregnancy-category D drugs. Of the newer azoles, voriconazole is usually avoided when patients are on treatment with protease inhibitors due to significant reduction of

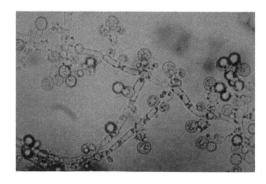

FIGURE 8 Potassium hydroxide preparation of oral smear showing fungal pseudohyphae and spores. *Source*: From Refs. 3, 11.

the area under the curve (AUC) of the antiretroviral agent, and posaconazole looks promising in cases of fluconazole-resistant strains. Intravenous amphotericin B deoxycholate can be used in cases of fluconazole-resistant strains; the lipid intravenous (IV) formulations of amphotericin B (Amphotec®, Abelcet®, and AmBisome®) have shown similar efficacy. The new antifungal class of echinocandins, with two agents available so far, is efficacious in treating azole-resistant candidiasis; caspofungin and micafungin are both available IV. Prognosis is usually good for mucocutaneous candidiasis, in contrast to invasive disease.

Cryptococcosis. The second most commonly encountered fungal OI in HIV after candidiasis, *Cryptococcus neoformans* infects 8.5% of patients at some stage of their disease and in its disseminated form represents by far the most common life-threatening fungal infection in this patient population. It is a ubiquitous fungus found throughout the world and can also infect immunocompetent hosts. The most commonly involved organ is the CNS, followed by the lungs. Patients present with days to months of malaise, fever, headaches, and nausea or vomiting, as well as altered mentation, personality changes, loss of memory, and cranial nerve palsies. Mucocutaneous involvement occurs in up to 10% of cases, usually in advanced HIV disease (CD4 cell count <50/mm^3), and skin lesions may occur weeks or months before presentation. Disseminated infection can present with cutaneous skin-colored or pink umbilicated lesions, which are, in general, asymptomatic, resembling molluscum contagiosum (Fig. 9) and are most often found in the head and neck area (14).

Other types of cutaneous lesions include pustules, cellulitis, ulceration, panniculitis, palpable purpura, subcutaneous abscesses, and vegetating plaques. Oral cavity nonhealing ulcers or nodules can be seen alone or along with cutaneous lesions (3). Hematogenous dissemination of *Histoplasma capsulatum* or *Coccidioides immitis* can produce identical skin lesions on the face. Biopsy of the lesion is usually necessary for definitive diagnosis, by demonstration of cryptococcal yeast forms with hematoxylin and eosin, PAS, or methenamine silver stain. Often, a Tzanck smear obtained by scraping the top of a lesion shows multiple encapsulated and budding yeast forms stained by Giemsa or by India ink preparation. *C. neoformans* can also be isolated on culture of the skin biopsy specimen. Histologically, all lesions reveal numerous encapsulated cryptococcal organisms. Cryptococcal meningitis is treated with IV amphotericin B and oral 5-flucytosine or with fluconazole. Mucocutaneous cryptococcal lesions resolve two to four weeks after beginning effective primary antifungal therapy, but relapses occur in over 50% of patients once primary induction therapy is stopped. Chronic prophylaxis with fluconazole is effective.

Histoplasmosis ("Ohio Valley fever"). Infection with *H. capsulatum* in HIV/AIDS is usually a systemic reactivation of primary infection in persons previously exposed to the fungus. *H. capsulatum* is endemic in the Midwestern United States, the Ohio and Mississippi river valley areas, and countries of South America, Southeast Asia, Africa, and Australia. In endemic areas, it can be the leading OI in HIV patients, usually with CD4 counts of less than

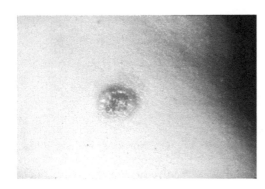

FIGURE 9 Cryptococcus neoformans, skin lesion. *Source*: From Ref. 22.

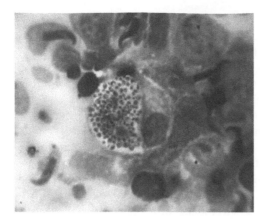

FIGURE 10 Histoplasma capsulatum organisms inside a macrophage, biopsy, Giemsa stain. *Source*: From Ref. 24.

100 cells/mm^3. It may present as persistent, large, nonhealing ulcers or ulcerated nodular or exophytic lesions of the oral cavity, esophagus, other areas of the gastrointestinal (GI) tract, the larynx, or the nose, (15) usually along with systemic manifestations such as fever, diarrhea, splenomegaly, and cytopenias from bone marrow infiltration. Meningitis, adrenal failure, or endocarditis may develop. Cutaneous dissemination occurs in about 10%, presenting as nodules, macules, or panniculitis. Often the lesions are suspicious for malignancy; biopsy for culture and fungal stains of a suspicious or nonhealing lesion closer to the periphery are helpful for diagnosis, demonstrating granulomatous infection and the characteristic fungal elements, often filling the macrophages (Fig. 10).

Detection of the fungal antigen in urine is another sensitive and specific test used for the diagnosis of active disease. Lipid formulations of IV amphotericin induction followed by oral itraconazole or fluconazole are often used for treatment, followed by secondary prophylaxis (16). Primary prophylaxis is considered in highly endemic areas if the CD4 count drops below 100 cells/mm^3. Prognosis varies with the degree of immunosuppression, extent of the infection, and response to treatment.

Coccidioidomycosis ("San Joaquin Valley fever"). The endemic dimorphic fungus *C. immitis* is found in the semiarid areas of the Sonora desert of the Southwestern United States, Mexico, and Central and South America and when in the mold form (arthroconidia) (Fig. 11) can cause pulmonary infection when inhaled. Disseminated infection usually represents reactivation and can include the CNS and bones in HIV/AIDS-infected persons or immunocompetent hosts (17).

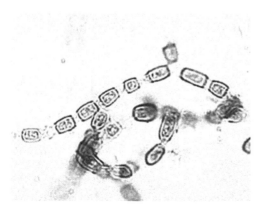

FIGURE 11 Coccidioides immitis infectious form (arthroconidia). *Source*: From Ref. 25.

Cutaneous lesions resemble molluscum and are often ulcerated. Any osseous head and neck structure can be infected by the fungus (maxilla, mandible, parietal, frontal, pre-, and paravertebral areas and temporal bone), and infections of the retropharyngeal space, trachea, larynx, lymph nodes, orbit, and thyroid have been reported (16). Diagnosis is usually made by biopsy for stains and culture and histopathology to rule out malignancy. Fungal stain of the tissue can reveal the characteristic *C. immitis* spherules of the yeast form (Fig. 12).

Serologic testing for specific antibodies by complement fixation is useful in establishing the diagnosis and following response to treatment. Fluconazole, posaconazole, and IV amphotericin B have been used for treatment. Surgery is sometimes necessary for debridement of the infected devitalized tissue. Prognosis varies and mostly depends on the site and extent of the infection.

Aspergillosis. The genus *Aspergillus* is another worldwide ubiquitous fungus, which has the ability to infect human hosts, and although invasive aspergillosis is rare in HIV disease, it can present as a primary cutaneous infection with pustular lesions, or as a necrotizing angioinvasive disseminated infection of the lungs, tracheobronchial tree, nasal cavity, sinuses, and other sites. Risk factors for invasive aspergillosis in HIV disease include leukopenia and therapy with corticosteroids, broad-spectrum antibiotics, and antineoplastic agents (16). Skin lesions appear as skin-colored to pink umbilicated papules resembling molluscum contagiosum. Diagnosis is established by biopsy for stains and culture. Serum antigen testing for *Aspergillus galactomannan* is useful in supporting the diagnosis of invasive disease. Despite treatment with newer azoles, such as voriconazole or posaconazole, or IV amphotericin B, prognosis remains grave.

Penicilliosis. The dimorphic fungus *Penicillium marneffei* is the third most common OI in HIV-infected residents of Southeast Asian countries and the southern part of China. The clinical presentation includes fever, weight loss, cough, anemia, and disseminated umbilicated papular skin lesions (in 71%), occurring most frequently on the face, pinna, upper trunk, and arms, and oral lesions including papules and ulcers. In addition, *P. marneffei* preferentially disseminates to the lung and liver. Diagnosis is usually by tissue or cytologic examination; treatment options include itraconazole and IV amphotericin.

Blastomycosis, Geotrichosis, and Sporotrichosis. Infections with *Blastomyces dermatitidis* are endemic to the Midwestern and south-central United States, presenting as localized pulmonary infection, or as disseminated disease, occasionally as crusted papular ulcerated facial lesions (Fig. 13).

Both Geotrichum *and* Sporothrix genera can cause skin lesions or oral nonhealing ulcers or erythematous lesions which resemble candidiasis (13).

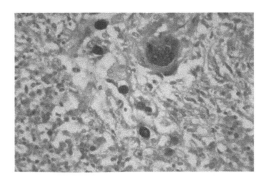

FIGURE 12 Coccidioides immitis spherule in tissue, PAS reaction. *Source*: From Ref. 26.

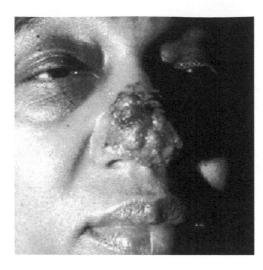

FIGURE 13 Blastomycosis, dissemination to the pinna. *Source*: From Ref. 28.

Viral Infections

Primary HIV Infection.   Primary infection with HIV usually presents as a mononucleosis-like syndrome after an incubation period of one to four weeks, as previously mentioned. The clinician should consider acute HIV infection in a mononucleosis-like presentation with negative serologies. The symptoms reported, by decreasing order of frequency, are fever (95%), lymphadenopathy, pharyngitis, maculopapular rash, myalgias/arthralgias, nausea, vomiting or diarrhea, headache, hepatosplenomegaly, neuropathy, oral or upper GI ulcerations, purpura, and conjunctivitis. Large painful oral ulcers are reported with acute HIV infection, which are associated with gram-negative bacterial colonization. Those are usually self-limited, but help in the differential diagnosis of acute PHI from other viral illnesses.

Herpes Simplex Virus.   Herpes simplex virus (HSV) Types 1 and 2 can cause both primary gingivostomatitis and recurrent labial, other skin area, or intraoral or esophageal ulcers in HIV-infected persons (Fig. 14). The lesions are more atypical and protracted with severe immunosuppression and CD4 counts less than 50 cells/mm^3 (18) and they can appear on the dorsal tongue as slit-like or dendritic ulcers. Herpetic keratitis is also reported. Persistent recurrent HSV infection is a marker of HIV disease progression. Diagnosis is made clinically, by biopsy of a skin or oral lesion, or via endoscopy. A smear can be sent to the laboratory for immunofluorescent stain or viral culture.

Usually the ulcers are self-limited, but can be persistent and accompanied by fever, malaise, dysphagia, and odynophagia. Treatment with oral acyclovir (200 or 400 mg up to five times daily) or oral valacyclovir (1 g twice daily) as soon as symptoms first appear and

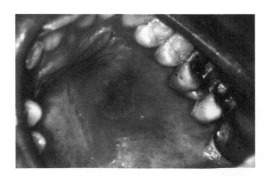

FIGURE 14 Herpes simplex virus of the palate. *Source*: Courtesy of the International AIDS Society-U.S.A. From Refs. 3, 4, 11.

for 7 to 10 days can sometimes shorten the duration or decrease the frequency of the outbreaks. IV treatment with foscarnet is reserved for rare cases of resistant HSV or poorly responsive cases. Prophylaxis with oral acyclovir or valacyclovir is sometimes given for frequently recurrent outbreaks.

Varicella Zoster Virus.   Orofacial herpes zoster infection usually follows the distribution of one of the three branches of the trigeminal nerve on one side of the face. It may also be disseminated. HIV infection has been associated with a 17-fold relative risk increase for zoster, which occurs at any CD4 count but becomes more severe as immunosuppression worsens (18) Involvement of the ophthalmic branch and the eye should be ruled out, and the patient presenting with suspicious lesions on the forehead or pinna should be referred for evaluation to an ophthalmologist, to rule out zoster ophthalmicus from involvement of the nasociliary branch of cranial nerve V (Fig. 15). Facial nerve involvement with facial palsy may occur (Ramsay-Hunt syndrome). Chronic forms and up to 20% recurrence rate have been reported.

Pain is usually the initial symptom, often referred to the teeth, followed by the characteristic eruption of papules, which quickly progress to vesicles and ulcers with crusts. Postherpetic neuralgia might be severe and require referral to a specialist. Oral ulcers have been reported.

Diagnosis is easily made clinically. Viral culture obtained from the base of a freshly opened vesicle often isolates the virus.

Treatment is most efficacious when started early. Oral acyclovir at high doses of up to 4 g in daily divided doses can be used (or alternatively, valacyclovir 1 g three times daily), both for 10 to 14 days. For more severe cases or ophthalmic branch involvement, IV acyclovir treatment is warranted. Oral steroids are recommended for facial nerve paralysis, but are better avoided in disseminated zoster.

Cytomegalovirus.   CMV disease in HIV is usually reactivation of a latent, previously acquired infection in patients with CD4 count of less than 100 cells/mm^3 (19) The typical primary CMV infection, presenting with a mononucleosis-like syndrome characterized by fever, pharyngitis, lymphadenopathy, and malaise, is not usually encountered in the setting of HIV infection. In the pre-HAART era, CMV reactivation disease could be asymptomatic or cause fever and constitutional symptoms or end organ disease, occurring in 40% of AIDS patients. The most common organ involved is the retina, in 85% of cases, with the GI tract accounting for another 10%. In the HAART era, incidence of new CMV-reactivation disease has decreased dramatically and is usually seen with CD4 counts less than 50 cells/mm^3. Oral and esophageal ulcers are the most common upper GI tract manifestation, CMV being the second most common cause of esophagitis after *Candida*, with HSV being the third. Necrotizing gingivitis and salivary gland involvement are also reported.

Diagnosis is made by biopsy, evidence of characteristic cytopathic changes on Giemsa stain and immunohistochemistry results. Quantitative polymerase chain reaction

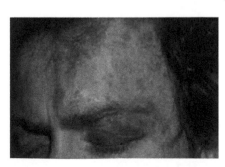

FIGURE 15 Herpes   zoster   ophthalmicus.
Source: From Ref. 29.

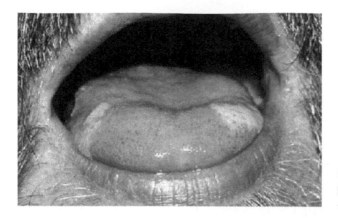

FIGURE 16   Oral hairy leukoplakia associated with EBV.
Source: From Ref. 30.

(PCR) for CMV viral load in serum can be used, but the clinical utility of the test is not yet
clear.

Whether treatment is beneficial for oral ulcers caused by CMV is not clear. Ulcerative
esophagitis-causing symptoms can be treated with IV antivirals such as ganciclovir,
foscarnet, or cidofovir, followed by oral maintenance, usually with oral valganciclovir.

Epstein–Barr Virus and Oral Hairy Leukoplakia.   OHL has been encountered
since the early epidemic and has been strongly linked to Epstein–Barr virus (EBV) (3). It
has a typical appearance of whitish thickening of the lateral tongue (Fig. 16), more
specifically of the foliate papillae on either or both sides, appearing corrugated or "hairy"
(Fig. 17); it is rarely found in other areas of the oral cavity. In contrast to pseudomembranous
oral candidiasis, the lesions cannot be scraped away with a tongue blade.

It is the most common oral lesion in HIV-infected persons, encountered in 20%
of asymptomatic patients and becoming more frequent with disease progression, with
pseudomembranous candidiasis the second most common, encountered in about 6%. It
does not, however, signify the presence of HIV infection, being infrequently found in solid
organ or bone marrow transplant recipients or patients undergoing chemotherapy. Presence
of OHL, regardless of the size of the lesion, signifies a more rapid progression to AIDS
even after adjusting for CD4 counts at a similar degree with oral candidiasis. Pathogenesis
is debated, but it seems the total EBV genome is invariably present in OHL lesions;
multiple strains or defective replication cycle have been speculated.

The diagnosis is usually made clinically, but can be confirmed only by biopsy, since
the involved epithelium shows characteristic changes and the presence of EBV can be
demonstrated by immunohistochemistry, in situ hybridization, or electron microscopy. This
can be useful for the differential diagnosis, which could include friction keratosis, smokers'
leukoplakia, leukoplakia associated with dysplasia and oral squamous cell carcinoma in situ,

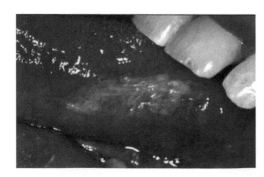

FIGURE 17   Oral   hairy   leukoplakia.
Source: Courtesy of the International AIDS
Society-U.S.A. From Refs. 3,4,11.

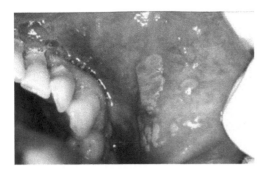

FIGURE 18 Oral warts. *Source*: Courtesy of the International AIDS Society-U.S.A. From Refs. 3, 4, 11.

lichen planus, hyperplastic candidiasis, geographic tongue, and certain genodermatoses. Of note, OHL is not associated with progression to malignancy, despite the well-known oncogenic association of EBV with other malignancies (Burkitt's lymphoma, nasopharyngeal carcinoma, and others).

Treatment is indicated for aesthetic or functional reasons; superinfection with *Candida* should be treated with fluconazole and the OHL lesion responds to high-dose acyclovir, but recurrence is the rule. Other agents, such as ganciclovir, foscarnet zidovudine, or topical podophyllum toxin, have been used with some success.

Human Papilloma Virus.   Lesions of human papilloma virus (HPV) in the oral cavity take the form of cauliflower-like, flat, or papilliferous warts (Fig. 18) and are usually caused by different HPV types from those causing genital lesions.

Flat oral warts are identical to the lesions of focal epithelial hyperplasia (Heck's disease). Rarely, dysplasia has been found in association with HPV lesions of the oral cavity. Large bulky lesions may be found in the larynx or tracheobronchial tree (respiratory papillomatosis), which can cause severe symptoms from hoarseness, dysphonia, or hemoptysis.

Diagnosis is made by the characteristic clinical appearance on physical examination or endoscopy.

Treatment for oral warts is usually by surgical or laser excision, fulguration, cryosurgery, or trichloroacetic acid application. Intralesional cidofovir injection has been used with varying degrees of success. Screening for other sites of infection (e.g., the genitourinary tract) and treatment of those areas are advised. Recurrence, however, is common.

Molluscum Contagiosum (Molluscipoxvirus).   The etiologic agent of molluscum contagiosum is a poxvirus of the family Poxviridae, which is encountered with increased frequency in HIV disease. Lesions are typically papular and umbilicated with a keratinized core that can be readily expressed. Lesions appear on the face and neck, sometimes in large numbers, and become aesthetically problematic. Treatment options include curettage, cryosurgery, and local trichloroacetic acid application. Immune restoration in cases of decreased CD4 count is helpful in controlling the extent of the lesions. Cidofovir has been used in recalcitrant cases, either topically or systemically.

Neoplastic Complications of HIV/AIDS

Kaposi's Sarcoma.   KS is a malignant vascular neoplasm usually arising in cutaneous tissues and lymph nodes. The incidence is higher in men who have sex with men; historically, it was one of the first features of the newly described syndrome in 1981, which was later termed AIDS. KS usually is seen with CD4 counts of less than 50 cells/mm^3. Lesions are typically red or purple macules coalescing to plaques, papules or nodules, but can be bluish or

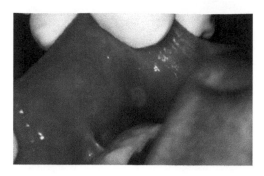

FIGURE 19 Aphthous ulcers. *Source*: Courtesy of the International AIDS Society-U.S.A. From Refs. 3, 4, 11.

the color of the surrounding skin or mucosa. Typically asymptomatic, they may become painful when ulcerated and secondarily infected. Oral mucosal lesions are the most common and usually occur in the palate (Fig. 19), gingiva, or lips; they can grow and become bulky, causing mechanical problems or bleeding.

Cutaneous lesions can be seen in the trunk, distal limbs, tip of the nose, and other areas of the head and neck. Due to the location and association with AIDS, they can be aesthetically embarrassing to the patient. The lungs, GI tract, and lymphatic system can also be involved.

KS has been strongly associated with human herpes virus Type 8 (HHV8), also known as KS-associated herpes virus, believed to be transmitted orally.

Diagnosis is made by biopsy. The differential includes purpura, bacillary angiomatosis, hematoma, pyogenic granuloma, and hemangioma.

If treatment is necessary, local excision, topical sclerotherapy, intralesional vinblastine, radiation therapy, or systemic chemotherapy with liposomal doxorubicin or other agents can be given for larger, aggressive lesions or systemic disease. In the HAART era, immune restoration can decrease or eliminate lesions.

Lymphoma. Oral localization of non-Hodgkin's lymphoma might be the initial symptom of this AIDS-defining complication.

Lymphoma can present as diffuse induration, nodule, or ulcers in the oral cavity (Fig. 20), mandibular or maxillary mass, or neck mass from lymph node involvement, but lymphadenopathy may be absent.

The vast majority of HIV-related lymphomas are of B-cell origin and many contain EBV DNA. The most common type is a large B-cell immunoblastic type, followed by Burkitt's, mantle cell, and plasmablastic lymphoma, which is frequently encountered in the oral cavity. OHL has been identified as a predictor of lymphoma. Spontaneous resolution of oral ulcers of lymphoma has been reported, followed by rapid recurrence. Therefore, biopsy of any suspicious oral lesion is recommended, even in the absence of lymphadenopathy or B type symptoms (fever, weight loss, malaise, and night sweats).

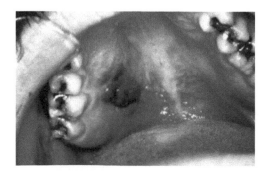

FIGURE 20 Kaposi's sarcoma of the palate. *Source*: Courtesy of the International AIDS Society-U.S.A. From Refs. 3,4,11.

Systemic chemotherapy after referral to an HIV oncology specialist is used in most cases, with varying degrees of prognosis.

A detailed discussion of lymphoma can be found in Chapter 17.

Oral Cancer.   Squamous cell carcinoma has not convincingly been associated with HIV; however, cases of oral cancer are reported and the incidence is expected to increase, given prolonged survival in the HAART era.

Idiopathic, Autoimmune, and Other Complications of HIV/AIDS

Oral Pigmentation.   Reported usually as palatal or buccal hyperpigmented melanotic macules, this HIV-related complication is frequently idiopathic or rarely associated with adrenal insufficiency (Addison's disease), oral zidovudine, or ketoconazole therapy. The exact significance of those idiopathic lesions is unclear.

Recurrent Aphthous Ulcers.   Aphthous ulcers of unknown etiology are relatively common in HIV disease, becoming more severe with worsening immunosuppression. Contrary to those found in the general population, aphthous ulcers (canker sores) are often large and not of the minor (herpetiform) type in HIV-infected persons. They can persist for weeks or even months, causing severe pain and disability with resultant malnutrition, which further complicates the problem. Empiric therapy with high-dose acyclovir usually fails. Most often, biopsy and cultures are performed to exclude specific treatable causes such as fungal or viral infection (especially CMV). In most cases, no etiologic agent is found (3). Topical treatment with steroid paste (Lidex) can sometimes be useful, but large lesions require more aggressive management, and oral thalidomide has been tested in clinical trials with very good results in healing these debilitating lesions.

Immune Thrombocytopenic Purpura.   Small clusters of purpuric lesions can be found in the oral cavity in HIV-related thrombocytopenia, which can progress to large ecchymoses. Spontaneous bleeding is not uncommon.

Lipohypertrophy and Facial Lipoatrophy.   A complication of HIV infection and antiretroviral therapy, loss or accumulation of adipose tissue in the head and neck area has been associated with the introduction of HAART.

Lipohypertrophy usually presents as soft subcutaneous tissue enlargement in the dorsal neck (dorsocervical fat pad) (Fig. 2D) lateral dorsal neck, or other areas. The primary treatment is surgical; open lipectomy combined with aggressive liposuction seems to be required.

Lipoatrophy is usually prominent around the cheeks and lateral frontal areas. This symptom is very embarrassing to many patients and various treatments have been employed. Removing the offending antiretroviral agent can be problematic if no other treatment options exist. Polylactic acid injections (Sculptra®) have been used for treatment, as have silicone implants to enhance the buccal area contour.

Benign Lymphoepithelial Cysts.   The most common location is the parotid, probably because of the presence of large lymphoid tissue inclusions within the gland (5); occasionally, lymphoepithelial cysts of the other salivary glands develop. In association with HIV infection, cysts are multiloculated, bilateral in 80% of cases, and contain clear serous liquid. They may need occasional aspiration, for functional or aesthetic reasons. Doxycycline sclerotherapy may prevent recurrence. Secondary infection can occur, usually by *Staphylococcus aureus,* in which case, incision, drainage, and appropriate antibiotics according to culture report should be prescribed.

Xerostomia.   Low salivary flow, reported often as a complication of salivary gland HIV infection, contributes to the infection risk of the periodontal and mucous membranes.

A Sjögren-like syndrome has been described. Saliva substitutes, fluoride applications, aggressive oral hygiene, and low sugar intake are all recommended.

Meth Mouth.   Use of crystal methamphetamine has escalated to an epidemic, especially on the West coast of the U.S. Associated xerostomia, bruxism, poor diet and hygiene, the drug itself, and sugar cravings all contribute to rapid dental decay known as "meth mouth."

Salivary Gland Enlargement.   Salivary gland enlargement has been associated with HIV infection. The enlargement is usually bilateral and most commonly involves the parotid glands. The glands feel soft, nonfluctuant, and nontender, with diffuse enlargement. Lymphomas can present as discrete unilateral masses within the major salivary glands and are accompanied by regional lymphadenopathy in 10% of cases. Other causes of salivary gland enlargement include CMV, *Pneumocystis jirovecii (carinii)*, adenovirus, KS, tuberculosis, *Mycobacterium avium* complex (MAC), and sarcoidosis.

Ear and Temporal Bone.   External otitis is seen in higher frequency in HIV infection and tends to be more aggressive and often necrotizing [necrotizing external otitis NEO)]. Preexisting external auditory canal dermatitis is common in HIV-related seborrheic dermatitis. The presentation can be atypical with less granulation tissue, and *Pseudomonas*, *Aspergillus*, and *Proteus* are often isolated. NEO can be complicated by temporal bone and skull base osteomyelitis. Most of the cases require hospital admission and parenteral antibiotics. Surgical debridement, as in malignant otitis externa, can be required. External auditory canal polyps from *P. jirovecii (carinii)* and KS lesions have been reported (5).

Otitis media (OM) in HIV has the same characteristics and pathogenic organisms as in the general population, but higher incidence due to the HIV-related lymphoid hyperplasia and obstruction. OM in HIV can be more often complicated by lateral sinus thrombosis, pseudoaneurysm of the internal carotid, or epidural abscess. OM which is refractory to common treatment or becomes invasive and fistulizing is likely due to mycobacteria or syphilis. OM from *Pneumocystis* has been reported.

Sensorineural hearing loss (SNHL) may be the first manifestation of AIDS, with a prevalence of about 35%. The causes include CNS infections by HIV (HIV encephalopathy), varicella zoster (Ramsay-Hunt syndrome), syphilis, tuberculosis, *P. jirovecii (carinii)*, *C. albicans*, *S. aureus*, *Toxoplasma gondii*, *C. neoformans*, CMV, and JC virus. CNS malignancies, depending on location (primary CNS lymphoma, KS, or metastatic disease), can be a cause (23–27). Use of HIV-related ototoxic medications (aminoglycosides, azidothymidine, dideoxyinosine, dideoxycytidine, pentamidine, acyclovir, erythromycin, flucytosine, pyrimethamine, trimethoprim-sulfamethoxazole, amphotericin B, and vincristine) can cause sudden or progressive SNHL, vertigo, nausea, and vomiting, or ataxia.

SNHL is discussed in detail in Chapter 28.

Rhinitis and Sinusitis.   Nasal congestion in HIV disease can have common causes, including viral or bacterial rhinosinusitis, allergic rhinitis (which is twice as common in HIV as in the general population), or other rhinitis. The common causes of sinusitis (*Streptococcus pneumoniae*, *Haemophilus influenzae*, and *Moraxella catarrhalis*) also account for most of the cases in HIV-infected persons. However, in HIV, infectious etiologies also include higher proportions of other gram-positive (*S. aureus*, *Staphylococcus epidermidis*, and *Propionibacterium acnes*), gram-negative (*Pseudomonas aeruginosa*), fungi (Aspergillus spp., *Rhizopus*, *Alternaria alternata*, *H. capsulatum*, and *Scedosporium apiospermum*), CMV, mycobacteria, and rarely parasites (cryptosporidium and microsporidium). Benign lymphoid hypertrophy, fungal or mycobacterial sinusitis, neoplasia (KS, lymphoma), and other causes should be included in the differential in HIV-infected persons (6). Chronic sinusitis, especially fungal sinusitis, can become aggressive and disseminate along perivascular and perineural spaces; in persistent cases, imaging is usually required to look for signs of advancement such as focal bone lysis, obliteration of the periantral fat and of the pterygopalatine fossa, and intracranial spread. Medical therapy consists of hypertonic, pulsatile nasal irrigation, combined with appropriate antibiotic treatment. When medical therapy fails, as is often the case, endoscopic sinus surgery followed by twice-daily nasal irrigations is recommended. Fungal sinusitis is discussed in detail in Chapter 13.

Benign lymphoid hypertrophy is encountered in up to 80% of cases in early HIV infection and can pose a differential diagnosis dilemma for lymphoma. Occasionally, the tissue can be bulky and cause secondary infectious complications such as OM and bacterial sinusitis from obstruction. Imaging will reveal a homogeneous smooth tissue bilaterally filling the nasal cavity and sinuses; biopsy or some degree of debulking might be required for flow cytometry and stains to rule out lymphoma.

KS can involve the nasal cavity and sinuses, presenting with obstruction and epistaxis. Lymphomas commonly involve the nasal cavity and biopsy can provide information on the lymphoma type and guide treatment.

Extranodal sinus histiocytosis (Rosai–Dorfman disease) can present as pedunculated nodules of the nasal cavity, which can cause obstruction and epistaxis, along with systemic signs and symptoms of bilateral cervical lymphadenopathy, low-grade fevers, leukocytosis, anemia, hypergammaglobulinemia, and an elevated erythrocyte sedimentation rate (6). Diagnosis is made by biopsy and management is expectant since spontaneous resolution might occur.

Larynx and Trachea. The larynx can be involved in bacterial (bacillary angiomatosis), mycobacterial (tuberculosis), fungal (candidiasis, histoplasmosis, and coccidioidomycosis), viral (HSV, varicella zoster virus (VZV), and HPV), and neoplastic (KS, lymphomas, and carcinomas) complications in HIV disease. Clinical presentations are described for each entity, but hoarseness, odynophagia, dysphagia, blood-streaked sputum, frank hemoptysis, and aspiration can be common manifestations of laryngeal and tracheal involvement. The otorhinolaryngologist should take respiratory precautions when examining a patient to avoid the risk of dissemination, especially of laryngeal TB or papilloma virus. Bacillary angiomatosis, and to a lesser extent, KS lesions, can bleed profusely if biopsied.

Esophagus. Other than candidiasis, HSV, and CMV, the esophagus can be involved in histoplasmosis and can be a site for KS, lymphoma, and squamous cell carcinoma. Idiopathic esophageal ulcers are described both in the chronic latent phase and in PHI. Esophageal motility disorders are common in HIV disease.

Neck Lymphadenopathy and Masses. Cervical lymphadenopathy affects 50% of HIV patients. The posterior cervical lymphatic chains are most commonly involved. When there is no obvious focus of infection, the differential diagnosis (Table 2) between reactive nodes, infected nodes, and neoplastic nodes is not always clear. When fine needle aspiration (FNA) fails to secure a diagnosis, open biopsy is indicated.

Special note should be made of two entities, which are encountered relatively often or exclusively in HIV infection.

Multicentric Castleman's Disease. Multicentric Castleman's disease (20) is a rare lymphoproliferative disorder, strongly associated with HHV8, the virus implicated in KS pathogenesis. The disease clinically presents with generalized malaise, night sweats, rigors, fever, anorexia, and weight loss; on physical examination, lymphadenopathy, hepatosplenomegaly, ascites, edema, and pleural as well as pericardial effusions predominate. Laboratory investigations may reveal thrombocytopenia, anemia hypoalbuminemia, and hypergammaglobulinemia. Treatment options are debated and include cytotoxic

TABLE 2   Differential Diagnosis of Lymphadenopathy in HIV
Disease Without an Obvious Primary Focus

Differential diagnosis of HIV-related lymphadenopathy
Acute HIV infection
Lymphoma
Tuberculosis
Mycobacterium avium complex and atypical mycobacteria
Immune reconstitution inflammatory syndrome
Kaposi's sarcoma
Histoplasmosis
Coccidioidomycosis
Castleman's disease
Syphilis
Epstein-Barr virus
Cytomegalovirus
Tularemia
Sarcoid

chemotherapy, immunotherapy with interferon or rituximab, and antivirals such as ganciclovir or foscarnet. Prognosis is poor.

Immune Reconstitution Inflammatory Syndrome. Immune reconstitution inflammatory syndrome (IRIS) presents as an adverse effect of HAART, usually within 8 to 12 weeks of initiation of treatment. It is believed to be due to immune restoration due to HAART, and intensification of the inflammatory reaction to a preexisting OI. Occasionally in IRIS, a new OI may present in the initial months of HAART treatment. Associated OIs can be tuberculosis (where paradoxical reactions after initiation of HAART have been seen even after many months of treatment), MAC disease, CMV end organ disease, hepatitis B or C flares, etc. Clinically, patients may present with fever, diffuse lymphadenopathy, and worsening of OI symptoms.

Although radiographic imaging can assist with diagnosis of lymphadenopathy since intense contrast enhancement suggests nodal increased vascularity, e.g., an acute infection, KS, and lymphomas, there is a definite need for excisional biopsy if FNA is not diagnostic.

PROGNOSIS AND THE ROLE OF THE SURGEON

The prognosis of this most potent 20th century epidemic has changed from a disease with an almost 100% fatality rate to a manageable syndrome within 20 years. This represents a change that is unprecedented in the history of medicine. Reports from around the developed world have documented the efficacy and safety of potent antiretroviral therapy and the huge impact (Fig. 22) this has had to the disease prognosis and survival. Unfortunately, as of 2006, the epidemic continues to be rampant in the poorest areas of the planet, although programs to deploy effective drugs may be under way.

The surgeon in 2006 is expected to encounter more and more survival success cases or new cases with a potential for control and long-term survival. Hence, philosophies that once discouraged certain therapies should be reevaluated. Effective treatment and collaborative work are the keys to the continuation of the survival benefits for HIV-infected persons.

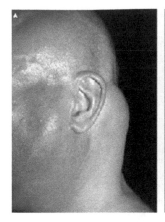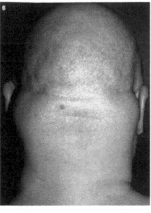

FIGURE 21 Lateral cervical fat pads in HIV-related lipody-strophy. *Source*: Courtesy of the Massachusetts Medical Society. From Ref. 30.

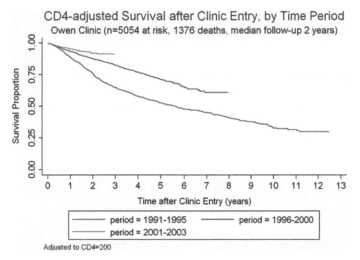

FIGURE 22 AIDS-related death proportions, UCSD Owen Clinic, by era. *Source*: Courtesy of Mathews WC, MD.

SUMMARY

As described in this chapter, HIV disease can present with many different head and neck manifestations. Both in the chronic latent stage and in the acute primary infection, any suspicious symptom should prompt testing for the presence of HIV infection. Since some of those symptoms have broad differential, require prompt diagnosis for improved outcomes, and have significant prognostic value, aggressive diagnostic workup and treatment are warranted.

REFERENCES

1. Flemming F. Oral manifestations. In: Fahey JL, Flemming DS, eds. AIDS/HIV Reference Guide for Medical Professionals. 4th ed. Baltimore, MD: Williams & Wilkins, 1997:189–193.
2. Silverman SS Jr, Migliorati CA, Lozada-Nur F, et al. Oral findings in people with or at high risk for AIDS: a study of 375 homosexual males. J Am Dent Assoc 1986; 112(2):187–192.
3. Greenspan JG. Oral manifestations of HIV infection and AIDS. In: Meringan B, eds. Textbook of AIDS Medicine. 2nd ed. Baltimore, MD: Williams & Wilkins, 1999:521–535.
4. Reznik DA. Oral manifestations of HIV disease. Top HIV Med JT 2005; 13(5):143–148.

5. Marsot-Dupuch K, Quillard J, Meyohas MC. Head and neck lesions in the immunocompromised host. Eur Radiol 2004; 14 (suppl 3):E155–E167.
6. Gurney TA, Murr AH. Otolaryngologic manifestations of human immunodeficiency virus infection. Otolaryngol Clin North Am 2003; 36(4):607–624.
7. 1993 revised classification system for HIV infection and expanded surveillance case definition for AIDS among adolescents and adults. MMWR Recomm Rep 1992; 41(RR-17):1–19.
8. WHO Reports on global HIV/AIDS situation. http://www.who.int/hiv/epiupdates/en/index.html (accessed Feb 2006)
9. Cases of HIV Infection and AIDS in the United States, 2004. http://www.cdc.gov/hiv/topics/surveillance/resources/reports/2004report/default.htm (accessed Feb 2006)
10. Guatelli J, Kuritzkes D. Richman D. Human immunodeficiency virus. In: Richman DD, Whitley RJ, Hayden FG, eds. Clinical Virology. 2nd ed. Washington, D.C.: ASM Press, 2002:685–729.
11. Greenspan JG. Oral complications of HIV infection. In: Sande MA, Volberding PA, eds. The Medical Management of AIDS. 6th ed. Philadelphia, PA: Saunders W.B., 1999:157–169.
12. Katz MH, Greenspan D, Westenhouse J, et al. Progression to AIDS in HIV-infected homosexual and bisexual men with hairy leukoplakia and oral candidiasis. AIDS 1992; 6(1):95–100.
13. Greenspan JS. Oral disease in human immunodeficiency infection. In: DeVita VT Jr, Hellman S, Rosenberg SA, eds. AIDS: Etiology, Diagnosis, Treatment and Prevention. 4th ed. Philadelphia, PA: Lippincott-Raven, 1997:355–363.
14. Johnson RA. HIV disease: mucocutaneous fungal infections in HIV disease. Clin Dermatol 2000; 18 (4):411–422.
15. Souza Filho FJ, Lopes M, Almeida OP, et al. Mucocutaneous histoplasmosis in AIDS. Br J Dermatol 1995; 133(3):472–474.
16. Johnson RA. HIV disease: mucocutaneous fungal infections in HIV disease. Clin Dermatol 2000; 18 (4):411–422.
17. Arnold MG, Arnold JC, Bloom DC, et al. Head and neck manifestations of disseminated coccidioidomycosis. Laryngoscope 2004; 114(4):747–752.
18. Rigopoulos D, Paparizos V, Katsambas A. Cutaneous markers of HIV infection. Clin Dermatol 2004; 22(6):487–498.
19. Springer KL, Weinberg A. Cytomegalovirus infection in the era of HAART: fewer reactivations and more immunity. J Antimicrob Chemother 2004; 54(3):582–586.
20. Waterston A, Bower M. Fifty years of multicentric Castleman's disease. Acta Oncol 2004; 43(8):698–704.
21. A Clinical Guide to Supportive & Palliative Care for HIV/AIDS 2003. http://hab.hrsa.gov/tools/palliative/chap8.html (accessed Feb 2006).
22. Cryptococcus neoformans. http://courses.washington.edu/medch401/infectiousdiseases/term15.htm (accessed Feb 2006).
23. Histoplasmosis. http://www.dental.mu.edu/oralpath/lesions/Histoplasmosis/histoplasmosis.jpg (accessed Feb 2006).
24. http://www.higiene.edu.uy/ciclipa/parasito/Histoplasma.jpg. (accessed Feb 2006).
25. http://www.cat.cc.md.us/courses/bio141/labmanua/lab10/images/arthroci.jpg (accessed Feb 2006).
26. http://timm.main.teikyo-u.ac.jp/pfdb/image/shibuya_k_1/1536x1024/30.jpg (accessed Feb 2006).
27. Blastomycosis. http://images.google.com/imgres?imgurl=http://www.mycology.adelaide.edu.au/gallery/photos/blasto1.gif&imgrefurl=http://www.mycology.adelaide.edu.au/gallery/photos/blasto1.html&h=391&w=288&sz=77&tbnid=sV0Q_s4MrKzAAM:&tbnh=120&tbnw=88&hl=en&start=4&pre (accessed Feb 2006).
28. IAPAC. http://www.iapac.org/home.asp?pid=77&toolid=2&itemid=3443 (accessed Feb 2006)
29. Oral Hairy Leukoplakia. http://depts.washington.edu/hivaids/oral/case2/fig1q.html (accessed Feb 2006).
30. Warren SM, May JW Jr. Images in clinical medicine. Lipodystrophy induced by antiretroviral therapy. N Engl J Med 2005; 352(1):63.
31. www.cdc.gov.

17

Lymphoma, Myeloproliferative Disorders, and Leukemia

Peter R. Holman
Division of Blood and Marrow Transplant, Moores Cancer Center, University of California, San Diego, California, U.S.A.

Robert A. Weisman
Division of Otolaryngology, Head and Neck Oncology Program, Moores Cancer Center, University of California, San Diego, California, U.S.A.

INTRODUCTION

Although hematologic malignancies and related disorders are not managed primarily by otolaryngologists, they represent an important group of serious illnesses that frequently express manifestations in the head and neck region. Among the hematological malignancies, lymphoma accounts for the majority of patients seen in a head and neck clinic. Lymphomas presenting in the head and neck region may be primary in that region, or, more frequently, may be part of a more widely disseminated process. In this chapter, lymphomas, in general, including both Hodgkin lymphoma (HL) and non-Hodgkin lymphoma (NHL), are discussed. The focus is on head and neck manifestations but systemic characteristics are also addressed.

DEFINITION

For the purposes of this review, a primary head and neck lymphoma is one arising from extranodal sites, such as Waldeyer's ring, nasal cavity, paranasal sinuses, oral cavity, salivary glands, thyroid gland, larynx, and orbit. The related disorders, solitary plasmacytoma and multiple myeloma (MM), are also included.

The myeloproliferative disorders (MPD) are a group of hematopoietic stem-cell diseases that include polycythemia rubra vera (PRV), chronic idiopathic myelofibrosis (MF), essential thrombocytosis (ET), and chronic myelogenous leukemia (CML). Each may occasionally present with head and neck manifestations and are included because of their and association with hematologic malignancies. PRV and ET are characterized by the overproduction of red blood cells and platelets, respectively. CML is often associated with extreme leukocytosis and splenomegaly. MF is characterized by marrow fibrosis resulting in marrow hypocellularity and extramedullary hematopoiesis.

Massive splenomegaly is common. All MPDs are characterized by an underlying tendency to transform into acute leukemia, greatest for CML and least for ET.

EPIDEMIOLOGY

Lymphoma

For unclear reasons, the incidence of NHL continues to rise. Only a small component of the increase relates to HIV-associated lymphomas. The incidence increases with older age. For HL, the peak incidence is in the second to third decade. A smaller peak occurs in the sixth decade. In the United States, approximately 64,000 cases of lymphoma occurred in 2005. Of these, approximately 7000 are HL. Of the NHL, 40% are indolent and 60% are aggressive. Nodal-based lymphomas very frequently present with lymphadenopathy involving head and neck locations. Anterior and posterior cervical, submandibular, and supraclavicular nodes are most commonly affected.

Approximately 25% of extranodal lymphomas affect head and neck sites. Almost always, these are NHL. In North America, sinonasal lymphomas comprise the single most frequent group, accounting for 25% of the cases. Waldeyer's ring sites as a group comprise 38% of patients with nasopharyngeal, tonsillar, and base-of-tongue involvement, accounting for 18%, 12%, and 8%, respectively (1). The aggressive natural killer (NK)-/T-cell NHL is rare in North America but occurs with an increased frequency in Southeast Asia. It is strongly associated with the Epstein–Barr virus (EBV). Burkitt's lymphoma is an aggressive malignancy that occurs in two forms. The endemic form frequently involves the jaw, orbit, and central nervous system (CNS) in addition to the abdomen and paraspinal region and accounts for approximately 50% of malignancies in parts of equatorial Africa. It is also strongly associated with EBV. The sporadic form occurs in North America and Western Europe and more frequently affects the nasopharynx in addition to nodal sites, often intra-abdominal.

MM accounts for 10% of hematological malignancies. It has an annual incidence of 4/100,000. It occurs at a similar rate in both males and females but affects blacks up to twice as often as whites.

Myeloproliferative Disorders

PRV affects approximately two persons per 100,000 each year. It has a median age of 60 years and affects twice as many males as females. ET affects approximately 2.5/100,000 people and has a female preponderance of 2:1. The median age at diagnosis is 60 years. MF has an incidence of 1.5/100,000 per year and a median age of onset of 67 years. CML affects 1 to 2/100,000 per year with a median age of onset of 50 to 60 years.

Leukemias

Leukemias are classified as acute and chronic. Acute lymphoblastic leukemia (ALL) is the most common malignancy affecting children. The incidence is approximately 3/100,000. In adults, acute myeloblastic leukemia (AML) accounts for the majority of cases. Approximately 12,000 new cases occur in the United States each year. There is a slight male predominance. Chronic lymphocytic leukemia (CLL) affects approximately 7000 people per year. Most are older than 50 years. CML is discussed in this chapter with the MPDs.

PATHOGENESIS

Lymphoma

Overall, the vast majority of NHLs are derived from B-cells. In Southeast Asia and the Caribbean, there is an increased incidence of T-cell lymphomas. The most current lymphoma classification is the World Health Organization (WHO) schema (2). It includes a large number of heterogeneous entities defined according to morphology, immunopheno-type, cytogenetics, molecular features, and clinical behavior. The resulting classification attempts to relate specific entities to their normal cellular counterparts. B-cell lymphomas can be categorized according to whether the cell of origin has transitioned through the lymph-node germinal center (GC). After undergoing heavy and light chain gene rearrange-ments and when selected by antigen binding within the GC, somatic hypermutation occurs. The use of somatic hypermutation as a marker allows the determination of whether a specific lymphoma is pre-GC, GC, or post-GC. Pre-GC lymphomas include most cases of CLL and mantle-cell lymphoma. GC or post-GC lymphomas include most cases of diffuse large B-cell lymphomas (DLBCLs), mucosa-associated lymphoid-tissue (MALT) lympho-mas, lymphoplasmacytic lymphomas [associated with Waldenstrom's macroglobulinemia (WM)], and follicular lymphoma. Extramedullary plasmacytomas are derived from a clone of pathologic plasmablasts that migrate from the bone marrow and become established in soft tissue with the assistance of adhesion molecules.

Gene microarrays are currently being evaluated to allow further discrimination within otherwise relatively homogeneous subtypes. This is best established for DLBCL, the most common lymphoma subtype seen in practice. DLBCL can be characterized into GC or activated subtypes (3). The GC subtype is associated with a better prognosis. It is expected that this technology will be more extensively adopted in general clinical practice to allow appropriate risk-adapted therapy. Currently, gene arrays are not widely available outside of clinical trials.

The latest comprehensive categorization of lymphomas is the WHO classification (Table 1), which evolved from the "working formulation" (WF) (4) and its successor, the Revised European-American Lymphoma (REAL) classification (5). Knowledge of the WF and its relationship to the WHO classification is helpful, because it can provide insight into both the nature and the expectations of treatment. Essentially, the WF categorized lymphomas according to the expected outcome with therapy and was thus a convenient tool for making therapeutic decisions. It grouped entities as low, intermediate, or high grade. The current, more precise WHO classification allows the inclusion of more homogeneous disease entities in clinical trials, which will lead to improved treatment outcomes.

Myeloproliferative Disorders

Recent studies have demonstrated the importance of the Jak-2 kinase, mutation in the pathogenesis of MPD. The mutation, a substitution of phenylalanine for valine at position 617 of the Jak-2 kinase results in transcriptional activation of cytokine receptor signaling pathways. It has been detected in 60% to 95% of patients with PRV, 55% of patients with MF, and 25% to 60% of patients with ET (6,7). CML is associated with the Philadelphia chromosome in most cases. In nearly all cases, the bcr-abl translocation is found using sensitive molecular techniques.

Leukemias

Most cases of leukemia are sporadic with no identifiable cause. Certainly, exposure to ionizing radiation and other carcinogens such as certain chemotherapeutic agents can be implicated in some cases. Many recurring genetic lesions have been described that result in the disruption of normal regulatory pathways. Autonomous proliferation may occur as a result of activating mutations. Increased self-renewal, loss of cell-cycle control, escape from apoptosis, and a block of cellular differentiation have all been reported (8). Acute promyelocytic leukemia (AML M3), which frequently presents with a low white blood cell (WBC) count and evidence, either laboratory, clinical, or both, of disseminated intravascular coagulation (DIC), is associated with the t(15;17) in most cases. The resulting fusion transcript promyelocytic leukemia-retioic acid receptor alpha (PML-RARα) predicts responsiveness to all-trans retinoic acid (ATRA), which has been used along with chemotherapy to manage this disorder successfully.

CLINICAL MANIFESTATIONS

Lymphoma

Most often, lymphoma is suspected following the finding of painless lymphadenopathy. Occasionally, with the more aggressive types, there may be associated pain and redness affecting the overlying skin. Differentiation from infection is important and patients have often received a course of antibiotics prior to undergoing a biopsy. Depending on the location, there may be symptoms related to organ compromise. Chest pain, pressure, or shortness of breath may occur with intrathoracic disease. The superior vena cava syndrome, with massive head and neck swelling, can occur with rapidly growing or bulky mediastinal adenopathy. Abdominal pain and swelling may occur with intra-abdominal lymphadeno-pathy. Splenomegaly may be associated with left upper quadrant discomfort and early satiety. Hydronephrosis may result from ureteral obstruction. Systemic symptoms, referred to as B symptoms, include fever, night sweats, and weight loss and generally are associated

TABLE 1   WHO Classification of Lymphoid Neoplasms

B-cell neoplasms
Precursor B-cell neoplasm
    Precursor B-lymphoblastic leukemia/lymphoma
    Precursor B-cell ALL
Mature (peripheral) B-cell neoplasms
    B-cell chronic lymphocytic leukemia/small lymphocytic lymphoma
    B-cell prolymphocytic lymphoma
    Lymphoplasmacytic lymphoma
    Splenic marginal zone B-cell lymphoma (±villous lymphocytes)
    Hairy cell leukemia
    Extranodal marginal zone B-cell lymphoma of MALT type
    Nodal marginal zone B-cell lymphoma (±monocytoid B-cells)
    Follicular lymphoma
    Mantle-cell lymphoma
    Diffuse large B-cell lymphoma
    Mediastinal large B-cell lymphoma
    Primary effusion lymphomas
    Burkitt's lymphoma/Burkitt cell leukemia
T-cell and NK-cell neoplasms
Precursor T-cell neoplasm
    Precursor T-lymphoblastic leukemia/lymphoma
    (Precursor T-cell ALL)
Mature (peripheral) T-cell neoplasms
    T-cell prolymphocytic leukemia
    T-cell granular lymphocytic leukemia
    Aggressive NK-cell leukemia
    Adult T-cell leukemia/lymphoma (HTLV-1+)
    Extranodal NK-/T-cell lymphoma, nasal type
    Enteropathy-type T-cell lymphoma
    Hepatosplenic γ-δ T-cell lymphoma
    Mycosis fungoides/Sèzary syndrome
    Anaplastic large-cell lymphoma, T-/null cell, primary cutaneous type
    Peripheral T-cell lymphoma, not otherwise specified
    Angioimmunoblastic T-cell lymphoma
    Anaplastic large-cell lymphoma, T-/null cell, primary systemic type
Posttransplantation lymphoproliferative disorders
Early lesions
    Reactive plasmacytic hyperplasia
    Infectious mononucleosis-like
PTLD, polymorphic
    Polyclonal (rare)
    Monoclonal
PTLD, monomorphic (classify according to lymphoma classification)
    B-cell lymphomas
    Diffuse large B-cell lymphoma (immunoblastic, centroblastic, anaplastic)
    Burkitt's/Burkitt-like lymphoma
    Plasma cell myeloma
T-cell lymphomas
    Peripheral T-cell lymphoma, not otherwise categorized
    Other types (hepatosplenic, γ-δ, T/NK)
Other types, rare
    Hodgkin's disease–like lesions (associated with methotrexate therapy)
    Plasmacytoma-like lesions

Abbreviations: HTLV1+, human T-cell lymphotropic virus 1; MALT, mucosa-associated lymphoid tissue; PTLD, posttransplantation lymphoproliferative disorders; NK, natural killer; WHO, World Health Organization; ALL, acute lymphoblastic leukemia.
Source: From Ref. 2.

with more aggressive disease. Skin involvement resulting in a rash that may be nodular may also occur. T-cell lymphomas have a greater propensity for skin involvement. Neurological involvement can present with focal findings, affecting both the central and the peripheral nervous system. In suspected cases, a magnetic resonance imaging scan in addition to spinal fluid sampling is mandatory (9).

WM, a syndrome that may accompany lymphoplasmacytic lymphoma, results from the presence of monoclonal immunoglobulin (Ig)M (macroglobulinemia). Symptoms can be related to the presence of the lymphoma, due to cytopenias related to marrow infiltration, or due to the monoclonal protein. Hyperviscosity related to the elevated IgM may be present, or the paraprotein may have self-directed antigenic specificity. Fatigue, headache, and weight loss are common. Bleeding is a common manifestation, with gum bleeding and epistaxis of concern in the head and neck. Neurological abnormalities, most commonly peripheral neuropathy, occur and focal cranial nerve abnormalities and mononeuritis multiplex may be seen. The hyperviscosity syndrome can result in confusion, lethargy, visual loss, deafness, ataxia, or diplopia. A sausage-like appearance of the retinal veins has been reported due to venous dilation and segmentation. This is a medical emergency that should be managed with rapidly instituted plasmapheresis.

The signs and symptoms of primary head and neck lymphoma depend on the site(s) of involvement. They are mostly related to either obstruction or mass effect. Systemic or B symptoms are present in the minority of patients (1). These tumors can mimic other neoplasms or can be mistaken for infections or other common head and neck disorders.

Sinonasal tumors typically present with nasal obstruction, which is most often unilateral. Epistaxis, hyposmia, nasal swelling, and mass are other common complaints. Tonsillar lymphomas present with unilateral enlargement, ulceration, dysphagia, and/or odynophagia. Lymphomas of the salivary glands and thyroid gland present as painless masses, and the diagnosis is rarely suspected initially. Laryngeal lymphomas, which are quite rare, present with voice change, airway obstruction, and, occasionally, with hemoptysis. Orbital lymphomas may present with a variety of ocular symptoms, with proptosis and diplopia being most common. Over 80% of all reported cases of extramedullary plasmacytoma occur in the head and neck, mostly in the upper aerodigestive tract. Clinically, they present as a mass and cause symptoms based on their location and by direct effect on adjacent structures, with upper airway obstruction, epistaxis, rhinorrhea, pain, and neck swelling being the most common.

Lymphoma Involving Specific Head and Neck Sites

Thyroid Lymphoma.   Lymphoma involving the thyroid gland is rare, accounting for only 2% to 3% of all cases of lymphoma and less than 10% of thyroid malignancies. Women are affected more frequently than men are by a ratio of 2.7:1. The median age at presentation is over 60 years. The most common subtypes are DLBCL and follicular Grade-3 lymphoma, accounting for at least 80% of cases. A rare but interesting subtype is marginal zone B-cell lymphoma, which arises from MALT. In many cases, this lymphoma arises from a background lymphocytic infiltrate occurring in the setting of Hashimoto's thyroiditis. MALT lymphomas are low grade and clinically indolent. Hodgkin's disease may rarely involve the thyroid gland (10), sometimes as the only site of disease. Burkitt's lymphoma and follicular Grade-1 and -2 lymphomas occur less frequently (11,12).

The presentation is most frequently a rapidly growing, painless neck mass, with or without adjacent lymphadenopathy (Fig. 1A and B). The more indolent lymphomas, such as follicular Grade-1 or -2 or the MALT lymphomas, generally are slower growing and may be confused with a goiter. The thyroid may be nodular or diffusely enlarged. Stridor, shortness of breath, hoarseness, and dysphagia may also occur. Although surgery plays no role in the

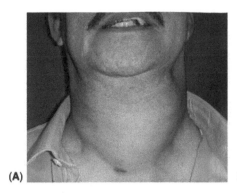
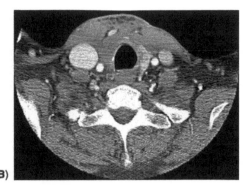

(A)   (B)

FIGURE 1 (A) Patient with enlarged thyroid gland simulating a goiter. FNA was nondiagnostic, and thyroidectomy was performed for compressive symptoms. (B) Computed tomography scan of the same patient showing infiltrative process involving the thyroid gland. *Abbreviation*: FNA, fine needle aspiration.

definitive treatment of lymphomas in general, the diagnosis in the thyroid may not be suspected preoperatively, and a thyroid lobectomy or even a total thyroidectomy may be performed inadvertently. A study comparing thyroid lymphomas that were debulked aggressively to those undergoing biopsy only, showed no difference in survival (13).

Fine needle aspiration (FNA), frequently performed for thyroid masses, is often nondiagnostic in cases of thyroid lymphoma. If the diagnosis is suspected, flow cytometry, immunohistochemical staining, and molecular markers can be performed on specimens obtained by FNA, provided that cellularity is adequate. Such specimens are best obtained with the assistance of a pathologist to ensure that an adequate amount of material has been obtained. Success rates for diagnosis of thyroid lymphoma from FNA range from 25% to 80%, but many authors state that open tissue biopsies may still be required to complete the diagnostic evaluation in the majority of cases. If the diagnosis is suspected but cannot be made on FNA, it is appropriate to perform an incisional biopsy without lobectomy.

Management depends primarily on the histology of the lymphoma. Localized aggressive lymphomas are treated with curative intent, currently with three cycles of CHOP-R chemotherapy (cyclophosphamide, doxorubicin, vincristine, and prednisone, + rituximab) followed by involved field irradiation; or with six cycles of CHOP-R, with or without involved field irradiation (11). Indolent lymphomas, if localized, should receive involved field irradiation, as this may be curative in a significant proportion of patients (14).

Waldeyer's Ring Lymphoma.   Lymphoma involving Waldeyer's ring accounts for more than 50% of all extranodal head and neck lymphomas. It most frequently involves the adenoids and tonsils. The base of the tongue is less commonly involved. Patients may present with a mass or evidence of compression with dysphagia, airway obstruction, or Eustachian tube blockage. Associated neck adenopathy may also be present. The overlying mucosa may be intact and diagnosis must be made by biopsy. The most frequent histology is the aggressive diffuse large-cell lymphoma, mostly of B-cell origin. This subtype accounts for 50% to 75% of cases (15,16). The indolent types, follicular and small lymphocytic lymphoma, also occur, but much less frequently (16). Extranodal marginal zone B-cell lymphoma does not commonly occur at this MALT site. Mantle-cell lymphoma has a particular propensity for the gastrointestinal (GI) tract and frequently may involve the nasopharynx (17). As is true for unsuspected GI involvement, blind nasopharyngeal biopsies will often demonstrate involvement in clinically unsuspected cases. Peripheral NK-/T-cell lymphomas are also rare at this site, in contrast to the higher incidence in the nasopharynx (16). Rare cases of Hodgkin's disease have been reported, affecting Waldeyer's ring. Most cases have been Stage 1 or 2 and the lymphocyte-predominant histology accounted for the majority (18).

Nasal Cavity and Paranasal Sinus Lymphoma. This region does not normally contain lymphoid tissue and NHL at these sites can be derived from B-cells, T-cells, or NK-cells. T-/NK-cell NHL is a specific entity, rare in the United States and Europe but seen most commonly in Asians and native Peruvians. It is associated with the EBV in the vast majority of cases and previously was termed lethal midline granuloma. Males are more frequently affected; the median age is 43 (19). It is an angiocentric, destructive lesion, with primary involvement of the nasal cavity. The paranasal sinuses are also frequently involved and can be associated with systemic disease (19). NK-/T-cell lymphomas have a predilection for relapse at distant extranodal sites. CNS prophylaxis should be included as a component of initial therapy. Additional sites where relapse is common include the skin, testes, orbit, and GI tract (20). Approximately 25% of maxillary sinus malignancies are lymphomas. In Caucasians, nasal lymphomas are most commonly diffuse large B-cell aggressive lymphomas. Most often, they are Stage 1 or 2 at diagnosis and frequently, primarily involve the paranasal sinuses (21). CNS relapse is not unusual, prompting some authors to recommend CNS prophylaxis as part of the initial therapy (22). Marginal zone B-cell lymphoma, Burkitt's and Burkitt-like lymphoma also occur. Nasopharyngeal lymphoma can present with nasal obstruction, sinus infiltration, pain, bloody nasal discharge, or facial swelling (Fig. 2A and B). Biopsy is required for diagnosis, and management is nonsurgical. Treatment options include radiation alone, but this is associated with a high local failure rate, especially in the T-/NK-cell type, and patients are generally treated with a combined modality approach utilizing adriamycin-based chemotherapy and irradiation (23).

Salivary Gland Lymphoma. The salivary gland is another site that normally does not contain lymphoid tissue, except for the intraparotid lymph nodes. In the setting of an autoimmune disease such as Sjögren's syndrome, lymphocytic infiltration occurs, and,

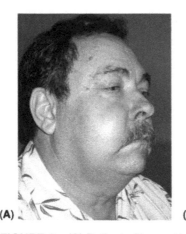 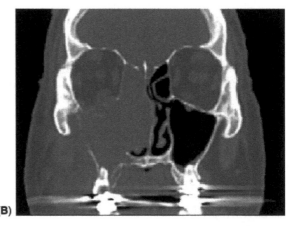

(A)   (B)

FIGURE 2 (**A**) Patient with non-Hodgkin's lymphoma of the maxillary sinus, presenting with right cheek swelling, pain, and nasal obstruction. (**B**) Computed tomography scan of patient in Figure 2A, showing opacification and expansion of right maxillary sinus, with possible bone erosion. At the time of biopsy by endoscopic sinus surgery, the orbital floor and lamina papyracea appeared to be dehiscent.

similar to Hashimoto's disease of the thyroid gland, can be a precursor to the development of lymphoma. In the absence of overt manifestations of lymphoma, monoclonal infiltrates demonstrated by polymerase chain reaction (PCR) have been reported. This finding has been reported in lymphoepithelial sialadenitis, also known as myoepithelial sialadenitis, a condition associated with lymphocytic infiltration of the salivary gland (24,25). Such patients are reported to have a 44-fold increase in the incidence of subsequent salivary or extrasalivary lymphoma, and they have a lifetime risk of 4% to 10% of developing lymphoma. The vast majority of lymphomas developing in this setting are of the MALT type, but more aggressive histologies also occur (26). Lymphocytic infiltrates are also described in the setting of HIV infection. In such cases, the infiltrate is generally polyclonal without an obvious increased risk for the development of lymphoma. Lymphoma arising in association with Warthin's tumor has also been described, albeit rarely (27).

Most salivary gland lymphomas occur in the parotid gland. Apart from the submandibular gland, other salivary gland sites are rarely affected. Diagnosis is made by biopsy and flow cytometry. Staging procedures include imaging and a bone marrow study. If localized, irradiation can result in excellent long-term control. If the diagnosis is suspected in a patient with Sjögren's syndrome where there is a background of chronic inflammation, an attempt should be made to obtain the diagnosis by FNA with flow cytometry. In some cases, a small open, incisional biopsy can be obtained from the extreme posterior inferior aspect, or tail, of the gland, well away from facial nerve branches. Parotidectomy in patients with Sjögren's syndrome, with or without associated lymphoma, carries a higher risk of temporary and permanent facial paralysis than surgery for abnormalities in noninflamed glands. A patient with concurrent Sjögren's and lymphoma in the parotid gland is shown in Figure 3.

Laryngeal Lymphoma. This is extremely rare and is the subject of case reports. Most cases described are DLBCL, but MALT lymphomas are also reported. The role of surgery is confined to biopsy and perhaps debulking or other measures to deal with airway compromise.

Hard Palate Lymphoma. These lymphomas are very rare. MALT lymphoma and mantle cell lymphoma (MCL) have been described. A mass may occur, resulting in difficulty with pronunciation (28,29). Plasmacytomas may also occur at this location.

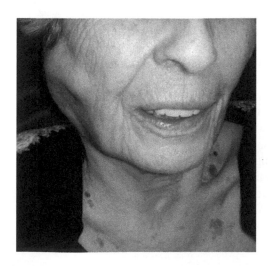

FIGURE 3 This elderly female had a long history of xerostomia and preexisting Sjögren's syndrome. She developed a rapidly enlarging right parotid mass that proved to be NHL on incision biopsy. The biopsy was performed on the posterior inferior portion of the mass, well away from the facial nerve. *Abbreviation*: NHL, non-Hodgkin's lymphoma.

Orbital Lymphoma. Orbital lymphomas account for approximately 1% of all NHL and up to 15% of extranodal NHL. Lymphomas involving the orbit most frequently affect elderly patients. Females are affected more commonly than males. In most cases, the orbit is the primary and only site of disease. Occasionally, it is involved as a secondary site. The most common histologic types are indolent, with marginal zone lymphoma being most common. Follicular and small lymphocytic lymphomas, lymphoplasmacytic lymphomas, and plasmacytomas also occur (30,31). Aggressive histologies, such as DLBCL, occur less frequently. Mantle-cell lymphoma may also be seen at this site. Most cases involve the orbit, often with lacrimal gland involvement. Conjunctival involvement may be seen, with eyelid involvement much less frequently. Bilateral disease is rare, occurring in up to only 5%.

Presenting symptoms most commonly include diplopia or blurred vision, proptosis, and excessive tearing. Eye pain may also be present (31).

For localized disease with low-grade histology, involved field radiation is the preferred treatment modality and very high rates of local control can be achieved (32). For aggressive histologies, combined modality therapy is generally recommended.

Myeloproliferative Disorders

PRV is frequently discovered incidentally when a complete blood count is performed for another reason. When symptoms are present, they are usually nonspecific. Fatigue, headache, and diaphoresis are common. Pruritis, often following a hot shower, is a frequent complaint. Up to 15% of patients may present with a thrombotic episode. Thrombotic cerebrovascular accidents, coronary artery thrombosis, Budd–Chiari syndrome, and pulmonary embolus all occur. Cavernous sinus thrombosis may also occur in untreated or poorly controlled disease. Erythromelalgia is specific to PRV and ET, and it is associated with an elevated platelet count and paradoxical vasodilation. It is characterized by redness, warmth, and a burning pain affecting the digits and responds promptly to aspirin. Gout may be a presenting manifestation of an MPD. There is an increased incidence of peptic ulcer disease in patients with PRV. Iron deficiency may occur and may initially mask the diagnosis. An elevated hematocrit with microcytosis is a clue to this possibility. Physical findings that may be present include a ruddy complexion, conjunctival injection, retinal vein engorgement, and spleen and/or liver enlargement. Splenomegaly is present in two-thirds of patients at presentation.

Apart from the ruddy complexion, specific head and neck manifestations are unusual. Epistaxis in addition to bleeding from other sites may occur in up to 40% of patients. Pyoderma gangrenosum is reported to occur with the MPD. This is a necrotizing skin ulceration that occurs most commonly on the limbs of patients with inflammatory bowel disease. It can also occur on the face. Manifestations of iron deficiency may include glossitis and cheilosis.

ET is also frequently an incidental finding. Once again, symptoms tend to be nonspecific. Bleeding and thrombotic manifestations occur with equal frequency, both being related to abnormal platelet function. In addition, when the platelet count is markedly elevated, acquired von Willebrand's disease may result from excessive binding of von Willebrand's factor to platelets. This results in mucosal bleeding such as purpura or epistaxis. Head and neck findings include transient visual disturbances such as monocular vision loss (amaurosis fugax) and mucosal or dental bleeding. Bleeding may be present in the presence or absence of concurrent von Willebrand's disease.

Chronic idiopathic MF usually presents with marked fatigue associated with anemia and a hypermetabolic state. Low-grade fevers and weight loss are frequent, as are symptoms related to a varying degree of splenomegaly, which may be massive. Hepatomegaly and splenomegaly occur due to extramedullary hematopoiesis.

Head and neck manifestations of MF are often a result of extramedullary hematopoiesis. This can result in tumors at any site. Lymph nodes may also be involved. Sweet's syndrome can occur in chronic idiopathic MF, presenting as cutaneous plaques or nodules at any site (33). This finding also occurs in a number of other hematological disorders, most commonly AML.

CML is diagnosed as an incidental finding in approximately one-third of patients. The most common symptoms are nonspecific and are related to anemia, bleeding, or infection. Early satiety due to splenomegaly is common.

Leukemias

Leukemias are classified as either acute or chronic. Within the acute category, the major types are AML and ALL. The equivalent chronic types are CML (discussed under MPDs) and CLL. CLL is the most common leukemia in adults, whereas in children, ALL is most frequently seen.

The acute leukemias are characterized by the proliferation and accumulation of immature blast cells. The blasts accumulate in the bone marrow, resulting in the failure of normal hematopoiesis. The WBC is usually elevated at presentation due to circulating blasts but a low WBC is not unusual. As a consequence of impaired hematopoiesis, symptoms and signs of anemia, thrombocytopenia and neutropenia are often present. Manifestations can include fatigue, pallor, bleeding or easy bruising, and infectious complications. Epistaxis or oozing from the gums related to dental procedures is frequently present. Purpura involving the buccal mucosa is also a relatively frequent observation in the setting of severe thrombocytopenia. DIC may contribute to bleeding, when present. Apart from manifestations related to pancytopenia, infiltration of tissues or organs including the skin may occur, especially in the setting of AML with monocytic differentiation. Gum infiltration is another relatively common feature of this leukemia subtype. Discrete violaceous lesions or a more generalized rash may occur. In such cases, a biopsy may show infiltration with myeloblasts.

Chloromas or granulocytic sarcomas are collections of blasts occurring as discrete masses. They can present as isolated masses at any site. Subcutaneous locations occur and may precede the development of systemic leukemia or another MPD. They have been frequently described involving a number of head and neck sites including the orbit, masseteric muscle, and maxillary sinus, but can occur at any location (34). They have been reported involving skin, bone, salivary glands, muscles, and mucosa and can be single or multiple. Cases of airway obstruction have been attributed to chloromas (35). Since they can represent the initial manifestation of leukemia, systemic manifestations or abnormal blood counts may not be present at diagnosis. A chloroma of the neck is shown in Figure 4. Biopsy of such lesions is essential for diagnosis and should result in an evaluation for systemic disease. Facial paralysis can also occur from infiltration of the nerve by malignant cells, as shown in Figure 5.

CLL, the most common leukemia, is often diagnosed incidentally as a result of a mature monoclonal lymphocytosis identified on a complete blood count. When signs or symptoms are present, they can include fatigue, fever, shortness of breath, weight loss, bleeding, and symptoms resulting from lymphadenopathy, often bulky. There is an increased risk of bacterial and fungal infections, partly related to hypogammaglobulinemia. An exaggerated response to insect bites can also occur. A skin rash due to cutaneous infiltration may sometimes be seen. Warm antibody-mediated autoimmune hemolytic anemia and immune thrombocytopenia occurs in up to 20% of patients with CLL (36).

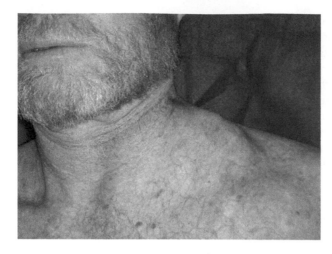

FIGURE 4 Swelling of the neck in a patient with ALL. Biopsy confirmed that this was a chloroma. *Abbreviation*: ALL, acute lymphoblastic leukemia.

DIAGNOSIS AND STAGING

Lymphoma

When lymphoma is suspected, a tissue diagnosis is required. Tissue biopsies should be large enough to provide adequate tissue for flow cytometry and molecular marker studies. For nodal lymphomas, excisional biopsy is recommended, although incisional biopsy is acceptable for large masses fixed to vital structures. For extranodal lymphomas, lymph nodes are not usually the source of material, and FNA and/or incisional biopsy are the preferred tissue-sampling methods. Frequently, an FNA will result in a tissue sample that is inadequate for definitive diagnosis and complete characterization. Flow cytometry should always be performed, especially if only an FNA is performed. Some very cellular aspirates may provide enough material to obviate the need for open biopsy. Care should be taken to handle the tissue gently, avoiding crush artifact. Specimens should be delivered fresh,

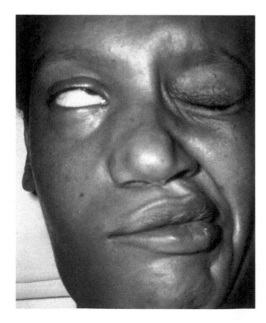

FIGURE 5 Patient with treated AML with complete right facial paralysis of eight months' duration. The paralysis did not improve after successful treatment of the leukemia. *Abbreviation*: AML, acute myeloblastic leukemia.

TABLE 2 Ann Arbor Staging Classification

Stage 1	Involvement of a single lymph node region or a single extralymphatic site (IE)
Stage 2	Involvement of two or more lymph node regions on the same side of the diaphragm, may have contiguous extralymphatic tissue involvement (IIE)
Stage 3	Involvement of lymph node regions on both sides of the diaphragm, possibly with spleen involvement (IIIS) or extralymphatic involvement (IIIE)
Stage 4	Diffuse extralymphatic involvement
A or B	B refers to the presence of systemic symptoms including fevers, night sweats, and significant weight loss (>10% body weight over 6 mo)

without fixative, promptly to the pathologist. Drying creates artifact that compromises an accurate reading of the histopathology.

Following tissue diagnosis, characterization of the extent of disease, or staging, is performed. The Ann Arbor staging system (Table 2) (37), originally devised for Hodgkin's disease, is also applied to NHL. The TNM system (tumor, nodes, and metastases) is not used for lymphomas, primarily due to the difficulty in specifying primary versus secondary sites. Additionally, the histology of the lymphoma is just as important as the anatomic distribution in dictating management and outcome. A bone marrow evaluation should be performed in all cases of lymphoma, with the exception of some very limited-stage cases of Hodgkin's disease. Computed tomography of the chest, abdomen, and pelvis completes the formal staging procedures. Increasingly, positron-emission tomography (PET scan) is performed because it can provide useful staging information at diagnosis or relapse and prognostic information during or following treatment. PET scans, when obtained pre- and post-treatment, allow differentiation of residual active disease from lymphadenopathy due to fibrosis (38).

A complete blood count and serum chemistry profile, including liver enzymes and serum lactate dehydrogenase (LDH), should also be obtained. Hepatic lymphoma involvement may be suggested by the finding of elevated transaminases, even in the setting of a normal-appearing liver. If dealing with a lymphoplasmacytic lymphoma and the possibility of WM, a serum protein electrophoresis, immunofixation, quantitative Igs, and serum viscosity should be obtained. The immunofixation will allow identification of the monoclonal protein as IgM. Most cases of MM are monoclonal IgG, with IgA and IgD occurring less frequently. Monoclonal IgG is also the most common paraprotein elaborated in plasmacytomas, although the non-IgG types are more likely to progress later to MM. Solitary plasmacytomas are diagnosed after excluding anemia and hypercalcemia. If present, a monoclonal paraprotein should resolve completely following therapy. Soft-tissue solitary plasmacytomas are much less likely to progress to MM, with approximately 70% remaining disease-free at 10 years (39).

Myeloproliferative Disorders

PRV is suspected when an elevated hematocrit is found. Confirmation of an elevated red blood cell mass has been advocated as necessary but is becoming increasingly difficult to obtain in most laboratories, and there are concerns regarding its sensitivity. For females and males, a hematocrit above 50% and above 56%, respectively, is associated with an elevated red-cell mass, and this measurement can sometimes be used as a proxy for the red-cell mass. Secondary causes of polycythemia must always be excluded in order to diagnose PRV. These include any conditions associated with chronic hypoxia. Infrequently, an erythropoietin-secreting tumor may be found. The measurement of endogenous erythropoietin may be helpful.

The diagnosis of ET is one of exclusion. On discovery of a consistently elevated platelet count of greater than 600,000, it is important to exclude iron deficiency anemia, infections, inflammatory disorders, and other neoplasms as the most common causes of secondary ET. The presence of the Jak-2 kinase mutation allows the diagnosis to be made in this and the other MPDs, apart from CML. However, a negative result does not exclude the diagnosis.

Chronic idiopathic MF is diagnosed by bone marrow examination. In the correct clinical situation of splenomegaly, cytopenias, nucleated red blood cells, teardrop-shaped red blood cells, and immature circulating WBCs, a diagnosis of marrow fibrosis is readily made. Cancer metastatic to the bone marrow can give a similar picture and needs to be excluded.

CML is diagnosed by the finding of the Philadelphia chromosome by conventional cytogenetics, preferably performed on a bone marrow sample or fluorescent in situ hybridization testing. PCR testing for the bcr-abl RNA transcript should also be obtained.

Leukemia

Acute leukemia is diagnosed by evaluation of the bone marrow. The presence of more than 20% blasts is diagnostic. Flow cytometry is helpful to further define the abnormal population of immature cells. Cytogenetic evaluation should always be performed, as it has important prognostic significance (40). CLL may be diagnosed by the finding of a monoclonal lymphocytosis in the peripheral blood. The typical cell is a mature lymphocyte seen with smudge cells on the peripheral blood smear. Variable numbers of prolymphocytes are often present. Flow cytometry demonstrates predominantly B-cells, expressing CD19 and CD20, with aberrant expression of the T-cell marker, CD5.

TREATMENT

Lymphoma

The treatment of lymphoma depends primarily on the histologic subtype and the stage. HL is treated with chemotherapy, or for more limited-stage disease, combination chemotherapy and radiotherapy. In this situation, the dose of both radiation and chemotherapy is less than if either modality is used alone. The advantage is a reduction in toxicity of each modality used alone. In some cases of very limited disease without B symptoms, radiation alone may be used. The current standard chemotherapy regimen is doxorubicin, bleomycin, vinblastine, dacarbazine (ABVD) (adriamycin, bleomycin, vinblastine, and dacarbazine), administered every two weeks for six months (one cycle equals one month). Two to four cycles of ABVD may be given, followed by involved field radiation, for more limited disease.

Of the NHL, indolent lymphomas, including follicular Grade-1 and -2 small lymphocytic lymphoma and lymphoplasmacytic lymphoma (sometimes associated with WM), are generally considered incurable. Although many active chemotherapeutic agents and combination regimens are available, in many cases, in the absence of symptoms, treatment is withheld until there is evidence of disease progression. Earlier treatment has not been shown to impact survival compared to the "watch and wait" approach (41). The anti-CD20 monoclonal antibody rituximab is a very active agent in this group of disorders, either as a single agent or combined with chemotherapy (42,43). It is noteworthy that lymphoma affecting head and neck sites in a localized fashion can be treated with involved field irradiation. Such an approach can be associated with low morbidity and prolonged disease-free intervals (44,45).

For the higher grade lymphomas, chemotherapy is indicated. The CHOP (cyclophosphamide, adriamycin, vincristine, and prednisone) regimen is generally administered with rituximab (46). For aggressive Stage-1 or -2 lymphomas involving most head and neck sites, localized irradiation used to be a reasonable option. However, a high rate of relapse has been observed, mostly at distant sites, probably due to the frequent occurrence of occult disease at presentation. For limited-stage disease, abbreviated (three to four cycles) combination anthracycline-based chemotherapy with monoclonal antibody therapy, followed by involved field radiotherapy, is administered with curative intent in most cases (47–53). This approach is modeled on data comparing combined modality therapy with radiation therapy alone for limited-stage nodal-based disease (54). For more extensive disease, six to eight cycles of immunochemotherapy are generally administered (46). For patients who relapse, a salvage chemotherapy regimen is indicated in appropriate candidates for further therapy. This is frequently a platinum-containing regimen, and for responsive patients, high-dose chemotherapy with autologous stem-cell transplantation may be curative (55).

Surgery when dealing with lymphoma is generally limited to biopsy, but, rarely, may have a role in debulking of particular sites for relief of symptoms. In the head and neck region, surgery is most often used to relieve airway obstruction, dysphagia, or bleeding. Plasmacytomas may be controlled by surgery alone when adequate margins can be obtained; however, when margins are close or tumor-free margins cannot be obtained, postoperative radiation therapy should be given. A large retrospective statistical analysis indicated that plasmacytomas treated with combined surgery and radiation had a better survival outcome than those treated with either of the modalities alone (56).

NK-/T-cell lymphomas are particularly aggressive and are also frequently managed with a combined modality approach. Recent Chinese studies suggest that involved field radiation as initial therapy may be sufficient, and, if given with chemotherapy, should be sequenced so that the irradiation is administered first (57,58).

The high-grade lymphomas, Burkitt's, Burkitt's-like, and lymphoblastic lymphoma, are treated with aggressive, intensive, multicycle chemotherapy, including CNS prophylaxis with intrathecal chemotherapy (59). Prophylaxis against tumor lysis syndrome is important when treating these aggressive tumors. Localized radiation therapy alone, even for limited-stage disease, is not appropriate for the high-grade tumors.

Solitary plasmacytomas are managed with localized irradiation. For involvement of head and neck sites, regional lymph nodes may be included.

Myeloproliferative Disorders

PRV is generally treated with phlebotomy with or without cytoreductive therapy, usually hydroxyurea. Low-dose aspirin also has benefits in terms of a reduction in the risk of thrombosis. ET is also managed with cytoreductive therapy in selected patients. Treatment is beneficial in high-risk patients, defined as those with extreme ET or those with cardiovascular or cerebrovascular risk factors. Patients with a prior history of thrombosis and those over 60 years of age should be treated (60). The current therapy of choice is hydroxyurea. An alternative is anagrelide, the specific megakaryocyte inhibitor. A recent randomized trial demonstrated a higher incidence of arterial thrombosis and a higher incidence of progression to chronic idiopathic MF with anagrelide when compared to hydroxyurea (61). Chronic idiopathic MF is managed with supportive care measures. Androgens and erythropoietin may be beneficial for the management of anemia. Splenectomy may be beneficial in selected patients but carries a high risk of morbidity and mortality and can result in transfusion independence. Thalidomide may also be beneficial in chronic MF (62). The only curative therapy is an allogeneic bone marrow stem-cell transplant, but this treatment has limited applicability given the advanced age of most patients and limited availability of a human leucocyte antigen–matched sibling donor. The introduction of reduced intensity regimens for preparation prior to transplant has opened up this option to a greater number of patients (63).

CML is currently managed with imatinib, the tyrosine kinase inhibitor. This is associated with very high rates of complete hematological response and also cytogenetic and molecular responses (64). Newer tyrosine kinase inhibitors that are effective in patients resistant to imatinib are in development. For suitable candidates who do not respond adequately to imatinib, an allogeneic transplant remains the only known curative option for this disorder.

Leukemia

AML is treated with intensive chemotherapy. The standard regimen is an anthracycline plus Ara-C (the three plus seven regimen). Following remission, consolidation, often with high-dose ARA-C, is administered. Depending on risk stratification, allogeneic or autologous transplant may be appropriate in selected patients. Acute promyelocytic leukemia (FAB M3) is treated with ATRA in addition to chemotherapy. Induction is followed by consolidation and then a maintenance regimen. There is no benefit from maintenance therapy in the other subtypes of AML.

ALL is treated with an intensive multiagent chemotherapy regimen. Up to six or eight months of intensive therapy is administered followed by maintenance therapy for up to a total of three years of therapy. CNS prophylaxis is an integral component of therapy. Allogeneic transplantation is indicated for patients with high-risk disease in first remission and for selected other patients at the time of relapse.

COMPLICATIONS AND PROGNOSIS

Prognosis for Lymphomas

Prognostic indices have been developed for the indolent and aggressive lymphomas. The International Prognostic Index (IPI) (65) is utilized to evaluate a patient's risk status for the aggressive lymphomas. The Follicular Lymphoma IPI (FLIPI) (66) is similarly utilized for the indolent follicular lymphomas. Using the IPI or FLIPI to determine therapy is the subject of ongoing clinical trials. The IPI and FLIPI criteria are shown in Tables 3 and 4, respectively. It is important to note that the IPI was validated using the conventional CHOP or similar chemotherapy regimen prior to the introduction of the widely used monoclonal antibody rituximab. Moreover, there is a lack of studies applying these prognostic indices to primary head and neck extranodal lymphomas.

Prognosis for MPDs and Leukemia

With appropriate management, prolonged survival (>12–15 years) is likely for PRV and ET. Many patients with ET may have a normal lifespan. Symptom control and prevention

TABLE 3A   International Prognostic Index

Prognostic factors
Age > 60 yr
Performance status >ECOG1
LDH > normal
Extranodal sites >1
Stage 3 or 4

Note: The table shows the identified prognostic variables.

TABLE 3B CR with Initial Therapy and the Chance of OS at Five Years

Risk group	Number of risk factors	CR%	OS%
Low	0–1	87	73
Low-intermediate	2	67	51
High-intermediate	3	55	43
High	4–5	44	26

Abbreviations: CR, complete response rate; OS, overall survival.

TABLE 4A Follicular Lymphoma International Prognostic Index[a]

Prognostic factors
Age >60
Ann Arbor Stage 3–4
Number of nodal sites >4
LDH > normal
Hemoglobin <12

[a]The table shows the identified risk factors.

TABLE 4B Five-Year and 10-Year Survival Probabilities According to the Number of Risk Factors

Risk group	Number of risk factors	5 yr OS (SE) (%)	10 yr OS (SE) (%)
Low	0–1	90.6 (1.2)	70.7 (2.7)
Intermediate	2	77.6 (1.6)	50.9 (2.7)
High	≥3	52.5 (2.3)	35.5 (2.8)

Abbreviation: OS, overall survival; SE, standard error.

of hemorrhagic and thrombotic manifestations are the goals of therapy. It is also important to limit therapy-related complications. In some situations, no therapy is indicated, as long as followup with a hematologist occurs. In PRV, eventually there may be progression to the postpolycythemic spent phase, a time during which increasing transfusion requirements develop. Additional complications that may develop include myeloid metaplasia with MF or AML (67). In appropriate circumstances, younger patients may be considered for a potentially curative allogeneic stem-cell transplant.

CML initial therapy is now imatinib mesylate (Gleevec) (64). The median duration of response has not yet been established and initial hematologic complete response rates are extremely high. Cytogenetic and molecular response rates are also high, but complete molecular responses are very rare. The only established curative therapy is an allogeneic transplant, but morbidity and mortality concerns remain. Currently, a trial of imatinib with consideration of an allogeneic transplant in appropriate candidates with a suboptimal initial response is indicated for most patients. Imatinib appears to alter the natural history of CML. Prior to imatinib, the median survival was four years, with typical progression from chronic phase to accelerated phase and ultimately, blast crisis.

CLL is a disorder with a widely variable prognosis. Many patients follow an asymptomatic course and may never require treatment. Others can be identified as higher risk based on the clinical presentation, course, or molecular features of the leukemic cells.

With conventional chemotherapy, the disorder is incurable, but an allogeneic transplant can be curative in selected patients.

AML and ALL can also be stratified in terms of risk status at the time of disease presentation. Cytogenetic abnormalities are particularly important in this regard. A risk-adapted approach to transplant is followed for eligible patients.

Complications

Complications relate to site-specific manifestations of the disorder and/or consequences of treatment with chemotherapy or radiation. Infectious complications are common, most often following treatment of acute leukemia. The most feared are fungal infections, especially with *Aspergillus* species (68) or mucormycoses (69). The incidence increases with prolonged periods of neutropenia or with immunosuppression given for the treatment of graft versus host disease following allogeneic stem-cell transplantation. Disease may be localized to head and neck structures including the nose, paranasal sinuses, or orbits (Fig. 6), or may be present at systemic sites, most frequently, the lung parenchyma. Intracranial spread may occur from direct extension of the rhinocerebral form of mucormycosis but can be seen in other opportunistic fungal infections. Invasive fungal infections of the head and neck in this setting have a very high case fatality rate and treatment includes high-dose systemic antifungal agents and early, aggressive surgical debridement. In addition to early medical and surgical intervention, neutrophil recovery and withdrawal of immunosuppressive medications, when possible, gives the best chance for a successful outcome. Complications that are related to the specific site of disease involvement are discussed under "Clinical Manifestations," above.

SUMMARY

This chapter includes a review of lymphomas, leukemias, and MPDs, and their head and neck manifestations. The head and neck symptoms and findings may lead to the initial diagnosis or may be local or systemic complications of the specific disorders. For head and neck specialists, involvement with patients who have these disorders requires fundamental knowledge of how these conditions appear in the head and neck region. The head and neck specialist who is familiar with the information in this chapter will be able to recognize many of these disorders through their head and neck manifestations and will be able to provide assistance in diagnosis by employing the appropriate techniques for procuring and handling biopsy specimens, especially when lymphoma is suspected. Infrequently, surgery may be required to relieve

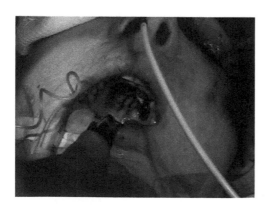

FIGURE 6 Extensive necrosis of facial, sinus, orbital, and oral structures occurred secondary to invasive *Aspergillus* infection in this patient with AML. Palate necrosis is shown here. Aggressive, early debridement, systemic antifungal therapy, and reversal of immunosuppression, when possible, are recommended. *Abbreviation*: AML, acute myeloblastic leukemia.

symptoms, including airway obstruction, or to assist in the management of complications of these disorders, which often require immediate attention and may be life threatening.

REFERENCES

1. Hanna E, Wanamaker J, Adelstein D, et al. Extranodal lymphomas of the head and neck. A 20-year experience. Arch Otolaryngol Head Neck Surg 1997; 123(12):1318–1323.

2. Harris NL, Jaffe ES, Diebold J, et al. World Health Organization classification of neoplastic diseases of the hematopoietic and lymphoid tissues: report of the Clinical Advisory Committee meeting-Airlie House, Virginia, November 1997. J Clin Oncol 1999; 17(12):3835–3849.

3. Rosenwald A, Wright G, Chan WC, et al. The use of molecular profiling to predict survival after chemotherapy for diffuse large-B-cell lymphoma. N Engl J Med 2002; 346(25):1937–1947.

4. National Cancer Institute sponsored study of classifications of non-Hodgkin's lymphomas: summary and description of a working formulation for clinical usage. The Non-Hodgkin's Lymphoma Pathologic Classification Project. Cancer 1982; 49(10):2112–2135.

5. Harris NL, Jaffe ES, Stein H, et al. A revised European-American classification of lymphoid neoplasms: a proposal from the International Lymphoma Study Group (see comments). Blood 1994; 84(5):1361–1392.

6. Baxter EJ, Scott LM, Campbell PJ, et al. Acquired mutation of the tyrosine kinase JAK2 in human myeloproliferative disorders. Lancet 2005; 365(9464):1054–1061.

7. Levine RL, Wadleigh M, Cools J, et al. Activating mutation in the tyrosine kinase JAK2 in polycythemia vera, essential thrombocythemia, and myeloid metaplasia with myelofibrosis. Cancer Cell 2005; 7(4):387–397.

8. Licht JD, Sternberg DW. The molecular pathology of acute myeloid leukemia. Hematology (Am Soc Hematol Educ Program) 2005:137–142.

9. Chamberlain MC, Nolan C, Abrey LE. Leukemic and lymphomatous meningitis: incidence, prognosis, and treatment. J Neurooncol 2005; 75(1):71–83.

10. Wang SA, Rahemtullah A, Faquin WC, et al. Hodgkin's lymphoma of the thyroid: a clinicopathologic study of five cases and review of the literature. Mod Pathol 2005; 18(12):1577–1584.

11. Ha CS, Shadle KM, Medeiros LJ, et al. Localized non-Hodgkin lymphoma involving the thyroid gland. Cancer 2001; 91(4):629–635.

12. Ansell SM, Grant CS, Habermann TM. Primary thyroid lymphoma. Semin Oncol 1999; 26(3):-316–323.

13. Pyke CM, Grant CS, Habermann TM, et al. Non-Hodgkin's lymphoma of the thyroid: is more than biopsy necessary? World J Surg 1992; 16(4):604–609; discussion 609–610.

14. Tsang RW, Gospodarowicz MK, Pintilie M, et al. Localized mucosa-associated lymphoid tissue lymphoma treated with radiation therapy has excellent clinical outcome. J Clin Oncol 2003; 21(22):4157–4164.

15. Kojima M, Tamaki Y, Nakamura S, et al. Malignant lymphoma of Waldeyer's ring. A histological and immunohistochemical study. APMIS 1993; 101(7):537–544.

16. Tan LH. Lymphomas involving Waldeyer's ring: placement, paradigms, peculiarities, pitfalls, patterns, and postulates. Ann Acad Med Singapore 2004; 33(4 suppl):15–26.

17. Zucca E, Fontana S, Roggero E, et al. Treatment and prognosis of centrocytic (mantle cell) lymphoma: a retrospective analysis of twenty-six patients treated in one institution. Leuk Lymphoma 1994; 13(1–2):105–110.

18. Quinones-Avila Mdel P, Gonzalez-Longoria AA, Admirand JH, et al. Hodgkin lymphoma involving Waldeyer's ring: a clinicopathologic study of 22 cases. Am J Clin Pathol 2005; 123(5):651–656.

19. Jaffe ES, Chan JK, Su IJ, et al. Report of the Workshop on Nasal and Related Extranodal Angiocentric T/Natural Killer Cell Lymphomas; definitions, differential diagnosis, and epidemiology. Am J Surg Pathol 1996; 20(1):103–111.

20. Cheung MM, Chan JK, Lau WH, et al. Primary non-Hodgkin's lymphoma of the nose and nasopharynx: clinical features, tumor immunophenotype, and treatment outcome in 113 patients. J Clin Oncol 1998; 16(1):70–77.

21. Cuadra-Garcia I, Proulx G, Wu C, et al. Sinonasal lymphoma: a clinicopathologic analysis of 58 cases from the Massachusetts General Hospital. Am J Surg Pathol 1999; 23(11):1356–1369.

22. Oprea C, Cainap C, Azoulay R, et al. Primary diffuse large B-cell non-Hodgkin lymphoma of the paranasal sinuses: a report of 14 cases. Br J Haematol 2005; 131(4):468–471.

23. Kim GE, Cho JH, Yang WI, et al. Angiocentric lymphoma of the head and neck: patterns of systemic failure after radiation treatment. J Clin Oncol 2000; 18(1):54–63.

24. Bahler DW, Swerdlow SH. Clonal salivary gland infiltrates associated with myoepithelial sialadenitis (Sjögren's syndrome) begin as nonmalignant antigen-selected expansions. Blood 1998; 91(6): 864–1872.

25. Harris N. Lymphoid proliferations of the salivary glands. Am J Clin Pathol 1999; 111(1 suppl)1: S94–S103.

26. Hsi E, Zukerberg L, Schnitzer B, et al. Development of extrasalivary gland lymphoma in myoepithelial sialadenitis. Mod Pathol 1995; 8(8):817–824.

27. Pescarmona E, Perez M, Faraggiana T, et al. Nodal peripheral T-cell lymphoma associated with Warthin's tumour. Histopathology 2005; 47(2):221–222.

28. Chang CC, Rowe JJ, Hawkins P, et al. Mantle cell lymphoma of the hard palate: a case report and review of the differential diagnosis based on the histomorphology and immunophenotyping pattern. Oral Surg Oral Med Oral Pathol Oral Radiol Endod 2003; 96(3):316–320.

29. Tauber S, Nerlich A, Lang S. MALT lymphoma of the paranasal sinuses and the hard palate: report of two cases and review of the literature. Eur Arch Otorhinolaryngol 2006; 263(1):19–22.

30. Coupland SE, Krause L, Delecluse HJ, et al. Lymphoproliferative lesions of the ocular adnexa. Analysis of 112 cases. Ophthalmology 1998; 105(8):1430–1441.

31. Ahmed, S, Shahid RK, Sison CP, et al. Orbital lymphomas: a clinicopathologic study of a rare disease. Am J Med Sci 2006; 331(2):79–83.

32. Martinet S, Ozsahin M, Belkacemi Y, et al. Outcome and prognostic factors in orbital lymphoma: a Rare Cancer Network study on 90 consecutive patients treated with radiotherapy. Int J Radiat Oncol Biol Phys 2003; 55(4):892–898.

33. Su WP, Alegre VA, White WL. Myelofibrosis discovered after diagnosis of Sweet's syndrome. Int J Dermatol 1990; 29(3):201–204.

34. Ferri E, Minotto C, Ianniello F, et al. Maxillo-ethmoidal chloroma in acute myeloid leukaemia: case report. Acta Otorhinolaryngol Ital 2005; 25(3):195–199.

35. Genet P, Pulik M, Lionnet F, et al. Leukemic relapse presenting with bronchial obstruction caused by granulocytic sarcoma. Am J Hematol 1994; 47(2):142–143.

36. Ward JH. Autoimmunity in chronic lymphocytic leukemia. Curr Treat Options Oncol 2001; 2(3): 253–257.

37. Carbone P, Kaplan H, Musshoff K, et al. Report of the Committee on Hodgkin's Disease Staging Classification. Cancer Res 1971; 31(11):1860–1861.

38. Israel O, Keidar Z, Bar-Shalom R. Positron emission tomography in the evaluation of lymphoma. Semin Nucl Med 2004; 34(3):166–179.

39. Dimopoulos MA, Hamilos G. Solitary bone plasmacytoma and extramedullary plasmacytoma. Curr Treat Options Oncol 2002; 3(3):255–259.

40. Mrozek K, Heerema NA, Bloomfield CD. Cytogenetics in acute leukemia. Blood Rev 2004; 18(2): 115–136.

41. Advani R, Rosenberg SA, Horning SJ. Stage I and II follicular non-Hodgkin's lymphoma: long-term follow-up of no initial therapy J Clin Oncol 2004; 22(8):1454–1459.

42. Czuczman MS, Grillo-Lopez AJ, White CA, et al. Treatment of patients with low-grade B-cell lymphoma with the combination of chimeric anti-CD20 monoclonal antibody and CHOP chemotherapy. J Clin Oncol 1999; 17(1):268–276.

43. McLaughlin P, Grillo-Lopez AJ, Link BK, et al. Rituximab chimeric anti-CD20 monoclonal antibody therapy for relapsed indolent lymphoma: half of patients respond to a four-dose treatment program. J Clin Oncol 1998; 16(8):2825–2833.

44. Guadagnolo BA, Li S, Neuberg D, et al. Long-term outcome and mortality trends in early-stage, Grade 1–2 follicular lymphoma treated with radiation therapy. Int J Radiat Oncol Biol Phys 2006; 64 (3):928–934.

45. Tsang RW, Gospodarowicz MK. Radiation therapy for localized low-grade non-Hodgkin's lymphomas. Hematol Oncol 2005; 23(1):10–17.

46. Coiffier B, Lepage E, Briere J, et al. CHOP chemotherapy plus rituximab compared with CHOP alone in elderly patients with diffuse large-B-cell lymphoma. N Engl J Med 2002; 346(4):235–242.

47. Hayabuchi N, Shibamoto Y, Nakamura K, et al. Stage I and II aggressive B-cell lymphomas of the head and neck: radiotherapy alone as a treatment option and the usefulness of the new prognostic index B-ALPS. Int J Radiat Oncol Biol Phys 2003; 55(1):44–50.

48. Sasai K, Yamabe H, Kokubo M, et al. Head-and-neck stages I and II extranodal non-Hodgkin's lymphomas: real classification and selection for treatment modality. Int J Radiat Oncol Biol Phys 2000; 48(1):153–160.

49. Nathu RM, Mendenhall NP, Almasri NM, et al. Non-Hodgkin's lymphoma of the head and neck: a 30-year experience at the University of Florida. Head Neck 1999; 21(3):247–254.

50. Tham IW, Lee KM, Yap SP, et al. Outcome of patients with nasal natural killer (NK)/T-cell lymphoma treated with radiotherapy, with or without chemotherapy. Head Neck 2006; 28(2):126–134.

51. Yu KH, Yu SC, Teo PM, et al. Nasal lymphoma: results of local radiotherapy with or without chemotherapy. Head Neck 1997; 19(4):251–259.

52. Frata P, Buglione M, Grisanti S, et al. Localized extranodal lymphoma of the head and neck: retrospective analysis of a series of 107 patients from a single institution. Tumori 2005; 91(6):456–462.

53. DiBiase SJ, Grigsby PW, Guo C, et al. Outcome analysis for stage IE and IIE thyroid lymphoma. Am J Clin Oncol 2004; 27(2):178–184.

54. Miller TP, Dahlberg S, Cassady JR, et al. Chemotherapy alone compared with chemotherapy plus radiotherapy for localized intermediate- and high-grade non-Hodgkin's lymphoma. N Engl J Med 1998; 339(1):21–26; comments N Engl J Med 1998; 339(20):1475–1477.

55. Philip T, Guglielmi C, Hagenbeek A, et al. Autologous bone marrow transplantation as compared with salvage chemotherapy in relapses of chemotherapy-sensitive non-Hodgkin's lymphoma. N Engl J Med 1995; 333(23):1540–1545.

56. Alexiou C, Kau RJ, Dietzfelbinger H, et al. Extramedullary plasmacytoma: tumor occurrence and therapeutic concepts. Cancer 1999; 85(11):2305–2314.

57. Li Y-X, Yao B, Jin J, et al. Radiotherapy as primary treatment for sIE and IIE nasal natural killer/T-cell lymphoma. J Clin Oncol 2006; 24(1):181–189.

58. Chim C-S, Ma S-Y, Au W-Y, et al. Primary nasal natural killer cell lymphoma: long-term treatment outcome and relationship with the International Prognostic Index. Blood 2004; 103(1):216–221.

59. Hoelzer D, Gokbuget N. Treatment of lymphoblastic lymphoma in adults. Best Pract Res Clin Haematol 2002; 15(4):713–728.

60. Finazzi G, Barbui T. Risk-adapted therapy in essential thrombocythemia and polycythemia vera. Blood Rev 2005; 19(5):243–252.

61. Harrison CN, Campbell PJ, Buck G, et al. Hydroxyurea compared with anagrelide in high-risk essential thrombocythemia. N Engl J Med 2005; 353(1):33–45.

62. Cervantes F. Modern management of myelofibrosis. Br J Haematol 2005; 128(5):583–592.

63. Rondelli D, Barosi G, Bacigalupo A, et al. Allogeneic hematopoietic stem-cell transplantation with reduced-intensity conditioning in intermediate- or high-risk patients with myelofibrosis with myeloid metaplasia. Blood 2005; 105(10):4115–4119.

64. O'Brien SG, Guilhot F, Larson RA, et al. Imatinib compared with interferon and low-dose cytarabine for newly diagnosed chronic-phase chronic myeloid leukemia. N Engl J Med 2003; 348(11):994–1004.

65. The International Non-Hodgkin's Lymphoma Prognostic Factors Project. A predictive model for aggressive non-Hodgkin's lymphoma. N Engl J Med 1993; 329(14):987–994; comments in N Engl J Med 1994; 330(8):574.

66. Solal-Celigny P, Roy P, Colombat P, et al. Follicular Lymphoma International Prognostic Index. Blood 2004; 104(5):1258–1265; comment in Blood 2005; 105(12):4892.

67. Spivak JL. Polycythemia vera: myths, mechanisms, and management. Blood 2002; 100(13):4272–4290.

68. Patterson TF, Kirkpatrick WR, White M, et al. Invasive aspergillosis. Disease spectrum, treatment practices, and outcomes. I3 Aspergillus Study Group. Medicine (Baltimore) 2000; 79(4):250–260; comments, 281–282.

69. Ferguson BJ. Mucormycosis of the nose and paranasal sinuses. Otolaryngol Clin North Am 2000; 33(2):349–365.

18

Malignant Melanoma

Maihgan A. Kavanagh and Donald L. Morton
John Wayne Cancer Institute at Saint John's Health Center, Santa Monica, California, U.S.A.

Robert A. Weisman
Division of Otolaryngology, Head and Neck Oncology Program, Moores Cancer Center, University of California, San Diego, California, U.S.A.

INTRODUCTION

Malignant melanoma of the head and neck region presents a unique set of diagnostic and treatment challenges. Melanoma can occur in the head and neck region as primary lesions of the skin (cutaneous), of the naso-oropharynx (mucosal), and of the eye (ocular). It can present as regional disease with anterior or posterior cervical lymphadenopathy. Melanoma can also form satellite lesions around the primary site or subcutaneous nodules in transit from the primary site to the draining lymph node basin. Melanoma is one of the few cancers that can metastasize virtually anywhere, but prefers lung, liver, brain, and small bowel.

EPIDEMIOLOGY

The overall incidence of malignant melanoma has increased dramatically over the last 30 years. According to the American Cancer Society, melanoma now comprises about 4% of all cancers in the United States. During 2005, almost 60,000 new cases of melanoma were diagnosed and it is estimated that more than 7500 people died of melanoma (1). Cutaneous melanoma is a disease of older patients; median age at diagnosis is 57 years and median age at death is 67 years. Although it can occur in infants and children, this is rare. Malignant melanoma is the fifth most common cancer in men and the sixth most common in women (1). Men are more likely to die of melanoma, usually because melanoma in men tends to occur on areas of the body associated with poorer prognosis, such as the torso, back, and head and neck regions. In contrast, females tend to develop melanoma of the extremity, which carries a better prognosis. Approximately 16% of all cases of melanoma occur in the head and neck regions (2).

PATHOGENESIS

Melanoma can occur as an autosomal-dominant familial syndrome in approximately 8% to 12% of all cases (3). These families are at overall increased risk of developing melanoma and will frequently develop multiple primary lesions at an earlier age. The cutaneous malignant melanoma–dysplastic nevi syndrome reflects a genetic abnormality located on the short arm of chromosome 1. Malignant melanoma cells frequently show this chromosomal 1 deletion, which results in loss of tumor suppression.

Like other skin cancers, melanoma has been associated with sun exposure. The incidence of melanoma is higher in regions of the world with higher ultraviolet light exposure. Increased rates of melanoma occur in populations with fair complexions. Blond or red-haired individuals with fair skin who sunburn easily are at greatest risk. People with multiple nevi also are more likely to develop melanoma. Areas of the body less protected by clothes, such as scalp, ears, and nose, are at increased risk. However, melanoma can occur on areas with minimal sun exposure and in individuals with darker skin tones; therefore, the actual etiology is thought to be multifactorial.

CLINICAL MANIFESTATIONS

Primary Lesion

A primary lesion is the most common manifestation of malignant melanoma of the head and neck region. This lesion can vary in appearance from the classical black-pigmented, raised lesion to an enlarging, skin-colored (amelanotic) mole (Fig. 1A and B). Melanoma can arise from a preexisting nevus or normal skin. The appearance of melanoma may be

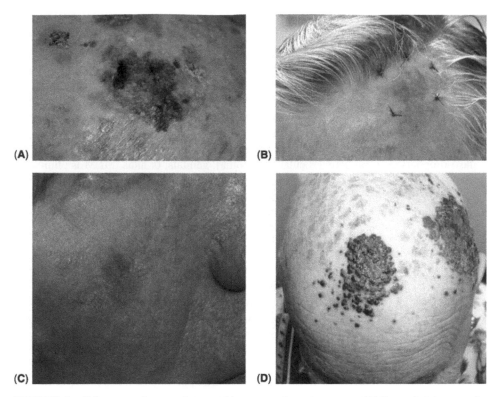

FIGURE 1   Primary melanoma has a wide range of appearances. (**A**) Superficial-spreading melanoma. (**B**) Amelanotic nodular melanoma of the scalp. (**C**) Lentigo maligna melanoma of the cheek. (**D**) Advanced cutaneous melanoma with satellite lesions of the scalp. *Source:* Courtesy of Dr. Mark Faries.

similar to other generally noninvasive skin cancers such as basal cell and squamous cell carcinoma, requiring biopsy for pathologic identification.

Primary cutaneous melanoma is identified in several ways. Classically, worrisome skin lesions that may be melanoma are described with the ABCDE mnemonic: Asymmetry, irregular Borders, variable Color, Diameter >6 mm, and Evolving lesions. Melanoma has two different growth phases: radial growth spreads laterally and superficially, whereas vertical growth penetrates deeply and has higher metastatic potential. Historically, melanoma is also identified by distinct histological subtypes.

Superficial spreading melanoma (SSM), the most common histological subtype, accounts for 70% of all primary melanomas and is most commonly seen in the head, neck, torso, and lower extremities. Frequently arising from an existing nevus, SSM is usually flat to slightly raised, with variable pigmentation and irregular borders (Fig. 1A). Growth of these tumors can be indolent initially; the radial growth phase may last for many years before signs of rapid vertical growth appear. Peak incidence of SSM occurs at a median age of 56 years (3).

The second most common histological subtype is nodular melanoma (NM). This subtype commonly occurs in the head, neck, and torso. It is characterized by a raised, frequently symmetric, darkly pigmented lesion with rapid onset and growth. Most of these lesions are pigmented, but a small percentage may be amelanotic (Fig. 1B). NM has no radial growth phase and a rapid vertical growth phase, resulting in a thicker lesion with higher risk of metastatic spread. The median age of onset is 49 years (3).

Accounting for about 10% of all melanomas, lentigo maligna melanoma (LMM) commonly occurs in the head and neck region like SSM, but arises from a preexisting lentigo maligna lesion that usually has been present for more than five years prior to diagnosis. LMM is frequently a large (>3 cm), flat lesion with brown to black pigmentation; it has an indolent course with a prolonged radial growth phase (Fig. 1C). LMM occurs in older individuals, with a median age of onset of 70 years (3).

Mucosal lentiginous melanoma (MLM) includes lesions occurring on the mucosa of the naso-oropharynx, conjunctiva (ocular melanoma), genitals, or anus. MLM is clinically aggressive and appears as a flat or ulcerated, pigmented, irregular lesion. It can frequently be missed on physical exam and then diagnosed retrospectively after the appearance of nodal metastases. Median age of onset is 56 years (3,4).

Regional Metastasis

On physical exam, the most common clinical manifestation of regional melanoma in the head and neck region is lymphadenopathy. This can involve the anterior and posterior cervical nodes, but can also include conventionally ignored nodal basins such as occipital, pre- and postauricular, intraparotid, and axillary basins. Prediction of the possibly involved nodal basin is complicated by the frequently unexpected lymph node drainage patterns of primary melanomas on the head, neck, and upper torso. Between 35% and 84% of patients have discordant drainage to unexpected lymph node basins (5,6). Almost 50% of patients with midline primary melanomas have lymph node drainage to both sides of the neck (6). Moreover, nonpalpable lymph nodes may contain significant melanoma metastases.

Another manifestation of regional spread is satellite and in-transit lesions. Satellite lesions are dermal or subcutaneous metastases within 2 cm of the primary lesion (Fig. 1D) (7). Melanoma can also form intralymphatic dermal or subcutaneous in-transit metastases extending from the primary lesion to the regional draining lymph node basin. These can be extensive and progressive, resulting in significant disease burden, particularly from primary melanomas on the scalp.

Systemic Disease

Unlike other cancers, melanoma can spread to any organ in the body. However, the most common metastatic sites are lung, liver, brain, small bowel, and lymph nodes. Clinical signs and symptoms correspond to the involved organ system. Because clinical presentation of melanoma metastases can be so variable, new symptoms such as pain, gastrointestinal distress, or seizures in a patient previously diagnosed with melanoma should prompt imaging and laboratory studies for the appropriate organ system. Metastases in nasal mucosal or paranasal sinuses may present with nasal obstruction, hemorrhage, or exophthalmos. Lymphadenopathy outside of the expected regional drainage basin may also be a sign of advanced systemic disease (7).

DIAGNOSIS

Staging

The diagnosis, staging, and treatment of primary melanoma are intimately related. Melanoma is staged by the characteristics of the primary tumor, nodes, and metastases (TNM). The TNM system for melanoma staging correlates with prognosis (Table 1) (7). Primary

TABLE 1 AJCC Staging for Melanoma and Corresponding Survival

Stage	TNM	Depth (mm)	Ulceration	No. of +LN	Metastasis	5 yr survival (%)	10 yr survival (%)
0	Tis	In situ	No	0	0	99.7	99.2
IA	T1aN0M0	≤1.0	No	0	0	95	88
IB	T1bN0M0	≤1.0	Yes, ≥level IV	0	0	91	83
	T2aN0M0	1.01–2.0	No	0	0	89	79
IIA	T2bN0M0	1.01–2.0	Yes	0	0	77	64
	T3aN0M0	2.01–4.0	No	0	0	79	64
IIB	T3bN0M0	2.01–4.0	Yes	0	0	63	51
	T4aN0M0	≥4.01	No	0	0	67	54
IIC	T4bN0M0	≥4.01	Yes	0	0	45	32
IIIA	T1-4aN1aM0	Any	No	1	0	70	63
	T1-4aN2aM0	Any	No	2–3	0	63	57
IIIB	T1-4bN1aM0	Any	Yes	1	0	53	38
	T1-4bN2aM0	Any	Yes	2–3	0	50	36
	T1-4aN1bM0	Any	No	1	0	59	48
	T1-4aN2bM0	Any	No	2–3	0	46	39
IIIC	T1-4bN1bM0	Any	Yes	1	0	29	24
	T1-4bN2bM0	Any	Yes	2–3	0	24	15
	any TN3M0	Any	Any	4	0	27	18
IV	any TanyNM1a	Any	Any	Any	Distant skin, SC, LN	19	16
	any TanyNM1b	Any	Any	Any	Lung	7	3
	any TanyNM1c	Any	Any	Any	Any, increased LDH	10	6

Abbreviations: AJCC, American Joint Committee on Cancer; TNM, primary tumor, nodes, and metastases; LN, lymph node; SC, subcutaneous; LDH, lactate dehydrogenase.
Source: From Refs. 8, 9.

melanoma is staged chiefly by histopathology or microstage, defined as depth of invasion and measured in millimeters. This is referred to as Breslow thickness, after the pathologist who developed this method. Thin melanomas (<1 mm) have less likelihood of metastatic spread, whereas thick melanomas (>4 mm) have a much higher metastasis rate.

Depth of invasion can also be measured by Clark's levels of invasion (7). This system relies on the pathological level of invasion from dermis to subcutaneous fat. Clark's level I extends through the epidermis but not into the basal lamina. Level II melanoma has entered the basal lamina. Melanoma extending through the papillary dermis is level III. Level IV tumors enter the reticular dermis and level V tumors reach the subcutaneous fat. Because of the challenge of distinguishing the various pathological levels, Clark's level of penetration is used less frequently than Breslow thickness. However, on body parts with overall thicker or thinner skin (i.e., ear and nose), Clark's levels can be more accurate than Breslow thickness. In general, melanoma of Clark's levels IV and V has a higher likelihood of metastatic spread.

In addition to depth of invasion, other important features of the primary melanoma are signs of regression and ulceration (7). Primary melanomas can elicit an immune response, resulting in tumor regression. Regression is seen pathologically by signs of fibrosis and pigment-containing macrophages in the upper dermis. Because the tumor may have been sufficiently deep to allow regional nodal metastasis prior to regression, signs of regression of the primary may prompt sentinel node biopsy (SNB) and closer followup. Ulcerated melanomas tend to be of the nodular histological type and behave more aggressively. Patients with ulcerated primaries have a decreased survival when compared with those with nonulcerated melanomas. Ulceration results in a tumor stage that is more advanced (Table 1).

Tissue Biopsy

Because of the variation in appearance of melanoma primary lesions, the only definitive diagnosis is with tissue biopsy. Since pathological staging is so important for prognosis and treatment planning, the initial biopsy must be a full-thickness punch biopsy rather than a shave biopsy. This preserves the lesion depth necessary for accurate pathological staging. For large lesions, small circumferential punch biopsies can be performed to judge the extent of lesion, which may extend beyond the visible pigmented lesion into normal-appearing skin (Fig. 1B). If possible, the entire pigmented area of the lesion should be removed in an excisional biopsy, because variation in depth across the lesion could affect the final stage. If the lesion diameter is greater than 2 cm or cannot be safely closed primarily, additional punch biopsies of suspicious areas may show more extensive or deeper tumor. Enlarged lymph nodes or possible metastatic masses seen on computed tomography or ultrasonography can be sampled by fine needle aspiration or core biopsy for tissue diagnosis; an experienced pathologist should assess the cytopathology.

TREATMENT

Loco-Regional Disease (Nodal Assessment)

After initial pathological assessment by punch or excisional biopsy, the next step is treatment of the primary site and staging of the regional lymph nodes. Treatment for the primary tumor consists of wide local excision. Local recurrence can be as high as 40% for primary melanomas that are not reexcised after biopsy (3). Melanoma-in-situ is treated by reexcision with at least 0.5-cm margins around the primary lesion or biopsy scar. When primary invasive melanomas are <1 mm thick or Clark's level II, adequate margins are 1 cm circumferentially. Melanomas that are 1.0 to 4 mm thick or extend to Clark's level III/IV are treated with 2-cm margins circumferentially. Because of the increased risk of microsatellites, melanomas thicker than 4 mm or extending to Clark's level V should be excised with 2- to 3-cm margins that include the underlying fascia (3). Wound closure is achieved primarily with local flaps or more rarely with skin grafting.

Some primary sites have special considerations. On areas of the face such as the nose, eyelids, and lips, where wide margins may cause significant morbidity, 1.0- to 2.0-cm margins are attempted. Moh's micrographic surgery has been performed for thin facial melanomas, but there is little long-term data on its efficacy. Melanoma on the helix of the ear is controlled with a wedge excision to permit cosmetic reconstruction.

Primary melanomas thinner than 0.75 mm, nonulcerated, and without signs of regression are generally treated by wide local excision of the primary site alone. Patients with deeper primary lesions (Breslow depth ≥1 mm or Clark's level IV/V), worrisome signs such as regression or ulceration, or incomplete biopsy with a positive deep margin, should undergo wide local excision with appropriate margins and staging with SNB.

SNB for melanoma was first described in 1990 by Morton, et al. as a way to obtain prognostic information about the spread of a primary melanoma and to avoid the morbidity of elective dissection for patients with no evidence of lymph node involvement on physical exam (10). Part of the American Joint Committee on Cancer (AJCC) staging of melanoma, SNB is now a standard of care, and, therefore, should be a routine part of the treatment offered patients with at-risk lesions. SNB is usually performed in conjunction with wide local excision of the primary lesion.

Prior to SNB, lymphoscintigraphy is used to map the nodal drainage from the primary melanoma site. This is performed preoperatively by injecting 300 to 1000 mCi of technetium-99m (Tc-99m) sulfur colloid intradermally around the primary biopsy site. Sequential images are then obtained to track the lymphatic drainage (Fig. 2A). Areas of increased radioactivity are confirmed with hand-held gamma probe and marked on the patient's skin (Fig. 2B). Lymphoscintigrams for primary lesions on the head and neck require interpretation by an experienced nuclear medicine physician, because drainage patterns in these lesions can be unexpected. Head and neck primaries drain to a mean of 2.5 sentinel lymph nodes (SLNs), requiring diligent tracking (6). The amount of Tc-99m sulfur colloid injected should be decreased in primaries overlying or directly adjacent to nodal basins, so that excess radioactivity does not result in "shine through" activity that obscures the SLN (5,11).

After lymphoscintigraphy, the patient is taken to the operating room and positioned to allow access to both primary and SLN sites. Approximately 0.5 mL of isosulfan blue dye is injected intradermally around the primary site (Fig. 2C). The primary site is then gently massaged for one to two minutes. The nodal drainage site marked by prior lympho-scintigraphy is confirmed with hand-held gamma probe and an incision is made over this area. Dissection is guided by the increased counts over background and blue lymphatic tracts, until a blue-stained and radioactive SLN is found (Fig. 2D). All SLNs seen on the lymphoscintigram should be biopsied in order to provide complete staging. Each SLN is bisected and then examined by hematoxylin and eosin and by immunoperoxidase staining. Patients whose SLNs contain melanoma usually undergo completion lymph node dissection of the involved basin.

For patients who have positive lymph nodes for melanoma (stage III), adjuvant treatment with high-dose interferon-α-2b is usually offered. In a large, randomized trial, a one-year course of treatment with interferon-α-2b showed an improved, relapse-free

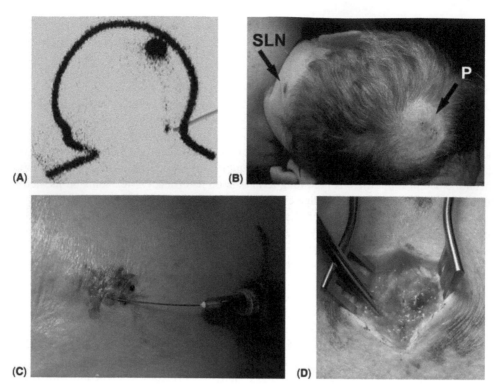

FIGURE 2 Treatment of primary melanoma. **(A)** Lymphoscintigraphy showing draining solitary sentinel lymph node. **(B)** Large pigmented primary (P) scalp melanoma (note healed central biopsy scar) with patient positioned laterally and sentinel node (SLN) marked on skin. **(C)** Injection of isosulfan blue dye intradermally around primary site. **(D)** Dissection over area with elevated counts reveals a radioactive, blue sentinel node with blue lymphatic tract. *Source*: Courtesy of Dr. Mark Faries.

survival, but no overall survival benefit compared to observation (12). Unfortunately, many patients cannot tolerate the toxicity of this treatment. Trials using low-dose interferon-α-2b have shown no difference in relapse-free or overall survival, and other forms of biotherapy and melanoma vaccines are being investigated.

Systemic Disease

Patients with metastatic melanoma may receive a number of treatment modalities. Solitary or few metastases in solid organs such as lung, small bowel, or liver can be treated with surgical excision. This is particularly effective for patients with a prolonged disease-free interval, characterized by a tumor doubling time of >60 days. Brain metastases can be managed with surgical excision or gamma knife radiation. Systemic immunotherapy and chemotherapy are options. Immunotherapy with interferon-α-2b has resulted in objective response rates in 7% to 23% of patients with stage IV disease (3). Interleukin-2–based regimens have had overall response rates of 21% to 24% (3). Responses to multiagent chemotherapy with dacarbazine (DTIC) are 10% to 53% in phase II trials (3), but combination treatments have not been superior in multicenter randomized trials (13,14). Metastatic melanoma continues to be an area of ongoing research for better systemic treatments.

COMPLICATIONS AND PROGNOSIS

Complications vary by treatment. The main complications from wide local excision are superficial: infection, wound dehiscence, and cosmetic defect. Risk of tumor recurrence after excision with appropriate margins is low. Complications of SNB are also local in nature: infection, seroma, injury to nerves, and dehiscence. The risk of lymphedema is minimal in the head and neck lymphatic basins.

The most important prognostic factors are primary tumor thickness, ulceration, and lymph node status. This is reflective of the AJCC TNM staging for melanoma (Table 1), where advancing stage corresponds with worsening prognosis (7). After biopsy and SNB, most patients can be given general prognostic counseling.

MUCOSAL MELANOMAS—SPECIAL CONSIDERATIONS

Mucosal melanomas of the head and neck are rare, with only about 1000 cases reported. Of more than 84,000 melanoma cases in the National Cancer Data Base, only 1.3% were mucosal, and 55% of that subgroup arose in the head and neck (15). The majority of head and neck mucosal melanomas are sinonasal in origin, and the others are primarily from the oral mucosa. Among the sinonasal tumors, 81% arise in the nose and 19% in the sinuses, although the size of some of these tumors makes it difficult to be sure of the site of origin. Most of the oral lesions arise from the hard palate and maxillary alveolar ridge. Melanomas arising in other head and neck mucosal sites such as the larynx, pharynx, and cervical esophagus have been reported, but are quite rare. A melanoma arising in the oropharynx is shown in Figure 3. The oral lesions are often detected by healthcare personnel as a dark spot in the mouth, but the sinonasal lesions are often only apparent after symptoms such as epistaxis or nasal obstruction occur. The sinonasal melanomas are often polypoid, which makes measuring their thickness problematic. Conjunctival melanomas are also mucosal in origin, and may come to the attention of head and neck specialists, both for surgical resection and treatment of the lymph nodes at risk, which are primarily in the parotid gland. A conjunctival melanoma is shown in Figure 4.

Staging of mucosal melanomas is not addressed in the TNM system. A simple and practical system used by most clinicians classifies tumors with localized primary disease as Stage I, those with regional disease as Stage II, and those with distant disease as Stage III. About 70% of patients with head and neck mucosal melanoma present with Stage I disease, about 15 to 20 % present with stage II disease, and the remainder present with Stage III

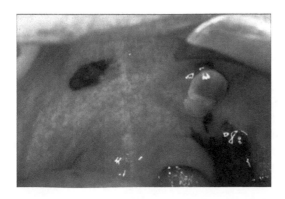

FIGURE 3 Mucosal malignant melanoma involving the palate. *Source*: Courtesy of Thomas Kennedy, MD.

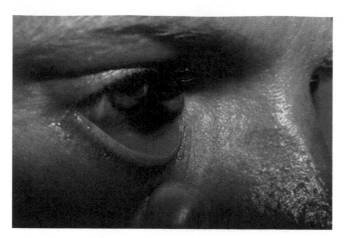

FIGURE 4 Malignant melanoma arising from the conjunctiva. This patient required orbital exenteration and parotidectomy. He eventually died from distant disease.

disease. The incidence of lymph node metastases is higher in oral mucosal melanomas than in sinonasal melanomas, as might be expected based on the higher density of lymphatic channels in the oral soft tissues. In a review of 59 patients seen over a 20-year span at Memorial Sloan-Kettering Cancer Center, the only independent predictors of outcome were clinical stage, thickness greater than 5mm, vascular invasion on histologic examination, and development of distant disease (16).

The infrequent occurrence of mucosal melanomas of the head and neck makes it difficult to evaluate different treatment approaches. Most authorities agree that surgery plays a primary role, and that postoperative radiation therapy is indicated in most cases (17). Radiation therapy is almost always used as an adjunct in the sinonasal melanomas because of the difficulty in obtaining wide margins in this anatomic location. A recent multicenter cooperative study concluded that postoperative radiotherapy has a positive effect on outcome in sinonasal melanomas invading the skull base (18). The mucosal melanomas also have a propensity for submucosal spread, making it difficult for surgeons to estimate the true tumor margin. Frozen section analysis of melanomas and their surgical margins is often difficult, which further hampers intraoperative assessment of the adequacy of the resection, resulting in close or positive margins that mandate postoperative radiotherapy. Although some mucosal melanomas of the head and neck have been reportedly cured by radiation treatment alone, there is a general consensus that radiation therapy should be used as a postoperative adjunct in most cases, with primary radiotherapy being used for palliation or in those patients in whom surgery is contraindicated for medical reasons. Some have suggested that because of the poor outcome for late stage disease, radiation should be reserved only for patients with potentially curable early stage disease (19).

Diagnostic measures for mucosal melanomas are similar to those for cutaneous melanomas, although imaging may play a greater role in evaluating the primary site, especially for the sinonasal melanomas. Biopsy, MRI, or CT of the primary site, and staging with PET and/or CT of the brain, chest, abdomen and pelvis, are performed in almost every case. Special stains, such as S-100 protein and HMB 45, may be required to make a histologic diagnosis. Treatment consists of surgery, which should encompass the primary site with as wide a margin as is feasible without creating inordinate functional or cosmetic deficits. Cervical node management is controversial, as it is with cutaneous melanomas. Because of the rarity of mucosal melanomas of the head and neck, no series has been reported evaluating sentinel node biopsy in this subgroup of melanomas. Prophylactic treatment of the neck should be considered for most oral cavity melanomas, but not for sinonasal melanomas. As noted above, radiation should be given post-operatively to almost all patients with mucosal melanoma of the head and neck. Adjunctive treatment with chemotherapy and biological agents such as interferon introduces additional toxicity, and has not been shown to impact patient survival.

Local recurrences are common after surgery for head and neck mucosal melanomas, occurring in more than half of patients in most reports (16, 17, 19). Nevertheless, local recurrence does not appear to be a good predictor of outcome. Lymph node metastases occur in as many as 42% of patients with oral mucosal melanomas, and in 15-20% of patients with sinonasal melanomas. Lymph node metastases can be controlled with neck dissection and postoperative radiation (in selected cases), but overall salvage is poor. This appears to be related to the strong correlation between lymph node metastases and distant failure. Distant metastases are most commonly seen in the lung, brain, bones, and liver, and death ensues in a mean of 5 months. The median time to relapse is about one year, although late relapses beyond 5 years are not unusual, as are seen with cutaneous melanomas. Cure rates have not improved much over the last several decades, and, as with all melanomas, improvement in disease control will probably rest with development of an effective systemic therapy.

SUMMARY

Melanoma of the head and neck regions presents a challenging clinical problem. The importance of full-thickness biopsy for pathological staging and surgical planning cannot be overemphasized. Improvements in staging conferred by SNB have increased our knowledge of the disease, while decreasing the possible complications. With its highly metastatic nature, melanoma is potentially life-threatening in all but its earliest stages, but with adequate surgical therapy, most patients with clinically localized disease will be salvaged.

REFERENCES

1. Jemal A, Murray T, Ward E, et al. Cancer statistics, 2005. CA Cancer J Clin 2005; 55:10–30. Erratum in: CA Cancer J Clin 2005; 55:259.
2. O'Brien CJ, Coates AS, Petersen-Schaefer K, et al. Experience with 998 cutaneous melanomas of the head and neck over 30 years. Am J Surg 1991; 162:310–314.
3. Morton DL, Essner R, Kirkwood JM, et al. Malignant melanoma. In: Kufe DW, Bast RC, Hait WN, et al., eds. Holland Frei Cancer Medicine. 7th ed. Hamilton, Ontario: BC Decker, Inc., 2006: 1644–1662.
4. Medina JE, Ferlito A, Pellitteri PK, et al. Current management of mucosal melanoma of the head and neck. J Surg Oncol 2003; 83(2):116–122.
5. Ollila DW, Foshag LJ, Essner R, et al. Parotid region lymphatic mapping and sentinel lymphadenectomy for cutaneous melanoma. Ann Surg Oncol 1999; 6(2):150–154.
6. de Wilt JH, Thompson JF, Uren RF, et al. Correlation between preoperative lymphoscintigraphy and metastatic nodal disease in 362 patients with cutaneous melanoma of the head and neck. Ann Surg 2004; 239(4):544–552.
7. Melanoma of the skin. In: Green FL, Page DL, Fleming ID, et al., eds. AJCC Cancer Staging Handbook. 6th ed. New York, NY: Springer-Verlag, 2002:209–217.
8. Surveillance, Epidemiology, and End Results (SEER) Program (www.seer.cancer.gov) SEER*Stat Database: Incidence - SEER 9 Regs Public-Use, Nov 2004 Sub (1973–2002), National Cancer Institute, DCCPS, Surveillance Research Program, Cancer Statistics Branch, released April 2005, based on the November 2004 submission.
9. Balch CM, Buzaid AC, Soong SJ, et al. Final version of the American Joint Committee on Cancer staging system for cutaneous melanoma. J Clin Oncol 2001; 19(16):3635–3648.

10. Morton D, Cagle L, Wong J, et al. Intraoperative lymphatic mapping and selective lymphadenectomy: technical details of a new procedure for clinical stage I melanoma. Proceedings of the Annual Meeting of the Society of Surgical Oncology, Washington, DC, 1990.

11. Morton DL, Wen DR, Foshag LJ, et al. Intraoperative lymphatic mapping and selective cervical lymphadenectomy for early-stage melanomas of the head and neck. J Clin Oncol 1993; 11 (9):1751–1756.

12. Eggermont A, Suciu S, MacKie R, et al. Post-surgery adjuvant therapy with intermediate doses of interferon α 2b versus observation in patients with stage IIb/III melanoma (EORTC 18952): randomised controlled trial. Lancet 2005; 366(9492):1189–1196.

13. Hauschild A, Garbe C, Stolz W, et al. Dacarbazine and interferon-α with or without interleukin 2 in metastatic melanoma: a randomized phase III multicentre trial of the Dermatologic Cooperative Oncology Group (DeCOG). Br J Cancer 2001; 84(8):1036–1042.

14. Ridolfi R, Chiarion-Sileni V, Guida M, et al. Cisplatin, dacarbazine with or without subcutaneous interleukin-2, and interferon alpha-2b in advanced melanoma outpatients: results from an Italian multicenter phase III randomized clinical trial. J Clin Oncol 2002; 20(6):1600–1607.

15. Chang AE, Karnell LH, Menck HR. The National Cancer Data Base report on cutaneous and noncutaneous melanoma: a summary of 84,836 cases from the past decade. The American College of Surgeons Commission on Cancer and the American Cancer Society. Cancer 1998; 83:1664–1678.

16. Patel SG, Prasad ML, Escrig M, et al. Primary mucosal malignant melanoma of the head and neck. Head and Neck 2002; 24:247–257.

17. Mendenhall WM, Amdur RJ, Hinerman RW, et al. Head and neck mucosal melanoma. Am J Clin Oncol 2005; 28:626–630.

18. Ganly I, Patel SG, Singh B, et al. Craniofacial resection for malignant melanoma of the skull base. Arch Otol Head Neck Surg 2006; 132:73–78.

19. Temam S, Mamelle G, Marandas P, et al. Postoperative radiotherapy for primary mucosal melanoma of the head and neck. Cancer 2005; 103:313–319.

19

Histiocytosis, Sickle Cell Anemia, and Rhabdomyosarcoma

Romaine F. Johnson
Department of Pediatric Otolaryngology, University of Texas, Dallas, Texas, U.S.A.

Shyan Vijayasekaran
Department of Pediatric Otolaryngology, Ear Science Institute, University of Western Australia, Perth, Australia

Charles M. Myer III
Department of Pediatric Otolaryngology, Cincinnati Children's Hospital and Department of Otolaryngology, University of Cincinnati, Cincinnati, Ohio, U.S.A.

LANGERHANS CELL HISTIOCYTOSIS

INTRODUCTION

Langerhans cell histiocytosis (LCH) is a hemopoietic disorder that can affect single or multiple sites simultaneously. It is a disorder that affects mostly children. The clinical course is variable and can range from isolated disease that resolves spontaneously to systemic disease that is rapidly progressive and lethal.

LCH was originally known as histiocytosis X. There were traditionally three categories: Letterer-Siwe syndrome, Hand-Schuller-Christian disease, and eosinophilic granuloma. Letterer-Siwe syndrome refers to a constellation of symptoms characterized by splenomegaly, hepatomegaly, lymphadenopathy, and bone lesions. Hand-Schuller-Christian disease included diabetes insipidus and exophthalmos in addition to the bone lesions. Eosinophilic granuloma typically involves a single bony lesion. Current terminology of LCH includes chronic unifocal LCH, multifocal LCH, and acute disseminated LCH. It is now known that all three disorders are part of a clinical spectrum of the same underlying disease (1).

EPIDEMIOLOGY

The exact incidence is unknown. Approximately two-thirds of patients will present with disease involving one site. The remaining patients present with multisystem LCH. The sites most commonly involved are bone (e.g., long bones and mandible), lung, and skin. Children with single-site lesions tend to have bone abnormalities, while whereas adults have lung disease (2).

PATHOLOGY

Langerhans cells are the pathognomonic cells for LCH and are located throughout the reticuloendothelial system. They express HLA-DR, S-100, and CD1a (Fig. 1A and B). The pathological hallmarks of these cells are "Birbeck" granules, which are rod-like structures with dilated terminal ends identified by electron microscopy (EM). The immunohistochemical identification of HLA-DR, S-100, and CD1a receptors has replaced EM identification. LCH appears to be a myeloproliferative disease due to changes in gene structure. The inciting events are unclear, but infection could be a contributing factor (3).

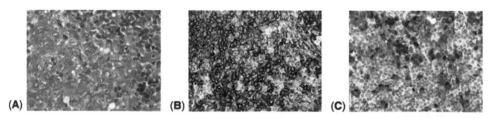

(A)   **(B)**   **(C)**

FIGURE 1   (A) Langerhans cell histiocytosis. H&E stain. (B) Langerhans cell histiocytosis. CD1 stain. (C) Langerhans cell histiocytosis. S-100 stain.

CLINICAL MANIFESTATIONS

LCH has a variable course. The use of the nomenclature of eosinophilic granuloma, Hand–Schuller-Christian disease, and Letterer-Siwe syndrome still plays a role in describing the disease, although there is significant overlap.

Eosinophilic granuloma (i.e., unifocal LCH) is characterized by the formation of solitary or multiple discrete nodules within bones and represents the majority of cases (60–80%). These lesions are typically found in children younger than 15 years. There is associated pain and tenderness with these lesions, and there may be difficulty with weight bearing (2).

Hand-Schuller-Christian disease (multifocal LCH) has similar bone "granulomas" along with other systemic manifestations. The skeletal anatomy of the head and neck is prominently involved. Mandibular defects include severe gingivitis, loss of mandibular height, and multiple loose teeth. The skull can have a "geographic skull" appearance on plain films secondary to multiple lesions. Involvement of orbital bones can result in changes in vision, and blindness can occur. Sellar involvement around the pituitary can lead to hypopituitarism, resulting in short stature and diabetes insipidus (2).

Otologic manifestations are particularly relevant to the otolaryngologist. Patients may present at any time during childhood. Mastoid disease may present in unifocal, multifocal, or systemic LCH. Patients typically present with otorrhea. The incidence of LCH ear disease (all types) is from 15% to 61%. It is usually unilateral, but bilateral disease may occur. The presence of polyps and granulation tissue in the external canal is highly suggestive of LCH. The middle ear is usually spared. Otitis externa can also be present. LCH can mimic cholesteatoma and should be kept in mind as a part of the differential of otorrhea, especially if bloody. A computed tomography (CT) scan typically shows aggressive lytic lesions similar to osteomyelitis, bone lymphoma, or sarcoma (4,5).

Letterer-Siwe disease (systemic LCH) is the rarest (approximately 10% of all LCH cases) and most severe form of LCH. Affected individuals are typically under the age of two years and present with diffuse eczema, draining ears, lymphadenopathy, and hepatosplenomegaly. Failure to thrive, weight loss, and pancytopenia are also present and portend a poor prognosis (2).

Another manifestation of LCH is primary pulmonary LCH, which affects both children and adults. Pulmonary LCH has been associated with cigarette smoking in adults, and the course tends to be severe. The childhood form of pulmonary LCH appears to be less severe but more chronic in nature (6).

DIAGNOSIS

The diagnosis of LCH can be challenging. A pathological diagnosis is needed for confirmation. Langerhans cells are present to varying degrees within individual specimens. Other inflammatory cells are also present. Over time, the primary site may show fibrosis predominating the lesion. The presence of the Langerhans cell on microscopy suggests the diagnosis, but immunohistochemical staining for S-100 or CD1a is needed to confirm the diagnosis. The presence of Birbeck granules, which can only be identified via EM, can also confirm the diagnosis. Once the diagnosis is made, a comprehensive evaluation, including a skeletal survey and basic laboratory evaluation, are important (2,3).

TREATMENT

Treatment of LCH depends on the site and extent of disease. Curettage and expectant management can be utilized for isolated bony disease (2,4,7). If the lesion is unresponsive or involves a critical site such as the orbit or vertebrae, low-dose radiation has been employed. More extensive lesions generally require systemic chemotherapy. Multiple regimens have been tried, including vincristine, methotrexate, and corticosteroids, with varying degrees of success. Currently, there are no standard treatment regimens for this disorder. Mastoid disease can be managed in several ways. Local otitis externa can respond to aural toilet and topical steroids. Mastoid disease can be treated with mastoidectomy for isolated disease, followed by systemic chemotherapy or radiation therapy if the disease is more problematic or widespread. There are reports of extensive resections for recalcitrant disease (8).

PROGNOSIS

The prognosis of LCH is variable (9). Most patients have excellent survival rates (77% at 20 years). The disease, however, can have a relapsing course. The long-term consequences of skeletal disease, mandibular disease, mastoid disease, hematological abnormalities, and the like can also produce significant comorbidity. These patients therefore require long-term followup.

SUMMARY

LCH is an uncommon disorder but has several manifestations of which the practicing otolaryngologist must be aware. It may present systemically, but it more often presents with isolated or multifocal bony lesions that cause local symptoms. Diagnosis is made by biopsy, and therapy can vary from simple curettage to systemic chemotherapy. The prognosis is good for most patients, although some progress to overwhelming systemic disease. Long-term followup is essential in all patients.

SICKLE CELL ANEMIA

INTRODUCTION

Sickle cell anemia is a hereditary blood dyscrasia that has worldwide distribution. In the United States, the disease primarily affects persons of African or Mediterranean descent. Despite the improving prognosis, this disorder still has the potential for significant morbidity and mortality, including cerebral vascular disease, pulmonary disease, and chronic anemia.

EPIDEMIOLOGY

The sickle cell trait offers genetic protection against *Plasmodium falciparum*, which is endemic in West Africa. Due to the trans-Atlantic slave trade and subsequent global migration, the trait has been distributed throughout the Western hemisphere. Sickle cell anemia affects up to 8% of African Americans. The majority of these patients have sickle cell trait. Sickle cell disease affects approximately 0.2% of African Americans. The prevalence of sickle cell disease in non-African Americans is approximately 0.08% (10,11).

PATHOPHYSIOLOGY

Sickle cell anemia is caused by a mutation in the β-globin chain of hemoglobin (Hb), replacing glutamic acid with valine at the sixth position of the chain. The association of two wild-type α-globin subunits with two mutant β-globin subunits forms Hb-S, which polymerizes under low oxygen conditions, causing distortion of red blood cells (RBCs) and a tendency for them to lose their elasticity. The gene for sickle cell disease has variable penetration. The sickle cell trait is largely asymptomatic, although patients are at risk of spleen infarction under extreme circumstances, such as exercise-induced exhaustion. Sickle cell disease has various genotypes, including sickle cell SS (homozygous), sickle cell thalassemia (sickle cell ST), and sickle cell C (Sickle SC) disease. In general, the most severe form is homozygous sickle cell (11).

Hb-S RBCs are inherently weak and error prone. The normal globulin molecule helps to protect the RBC membrane from the negative effects of utilizing iron to facilitate its oxygen-carrying capacity. The normal RBC tends to carry iron in the more stable ferrous (Fe^{2+}) state, while the sickle cell globulin molecule promotes iron to rest in the more unstable ferric (Fe^{3+}) state. The ferrous state of heme accelerates the formation of oxygen-free radicals that subsequently damage the erythrocyte's cell membranes. Chronic cell dehydration is critical for sickle deformation. These sickled cells have increased adherence to endothelium, exposing it to shear damage and free radical damage. Additionally, affected individuals have a higher number of immature erythrocytes to compensate for sickled RBCs. These immature cells also tend to adhere to endothelium, leading to further damage. Persistent endothelial damage induces inflammatory change that perpetuates further endothelial damage, leading to a destructive cycle that results in the end-organ damage that affects many patients (12).

CLINICAL MANIFESTATIONS

The clinical manifestations of sickle cell disease involve every organ system (Table 1). The most common presentations are acute pain crises, cerebral vascular accidents (CVA), acute chest syndrome (ACS), cholelithiasis, and splenic infarctions. Acute pain crisis is an episode of acute pain not caused by any other factor than sickle cell. It occurs in the vast

TABLE 1 Systemic Features of Sickle Cell Anemia

Organ system	Manifestations
Neurologic	Acute pain crisis
	Cerebral vascular disease
	Chronic pain syndrome
Pulmonary	Acute chest syndrome
	Reactive airway disease
	Chronic restrictive lung disease
Gastrointestinal	Cholelithiasis
	Dyspepsia
	Chronic hepatitis (secondary to multiple blood transfusions)
Hematological	Hemolytic anemia
	Acute aplastic anemia
	Splenic enlargement/autoinfarction
Orthopedic	Osteonecrosis
	Osteomyelitis
	(Salmonella and *Staphylococcus aureus*)
Immunologic	Immunodeficiency
	Erythrocyte auto/alloimmunizations
	Transfusion reactions

majority of these patients. The most common sites affected are the abdomen, femoral shaft, knee, and lower back. The etiology remains unclear. There appears to be an inciting factor in many cases. Inciting factors may include emotional stress, physical exertion, and alcohol consumption. Pain probably results from microinfarction of the end organ, for example, medullary infarction resulting in bone pain. About 1% of sickle cell patients have more than six episodes per year (12).

ACS is another common presentation of sickle cell crisis. Patients present with a new infiltrate on chest films, chest pain, fever, and tachypnea. The causes include infections (e.g., parvovirus), fat embolism from bone infarction, and surgery. This condition also causes chronic lung inflammation not unlike asthma in the early stages and restrictive lung diseases in the late stages (13).

CVA can be a devastating consequence of sickle cell. They may be thromboembolic or hemorrhagic. CVA associated with sickle cell disease may occur at any age, and often the first episode occurs in the first decade of life. Risk factors for CVA include being a homozygous genotype, history of transient ischemic attacks, and previous ACS episodes (14,15).

Splenic autoinfarction is another important clinical manifestation. This leads to increased susceptibility to infections from encapsulated organisms such as *Haemophilus influenzae* and *Streptococcus pneumoniae* (11).

Although these patients are at increased risk of infections due to pneumococcus and *H. influenzae*, there does not appear to be an increased risk of otitis media or sinusitis. Sickle cell patients do appear to be at increased risk for sleep-related breathing disorders. Sleep disturbance can be due to adenotonsillar hypertrophy or chronic lung disease.

DIAGNOSIS

Sickle cell is diagnosed by Hb electrophoresis. The sickle cell solubility test is another test that detects the presence of sickle Hb; however, it does not distinguish between sickle cell trait and other sickle cell disorders. Family studies and the measurement of Hb-A2 and Hb-F are used to complete the diagnosis of sickle cell disease (16). In the United States, there is universal screening for sickle cell disease. Therefore, the diagnosis should be well established in most clinical encounters.

TREATMENT

The treatment of sickle cell depends in large part on the severity of the phenotype. Patients with known sickle cell trait should undergo genetic counseling to help assess the risk to any offspring. Patients who exhibit clinical manifestations are managed expectantly. All symptomatic patients should have their care managed by a multidisciplinary hematology team.

Management of acute pain crisis is one of the more problematic areas of sickle cell treatment. As previously stated, these patients present with severe pain without a clear etiology. The mainstay of pain treatment is the use of anti-inflammatory medications and opioid analgesics. Nonpharmacologic treatment includes cutaneous stimulation, hot and cold packs, massage, and relaxation techniques. A consistent pain scale instrument (e.g., visual pain analog scale) is helpful to quantify the amount of pain present. Liberal use of analgesia is recommended. Side effects are the only limiting factor with opioid administration (16).

ACS is the second most common cause of hospital admission in sickle cell disease. In addition to adequate analgesia and broad-spectrum antibiotic therapy, exchange transfusion has been shown to modulate the severity of the disorder. Hydroxyurea has been shown to prevent recurrences of ACS as well as acute pain crisis. The drug appears to work by reducing the number of sickled RBCs in circulation (17). The indications for this therapy are controversial. Due to adverse reactions, use of hydroxyurea in children is also debated.

Treatment of CVA centers primarily on prevention. In the event of acute stroke, immediate transfusion therapy is undertaken. The goal of transfusion is to reduce the Hb-S concentration to less than 30%. Patients thereafter are maintained on continual transfusion therapies with chelation therapy for five years. CVA prevention utilizes noninvasive transcranial Doppler to monitor high-risk vasculature (e.g., internal carotids). Patients with abnormal Doppler velocities are treated with blood transfusions to reduce Hb-S concentrations. Patients aged 2 to 16 years with sickle cell should be screened yearly for vessel disease (11,12,14,15).

Other treatments for sickle cell disease include prophylactic transfusion therapy, glucocorticoids, nitric oxide, and bone marrow transplants. The efficacy of many of these treatments is still being evaluated.

PERIOPERATIVE MANAGEMENT

The stress of surgery, even if minor, may induce a sickle crisis. It is therefore important for the otolaryngologist to be aware of the perioperative management of a patient with sickle cell disease.

Sickle cell trait does not cause an increase in operative morbidity. On the other hand, sickle cell disease has a high incidence of perioperative problems. Complications related to sickle cell events, such as acute pain syndrome, are increased after surgery. Sickle cell disease may not increase the risk of common complications such as fever, infection, and bleeding; however, these events may increase stress such that they may in themselves induce sickle crises.

Preoperative assessment is critical for these patients. They should be managed in the perioperative period by the primary hematologist as well as an anesthesiologist. Predictors of perioperative complications include type of surgery, increased age, previous history of complications, history of ACS, and preexisting infection (11,13,16).

Tonsillectomies and ventilating tubes are considered low-risk procedures. High-risk procedures include intra-abdominal and neurological surgery. The incidence of perioperative events for tonsillectomy and for myringotomy tube insertion were 0% and 2.9%, respectively, compared with 16% for cesarean section (18). History of several acute pain crises within the last year and/or ACS appears to be among the most significant findings of perioperative risk. Patients with end-organ damage (e.g., lung, kidney, etc.) would also be at a higher risk for complications (12).

Preoperative assessment of patients with sickle cell should include hematocrit, blood urea nitrogen, creatinine, urine dipstick, chest film, and pulse oximetry. One may also consider blood cross match, pulmonary function testing, and liver function tests, if clinically warranted.

The adage "an ounce of prevention is worth a pound of cure" is especially true in the perioperative management of these patients. Interestingly, there is mixed evidence regarding the efficacy of various treatments for prevention of sickle cell events. Prophylactic blood transfusion to prevent sickle cell events was once popular; however, evidence-based reviews of the literature did not support this practice. The current recommendations for transfusion are based on the patient's preoperative risk. Patients undergoing low-risk operations such as tonsillectomy do not routinely need transfusion therapy. High-risk operations require a thorough assessment of the risk and benefits of transfusion therapy with a multidisciplinary hematology team. If indicated, the transfusion goal is to reduce the Hb-S concentration to less than 30% (19).

Other measures to reduce perioperative risk include increasing oxygen-carrying capacity, hydration, body temperature, and anesthetic technique, all of which are controversial. Patients with anemia should probably be transfused, although a concentration of Hb that should initiate transfusion is not agreed upon in the literature (12).

Events that are presumed to cause dehydration, for example, exposure to high altitude, are associated with sickle cell events; therefore, it is recommended that sickle cell patients be kept well hydrated. This issue can be especially problematic for patients undergoing tonsillectomy, which can cause severe dehydration. These patients should be hospitalized to ensure adequate hydration before discharge (12).

Theoretically, hypothermia may cause a sickle cell event; however, there is insufficient evidence in clinical practice to support this concept. Also, hyperthermia (pyrexia) is common after surgery in sickle cell patients. It does not appear to increase their risk of acute events and should be managed in a manner similar to that for a non–sickle cell patient.

SUMMARY

Sickle cell disease is a blood disorder commonly seen in otolaryngology. The disease has a chronic course and can cause significant morbidity. The otolaryngologist is often asked to evaluate and treat these patients for common head and neck abnormalities. Although the prevalence of head and neck disorders is not greatly increased in sickle cell disease, these patients present special perioperative problems. Comprehensive multidisciplinary management is essential in these cases.

*R*HABDOMYOSARCOMA

INTRODUCTION

Rhabdomyosarcoma is primarily a disease of childhood and accounts for up to 5% of all malignancies in children aged 5 to 14 years. It is the most common sarcoma of childhood. Skeletal muscle is the cell origin. Tumors may be present in any area of the body, although they most frequently occur in the head and neck, followed by the genitourinary (GU) system and extremities.

EPIDEMIOLOGY

Rhabdomyosarcoma has several subtypes, including embryonal and alveolar rhabdomyosarcoma. The prevalence of these subtypes differs by age. The embryonal subtype occurs more commonly in young children (age less than four years), while alveolar subtype occurs in children of all ages. The incidence of sarcomas appears to be stable over the last 20 years (20–22).

PATHOLOGY

Rhabdomyosarcoma is classified into three cell types: embryonal, alveolar (which has botryoid and spindle cell variants), and pleomorphic. The embryonal subtype accounts for 60% to 70% of childhood cases and is the most common subtype. It is also the most common subtype presenting in the head and neck (20–22).

Rhabdomyosarcomas are malignant tumors of skeletal muscle. They are part of the larger group of soft-tissue sarcomas. Sarcomas of bony origin are classified separately. Like most malignant tumors, the etiology is probably multifactorial. Studies have suggested that maternal exposure to ionizing radiation during pregnancy increases the risk of sarcoma development. There is also evidence that socioeconomic status and maternal use of recreational drugs during pregnancy play a role in soft-tissue sarcoma development. Chromosomal abnormalities probably play a role in sarcoma development (20), especially translocation of chromosomes 2,13 and 1,13. The associated chromosome abnormalities can be used for diagnostic confirmation and have a role in residual tumor diagnosis and monitoring. An example is the use of chromosomal confirmation to assess a residual mass for viable tumors cells. Several syndromes have been associated with the development of rhabdomyosarcoma. Among them are Li-Fraumeni, neurofibromatosis type I, and Beckwith–Wiedemann syndrome (22).

CLINICAL MANIFESTATIONS

Patient presentation depends on the tumor location and size. Head and neck presentations mimic other head and neck neoplasms and depend on the site and extent of the mass. These tumors occur along the anterior skull base, parameningeal surfaces, temporal bone, and within the orbit.

Temporal bone and middle ear tumors often present with unilateral otorrhea and conductive hearing loss. As the tumor progresses, facial nerve paralysis and other cranial nerve neuropathies occur. Other head and neck manifestations include nasal obstruction, facial swelling, oropharyngeal mass, and unilateral proptosis. Metastatic rhabdomyosarcoma is part of the differential diagnosis for pediatric neck masses (23).

Rhabdomyosarcomas may occur in multiple other locations. Common areas include the kidney, biliary tract, extremities, and spinal cord. The symptoms will depend on the site and severity of the disease.

DIAGNOSIS

Diagnosis is made by biopsy (fine needle or open biopsy). If rhabdomyosarcoma is strongly suspected, comprehensive imaging should be done prior to open biopsy to accurately delineate tumor extent. Once a diagnosis is established, a multidisciplinary approach is required for all patients. CT scan of the chest and bone marrow aspirate should always be performed. Further imaging is based upon tumor location, i.e., magnetic resonance imaging (MRI) scans of the skull base for parameningeal disease and a CT scan of the abdomen and pelvis for GU and lower extremity primaries (21,22,24).

TABLE 2 Grouping of Rhabdomyosarcoma

Group	Subgroup	Description
I: Localized disease or completely resected *(low risk)*	Ia Ib	Ia: Tumor limited to muscle of origin Ib: Local spread beyond muscle of origin
II: Gross total resection	IIa IIb	IIa: Residual microscopic tumor IIb: Microscopic tumor cells in local lymph nodes
III: Incomplete resection *(intermediate risk)*	IIIa IIIb	IIIa: Biopsy only IIIb: 50% resection
IV: *(High risk)*	–	Distant metastatic disease present at onset

TABLE 3 Tumor, Node, and Metastasis Staging

Tumor	T1	Tumor <5 cm
	T2	Tumor >5 cm
Node	N0	Negative nodes
	N1	Any positive nodes
Metastasis	M0	–
	M1	Any metastasis
Stage I	–	Favorable sites, any size, any nodal status [orbit, GU (not bladder or prostate), head and neck]
Stage II	–	Unfavorable sites, but small and negative lymph nodes (extremities, bladder, prostate, and parameningeal)
Stage III	–	Unfavorable sites, small or large and positive lymph nodes
Stage IV	–	Distant metastatic disease

Abbreviations: GU, genitourinary.

The Intergroup Rhabdomyosarcoma Study Group has established prognostic indicators for rhabdomyosarcoma. This group, along with the National Wilms Tumor Study Group and the Children's Oncology Group, produced a staging system based on tumor size, nodal involvement, and presence or absence of metastases (Tables 2 and 3). These staging systems help determine the level of risk of individual patients and can help tailor treatment options (Fig. 2A and B) (24).

TREATMENT

The management of previously untreated childhood rhabdomyosarcoma has been well studied. All patients are treated with multimodality therapy and are considered to have micrometastases. Therefore, all patients receive chemotherapy (22). The principles of

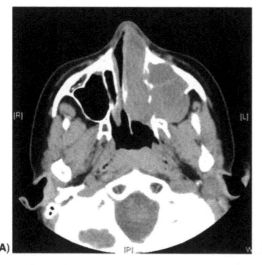
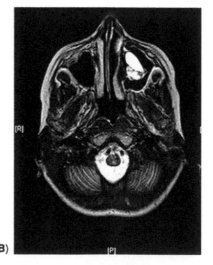

FIGURE 2 (**A**) Nasal rhabdomyosarcoma before treatment, staged as group III (biopsy only), T2N0M0 (Stage II–orbit involvement). (**B**) MRI of tumor after treatment with course of chemotherapy. Patient underwent medical maxillectomy and additional radiation therapy. *Abbreviation*: MRI, magnetic resonance imaging.

surgical treatment are to preserve all vital cosmetic and functional structures to accept close margins, and to reserve radical surgery for recurrence following radiotherapy and chemotherapy.

Orbital tumors require biopsy for diagnosis, followed by chemotherapy and radiation therapy. If a tumor persists after primary therapy, orbital exenteration should be considered (22).

Extraorbital head and neck tumors are treated with wide local excision and neck lymph node sampling of clinically involved lymph nodes. Close margins (<1 mm) are reasonable if anatomic restrictions are present. Anterior skull base tumors can be resected in cases of children with recurrent locoregional disease and residual disease following chemotherapy and radiation therapy. Tumors that are considered unresectable should undergo radiation and chemotherapy, with surgery to remove any residual masses, if feasible.

As previously mentioned, chemotherapy is used in the treatment of all patients with rhabdomyosarcoma (22). The regimen depends on the risk status of the patient (Table 2). "Low-risk" patients receive vincristine and dactinomycin. "Intermediate-risk" patients receive additional doses of cyclophosphamide. "High-risk" patients have poor response rates to current chemotherapeutic options. High-dose chemotherapy with stem cell rescue is under investigation. In general, patients in this group receive the standard therapy plus additional drugs such as ifosfamide and doxorubicin.

Radiation therapy is tailored to the specific disease. Patients who do not have residual disease after primary treatment do well without radiation. Patients with gross residual disease receive a standard dose of 5000 cGy. Radiation is given after chemotherapy (20,22).

Patients with middle-ear rhabdomyosarcoma deserve special mention due to the potential role the otolaryngologist plays in early diagnosis and intervention. As mentioned, these patients can present with bloody otorrhea not responsive to conservative management. Middle-ear rhabdomyosarcoma tends to present in a parameningeal location and often is unresectable (Groups III and IV) (25). However, most tumors are small (<5 cm) and do not involve lymph nodes. These patients are usually treated with chemotherapy and radiation. Five-year survival rates are 67% for all patients and have improved over time (25).

PROGNOSIS

Recurrent rhabdomyosarcoma presents the most favorable prognosis if it is local or regional. Most children, however, present with advanced disease (distant metastasis or unresectable disease) and have a poor prognosis. These patients are generally treated with combinations of chemotherapeutics that have not been given to them previously.

The prognosis of low-risk patients is good, with greater than 95% five-year survival rates with standard therapies. Intermediate-risk patients have between 50% and 70% survival rates. High-risk patients have poor outcomes, with survival rates from 22% to 34% (22,26,27).

SUMMARY

In general, pediatric rhabdomyosarcoma is a soft-tissue malignancy commonly seen in the head and neck. Its presentation depends on the site and extent of the disease. Surgical management is an important part of treatment. Complete resection can place a patient in the low-risk group with a more favorable prognosis. A multidisciplinary approach is imperative in the management of this disease. As with most malignant tumors, early diagnosis and treatment can make a significant difference in outcomes.

REFERENCES

1. Coppes-Zantinga A, Egeler RM. The langerhans cell histiocytosis X files revealed. Br J Haematol 2002; 116(1):3–9.
2. Lipton JM, Arceci RJ. Dendritic cell disorders. In: Hoffman R, ed. Hematology: Basic Principles and Practice. 4th ed. Philadelphia, PA: Churchill Livingstone (Elsevier), 2005:857–868.
3. Aster JC. Diseases of white blood cells, lymph nodes, spleen, and thymus. In: Kumar V, Abbas AK, Fausto N, eds. Robbins & Cotran Pathologic Basis of Disease. 7th ed. Philadelphia, PA: Elsevier Saunders, 2004:661–710.
4. Azouz EM, Saigal G, Rodriguez MM, et al. Langerhans' cell histiocytosis: pathology, imaging and treatment of skeletal involvement. Pediatr Radiol 2005; 35(2):103–115.
5. Irving RM, Broadbent V, Jones NS. Langerhans' cell histiocytosis in childhood: management of head and neck manifestations. Laryngoscope 1994; 104(1 Pt 1):64–70.
6. Vassallo R, Ryu JH. Pulmonary langerhans' cell histiocytosis. Clin Chest Med 2004; 25(3): 561–571, vii.
7. Davis SE, Rice DH. Langerhans' cell histiocytosis: current trends and the role of the head and neck surgeon. Ear Nose Throat J 2004; 83(5):340, 342, 344 Passim.
8. Merchant S, Nadol JB Jr. Otologic manifestations of systemic disease. In: Cummings CW, ed. Cummings Otolaryngology–Head and Neck Surgery. 4th ed. Philadelphia, PA: Elsevier, 2005: 2881–2905.
9. Lahey ME. Prognostic factors in histiocytosis X. Am J Pediatr Hematol Oncol 1981; 3(1): 57–60.
10. Uddin DE, Dickson LG, Brodine CE. Screening of military recruits for hemoglobin variants. JAMA 1974; 227(12):1405–1407.
11. Stuart MJ, Nagel RL. Sickle cell disease. Lancet 2004; 364(9442):1343–1360.
12. Firth PG, Head CA. Sickle cell disease and anesthesia. Anesthesiology 2004; 101(3): 766–785.
13. Stuart MJ, Setty BN. Sickle cell acute chest syndrome: pathogenesis and rationale for treatment. Blood 1999; 94(5):1555–1560.
14. Ohene-Frempong K, Weiner SJ, Sleeper LA, et al. Cerebrovascular accidents in sickle cell disease: rates and risk factors. Blood 1998; 91(1):288–294.
15. Adams RJ, McKie VC, Carl EM, et al. Long-term stroke risk in children with sickle cell disease screened with transcranial Doppler. Ann Neurol 1997; 42(5):699–704.
16. Ballas SK. Sickle cell anaemia: progress in pathogenesis and treatment. Drugs 2002; 62(8): 143–1172.
17. Charache S, Terrin ML, Moore RD, et al. Effect of hydroxyurea on the frequency of painful crises in sickle cell anemia. Investigators of the Multicenter Study of Hydroxyurea in Sickle Cell Anemia. N Engl J Med 1995; 332(20):1317–1322.
18. Koshy M, Weiner SJ, Miller ST, et al. Surgery and anesthesia in sickle cell disease. Cooperative Study of Sickle Cell Diseases. Blood 1995; 86(10):3676–3684.
19. Davies SC. Blood transfusion in sickle cell disease. Curr Opin Hematol 1996; 3(6):485–491.
20. Gurney JG, Young JL Jr, Roffers SD, et al. Soft tissue sarcomas. In: Ries LA, Smith MA, Gurney JG, et al., eds. Seer Pediatric Monograph. Bethesda, MD: National Cancer Institute, Seer Program, 1999:111–123.
21. Rosenberg AE. Bone, joints, and soft tissue tumors. In: Kumar V, Abbas AK, Fausto N, eds. Robbins & Cotran Pathologic Basis of Disease. 7th ed. Philadelphia, PA: Elsevier Saunders, 2005:1321–1322.
22. National Cancer Institutes PDQ Cancer Information Database. Childhood Rhabdomyosarcoma. http://www.cancer.gov/cancertopics/pdq/treatment/childrhabdomyosarcoma/Healthprofessional (Accessed October 2005).
23. Van De Graaf RL, Cass SP. Tumors of the ear and temporal bone. In: Bluestone CD, ed. Pediatric Otolaryngology. 4th ed. Philadelphia, PA: Saunders, 2004:849–859.
24. Breitfeld PP, Meyer WH. Rhabdomyosarcoma: new windows of opportunity. Oncologist 2005; 10 (7):518–527.
25. Hawkins DS, Anderson JR, Paidas CN, et al. Improved outcome for patients with middle ear rhabdomyosarcoma: a children's oncology group study. J Clin Oncol 2001; 19(12):3073–3079.
26. Gurney JG, Severson RK, Davis S, et al. Incidence of cancer in children in the United States. Sex-, race-, and 1-year age-specific rates by histologic type. Cancer 1995; 75(8):2186–2195.
27. Crist W, Gehan EA, Ragab AH, et al. The third intergroup rhabdomyosarcoma study. J Clin Oncol 1995; 13(3):610–630.

20

Crohn's Disease and Ulcerative Colitis

Maria T. Abreu and Junsuke Maki
Department of Medicine, Division of Gastroenterology, Inflammatory Bowel Disease Center, Mount Sinai School of Medicine, New York, New York, U.S.A.

INTRODUCTION

Crohn's disease (CD) and ulcerative colitis, collectively part of the inflammatory bowel diseases (IBD), are both diseases of the gastrointestinal tract that arise in genetically susceptible individuals. Both CD and ulcerative colitis, though clinically different entities, are thought to be part of a spectrum of diseases where environmental and immunologic factors determine the extent and severity of clinical manifestations.

DEFINITION

These disorders are characterized by a loss of controlled mucosal immune responses, leading to acute and chronic inflammation within the gut. Ulcerative colitis is restricted to the mucosa of the colon and a colectomy is curative. CD can manifest in any portion of the intestinal tract but predominantly affects the distal ileum and colon.

EPIDEMIOLOGY

The incidence and prevalence of both CD and ulcerative colitis depend significantly on geographic locations and ethnic background. The countries of North America and northern Europe, which include most of the industrialized nations, encompass the highest rates of disease activity. In North America, the incidence of CD and ulcerative colitis ranges from 3.1 to 14.6 and 2.2 to 14.3 cases per 100,000 person-years, respectively. The prevalence rates range from 26 to 199 cases for CD and 37 to 246 cases for ulcerative colitis per 100,000 persons (1). Comparatively, South America, Asia, and Africa represent regions of low incidence and prevalence of IBD, although there seems to be an increasing incidence in these areas, as well. Within these geographic variations, there are also ethnic and racial differences in the incidence of IBD. CD and ulcerative colitis are estimated to be four to eight and two to four times higher in Jewish populations, respectively (2). Even within the Jewish population, IBD is seen more frequently in Americans and Europeans of Ashkenazi descent, compared with those of Sephardic and Oriental Jews of Asian or African origin. In the United States, the African American population has remained significantly lower in overall incidence and prevalence compared with Caucasians, but the differences seem to be diminishing.

Studies indicate that over the past few decades, the incidence of ulcerative colitis and CD has stabilized in areas of high incidence but continues to rise in other geographic locations (1). It is hard to say if these overall increases are true increases in incidence related to changes in environmental factors, or whether there is increased reporting and better diagnostic techniques used for diagnosis.

The age of onset for both CD and ulcerative colitis ranges from 15 to 40 years. Some studies further suggest a bimodal age distribution with a lesser peak between the ages of 55 and 65 years (3). The etiology of the second peak remains to be elucidated. Some data also indicate a higher incidence of ulcerative colitis among men and a higher incidence of CD among women. It is unclear whether environmental factors play a role in the differences found between the two genders.

PATHOGENESIS

A family history of IBD increases the risk of developing CD or ulcerative colitis. Roughly, 15% of IBD patients have had at least one first-degree relative affected by IBD (4). It is now believed that IBD is a heterogeneous disease involving genetic, immunologic, and environmental factors. Research models have suggested an inappropriate immunologic response at the mucosal level against normally symbiotic gut bacterial flora. *CARD15*, a gene found on the IBD1 loci on chromosome 16, was the first gene to be associated with CD. It is a cytosolic protein expressed in monocytes that functions as a receptor for intracellular liposaccharides and is an activator of nuclear factor kappaB. In approximately 15% of Crohn's patients, there is a mutation of *CARD15*, resulting in an aberrantly functioning protein that may lead to chronic gut inflammation. Since only a small portion of the Crohn's population has this defective gene mutation, it is assumed that several other mechanisms are involved in the activation of the mucosal immune response.

CLINICAL MANIFESTATIONS

Extraintestinal manifestations associated with IBD may occur months to years before the onset of intestinal disease. Approximately 25% to 33% of patients with IBD are reported to have some type of extraintestinal manifestation (5). In most cases, however, these manifestations are found concurrently with or after the diagnosis of disease. Although CD and ulcerative colitis are found under the heading of IBD, the associations of extraintestinal manifestations are not equally distributed between the two diseases. The majority of these manifestations are associated with CD, but there are certain disorders that affect both diseases equally.

Pathophysiology of Extraintestinal Manifestations

The etiology of extraintestinal manifestations is a topic that is still not well understood; however, there is data supporting the concept of a dysregulation of mucosal defenses in the intestinal tract of IBD, leading to a systemic inflammatory response in extraintestinal sites. There is also evidence suggesting that an important initiating factor in the pathogenesis of IBD resides in intestinal bacterial products and foreign proteins interacting with local mucosal defenses. Interestingly, animal studies in HLA B-27 transgenic mice grown in germ-free environments do not exhibit either intestinal or extraintestinal pathology (6). There are also genetic considerations that go hand in hand with these immunologic factors. Connections between certain major histocompatibility complexes (MHC) and IBD have been well known, but studies also indicate that certain extraintestinal manifestations are also associated with specific MHC loci. HLA-A2, HLA-DR1, and HLA-DQw5 are all associated with extraintestinal manifestations related to CD, and HLA-DR103 has been associated with patients with ulcerative colitis (7).

Ocular Manifestations

Although ocular manifestations in IBD are found in less than 10% of patients with CD and ulcerative colitis (8), they are often overlooked or mistaken for other ocular disorders and can cause significant morbidity in patients who do not receive proper therapy. Many of the ocular complaints are nonspecific and may include tearing, burning, pruritis, ocular pain, photophobia, blurry vision, and blindness. Ocular pathology associated with IBD has also been linked to other extraintestinal manifestations, especially those involving joints.

Conjunctivitis is a common cause of red eyes in the general population, and it may share many of the symptoms of IBD-related ocular disease; however, conjunctivitis is never acutely painful. Although conjunctivitis is common in IBD populations, there is no known correlation between conjunctivitis and IBD. Since eye pathology in IBD can mimic benign eye conditions, physicians must take extra care in making correct diagnoses.

Episcleritis.   Inflammation of the episclera is the most common ocular manifestation of IBD and is found in roughly 2% to 5% of IBD patients (9). It is more commonly seen in patients with CD, especially when the colon is involved. Episcleritis is usually seen during flares of systemic IBD and generally subsides with resolution of intestinal symptoms. Episcleritis should be suspected in patients with complaints of eye irritation, burning, or redness in one or both eyes during an IBD flare. The eye examination may reveal areas of focal or diffuse redness interspersed with patches of white sclera between the dilated episcleral vessels. Treatment is dependent on the severity of eye disease and its associated intestinal disease activity. Cold compresses and topical steroids in conjunction with appropriate intestinal treatment are usually sufficient and resolve the problem rapidly. There have been recent case reports in patients with active CD and refractory episcleritis, who have responded to infliximab (Fig. 1) (11).

Uveitis.   Uveitis is not seen as commonly as episcleritis, only occurring in 0.5% to 3% of the IBD population; however, the morbidity associated with uveitis is far greater than that of episcleritis. It is associated with arthralgias and skin manifestations; therefore, in any patient presenting with ocular findings along with skin or joint symptoms, uveitis must be considered. Unlike episcleritis, uveitis can occur during periods of gastrointestinal flares or quiescence and may sometimes even precede the initial IBD symptoms. It is therefore vital to elicit any type of eye symptom when evaluating a patient with IBD. Affected individuals complain of eye pain, blurry vision, photophobia, and headaches caused by an inflammatory reaction of the vascular coat of the eye. In anterior uveitis, the iris and ciliary body are affected. These patients often exhibit painful eyes with photophobia and blurry vision. In a seriously affected eye, there may be an abnormal pupillary light reflex due to a fixed miotic eye. Although less common than anterior uveitis, posterior segment uveitis does occur. Posterior uveitis includes areas affected from the vitreous to the retina; therefore, these patients present differently from those patients affected with anterior uveitis (8). The patient with posterior uveitis presents with acute changes in visual acuity and should be evaluated with a slit lamp for a definitive diagnosis. Untreated long-term complications of uveitis include glaucoma and cataracts secondary to intraocular adhesions, macular dysfunction, and papillary abnormalities. Treatment of uveitis includes topical steroids and cycloplegics, but systemic corticosteroids and other immunosuppressants are often

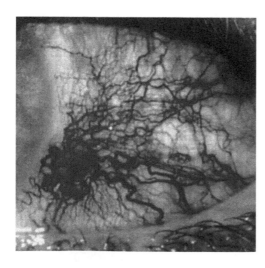

FIGURE 1   Episcleritis. *Source*: From Ref. 10.

required. Recent case reports have shown the success of infliximab for the treatment of acute uveitis (Fig. 2) (12). Chapter 6 contains a detailed discussion of uveitis.

Scleritis. Scleritis is an uncommon but severe ocular finding in IBD and may cause deterioration of vision. The diagnosis may precede or occur after onset of intestinal symptoms. These patients often complain of severe eye pain that is tender to palpation. Unlike conjunctivitis or episcleritis, the deeper vascular beds are affected in scleritis, causing dilated vessels set on a pink sclera. This condition, if left untreated, can cause retinal detachment and optic nerve edema, and therefore requires prompt evaluation by an ophthalmologist. Treatment includes aggressive therapy with systemic corticosteroids, immunosuppressants, and Non-Steroidal Anti-Inflammatory Drug to deter loss of vision.

Other Ocular Conditions. Although rare, there are other ocular pathologies associated with IBD. Some of these include par planitis, keratitis, retinitis, central and retinal artery occlusions, central retinal vein occlusions, optic neuritis, and retinal vasculitis (13). Side effects from IBD treatment, especially systemic corticosteroids, also cause ocular pathology. Chronic use of steroids can cause cataracts, increased intraocular pressure, and open-angle glaucoma (this is more often caused by topical steroids) (14). It is important that patients on chronic steroid usage be evaluated regularly by an ophthalmologist.

Oral Manifestations

Oral lesions are common in both CD and ulcerative colitis. Intraoral pathology is seen in roughly 9% of patients diagnosed with CD (15). Aphthous ulcers and angular stomatitis are findings frequently seen in IBD patients. Aphthous ulcerations in CD tend to be widespread and severe, and they may present prior to intestinal disease activity or result as a consequence of intestinal pathology. It should be noted, however, that these conditions are also found commonly in the general population and therefore are nonspecific for IBD. Pyostomatitis vegetans, a pustular lesion with cobblestoning appearance, mucosal tags, mucogingivitis, and persistent rubbery lip swelling are some of the specific findings associated with CD. In a retrospective study done in children with CD, inspection of the oral cavity by a dentist yielded an increased number of oral CD, suggesting an underestimated percentage of patients with extraintestinal (oral) CD (16). In addition, a recent study involving 49 children with CD found roughly 40% of patients with oral disease specific to CD when evaluated by a pediatric dental surgeon. Of the 30 patients with oral CD, only nine patients (45%) were identified to have oral CD by gastroenterologists. Interestingly, patients with oral CD were more likely to have perianal disease compared to those with nonoral CD (50% vs. 17%, $p = 0.023$) (Fig. 3) (18).

Orofacial granulomatosis is a syndrome comprised of a spectrum of conditions with possibly numerous etiologies that all contain noncaseating granulomas in the oral cavity

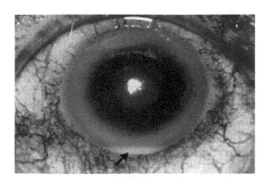

FIGURE 2 Acute anterior uveitis.
Source: From Ref. 10.

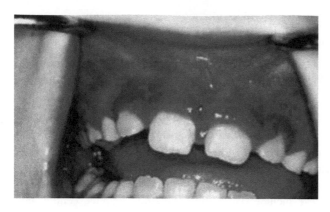

FIGURE 3 Mucogingivitis in relation to the maxillary permanent incisors. *Source*: From Ref. 17.

and face similar or identical to lesions found in CD. It is a clinical finding that includes cheilitis granulomatosis, Melkersson–Rosenthal syndrome, and sarcoidosis (19). Cheilitis granulomatosa is an idiopathic inflammatory disorder and is considered a variant of Melkersson–Rosenthal syndrome. It is associated with swelling of one or both lips, angular cheilitis, and noncaseating granulomatous lesions on histology. A rare extraintestinal manifestation, the diagnosis of cheilitis granulomatosa often precedes the diagnosis of Crohn's by several years. Treatment of cheilitis granulomatosa consists of local intralesional injections of triamcinolone or systemic corticosteroids (20).

In ulcerative colitis, oral manifestations, including ulcers similar to pyoderma gangrenosum and other hemorrhagic lesions, may be present. In over 50% of oral ulcers found in IBD, topical steroids have proven successful. With refractory oral lesions, systemic corticosteroids, azathioprine, and methotrexate have been used with good results (21).

Aural Manifestations

Sensorineural hearing loss (SNHL) has been reported in both CD and ulcerative colitis. Although there is no clear-cut association between IBD and SNHL, there have been numerous case reports in other types of autoimmune diseases such as rheumatoid arthritis (Chapter 1), systemic lupus erythematosus (Chapter 1), Wegener's granulomatosis (Chapter 8), and primary Sjögren's disease (Chapter 2). In 1979, McCabe reported 18 patients with progressive bilateral hearing loss, which he coined autoimmune SNHL (22). Since then, there have been a few case reports of SNHL with IBD, and growing evidence reveals a higher incidence found in ulcerative colitis than in CD. Notably, however, a study in 1982 found a higher incidence of SNHL in patients with Crohn's colitis (11/20) than in those with CD of the small bowel (0/5) (23).

In ulcerative colitis, there seem to be two types of hearing loss: a mild subclinical type and a severe type that leads to deafness. The pathogenesis of SNHL in both ulcerative colitis and CD is still unknown, but is postulated that a T lymphocyte mediated response, an immune complex deposition, or a vasculitis affecting the inner ear is responsible. SNHL at this point is a clinical diagnosis, because there is very little laboratory data to confirm the diagnosis; however, recent studies have reported certain antibodies that link SNHL with IBD. In one case report, antibodies directed against collagen type II, located in the inner ear, were found in a patient with CD (24). There is also growing evidence for an anti-68 kDa antibody found in patients with rapidly progressive SNHL in ulcerative colitis. Recent studies have focused on the utility of bovine heat shock protein (bHSP) 70 in treatment of corticosteroid-responsive SNHL. A bHSP assay study found that sera taken from patients with suspected autoimmune inner ear disease was low in sensitivity (42%) but highly specific (92%) with a positive predictive value of 91% (25). These findings suggest a possible immune-mediated response with SNHL, especially with ulcerative colitis. Most of these patients respond well to systemic corticosteroids, with or without the addition of immunosuppressants, as long as therapy is initiated rapidly. Given the treatable nature of SNHL, along with the complications associated with use of corticosteroids and immunosuppressants, it is important to find a useful diagnostic tool for this condition. SNHL is discussed in detail in Chapter 28.

Nasal Manifestations

There has been limited information regarding the connection between IBD and sinonasal disease. Case reports have described patients with parasinusitis with polypoidal changes, bilateral nasal congestion without ulceration or polyposis, nasal stenosis, and chronic nasal congestion with crusting, all of which resolved with oral corticosteroid treatment. A cross-sectional study in IBD patients at a tertiary care outpatient clinic explored the possible relationship between IBD and chronic sinonasal disease. The study concluded there was an elevated prevalence of sinonasal disease in IBD, especially in those patients with CD, who had experienced obstructive bowel complications (26). Although the increased prevalence of sinonasal disease in IBD could be an extraintestinal manifestation of IBD, there is little data at this time to suggest a relationship between the two.

Laryngeal Manifestations

Although rare extraintestinal manifestations of IBD, upper airway disease has been described in association with IBD. In most cases of laryngeal pathology, the disease is found after gastrointestinal diagnosis, but there have been some cases where it has preceded the development of IBD. Subglottic stenosis has been associated with other granulomatous diseases such as sarcoidosis and tuberculosis, but there have been case reports linking it to IBD (27). Cough and voice hoarseness are some of the symptoms associated with subglottic stenosis. Nonspecific edema with ulcerations of the larynx has also been found in patients with CD and ulcerative colitis (28). Treatment includes intravenous steroids for patients with airway compromise from subglottic stenosis and oral corticosteroids for most other forms of laryngeal pathology. For refractory cases of laryngeal disease, infliximab has been used with good results (29).

Dermatologic Manifestations

Erythema Nodosum and Pyoderma Gangrenosum. Skin disorders associated with IBD occur in roughly 15% of the population (30). The two most common skin manifestations associated with IBD are erythema nodosum and pyoderma gangrenosum. The former parallels intestinal disease activity and treatment is usually directed at controlling bowel symptoms. Erythema nodosum is usually located on the extensor surfaces of the extremities, especially the anterior tibial surface. Pyoderma gangrenosum parallels IBD activity in 50% of cases and typically is seen in the lower extremities but can develop anywhere on the body.

Metastatic Crohn's Disease. Metastatic Crohn's disease (MCD) is a rare condition that involves cutaneous noncaseating granulomatous lesions distant from the affected intestinal tract. It is considered a primary inflammatory process seen outside of the gut. The lesions are typically dermal inflammatory reactions with multinucleated giant cells, histiocytes, and epithelioid cells. These lesions usually present in patients with established disease. MCD is often observed in patients in their forties or older with colonic and rectal involvement where granulomatous lesions are seen most commonly in the anterior abdominal wall. There have, however, been some case reports involving the malar area, retroauricular folds, and forehead (31,32). MCD responds well to mesalmine and oral corticosteroids, and some case reports show good response with infliximab (33).

Sweet's Syndrome. Sweet's syndrome, or acute febrile neutrophilic dermatosis, is a rare condition associated with both CD and ulcerative colitis, although it is seen with certain types of cancer, as well. It is classically characterized by fever, tender red plaques, leukocytosis, and neutrophilic infiltrate with leukocytoclasis on histology. The tender plaques usually involve all extremities and the face, including ocular symptoms such as conjunctivitis and iridocyclitis. Women are commonly more affected than men, and symptoms usually coincide with intestinal disease activity (34). Most patients respond to systemic corticosteroids. There has been one case report of a patient who developed Sweet's syndrome after use of azathioprine in Crohn's colitis (35).

TREATMENT

Treatment of each manifestation in this chapter is discussed in the individual section for that manifestation.

COMPLICATIONS

Several different types of medications are used to treat a range of disease pathology in both CD and ulcerative colitis. The common complications resulting from medical therapy are listed in Table 1. The most frequent head and neck side effects are caused by steroid therapy. Patients who use steroids for ocular pathology are at risk for increased intraocular pressure. Although the exact mechanism is unknown, it is believed there is activation of steroid receptors in the trabecular meshwork, resulting in increased deposition of extracellular material (36,37). One study has reported that a six-week course of potent topical steroid therapy increased intraocular

TABLE 1 Head and Neck Complications Associated with Medical Therapeutics in Inflammatory Bowel Diseases

Medications	Complications	Frequency
Mesalamine	Rhinitis	5%
	Tinnitus	<1%
	Conjunctivitis	<2%
	Eye pain and blurry vision	<1%
	Alopecia	<1%
Corticosteroids	Cataracts	2.5–60%
	Increased intraocular pressure (topical)	20%
Methotrexate	Alopecia	3–10%
	Photosensitivity	3–10%
	Stomatitis	3–10%
Cyclosporine	Hirsutism	0–2%
	Gingival hyperplasia	4–6%

Source: Data extracted from various sources including Micromedex and Moseby's Drug Consult 2005.

pressure by >5 mmHg in roughly 20% of the study population (17). In most cases, discontinuation of steroid therapy decreases intraocular pressure to normal levels.

REFERENCES

1. Loftus EV Jr. Clinical epidemiology of inflammatory bowel disease: incidence, prevalence, and environmental influences. Gastroenterology 2004; 126(6):1504–1517.
2. Gilat T, Grossman A, Fireman Z, et al. Inflammatory bowel disease in Jews. In: McConnell R, Rosen P, Langman M, et al., eds. The Genetics and Epidemiology of Inflammatory Bowel Disease. Basel, Switzerland and New York, NY: Karger, 1986:135–140.
3. Ekbom A, Helmick C, Zack M, et al. The epidemiology of inflammatory bowel disease: a large, population-based study in Sweden. Gastroenterology 1991; 100(2):350–358.
4. Weterman IT, Pena AS. Familial incidence of Crohn's disease in The Netherlands and a review of the literature. Gastroenterology 1984; 86(3):449–452.
5. Lichtenstein DR, Park PD, Lichtenstein GR. Extraintestinal manifestations of inflammatory bowel disease. Probl Gen Surg 1999; 16(2):23–39.
6. Rath HC, Herfarth HH, Ikeda JS, et al. Normal luminal bacteria, especially Bacteroides species, mediate chronic colitis, gastritis, and arthritis in HLA-B27/human β2 microglobulin transgenic rats. J Clin Invest 1996; 98(4):945–953.
7. Roussomoustakaki M, Satsangi J, Welsh K, et al. Genetic markers may predict disease behavior in patients with ulcerative colitis. Gastroenterology 1997; 112(6):1845–1853.
8. Mintz R, Feller ER, Bahr RL, et al. Ocular manifestations of inflammatory bowel disease. Inflamm Bowel Dis 2004; 10(2):135–139.
9. Petrelli EA, McKinley M, Troncale FJ. Ocular manifestations of inflammatory bowel disease. Ann Ophthalmol 1982; 14(4):356–360.
10. Leibowitz H. Primary care: the red eye. NEJM 2000; 343:345 © 2000 Massachusetts Medical Society.
11. Finkelstein W. Treatment of acute episcleritis associated with Crohn's disease with Infliximab. Am J Gastroenterol 2002; 97:S152.
12. Fries W, Giofre MR, Catanoso M, et al. Treatment of acute uveitis associated with Crohn's disease and sacroileitis with infliximab. Am J Gastroenterol 2002; 97(2):499–500.
13. Matsuo T, Yamaoka A. Retinal vasculitis revealed by fluorescein angiography in patients with inflammatory bowel disease. Jpn J Ophthalmol 1998; 42(5):398–400.
14. Renfro L, Snow JS. Ocular effects of topical and systemic steroids. Dermatol Clin 1992; 10(3):505–512.
15. Asquith P, Thompson RA, Cooke WT. Oral manifestations of Crohn's disease. Gut 1975; 16(4):1249–1254.
16. Pittock S, Drumm B, Fleming P, et al. The oral cavity in Crohn's disease. J Pediatr 2001; 138(5):767–771.
17. Wordinger RJ, Clark AF. Effects of glucocorticoids on the trabecular meshwork: towards a better understanding of glaucoma. Prog Retin Eye Res 1991; 18(5):629–667.
18. Harty S, Fleming P, Rowland M, et al. A prospective study of the oral manifestations of Crohn's disease. Clin Gastroenterol Hepatol 2005; 3(9):886–891.
19. van de Scheur MR, van der Waal RI, Volker-Dieben HJ, et al. Orofacial granulomatosis in a patient with Crohn's disease. J Am Acad Dermatol 2003; 49(5):952–954.
20. van de Scheur MR, van der Waal RI, Bodegraven AA, et al. Cheilitis granulomatosa and optic neuropathy as rare extraintestinal manifestations of Crohn's disease. J Clin Gastroenterol 2002; 34(5):557–559.
21. Bradley PJ, Ferlito A, Devaney KO, et al. Crohn's disease manifesting in the head and neck. Acta Otolaryngol 2004; 124(3):237–241.
22. McCabe BF. Autoimmune sensorineural hearing loss. Ann Otol Rhinol Laryngol 1979; 88(5 Pt 1):585–589.
23. Loft DE, Dowd AB, Khan MZH, et al. Auditory dysfunction in inflammatory bowel disease. Eur J Gastroenterol Hepatol 1989; 1:129–132.
24. Bachmeyer C, Leclerc-Landgraf N, Laurette F, et al. Acute autoimmune sensorineural hearing loss associated with Crohn's disease. Am J Gastroenterol 1998; 93(12):2565–2567.
25. Bloch DB, Gutierrez JA, Guerriero V Jr, et al. Recognition of a dominant epitope in bovine heat-shock protein 70 in inner ear disease. Laryngoscope 1999; 109(4):621–625.

26. Book DT, Smith TL, McNamar JP, et al. Chronic sinonasal disease in patients with inflammatory bowel disease. Am J Rhinol 2003; 17(2):87–90.
27. Camus P, Piard F, Ashcroft T, et al. The lung in inflammatory bowel disease. Medicine (Baltimore) 1993; 72(3):151–183.
28. Yang J, Maronian N, Reyes V, et al. Laryngeal and other otolaryngologic manifestations of Crohn's disease. J Voice 2002; 16(2):278–282.
29. Ottaviani F, Schindler A, Capaccio P, et al. New therapy for orolaryngeal manifestations of Crohn's disease. Ann Otol Rhinol Laryngol 2003; 112(1):37–39.
30. Greenstein AJ, Janowitz HD, Sachar DB. The extra-intestinal complications of Crohn's disease and ulcerative colitis: a study of 700 patients. Medicine (Baltimore) 1976; 55(5):401–412.
31. Gilson MR, Elston LC, Pruitt CA. Metastatic Crohn's disease: remission induced by mesalamine and prednisone. J Am Acad Dermatol 1999; 41(3 Pt 1):476–479.
32. Biancone L, Geboes K, Spagnoli LG, et al. Metastatic Crohn's disease of the forehead. Inflamm Bowel Dis 2002; 8(2):101–105.
33. Van Dullemen HM, de Jong E, Slors F, et al. Treatment of therapy-resistant perineal metastatic Crohn's disease after proctectomy using anti-tumor necrosis factor chimeric monoclonal antibody, cA2: report of two cases. Dis Colon Rectum 1998; 41(1):98–102.
34. Kemmet D, Hunter JA. Sweet's syndrome: a clinicopathologic review of twenty-nine cases. J Am Acad Dermatol 1990; 23(3 Pt 1):503–507.
35. Padda S, Ramirez F, Berggreen PJ. Sweet's syndrome associated with the use of azathioprine in a patient with Crohn's colitis. Am J Gastroenterol 1998; 93:A1735.
36. Weinreb RN, Bloom E, Baxter JD, et al. Detection of glucocorticoid receptors in cultured human trabecular cells. Invest Ophthalmol Vis Sci 1981; 21(3):403–407.
37. Wordinger RJ, Clark AF. Effects of glucocorticoids on the trabecular meshwork: towards a better understanding of glaucoma. Prog Retin Eye Res 1991; 18(5):629–667.

21

Paget's Disease of Bone and Fibrous Dysplasia

Edwin M. Monsell and Geetha Subramanian
Department of Otolaryngology-Head and Neck Surgery, Wayne State University School of Medicine, Detroit, Michigan, U.S.A.

PAGET'S DISEASE

INTRODUCTION

Paget's disease is a progressive disease of bone affecting primarily the middle aged and elderly.

The most common otolaryngic manifestation is hearing loss, which is related to involvement of the skull (1,2).

DEFINITION

Paget's disease of bone (PDB) is a focal or multifocal disease of bone remodeling in which transformed, multinucleated osteoclasts excavate bone at a greatly accelerated rate. Cycles of osteolysis and repair continue to remodel affected bone as the lesion slowly enlarges. Pagetic bone becomes highly vascular and thicker but structurally weaker.

EPIDEMIOLOGY

PDB occurs mainly in middle and later years. The disease is more prevalent in men than in women, ranging from 1.4 to 1.9:1 in various surveys. PDB is most common in North America, Europe, Australia, and New Zealand. It is more common in the United Kingdom, the Low Countries, France, and Germany and less prevalent in Scandinavia. It is relatively uncommon in Africa and Asia (3).

PATHOGENESIS

Evidence supports viral and genetic etiologies for PDB. Pagetic osteoclasts contain viral mRNA and inclusions that resemble paramyxoviruses. Vectors containing measles virus genes can convert osteoclast precursors to pagetic-like osteoclasts.

A positive family history of PDB has been reported in 1% to 40% of cases in various clinical series. Familial occurrence supports a dominant inheritance pattern with variable penetrance. Susceptibility loci have been mapped to chromosomes 18q21-22, 18q23, 6p21.3, and other locations. *SQSTM1*, a gene on chromosome 5q35 also associated with PDB, encodes a protein, p62 (sequestosome 1), which is involved in several signaling pathways important in osteoclast differentiation and activation. No single locus is associated with a large proportion of familial cases.

Normal bone undergoes continuous remodeling in an organized focal process. Osteoclasts excavate existing bone, creating a channel up to 40 to 60 mm deep within 4 to 12 days. This channel is repaired by osteoblasts in a coupled process over a period of two to three months. A feature unique to remodeling in the normal mammalian otic capsule is the sparing of a 400-μm wide zone surrounding the perilymphatic space.

Pagetic osteoclasts are larger, contain many more nuclei, and are far more active resorbers of bone than normal osteoclasts. The pattern of resorption in PDB is unrelated to the structural requirements of bone. Pagetic bone has a mosaic appearance of multiple cement lines that develop as pagetic osteoclasts and reactive osteoblasts repeatedly break down and repair areas of bone (3).

Paget's disease typically results in thickening and enlargement of the skull (Fig. 1), which expands outward, so the intracranial space is not compromised. Later, thickening

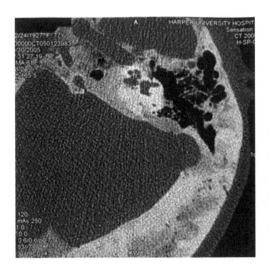

FIGURE 1 High-resolution axial computed tomography scan of the left temporal bone in a 78-year-old woman showing extensive Paget's disease of bone. The pattern of involvement shows the classic "cotton wool" appearance of Paget's disease. Audiometry showed profound deafness in this ear. *Source*: Courtesy of Edwin M. Monsell, MD, PhD.

and sclerosis predominate, often producing a characteristic "cotton wool" appearance on radiographs (Fig. 1).

Histologic studies in cases with pagetic hearing loss have demonstrated that hair cells and spiral ganglion cells remain intact (2). Auditory-evoked potentials are normal. The internal auditory canal lumen is not compromised. Conversely, both the sensorineural hearing loss and the air-bone gap in PDB are closely associated with the loss of bone mineral density in the cochlear capsule (1).

CLINICAL MANIFESTATIONS

Paget's disease may affect any bone in the body, but it most commonly involves the skull (about 30% of cases), pelvis, long bones, and spine. Often, patients are asymptomatic, and the diagnosis is made incidentally from radiographs, bone scans, or an elevated serum alkaline phosphatase level.

PDB may present with bone pain, hearing loss, fracture, nerve root compression, or headache. Pagetic bone pain is usually constant, dull, and poorly localized. Pain may also result from osteoarthritis in the joints adjacent to the affected bones.

Hearing loss is usually bilaterally symmetrical and progressive. A high-frequency sensorineural loss and low-frequency air-bone gap are characteristics (1).

DIAGNOSIS

Hearing loss is one of the most common complications. Pagetic hearing loss may be suspected in any middle-aged or elderly person showing characteristic auditory features [high-frequency sensorineural hearing loss and low-frequency air-bone gap (1)] or any level of hearing loss with a positive history of PDB. Patients can be screened with a serum alkaline phosphatase test; levels of bone-specific alkaline phosphatase are often several times normal in active PDB.

Computed tomography (CT) scans are confirmatory (1). Technetium bone scans will demonstrate the areas of the skeleton that are involved. Confirmatory biopsy is rarely indicated. Radiographs may show lytic lesions that need to be differentiated from cancer metastases and other lesions. Sclerosing appearances develop later in the course of the disease.

TREATMENT

The emphasis has shifted from treatment of symptoms to treatment for prevention of complications. Lesions should be treated to prevent hearing loss, pathologic fractures, secondary arthritis, and neurologic complications. Patients should be treated before surgical procedures involving pagetic bone to reduce bleeding and risk of infection. Thus, according to current thinking, nearly every patient should be treated.

Calcitonin and etidronate were the most commonly used medications for treatment of Paget's disease in the past. These have declined in usage since the arrival of newer bisphosphonates (pamidronate, alendronate, and risedronate), which are more successful in controlling the disease with limited side effects. When the rate of bone resorption is controlled by medication, the rate of bone formation is gradually reduced. Lytic areas are at least partially repaired, and the new bone formed has a more normal lamellar appearance. Serum alkaline phosphatase levels and urinary hydroxyproline excretion approach normal values. Patients need to be followed indefinitely because the pagetic process usually resumes if treatment is discontinued (3).

Treatment may slow the progression of hearing loss but does not reverse the deficit or correct deformities of bone, even if biochemical markers are normalized. Surgical exploration, stapedotomy, and ossicular chain repair are generally not indicated because ossicular function is not impaired, even when the characteristic air-bone gap is present (1).

COMPLICATIONS AND PROGNOSIS

Involvement of the temporal bone qualitatively by CT is highly correlated with involvement of the otic capsule in quantitative CT studies, even when the otic capsule appears to be uninvolved by clinical CT.

Bilateral involvement of the otic capsules is typical when Paget's disease involves the skull. The pagetic process and associated hearing loss are established well before signs appear in the facial skeleton.

Treatment can halt the progression of the disease but does not result in improved hearing. Patients usually respond well to amplification or cochlear implantation, when indicated.

Bowing of weight-bearing bones, increased skull size, and other deformities occur in advanced disease. The maxilla and other facial bones may be involved, producing deformity. Osteosarcoma is a rare complication of the disease. It typically occurs in a setting of long-standing, widespread disease. Patients should be treated to stabilize the disease before elective surgery in affected areas to minimize intraoperative blood loss and risk of infection.

SUMMARY

Paget's disease is a progressive disease of bone remodeling. Its systemic manifestations include bone pain and deformity. Pagetic hearing loss due to skull involvement is common and occurs before the development of obvious deformity. Treatment is usually successful in controlling the disease and reducing complications. Hearing levels are stabilized with effective treatment, but do not improve.

*F*IBROUS DYSPLASIA

INTRODUCTION

Fibrous dysplasia (FD) is a genetic disease that causes deformities in soft tissue and bone.

DEFINITION

FD is a benign, usually self-limited, focal fibro-osseous disease of bone. Lesions may be single (monostotic) or multiple (polyostotic), or may occur as part of the McCune-Albright syndrome (MAS). MAS is a rare disorder characterized by a classic triad of polyostotic FD, café-au-lait spots, and peripheral precocious puberty. Other endocrine disorders, including hyperthyroidism and hypophosphatemia, may accompany MAS. Malignant transformation is rare (4).

EPIDEMIOLOGY

FD can occur at any age but primarily affects adolescents and young adults, without gender predilection. MAS occurs primarily in females.

PATHOGENESIS

FD has been linked to activating mutations in the α subunit of stimulatory G protein, which is active in cell signaling. This mutation appears to occur after fertilization in somatic cells and has been located at 20q13.2-13.3. Mutations that occur early in embryonic development may result in more widespread or severe disease, including MAS and Mazabraud's syndrome. As a result of this mutation, GTPase activity is inhibited. There is a constitutive activation of adenylate cyclase and increased formation of cyclic adenosine monophosphate. G protein is produced by *GNAS*, a complex imprinted gene. Defects in this gene or its imprinting have been associated with various human diseases. Hormone hypersecretion in MAS appears to result from such "gain of function" mutations. Fibroblast growth factor 23 (FGF-23) may be involved in the mechanism of renal phosphate wasting, hypophosphatemia, and abnormal vitamin D metabolism in isolated FD and MAS.

CLINICAL MANIFESTATIONS

Monostotic FD is most common and usually is identified in the third decade of life. Polyostotic disease usually is diagnosed in the first decade. Most lesions of FD are detected as asymptomatic, incidental findings. Deformity of the maxilla, face, or skull may occur. FD may present in the spine or appendicular skeleton with a pathologic fracture. Involvement of the paranasal sinuses (Fig. 2) is usually asymptomatic. Active lesions may cause pain or nerve entrapment.

Temporal bone involvement is uncommon. The most common presentations are hearing loss (80%), mass (26–50%), draining ear (14–30%), otalgia (7–10%), and trismus (2.3–10%) (1). A conductive hearing loss or canal cholesteatoma may result from collapse of the external auditory canal, if it is extensively involved. The otic capsule and/or internal auditory canal are rarely involved. This involvement is associated with sensorineural hearing loss, which may be profound (5). Facial nerve involvement is not unusual (5–10%).

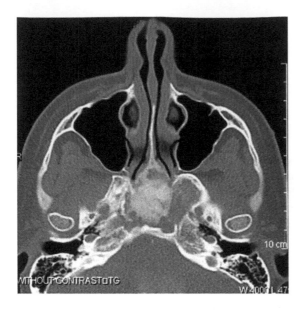

FIGURE 2 High-resolution axial computed tomography scan showing a biopsy-proven lesion of fibrous dysplasia in the sphenoid sinus. The center of the lesion has the classic "ground glass" appearance. *Source*: Courtesy of Edwin M. Monsell, MD, PhD.

Precocious puberty, thyroid disease, and secreting pituitary microadenomas predominate among the endocrinopathies in MAS. Clinical presentations include thyrotoxicosis, acromegaly, and Cushing syndrome (6).

DIAGNOSIS

Lesions are best evaluated by CT. Radiological studies show a characteristic "ground glass" appearance (Fig. 2). Radiolucent (lytic), radiopaque (sclerotic), and mixed types of radiographic appearances occur. A lesion might also be cystic or might have a thin bony cortex. A technetium bone scan will identify other areas of skeletal involvement. The serum alkaline phosphatase level will provide insight into the level of disease activity.

The differential diagnosis includes ossifying and nonossifying fibroma, well-differentiated osteogenic sarcoma, simple bone cyst, osteofibrous dysplasia, adamantinoma, and PDB. A tissue diagnosis (biopsy) is recommended in nonclassical presentations; ossifying fibroma and osteogenic sarcoma, in particular, would be treated differently. Sequencing the $G(s)\ \alpha$ gene has been suggested as a way to confirm the diagnosis of FD in selected cases.

The café-au-lait spots of MAS are described as having an irregular, trabecular ("coast of Maine") appearance, as opposed to the smoother ("coast of California") outline of café-au-lait spots in neurofibromatosis (6). Suspected endocrinopathies are pursued with appropriate evaluations.

TREATMENT

Most lesions are observed. The rationale for the use of bisphosphonates (pamidronate) to treat active, symptomatic lesions is that lesions have active osteolysis, and sometimes pain can be relieved. Treatment with pamidronate has been associated with a decrease in the elevated plasma FGF-23 levels in a few cases. Nevertheless, there are insufficient longitudinal data on safety and efficacy, especially in children, to make evidence-based recommendations for treatment of FD with bisphosphonates at this time.

COMPLICATIONS AND PROGNOSIS

Canaloplasty for collapse of the external auditory canal in FD has a high failure rate (6). Appendicular abnormalities are usually corrected after skeletal maturity is achieved. Results are usually satisfactory. It is unclear whether preoperative treatment reduces the vascularity of the lesion sufficiently to be beneficial in surgery.

SUMMARY

FD is a genetic disease of soft tissue and bone. Lesions are usually self-limited. Medical treatment is available but not well validated. Surgery in the head and neck is indicated to resolve questions of diagnosis or correct deformity.

REFERENCES

1. Monsell EM. Mechanism of hearing loss in Paget's disease of bone. Laryngoscope 2004; 114 (4):598–606.
2. Khetarpal U, Schuknecht HF. In search of pathologic correlates for hearing loss and vertigo in Paget's disease. A clinical and histopathologic study of 26 temporal bones. Ann Otol Rhinol Laryngol Suppl 1990; 145:1–16.
3. Kanis JA. Pathophysiology and Treatment of Paget's Disease of Bone. 2nd ed. London, England: Martin Dunitz Lt., 1998.
4. Megerian CA, Sofferman RA, McKenna MJ, et. al. Fibrous dysplasia of the temporal bone: ten new cases demonstrating the spectrum of otologic sequelae. Am J Otol 1995; 16(4):408–419.
5. Nager GT, Kennedy DW, Kopstein E. Fibrous dysplasia: a review of the disease and its manifestations in the temporal bone. Ann Otol Rhinol Laryngol Suppl 1982; 92:1–52.
6. DiCaprio MR, Enneking WF. Fibrous dysplasia. Pathophysiology, evaluation, and treatment. J Bone Joint Surg Am 2005; 87(8):1848–1864.

22

Systemic Allergic Disorders: IgE-Mediated Disorders, Angioedema, Nonsteroidal Anti-Inflammatory Drug Sensitivity, and Stevens-Johnson Syndrome

Michelle Hernandez and Stephen I. Wasserman
Department of Medicine, Division of Rheumatology, Allergy, and Immunology, University of California, San Diego, California, U.S.A.

INTRODUCTION

By their very nature, allergic and immunologic disorders are systemic, and their effects manifest in many organ systems, including the structures of the head, neck, and upper airway. The disorders that are discussed in this chapter are the consequence of the generation of allergen-specific IgE antibodies, generally to inhaled allergen. Additionally, there are a number of disorders that clinically mimic IgE-mediated processes, and their pathophysiology, recognition, and treatment are also included here.

IgE-MEDIATED DISORDERS

In most instances, IgE-mediated processes are expressed in the eye, nose, upper and lower airways, and skin. They are the underlying processes for the disorders known as allergic conjunctivitis, allergic rhinosinusitis, asthma, urticaria/angioedema, and anaphylaxis. In this chapter, we focus on the effects of IgE-mediated processes on the nose and upper airway, including rhinosinusitis and angioedema and those processes that might be confused with them.

ALLERGIC RHINOSINUSITIS

DEFINITION

Allergic rhinosinusitis is a disorder expressed in the tissues of the nares and upper airway, manifested by local edema and inflammatory infiltration of the submucosa and mucosa, and associated with increased secretion of mucoid materials with accompanying inflammatory leukocytes. These processes lead to obstruction of airflow and of mucus drainage, and, therefore, may be complicated by postobstructive infectious complications.

By definition, allergic disease is dependent on the host generation of allergen-specific IgE antibodies.

EPIDEMIOLOGY

Allergic rhinosinusitis is a diagnosis made clinically, as there are no definitive objective tests available for routine clinical use to confirm this entity. There are two major forms of this disorder: seasonal and perennial. Thus, it is a diagnosis based on history (often by questionnaire) and physical examination. In some epidemiological studies, the presence of allergy is confirmed by results of skin prick tests or in vitro allergy testing. The prevalence of this disorder varies widely in the literature, based upon the different sources of the data (i.e., questionnaires, phone interviews, and direct examination), but the majority of the literature suggests that 20% to 25% of children and about 15% of adults suffer from this condition (1). Peak prevalence is between 10 and 30 years in most countries (2). Atopic individuals are at much increased risk for this disorder and there is a significant correlation between the report of nasal symptoms and the prevalence of allergen-specific IgE. There is a strong genetic component to allergic rhinosinusitis, and children whose parents are both allergic have a high likelihood (>50%) of manifesting allergic rhinosinusitis before school age. Also, the presence of other allergic manifestations (e.g., eczema) foreshadows the presentation of allergic rhinosinusitis. Allergic disease must be differentiated from other causes of rhinitis, including infection, genetic disorders (cystic fibrosis and ciliary defects), and drug-induced, hormonal, occupational, anatomic, neoplastic, and irritant causes.

PATHOGENESIS

The fundamental cause of allergic rhinosinusitis is the generation of allergen-specific IgE antibodies to inhalant materials normally immunologically ignored. The presence of allergen-specific IgE can be determined either by prick puncture skin testing or by in vitro testing. Recent work indicates that intradermal skin testing does not add to the diagnostic armamentarium for this problem, and in the face of a negative prick puncture skin test, intradermal testing adds nothing to the diagnosis (3). The specific allergen to which an individual is sensitized is based, to some degree, on genetics, and, to a larger degree, on environment. The most important allergens for perennial symptoms are house dust mites, furred animals, and cockroaches. Seasonal allergens include molds and the pollens of grasses, trees, and weeds.

The generation of IgE is regulated by the interaction of T-lymphocytes and antigen-presenting cells and is facilitated by the cytokines Interleukin (IL)-4 and IL-13. Complex interactions between allergen-specific T-lymphocytes and B-lymphocytes, including binding of CD40/CD40 ligand, eventuate in the immunoglobulin gene switch/recombination to IgE (4). IgE may be synthesized locally within the nasal mucosa as well as systemically, although the importance of local IgE production is uncertain. Secreted IgE is then bound tightly to high-affinity receptors on the surface of tissue mast cells and circulating peripheral blood basophils. These cells possess, preformed, a number of inflammatory mediators exemplified by histamine, and upon activation, generate and release a variety of vasoactive and inflammatory molecules including leukotrienes (LTs), chemoattractants, and active enzymes. Activation occurs when an allergen cross-links two adjacent IgE molecules on the surface of mast cells or basophils, and this causes release of preformed mediators and the generation and release of unstored ones. These mediators alter the control of the nasal vasculature and activate nasal neuronal reflexes to induce airflow obstruction, nasal itch/sneezing, and vasodilatation. In addition, they augment nasal mucus secretion, stimulate vascular leakage, and promote plasma protein transudation. In addition to these direct effects, inflammatory mediators generated by the IgE–allergen interaction support eosinophilic polymorphonuclear leukocyte migration and survival and activate endothelial cells to express adhesion molecules relevant to the local influx of eosinophils and basophils to generate a characteristic allergic inflammatory state. Much of this cascade has been verified in human studies of allergen deposition into the nasal cavity followed by measurement of physiologic changes accompanied by histopathological analysis of the nasal tissue and the direct measurement of inflammatory mediators and cytokines in nasal tissue and secretions (5).

CLINICAL MANIFESTATIONS

The most important and prevalent nonrhinitic symptoms expressed by patients with allergic rhinosinusitis are ocular, otic, and respiratory: patients note itchy and watery eyes and manifest injection of the conjunctivae. The palpebral conjunctivae may demonstrate cobblestoning, indicating lymphocytic infiltration. Otic manifestations include patient-reported sensations of fullness or clicking sensations and decreased auditory acuity. Nonnasal respiratory effects are manifest as asthma with cough and wheezing dyspnea. While not all patients with allergic rhinosinusitis have asthma, most asthmatic patients experience rhinitis, and importantly, studies indicate that appropriate management of rhinosinusitis improves the efficacy of asthma treatment. The local head and neck manifestations of allergic rhinosinusitis include pale and boggy nasal mucosae and swollen turbinates, resulting in obstruction of airflow. Additionally, copious nasal secretions, generally described as watery, but often containing mucoid materials and plasma proteins, are present. There may be tenderness over the sinuses and in uncomplicated allergic rhinosinusitis, sinus radiographs may demonstrate mucosal thickening. Some patients may appreciate nasal congestion as headache rather than as facial pressure/pain. Abnormal mobility of the tympanic membrane and the presence of otitis media commonly are noted. Fatigue, perhaps due to sleep disturbances caused by nasal airflow obstruction, commonly accompanies allergic rhinosinusitis (6).

DIAGNOSIS

The diagnosis of allergic rhinosinusitis is based first upon clinical presentation. Thus, the presence of itchy/watery eyes, sneezing, palatal itching, clear watery rhinorrhea, and sinus/facial pressure suggest this disorder. In addition, the presence of other allergic manifestations such as asthma, eczema, or urticaria/angioedema, and a family history of atopic disorders, provide further support. Exacerbation of symptoms during specific seasons of the year (spring = trees, late spring to early summer = grasses, and fall = weeds and molds), or with certain exposures (e.g., cat), is additional evidence of an allergic etiology. Physical examination may be relatively unremarkable or may reveal pale and swollen nasal mucosa, sometimes described as a bluish discoloration, enlarged turbinates, and copious nasal secretions. Profound erythema of the mucosa and/or the presence of purulent nasal discharge should suggest other diagnoses or the presence of complications of underlying allergic disease. Specialized tests of nasal airway resistance, nasal airway caliber, and nasal provocation testing with specific allergens have been used in research settings but are not widely available for clinical use. Supporting laboratory tests include assessment of peripheral blood eosinophilia that may reach 10% to 12%, but may be normal, and the quantitation of total serum IgE. Total IgE may be normal or moderately elevated in allergic rhinosinusitis but is not a conclusive diagnostic test for this disorder. Specific diagnosis is made by the demonstration of elevated amounts of allergen-specific IgE antibody. This may be done by performing allergy prick puncture skin testing, or in vitro, using a modification of the radioallergosorbent technology. There is good correlation between these two testing modalities, and the choice of test is based on availability of the test, the presence or absence of dermatographism, the ability to withhold antihistaminic medications, and the cost. Recent studies indicate that a negative prick puncture skin test essentially rules out allergic nasal disease, and therefore no additional information is to be gained by performing intradermal skin tests for inhalant allergens in this setting (3). A positive reaction to a prick puncture skin test, or an in vitro test, must be correlated with the clinical situation to verify the diagnosis. For example, in a patient with springtime rhinitis, a reaction to ragweed (a fall allergen) is unlikely to be relevant.

TREATMENT

Therapy for allergic rhinosinusitis is directed initially at the symptomatic manifestations. Thus, rhinorrhea, sneezing, and nasal obstruction are the targets of therapy, based on the patient's presenting problems.

Antihistaminics
Histamine is a major contributor to all of these symptoms; therefore, its blockade is the initial treatment of choice (7). Generally an H-1 antagonist, either a first-generation molecule such as chlorpheniramine, or, if soporific effects are a problem, a second-generation antihistaminic such as loratidine, cetirizine, or fexofenadine, is the treatment of choice. Alternatively, an antihistaminic agent (azelastine) can be applied directly to the nasal mucosa via inhalation.

Antihistaminics may help diminish nasal obstruction but are often not fully effective against this symptom.

Vasoconstrictors

To decrease congestion, two strategies are available. The one often employed first by patients is the use of vasoconstrictor agents. These may be used topically, with the problem of rhinitis medicamentosa, rebound vasodilatation that is often worse than the presenting problem. Oral use of decongestants may be effective in ameliorating congestion in some patients but their use may be associated with hypertension and sleep disorders.

Corticosteroids

A more effective approach to nasal congestion and inflammation is the use of a topical nasal corticosteroid spray. This class of agent is the most potent and effective modality for the treatment of allergic rhinitis and is effective against all of the manifestations of this disorder (8). Common side effects include local nasal irritation and occasional thrush. Less common, but possibly important in the case of long-term use, are an increase in incidence of glaucoma, cataracts, and osteoporosis. These drugs diminish the inflammatory influx of cells into the nasal mucosa and diminish the strength of the local allergic response.

Cromones

An alternative anti-inflammatory agent available for topical nasal usage is cromolyn, a drug that is less potent than inhaled steroids but virtually free of side effects.

LT Receptor Antagonists

The use of an LT receptor antagonist (montelukast and zafirlukast) has been shown to augment the effect of an antihistaminic agent in control of nasal obstruction (9); however, those two drugs together are less effective in controlling nasal symptoms than inhaled glucocorticoids.

Allergen Avoidance

Another strategy for the control of allergic nasal disease is allergen based. The first is allergen avoidance and is best based on direct knowledge of the specific allergen in question. Removal of furred animals, control of cockroaches or mold, and use of impervious bed covers to diminish mite exposure have all been shown to be effective in controlling allergen-induced symptoms in sensitized patients. Closure of windows and use of air conditioning and air filtration can help decrease pollen exposure during pollination seasons.

Immunotherapy

The only specific and potentially curative therapy currently available for the treatment of allergic rhinosinusitis is allergen immunotherapy (10). This modality consists of providing incrementally increasing amounts of allergen to which the patient is sensitive, until a fixed maintenance dose is reached. It is essential for high doses of allergen to be provided if a therapeutic immune response is to occur. Successful immunotherapy results in the generation of allergen-specific IgG antibodies and a modified T-lymphocyte response characterized by the generation of regulatory T-lymphocytes. Immunotherapy should be reserved for those patients failing medical therapy.

COMPLICATIONS

Generally, allergic rhinosinusitis is a benign condition readily responsive to therapeutic intervention.

Sinusitis

The major complications of this disorder are due to inflammatory obstruction of the osteomeatal complex. Such obstruction leads to the prevention of normal clearance of the sinuses, diminishes gas exchange leading to lowered oxygen tension, and predisposes one to sinus infection. In this setting, infection is generally due to aerobic bacteria including *Streptococcus pneumoniae*, *Haemophilus influenzae*, and *Moraxella catarrhalis*. In some patients, fungal superinfection may also occur, most commonly due to *Alternaria* or *Aspergillus* species. In some patients, aberrant allergic or immunologic responses to the fungi have been presumed to contribute to the histopathologic manifestations of the disease. Acute sinusitis is generally manifest by fever, local pain, and purulent nasal drainage. Symptoms in subacute or chronic sinusitis are generally less specific and include nasal obstruction, diminished sense of smell, halitosis, and postnasal discharge.

Otitis

Although the direct contribution of allergic mechanisms to otitis media remain controversial, it is clear that obstruction to Eustachian tube drainage and resultant dysfunction can result in symptoms of ear fullness and diminished hearing and may contribute to the severity and persistence of otitis media.

Nasal Polyposis

Another complication of untreated IgE-mediated nasal disease is the development of nasal polyps. Because they are a characteristic finding in the syndrome of nonsteroidal anti-inflammatory drug (NSAID) hypersensitivity, this topic will be dealt with in that section below.

PROGNOSIS

Allergic rhinosinusitis is generally a benign, albeit chronic, condition that responds well to therapy. Epidemiologic studies suggest that its highest incidence is in young adulthood, suggesting a waning of symptoms as one ages; however, allergic rhinosinusitis can persist for many decades. Some patients with this condition develop asthma; this is particularly true in children (the so-called "allergic march").

SUMMARY

Allergic rhinosinusitis is an extremely common disorder. It is generally easily treated but may be complicated by sinusitis (acute or chronic) and otitis. Additionally, as for all allergic diseases, patients must be evaluated for non–head-and-neck manifestations, including ocular and lower respiratory dysfunction.

*A*NGIOEDEMA

INTRODUCTION

Angioedema is an uncommon and usually self-limited swelling of the deep dermis. It can, however, be complicated by potentially serious adverse consequences, including death. Although IgE-mediated mechanisms are not the major cause of angioedema, they are among the few that can be clearly identified, and thus this topic will be discussed here. Angioedema occurs together with urticaria approximately 85% of the time; in 15% of instances, it occurs alone.

DEFINITION

Angioedema (Fig. 1) is the abrupt and transient swelling of the skin, mucous membranes, or both, including the upper respiratory and intestinal epithelial linings (11). In some cases, angioedema and urticaria should be viewed as varying manifestations of the same pathologic process, and they are common components of anaphylactic reactions. Angioedema involves the reticular dermis and subcutaneous or submucosal tissue, particularly of acral areas, while urticaria involves the papillary dermis and mid-dermis throughout the body. The depth of involvement will result in different clinical presentations. Urticarial lesions are erythematous, short lived (<24 hours) and intensely pruritic, while the swelling of angioedema is nonpitting, pink or skin colored, more persistent and described as burning, stretching, or painful, rather than pruritic.

EPIDEMIOLOGY

The prevalence of angioedema is not well characterized. It is said that up to 20% of individuals experience urticaria at some point in life and that half of such patients also have angioedema; however, chronic urticaria/angioedema (persisting more than six weeks) is much less common (approximately 0.1% of the population). Anaphylaxis occurs at a rate of approximately 30/100,000 person-years. Urticaria/angioedema are among the most common manifestations of anaphylaxis, appearing in about half of all such occurrences. IgE-mediated mechanisms have been shown to cause approximately 60% of anaphylactic reactions and are common causes of acute urticaria/angioedema. Its role as the cause of chronic angioedema, however, is much less clear, and in most instances of chronic angioedema, no causative factor is identified. In some of these patients, physical urticaria/ angioedema such as that caused by exposure to cold, or exercise-induced anaphylaxis, has been demonstrated to be responsible.

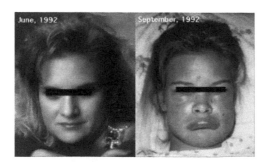

FIGURE 1   Facial angioedema.

Less common but clearly identifiable causes of angioedema include drug use and alteration of complement metabolism. A recent prospective study noted that angioedema due to angiotensin-converting enzyme inhibitor (ACE-I) use occurred in 86 of 12,557 patients (0.68%) (12). ACE-I–induced angioedema was about three times more likely to occur among black patients (1.62% vs. 0.55% for white patients), and slightly more likely in women (0.84% vs. 0.54% for men). Approximately 50% of patients with ACE-I–induced angioedema experience their first episode within the first week of treatment; however, some patients may have ACE-I for months before angioedema develops.

The prevalence of hereditary angioedema (HAE), an autosomal-dominant disease, is about 1:50,000 persons (13). This disease has been reported in all races. It is due to a mutation in one copy of the inhibitor of the first component of complement. A disorder with similar pathogenesis can be acquired in patients with an unusual complement consumption profile due to lymphoma or in patients generating an IgG autoantibody to the inhibitor itself.

PATHOGENESIS

The swelling of angioedema is caused by local plasma extravasation. This occurs after a rapid increase in the permeability of submucosal and postcapillary venules.

Although angioedema may be precipitated by both immune-mediated and non–immune-mediated mechanisms, it is more easily classified into those mediated by mast cell degranulation and those mediated by bradykinin.

Immune-mediated mechanisms include those dependent on IgE (food allergy, drug allergy, hymenoptera sting, and inhaled/contact allergens) and those that are immune-complex-mediated (mononucleosis, other viral syndromes, and systemic lupus erythematosus). Inhibition of prostaglandin synthesis through cyclo-oxygenase (COX)-1 may cause angioedema as substrates are redirected to the lipo-oxygenase pathway, resulting in the production of cysteinyl LTs and vasoactive hydroxyl fatty acids, which presumably act on mast cells. (See also below.) Chronic angioedema (episodes that are recurrent over a greater-than-six-week period) may be idiopathic, accompany presumed mast-cell–dependent physical urticarias (cholinergic, cold, solar, and heat urticaria) or exercise anaphylaxis, or be associated with autoantibodies affecting mast-cell function. Anti-IgE and anti-FC epsilon receptor 1 (on mast cells) antibodies have been identified; these are found to occur quite commonly along with antithyroglobulin and antimicrosomal antibodies (14).

Bradykinin is the mediator responsible for ACE-I–associated angioedema and HAE. ACE inactivates bradykinin, a powerful vasoactive peptide in human skin. Inhibition of ACE results in slow bradykinin inactivation, with consequent bradykinin accumulation and vasodilatation (13).

Patients with HAE have defects in C1 inhibitor function (15). C1 is the first component of the complement cascade. Type 1 HAE patients have a quantitative defect in C1 inhibitor due to a truncating mutation that prevents synthesis, while Type 2 HAE patients have a functional defect due to an inactivating mutation that does not prevent protein secretion. In both, one normal gene is present. Recently, Type 3 HAE has been described, where both the C1 inhibitor levels and function are normal. This occurs exclusively in women and is suspected to be associated with estrogen activity. C1 inhibitor levels may be exhausted in situations of rapid complement utilization (lymphoma) or in the presence of an autoantibody to the inhibitor itself.

C1 inhibitor deficiency causes excessive formation of the enzyme kallikrein, resulting in increased production of bradykinin. C1 inhibitor is also responsible for keeping the complement cascade in check; thus, deficiency leads to increased spontaneous activation of C1 with secondary consumption of C2 and C4.

CLINICAL MANIFESTATIONS

Angioedema preferentially affects the face, hands, arms, legs, and genitalia.

Acute allergic angioedema is often (about half the time) accompanied by urticarial lesions. Mucosal or cutaneous angioedema can occur within minutes of ingestion or injection of an offending agent. Swellings typically subside within 24 to 48 hours, although relapses may occur. The areas of swelling do not leave any residual bruising unless vigorously rubbed. Some episodes of acute allergic angioedema are accompanied by symptoms of anaphylaxis, including bronchospasm and hypotension.

Angioedema due to ACE-I has a predilection for the head, neck, lips, mouth, tongue, larynx, pharynx, and subglottic areas, without urticaria (16).

Patients with HAE are usually asymptomatic until the second decade of life. Some episodes may be preceded by a nonpruritic urticarial eruption, but generally, such episodes occur in the absence of urticaria. Swellings may be precipitated by exercise, stress, alcohol consumption, hormonal factors, and even minor trauma such as dental procedures (13). In contrast to angioedema due to other factors, the swelling in HAE patients may slowly spread and persist for up to three to four days. Angioedema can also mimic an acute intestinal obstruction with associated abdominal pain and vomiting.

The most feared and potentially fatal presentation of angioedema involves the mucosae of the pharynx, larynx, and subglottic areas. Stridor and dyspnea may precede respiratory obstruction, asphyxia, and sometimes death. ACE-I angioedema is the most common cause of acute angioedema presenting to emergency departments (17–38%) (17), and up to 20% may be life threatening. In a series of 225 patients with both hereditary and acquired angioedema, 10% required intubation or tracheostomy at least once. Thus, prompt identification and management of airway angioedema is essential in preventing mortality (18).

DIAGNOSIS AND DIFFERENTIAL DIAGNOSIS

The differential diagnosis of angioedema includes superior vena cava syndrome, facial cellulitis, allergic contact or photodermatitis, Crohn's disease of the mouth and lips, dermatomyositis, facial lymphedema, tumid or discoid lupus erythematosus, Ascher syndrome, and Melkersson–Rosenthal syndrome (13). A complete history, including symptoms of associated urticaria, duration, location, potential precipitants, medication history (particularly of ACE-I and B-adrenergic blocking agents), and systemic manifestations, is essential. Physical exam must focus on airway evaluation and visualization of the lesion(s) and other associated disease processes. Historical factors should lead to directed blood work. Epicutaneous or radioallergosorbent testing (RAST) testing may be used for suspected allergens. Laboratory studies for evaluation of HAE include C1 inhibitor levels and function, C4 level, and C1q (if decreased, this would indicate acquired C1 inhibitor).

TREATMENT

If the respiratory tract is involved, securing the airway is the top priority. Approaches to consider include nasopharyngeal intubation, endotracheal intubation (which is often difficult), nasotracheal intubation, and cricothyrotomy. IV access should be obtained. IM epinephrine (0.3 mL of 1:1000) should be given to reduce the edema and may be repeated every 10 minutes. Admission to the hospital with careful observation for 24 hours is suggested for patients with laryngeal edema.

In cases of idiopathic angioedema, or in anaphylaxis with angioedema, use of epinephrine is critical. Diphenhydramine (50 mg) IM or IV and solumedrol IV (40 mg) may be helpful acutely, and chronic angioedema should be treated with daily anti-histaminics. In some situations, LT receptor antagonists, or even immunosuppressants, may be helpful in controlling chronic angioedema.

Patients with HAE will not respond to these measures. Intravenous fresh frozen plasma or C1 inhibitor concentrate (not yet available in the United States except in clinical trials) are effective by raising serum levels of C1 inhibitor sufficiently to prevent ongoing bradykinin and complement activation (19). In HAE, fibrinolytic inhibitors have been employed to ameliorate acute angioedema. Discontinuing any offending medication is essential. Preventive medications for patients with both Type 1 and Type 2 HAE include anabolic steroids (danazol and stanazolol) and antifibrinolytic agents. Anabolic steroids have been shown to increase the circulating levels of C1 inhibitor by decreasing consumption of the product of the normal C1-inhibitor gene (15).

COMPLICATIONS AND PROGNOSIS

Relapses can occur after an episode of ACE-I angioedema apparently resolves, despite discontinuing the offending drug. If unidentified, episodes of angioedema after repeated ACE-I exposure may lead to more severe attacks (20). A series evaluating patients with HAE noted that the average time between onset of laryngeal edema and asphyxiation was seven hours (18). The interval between onset of the laryngeal edema and asphyxiation was 20 minutes in a nine-year-old boy with no previous clinical signs of HAE. The retrospective survey of 58 patients with HAE revealed 40% of deaths by asphyxiation. A case fatality rate for anaphylaxis is difficult to determine and is not known for angioedema associated with urticaria or that which occurs independently in the absence of a known inciting cause.

The prognosis for known instances of HAE and for ACE-I–mediated angioedema is excellent with proper treatment. In cases of anaphylaxis in which the inciting agent is known, prognosis is good if the offending agent can be avoided, and if IM adrenaline (Epi-pen®) is available for immediate use. Such patients should avoid ACE-I and B-adrenergic inhibitory agents. In idiopathic chronic angioedema, maintenance treatment is built on use of antihistaminics, and the natural history is that many patients become free of angioedema after 5 to 20 years.

SUMMARY

Multiple mechanisms may produce the end result of angioedema. After evaluation of the airway, a thorough history may provide the necessary clues to guide the appropriate management of this disorder.

ASPIRIN (NSAID) HYPERSENSITIVITY

INTRODUCTION

Three manifestations of sensitivity to NSAIDs are of importance to the head and neck. They include urticaria/angioedema, anaphylaxis, and rhinoconjunctivitis/asthma. These appear to occur separately, and, in most instances, cross-reaction with other drugs in the class is common.

DEFINITION

By definition, NSAID hypersensitivity is present in patients who react adversely to the administration of this class of drug. It was originally described by Widal as a symptom complex of aspirin sensitivity, asthma, and nasal polyposis, and is now known to be associated with chronic pansinusitis and tissue and peripheral blood eosinophilia. Another group of patients react to the ingestion of these drugs with acute urticaria/angioedema, or, more controversially, with exacerbation of underlying urticaria/angioedema. Finally, a small group of patients have immediate anaphylactic reactions to the ingestion of this class of drug. Only in the latter group does selectivity for a particular agent within the class appear to be common (21).

EPIDEMIOLOGY

NSAID hypersensitivity tends to present in early adult years as rhinorrhea, nasal congestion, and hyposmia. In patients with asthma, NSAID hypersensitivity may develop concurrently or some years after the diagnosis of asthma has been established. In both groups, peripheral blood and tissue eosinophilia and pansinusitis with nasal polyposis are common. Approximately 10% of patients with steroid-dependent asthma have been found to be NSAID hypersensitive, whereas one-third of asthmatics with associated nasal polyposis and chronic sinusitis are sensitive to this class of drug. Although most normal patients tolerate these drugs, epidemiological studies suggest adverse reaction rates of up to 1%.

Cutaneous manifestations of NSAID hypersensitivity have been subclassified as urticaria/angioedema in normal individuals (an uncommon occurrence), single-drug–induced urticaria/angioedema/anaphylaxis in normal individuals (also rare, and possibly IgE mediated), and exacerbation of underlying urticaria/angioedema (in approximately 25% of patients with chronic urticaria).

PATHOGENESIS

In the vast majority of cases of NSAID hypersensitivity (asthma, rhinosinusitis, and polyposis), the pathogenetic mechanism behind the reaction is inhibition of the constitutively active enzyme COX-1 responsible for the generation of prostaglandins. In these instances, patients tolerate use of COX-2 inhibitors but cannot tolerate most or any of the COX-1 inhibitory agents. Dietary salicylates, or salicylates such as magnesium or choline salicylates, are tolerated by the vast majority of such patients. Acetaminophen at low doses is generally tolerated, but some patients do react adversely to high doses (1 g) of this agent. The precise mechanism by which these drugs induce respiratory manifestations remains uncertain but is thought to include alteration of prostaglandin production, enhanced LT synthesis, induction of Th-2 lymphocyte inflammation, and tissue eosinophilia. The latter event substantially enhances local production of LTs, further exacerbating upper and lower airway symptoms. Although genetic abnormalities in the LT synthetic pathway or in LT receptors have been found, to date, no single explanation for this syndrome has been established (22).

In the smaller group of patients experiencing immediate anaphylactic symptoms, the presence of drug-specific IgE has been suggested but not yet proven.

CLINICAL MANIFESTATIONS

In patients with respiratory manifestations of NSAID hypersensitivity, the most common findings are nasal obstruction, watery rhinorrhea, hyposmia, and asthma. A high proportion of these patients suffer from nasal polyposis and chronic and recurrent sinus infection. In patients with this syndrome, pansinusitis is common. Although nasal polyps may complicate ordinary allergic rhinitis (approximately 1–2% in some studies) and are a common manifestation of cystic fibrosis (up to 50% of such patients), the highest incidence of nasal polyps occurs in the patients with NSAID hypersensitivity (up to 90%). Such polyps often respond to systemic steroid treatment but may recur within days of its cessation.

In patients with nonrespiratory manifestations, the usual presentation is that of acute or chronic urticaria/angioedema (see above). Patients occasionally present with anaphylaxis, and retrospective reviews of drug-induced anaphylactic episodes treated in emergency departments suggest that such drugs comprise a greater proportion of adverse drug reactions than previously thought.

DIAGNOSIS

The clinical diagnosis of NSAID hypersensitivity can be made from the above-noted manifestations, particularly in patients with rhinorrhea, eosinophilia, nasal polyps, pansinusitis, and asthma. It may be suspected in patients with urticaria/angioedema and considered in patients experiencing anaphylaxis. Unfortunately, no easily administered test or laboratory procedure can make this diagnosis. Currently, in the United States, the only test reagents available for diagnosis are the COX-1 inhibitors. Challenge via the oral route, in a graded manner beginning with doses of aspirin as low as 5 mg and increasing to a top dose of 650 mg, has been used to define the patient population reactive to NSAIDs (23). Patients undergoing such challenges generally develop rhinorrhea and asthma within 30 minutes of the inciting dose, and these manifestations usually require aggressive therapy for control. Urticaria/angioedematous responses usually occur two to six hours after an inciting dose. If a patient tolerates a graded challenge to 650 mg of aspirin, the diagnosis of NSAID hypersensitivity cannot be established. In Europe, an inhaled form of lysyl-aspirin is available for testing, and this modality appears to be associated with fewer systemic side effects.

TREATMENT

Treatment of NSAID hypersensitivity consists of avoidance of the inciting drug(s) and pharmacological treatment of the presenting problem. For patients with nasal polyposis/pansinusitis, treatment with oral glucocorticoids is frequently required to gain control of the clinical situation, and many patients later will tolerate topical steroids with good results. Some patients require continued systemic steroids, albeit often on alternate days. Surgical care of sinus symptoms is often required, and many patients have had repeated surgeries (24). In patients with asthma, inhaled steroids are almost always required. LT receptor antagonists have proven beneficial to a large proportion of patients with NSAID hypersensitivity (25).

Despite the use of steroids and LT receptor antagonists, many patients remain symptomatic. In these patients, NSAID desensitization should be considered. Desensitization is accomplished by graded administration of increasing doses of aspirin (or other NSAID) until tolerance of the dose is achieved. Doses are then increased to 650 mg aspirin. Such desensitization usually produces a refractory period of 24 to 72 hours, during which NSAID ingestion is tolerated. To continue the refractory period, the patient must be maintained on chronic aspirin therapy, generally 650 mg twice daily. It is currently unknown how this treatment works. After desensitization, many patients not only can tolerate NSAIDs but also note improvement of respiratory symptoms with improved sense of smell, decreased numbers of sinusitis episodes and sinus surgeries, decreased asthma exacerbations, and reduced need for corticosteroid medications (26).

COMPLICATIONS AND PROGNOSIS

The major complications of NSAID hypersensitivity are the manifestations of the disorder itself, when sinusitis, asthma, and, if pertinent, urticaria/angioedema/anaphylaxis, with their consequent morbidities and mortalities, ensue. Side effects from chronic use of glucocorticoids, risks from repeated surgeries, and, in patients desensitized to NSAIDs and taking aspirin, gastrointestinal bleeding, are also problems.

The prognosis of NSAID hypersensitivity must be guarded. To date, no procedure clearly alters the course of the disease. Some studies suggest that early conservative operative intervention in the case of pansinusitis/polyposis may slow disease progression, but many patients continue to require corticosteroids and repeat operative intervention. Asthma in this population is almost always steroid dependent and can be quite severe. Desensitization offers some hope of controlling the disease, but if aspirin is discontinued, even after years of use, the hypersensitivity may recur within days.

SUMMARY

Many patients respond to the ingestion (or intravenous administration) of NSAIDs with a hypersensitivity response manifest as anaphylaxis or as a cutaneous or respiratory reaction. Avoidance of causative class of drug, use of glucocorticoids and LT receptor antagonists, and surgical intervention are often necessary. Desensitization offers some hope for partial control of this difficult problem.

*S*TEVENS–JOHNSON SYNDROME

INTRODUCTION

In 1922, Stevens and Johnson described two boys who had "an extraordinary, generalized eruption with continued fever, inflamed buccal mucosa, and severe purulent conjunctivitis" (27). Stevens–Johnson syndrome (SJS) (Figs 2 and 3) is a severe mucocutaneous disorder that is usually drug induced and associated with high morbidity and poor prognosis. Identifying patients with SJS is crucial, because these patients should be referred to intensive care units or burn centers for management.

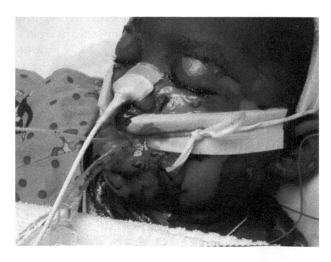

FIGURE 2   Stevens–Johnson syndrome face.

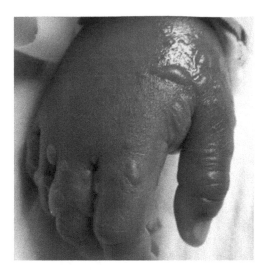

FIGURE 3 Stevens–Johnson syndrome hand.

DEFINITION

SJS is one clinical presentation of a severe cutaneous drug reaction. Experts in the field utilize a classification in which erythema multiforme (EM), SJS, and toxic epidermal necrolysis (TEN) represent severity variants of the same process (28,29). EM-minor is usually self-limited and caused by infections. Drug-induced EM, termed EM-major, can progress into SJS or, when very severe, TEN. SJS is a bullous disorder, with ulceration, purpura, fever, and involvement of mucous membranes in more than two locations, as well as the skin. TEN is used to describe more severe SJS-like disease, with sloughing of the skin resembling a third-degree burn.

EPIDEMIOLOGY

SJS and TEN show no predilection for race, gender, or age. Both are rare, with an estimated incidence of SJS ranging from one to two cases per million person-years and 0.4 to 1.2 cases per million person-years for TEN. Drug-induced SJS and TEN typically begin two to three weeks after the initiation of therapy but may occur more rapidly with drug rechallenge. In a retrospective case control study, sulfonamides showed a relative risk of 172, followed by other antibiotics, imidazole antifungals, anticonvulsants, NSAIDS, and then allopurinol and others (30). The risk for developing SJS/TEN with antiepileptic therapy typically occurs within the first eight weeks of therapy. Patients with HIV have a higher incidence of SJS and TEN, with a combined incidence of 1 per 1000 person-years. Sulfonamides are the major culprit, with the risk of reaction 10 to 100 times higher among HIV-positive patients than among other persons (31).

PATHOGENESIS

The exact mechanism producing SJS and TEN is unclear. Patients with SJS and TEN induced by anticonvulsants or sulfonamides may have an alteration in the detoxification of reactive drug metabolites. CD8 cells predominate in the lesions of blistering reactions, suggesting a cell-mediated cytotoxic reaction against epidermal cells (32). Tumor necrosis factor-α, perforin, granzyme B (GrB), and Fas Ligand (FasL) have been shown to be increased in the early stage of disease, further supporting a cytotoxic mechanism (33).

CLINICAL MANIFESTATIONS

SJS is characterized by the presence of widely distributed purpuric macules and blisters that predominate on the trunk and face. The lesions may be preceded one to three days by fever and influenza-like symptoms. The rash can spread within hours and is usually maximal within four days. About 90% of patients have painful erosions or crusts on mucous membranes. Widespread mucosal erosions result in impaired alimentation, photophobia, and painful micturition. Gastrointestinal epithelia can be involved, resulting in profuse diarrhea. Diffuse interstitial pneumonitis and tracheobronchial epithelial involvement can occur, resulting in respiratory distress. About 85% of patients have conjunctival lesions, ranging from hyperemia to pseudomembrane formation. Mild elevation of hepatic enzymes may occur, with overt hepatitis in 10% of cases (34).

The extent of epidermal detachment differentiates SJS from TEN. In SJS, confluence of blisters may lead to detachment of the skin below 10% of body surface area (BSA). TEN is characterized by the same lesions as SJS, but detachment of large epidermal sheets occurs on more than 30% of BSA, leading to a positive Nikolsky's sign. Cases with detachment between 10% and 30% of BSA are labeled overlap SJS–TEN (28).

Fluid losses occur with skin detachment, leading to prerenal azotemia and electrolyte imbalances. The skin lesions are usually first colonized by *Staphylococcus aureus*, followed by gram-negative rods. Patients also enter a hypercatabolic state with insulin resistance, and thermoregulation is impaired. Immunologic function is altered, as well, predisposing these patients to sepsis.

Laboratory abnormalities include anemia, lymphopenia in 90% of patients due to depletion of CD4+ T-lymphocytes, and neutropenia, a poor prognostic indicator. Approximately 30% of patients have elevation of transaminases and amylase/lipase without other evidence of pancreatic involvement. Mild proteinuria is common.

DIAGNOSIS AND DIFFERENTIAL DIAGNOSIS

Skin disorders presenting with desquamation, exfoliation, or blistering are sometimes misdiagnosed as SJS or TEN. The differential diagnosis of SJS/TEN includes exfoliative dermatitis, staphylococcal scalded skin syndrome, acute exanthematous pustulosis, paraneoplastic pemphigus, thermal burns, phototoxic reactions, and pressure blisters.

TREATMENT

Prompt recognition of SJS and TEN can be lifesaving. Early recognition and withdrawal of all potential causative drugs has been shown to produce favorable outcomes (35). Drugs introduced within one month of the reaction should be considered suspicious.

The remaining interventions are similar to those of patients suffering thermal burns: thermal environmental control, fluid replacement, pain control, nutritional support, and antibacterial treatment when needed. Intubation and mechanical ventilation are needed when the trachea and bronchi are involved. Anticoagulation has been recommended, because thromboembolism and disseminated intravascular coagulation (DIC) are important causes of morbidity and mortality. Aggressive management by an ophthalmologist is necessary.

Corticosteroids, cyclosporine, and intravenous immunoglobulin (IVIg) have been used for treatment of SJS/TEN. Clinical studies with IVIg treatment both support its use and show no effect (36). The indication and mode of usage for immunomodulatory drugs in the routine management of SJS or TEN remain unclear.

COMPLICATIONS AND PROGNOSIS

Mortality rates for SJS range from 5% to 10% and increase to 30% to 40% for cases of TEN. Most patients die of sepsis or pulmonary involvement. SJS and TEN can produce significant ocular sequelae, including severe visual loss in a significant number of patients, requiring intensive involvement of an ophthalmologist. Residual skin discoloration, persistent erosions of the mucous membranes, phimosis, abnormal nail regrowth, and synechiae of the genital mucosae can also occur.

SUMMARY

SJS and TEN are severe skin reactions, usually to drugs, associated with widespread epidermal destruction. Prompt identification and appropriate management are essential to minimize disease-related morbidity and mortality.

REFERENCES

1. Strachan DP. Epidemiology of hayfever: towards a community diagnosis. Clin Exp Allergy 1995; 25 (4):296–303.
2. Broder I, Higgins MW, Mathews KP, et al. Epidemiology of asthma and allergic rhinitis in a total community, Tecumsah, Michigan. 3. Second survey of the community. J Allergy Clin Immunol 1974; 53(3):127–138.
3. Schwindt CD, Hutcheson PS, Leu SY, et al. Role of intradermal skin tests in the evaluation of clinically relevant respiratory allergy assessed using patient history and nasal challenges. Ann Allergy Asthma Immunol 2005; 94(6):627–633.
4. Howarth PH. Allergic and nonallergic rhinitis. In: Adkinson NF, Yuninger JF, Busse WW, et al., eds. Allergy; Principles and Practice. 6th ed. Philadelphia, PA: Mosby, Inc., 2003:1391–1410.
5. Rajakulasingam K, Anderson DF, Holgate ST. Allergic rhinitis, nonallergic rhinitis, and ocular allergy. In: Kaplan AP, ed. Allergy. 2nd ed. Philadelphia, PA: WB Saunders Co., 1997:421–447.
6. Craig TJ, Teets S, Lehman EB. Nasal congestion secondary to allergic rhinitis as a cause of sleep disturbance and daytime fatigue and the response to topical nasal corticosteroids. J Allergy Clin Immunol 1998; 101(5):633–637.
7. Simons FER. Antihistimines. In: Adkinson NF, Yuninger JF, Busse WW, et al., eds. Allergy; Principles and Practice. 6th ed. Philadelphia, PA: Mosby, Inc., 2003:834–869.
8. Nelson HS. Mechanisms of intranasal steroids in the management of upper respiratory allergic diseases. J Allergy Clin Immunol 1999; 104(4 Pt 1):S138–S143.
9. Philip G, Malmstrom K, Hampel FC, et al. Montelukast for treating seasonal allergic rhinitis: double-blind, placebo-controlled trial performed in the spring. Clin Exp Allergy 2002; 32(7):1020–1028.
10. Durham SR, Walker SM, Varga EM, et al. Long term clinical efficacy of grass-pollen immunotherapy. N Engl J Med 1999; 341(7):468–475.
11. Greaves M, Lawlor F. Angioedema: manifestations and management. J Am Acad Dermatol 1991; 25 (1 Pt 2):155–161; discussion 161–165.
12. Kostis JB, Kim HJ, Rusnak J, et al. Incidence and characteristics of angioedema associated with enalapril. Arch Intern Med 2005; 165(14):1637–1642.
13. Kaplan AP, Greaves MW. Angioedema. J Am Acad Dermatol 2005; 53(3):373–388.
14. Kaplan A. Urticaria and angioedema. In: Adkinson NF, Yuninger JW, Busse WW, et al., eds. Allergy; Principles and Practice. 6th ed. Philadelphia, PA: Mosby, Inc., 2003:1537–1558.
15. Gompels MM, Lock RJ, Abinun M, et al. C1 inhibitor deficiency: consensus document. Clin Exp Immunol 2005; 139(3):379–394; erratum in 2005; 141(1):189–190.
16. Sabroe RA, Black AK. Angiotensin converting enzyme (ACE) inhibitors and angio-oedema. Br J Dermatol 1997; 136(2):153–158.
17. Pigman EC, Scott JL. Angioedema in the emergency department: the impact of angiotensin-converting enzyme inhibitors. Am J Emerg Med 1993; 11(4):350–354.
18. Bork K, Siedlecki K, Bosch S, et al. Asphyxiation by laryngeal edema in patients with hereditary angioedema. Mayo Clin Proc 2000; 75(4):349–354.

19. Bork K, Barnstedt SE. Treatment of 193 episodes of laryngeal edema with C1 inhibitor concentrate in patients with hereditary angioedema. Arch Intern Med 2001; 161(5):714–718.
20. Brown NJ, Snowden M, Griffin MR. Recurrent angiotensin-converting enzyme inhibitor—associated angioedema. JAMA 1997; 278(3):232–233.
21. Simon RA, Namazy J. Adverse reactions to aspirin and nonsteroidal antiinflammatory drugs (NSAIDs). Clin Rev Allergy Immunol 2003; 24(3):239–252.
22. Stevenson DD, Zuraw BL. Pathogenesis of aspirin-exacerbated respiratory disease. Clin Rev Allergy Immunol 2003; 24(2):169–188.
23. Nizankowska E, Bestynska-Krypel A, Cmiel A, et al. Oral and bronchial provocation tests with aspirin for diagnosis of aspirin-induced asthma. Eur Respir J 2000; 15(5):863–869.
24. McFadden EA, Woodson BT, Fink JN, et al. Surgical treatment of aspirin triad sinusitis. Am J Rhinol 1997; 11(4):263–270.
25. Dahlen B. Treatment of aspirin-intolerant asthma with antileukotrienes. Am J Respir Crit Care Med 2000; 161(2 Pt 2):S137–S141.
26. Berges-Gimeno MP, Simon RA, Stevenson DD. Long-term treatment with aspirin desensitization in asthmatic patients with aspirin-exacerbated respiratory disease. J Allergy Clin Immunol 2003; 111 (1):180–186.
27. Stevens AM, Johnson FC. A new eruptive fever associated with stomatitis and ophthalmia: report of two cases in children. Am J Dis Child 1922; 24:526–533.
28. Bastuji-Garin S, Rzany B, Stern RS, et al. Clinical classification of cases of toxic epidermal necrolysis, Stevens-Johnson syndrome, and erythema multiforme. Arch Dermatol 1993; 129(1): 92–96.
29. Wolf R, Orion E, Marcos B, et al. Life-threatening acute adverse cutaneous drug reactions. Clin Dermatol 2005; 23(2):171–181.
30. Auquier-Dunant A, Mockenhaupt M, Naldi L, et al. Correlations between clinical patterns and causes of erythema multiforme majus, Stevens-Johnson syndrome, and toxic epidermal necrolysis: results of an international prospective study. Arch Dermatol 2002; 138(8):1019–1024.
31. Porteous DM, Berger TG. Severe cutaneous drug reactions (Stevens–Johnson syndrome and toxic epidermal necrolysis) in human immunodeficiency virus infection. Arch Dermatol 1991; 127(5):740–741; comment 714–717.
32. Correia O, Delgado L, Ramos JP, et al. Cutaneous T-cell recruitment in toxic epidermal necrolysis: further evidence of CD8+ lymphocyte involvement. Arch Dermatol 1993; 129(4):466–468; comment Arch Dermatol 1994; 130(1):116–117.
33. Posadas SJ, Padial A, Torres MJ, et al. Delayed reactions to drugs show levels of perforin, granzyme B, and Fas-L to be related to disease severity. J Allergy Clin Immunol 2002;109(1):155–161.
34. Soter NA. Erythema Multiforme and Stevens-Johnson syndrome. In: Kaplan AP, ed. Allergy. 2nd ed. Philadelphia, PA: W. B. Saunders, Inc., 1997:643–651.
35. Garcia-Doval I, LeCleach L, Bocquet H, et al. Toxic epidermal necrolysis and Stevens-Johnson syndrome: does early withdrawal of causative drugs decrease the risk of death? Arch Dermatol 2000; 136(3):323–327; comment 410–411.
36. Bachot N, Revuz J, Roujeau JC. Intravenous immunoglobulin treatment for Stevens-Johnson syndrome and toxic epidermal necrolysis: a prospective noncomparative study showing no benefit on mortality or progression. Arch Dermatol 2003; 139(1):33–36.

23

Migraine Syndrome

Robert W. Baloh
Department of Neurology, David Geffen School of Medicine, University of California, Los Angeles, California, U.S.A.

INTRODUCTION

Migraine is a syndrome characterized by periodic headaches. Often, however, patients experience other symptoms, including hearing loss, tinnitus, and dizziness; and in some cases, these can be the only symptoms. Migraine is nearly always familial and occurs in complex patterns and settings. The association of migraine and dizziness dates back to the nineteenth century when Liveing noted their connection in his book *On Megrin: Sick Headaches and Some Allied Health Disorders*. Overall, episodic vertigo occurs in about one-quarter of patients with migraine headaches—approximately the same frequency as that of the classical migraine visual aura. In addition, patients with migraine frequently report sensitivity to motion, with bouts of carsickness in childhood and motion sickness as adults. Auditory symptoms are generally considered less common than vestibular symptoms with migraine, but phonophobia occurs in more than two-thirds of patients, usually in association with headache. Tinnitus is also very common and sudden deafness occurs in a small percentage of patients with migraine. Recent advances in exploration of the genetics and pathophysiology of migraine provide new hope for understanding the link between dizziness, tinnitus and hearing loss, and the periodic headaches characteristic of the disorder.

DEFINITION

An abbreviated version of the classification of migraine developed by the International Headache Society (IHS) is shown in (Table 1) (1). Migraine without aura (MO) is by far the most common variety and is best described as a sick headache. Rigid criteria for the diagnosis of MO have been established by the IHS (see "Diagnosis"). Migraine with aura (MA) is defined as "an idiopathic recurring disorder manifesting with attacks of neurological symptoms unequivocally localizable to cerebral cortex or brainstem, gradually developed over 5 to 20 minutes, and usually lasting less than 60 minutes." The visual symptoms, including the classic scintillating scotoma and fortification spectra, are the most commonly recognized aura phenomena, but somatosensory and vestibular symptoms are probably equally common. Although less common, basilar migraine and migraine aura without headache are of particular interest from a neurotologic point of view.

The occurrence of migraine aura without headache has been recognized for many years, although the concept is often difficult for both patients and physicians to deal with. Patients can have isolated aura symptoms at one point in life and typical migraine headaches at another. In some patients, there are symptoms that occur alone on some occasions and with typical headaches on other occasions. Some have only aura symptoms and never experience a headache. Terms such as "migraine equivalent" and "migraine accompaniment" have been used to describe these isolated aura symptoms (such as benign

TABLE 1 Abbreviated International Headache Society Classification of Migraine

Migraine without aura
Migraine with aura
   Migraine with typical aura
   Migraine with prolonged aura
   Familial hemiplegic migraine
   Basilar migraine
   Migraine aura without headache
   Migraine with acute-onset aura
Ophthalmoplegic migraine
Retinal migraine

recurrent vertigo), but a diagnosis is difficult to obtain without the presence of typical headaches at some time during the course.

Basilar migraine is a subtype of MA characterized by recurrent headaches, preceded by multiple neurological symptoms such as vertigo, ataxia, dysarthria, tinnitus, and visual phenomena consistent with ischemia in the distribution of the vertebrobasilar system (1). Motor and sensory symptoms such as circumoral and extremity paresthesias, weakness, and drop attacks are occasionally seen, as well. When vertigo occurs, it usually has an abrupt onset and lasts 5 to 60 minutes. Headache following the aura is usually occipital and can be unilateral or bilateral, but it can occur anywhere, especially in children.

EPIDEMIOLOGY

Migraine is among the most common reasons for outpatient visits to physicians, resulting in more than 18 million visits annually in the United States. It is estimated to affect approximately 15% of women and 5% of men. Approximately 20% of adults with migraine indicate that their headaches began before the age of 10. In the prepubertal period, boys and girls are approximately equally affected, but at puberty, migraine decreases in boys and increases in girls so that a 2.5:1 female preponderance is established by adulthood. Although migraine usually begins before the age of 40, a substantial number of adults are affected later in life.

Basilar migraine is estimated to affect 10% to 24% of patients suffering from migraine. One must be alert to the possibility of basilar migraine in any patient presenting with transient vertigo and other posterior fossa symptoms. Some patients are unaware that migraine is the cause of their headaches and are much more concerned about the aura symptoms.

PATHOGENESIS

Probably the most common characteristic of migraine symptoms is the classical visual aura. It typically begins with a small scintillating scotoma that gradually enlarges over 20 to 30 minutes. There is convincing evidence that the visual aura is secondary to a spreading wave of cortical depression beginning at the occipital pole and then gradually spreading across the cortex before stopping at the central sulcus (1). Although decreased cerebral perfusion is associated with the spreading wave of depression, it is probably a secondary phenomenon rather than a primary process. The spreading wave of cortical depression is associated with marked accumulation of extracellular potassium that must be cleared before neuronal activity can return to normal. Although the exact mechanism for the spreading wave of depression is not known, most agree that the initial event is local buildup of potassium in the extracellular space.

The spreading wave of depression and associated increased extracellular potassium can lead to a typical migraine headache. Trigeminal nerve fibers surrounding pial arteries on the ventral surface of the brain are depolarized by the high potassium concentration. This in turn leads to a release of neurotransmitters such as substance P and calcitonin gene-related peptide by both orthodromic and antidromic conduction. The result is an increase in vascular permeability, dilatation of cerebral vessels, and a local inflammatory response, further activating pain-provoking fibers of the trigeminal vascular system. Thus, the headache of migraine could be a secondary phenomenon, the end result of a local increase in extracellular potassium concentration.

Vasomotor abnormalities have long been considered in the pathophysiology of migraine symptoms. Vasodilatation of extracranial vessels accompanies the typical migraine headache. Vasospasm occurs in some intracranial vessels with migraine, although, as mentioned above, there is controversy regarding its role in the production of symptoms. Although vasospasm is associated with classical migraine visual aura, it is most likely that vasospasm results from a metabolic defect slowly spreading across the cerebral cortex and is secondary to hypometabolism. Vasospasm is, however, more likely a cause of retinal and labyrinthine migraine. Some patients experience episodes of monocular blindness, and when examined during these episodes, there is vasospasm of the retinal arteries. Furthermore, such patients respond to antispasmodic agents. Sudden episodes of hearing loss and vertigo associated with migraine may be secondary to vasospasm of the cochlear and/or vestibular branches of the internal auditory artery. These disorders also often respond to antispasmodic agents.

One way to explain the heterogeneity of migraine syndromes is to postulate a group of defects in genes that code for a family of proteins with similar properties and functions. A family of ion channels is appealing in this regard, because many of the migraine syndromes share the clinical features of the known inherited ion channel disorders. With the finding of an abnormal voltage-gated calcium channel gene and a sodium–potassium ATPase gene in familial hemiplegic migraine syndromes, mutations in other channel genes are a prime candidate for other migraine syndromes, including migraine with and without aura (1,2). These channels are remarkably diverse in their conductance and gating mechanisms, and most neurons express several subtypes that are characterized by different functional and pharmacological properties.

A defective channel protein could explain the local buildup of extracellular potassium that initiates a spreading wave of depression in migraine. Since protein channels in the inner ear are critical for maintaining the potassium-rich endolymph and neuronal excitability, a defective channel shared by the brain and inner ear could lead to a reversible hair-cell depolarization and auditory and vestibular symptoms. The headache of migraine could be a secondary phenomenon, the end result of a local increase in extracellular potassium concentration. Many of the well-known triggers for migraine symptoms, including stress and menstruation, could result from hormonal influences on defective channels.

Numerous studies over the years have documented familial aggregation of migraine, and some have suggested that a positive family history should be part of the diagnostic criteria. In nearly all studies, the incidence of a positive family history in patients with migraine headaches was significantly greater than in controls (the incidence of a positive family history varies from approximately 40% to 90%, compared with approximately 5–20% in controls). The percentage of positive family histories tends to be greater in those studies in which family members were individually interviewed than in studies that relied on questionnaires or the recall of the proband. Studies in monozygotic and dizygotic twins have also supported a strong genetic component for migraine, particularly for MA (2). Also, the fact that the prevalence of migraine in African and Asian populations is lower than in European and North American populations favors a major genetic component.

CLINICAL MANIFESTATIONS

As noted above, MO can best be described as a "sick headache." Vague prodromal symptoms precede it, but aura phenomena are absent. The headache, unilateral or bilateral, builds slowly in intensity and may go on for several days. Nausea, vomiting, diarrhea, chills, and prostration can all accompany the headache. Nonspecific dizziness is a common complaint, and patients frequently report visual blurring and a sense of unsteadiness during the entire headache phase. Vertigo can occur before, during, or entirely separate from the episodes of headache (3).

In MA, the aura typically precedes the onset of severe, throbbing, unilateral headaches. The aura symptoms slowly progress over several minutes, last 15 to 60 minutes, and then gradually abate. In about 25% of patients, however, onset is abrupt. The headache begins as the aura diminishes, usually reaching its peak in about an hour and gradually subsiding over the next four to eight hours. Nausea and vomiting typically accompany the onset of head pain. The migraine aura consists of transient neurologic dysfunction, often with visual disturbances, but it also commonly includes prominent vertigo or somatosensory symptoms. A characteristic feature of migrainous paresthesia is a gradual spread over the face or extremity, sometimes migrating from face to extremity on the same side or sometimes crossing over to the face and extremity on the opposite side. When focal neurologic symptoms such as hemianopsia, hemiparalysis, or unilateral paresthesias occur in an aura, they usually occur on the side opposite that of the headache. Only about 12% of patients with migraine regularly experience aura with their headaches, but as many as two-thirds have occasional attacks with aura.

Speculation on a relationship between migraine and Ménière's syndrome dates back to the initial description of the syndrome by Prosper Ménière in 1861 (4). He noted that both conditions commonly manifested episodes of vertigo, fluctuating hearing levels, and recurring vomiting. Although many subsequent authors also have speculated on the relationship between migraine and Ménière's disease, there is still no generally accepted mechanism to explain the connection. Numerous studies have documented that migraine can lead to permanent auditory and vestibular deficits. Asymmetries on caloric examination occur with a higher frequency in patients with migraine than in control populations. Vasospasm could lead to ischemic damage to the endolymphatic duct and sac, resulting in impaired fluid circulation and the eventual development of endolymphatic hydrops (Fig. 1) (5).

MIGRAINE EQUIVALENTS

Benign paroxysmal vertigo of childhood, benign recurrent vertigo of adulthood, and vestibular Ménière's syndrome are all probably migraine equivalents. In benign paroxysmal vertigo of childhood, vertigo typically begins before the age of four and occurs up to several times a month. After a period of two or three years, the spells decrease in number and gradually disappear. Most children have no further spells after age seven or eight. Follow-up studies of patients with typical benign paroxysmal vertigo during childhood showed that most eventually develop typical migraine headaches. Benign recurrent vertigo of adulthood can begin

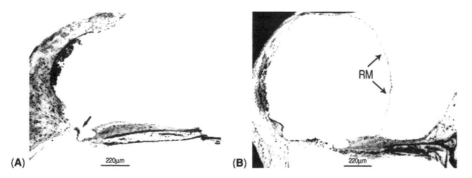

FIGURE 1 Patient with long-standing migraine with aura developed sudden deafness in the left ear at age 50 and Ménière's syndrome on the right side at age 73. Postmortem examination of the inner ears showed the following. (**A**) Loss of the organ of Corti (*arrow*) and prominent fibrosis of the left cochlea consistent with old infarction and (**B**) Hydrops in the right cochlea (RM). Presumably, the right inner ear suffered only minimal damage with the original ischemic event, but the damage later led to the development of delayed endolymphatic hydrops. *Abbreviation*: RM, Reisoner membrane.

anywhere from age seven to 55 and is typically associated with nausea, vomiting, and diaphoresis. The attacks often occur on awakening in the morning, being particularly common around menses in women. The duration varies from minutes to hours, and patients are asymptomatic between the spells. Several studies have shown that patients with benign recurrent vertigo have either migraine themselves or strong family history of migraine. Furthermore, the episodes of vertigo have several features in common with migraine, including precipitation by alcohol, lack of sleep, emotional stress, and female preponderance. In their initial recommendations on criteria for the diagnosis of Ménière's disease, the American Academy of Ophthalmology and Otolaryngology Committee on Hearing and Equilibrium defined vestibular Ménière's disease as recurrent attacks of vertigo without associated auditory symptoms. It was assumed that most of these patients would progress to manifest all of the symptoms of classical Ménière's syndrome; however, because there are so many causes of recurrent episodes of vertigo other than Ménière's disease, more recently, the American Academy of Otolaryngology Head & Neck Surgery Committee on Hearing and Equilibrium recommended discarding the term "vestibular Ménière's syndrome." Furthermore, follow-up studies of patients with vestibular Ménière's disease have found that only a small minority of these patients ever go on to develop the typical features of Ménière's syndrome.

DIAGNOSIS

The diagnosis of migraine is relatively easy when headaches are the major feature and there is a strong family history. In patients for whom headache is less prominent, and in patients with migraine equivalents, the diagnosis can be missed if one is not aware of the diversity of this syndrome (6). Often, patients will present with aura symptoms such as vertigo and will only mention associated headache after being questioned.

The criteria for the diagnosis of MO established by the IHS are summarized in Table 2. The patient must have at least five headache attacks that meet the criteria, and other causes of headache must be ruled out. No laboratory or radiological findings are specific for migraine. The physical and neurological examinations are normal and serve primarily to exclude other causes of headache. A classic migraine attack typically has five phases: a prodrome (e.g., depression, cognitive dysfunction, and food cravings), aura (e.g., visual, sensory, or motor phenomena), headache (usually unilateral and throbbing), resolution (when pain wanes), and recovery. None of these phases is obligatory for the migraine diagnosis, however. Symptoms (severity, duration, nature of prodrome or aura) also vary considerably between individuals. Thus, the diagnosis of migraine is based on a combination of sequentially occurring symptoms and paroxysmal attacks. Motion sickness is often the first symptom of migraine in children and has been recommended for inclusion as a minor criterion for the diagnosis.

TABLE 2 Diagnostic Criteria for Migraine Without Aura

1) At least five attacks fulfilling A–C
   A) Headache lasts 4–72 hr (untreated)
   B) Headache has at least two of the following features:
      Unilateral
      Pulsating
      Moderate or severe (inhibits or prohibits daily activities)
      Aggravated by walking, stair-climbing, or similar physical activities
   C) During headache at least one of the following exists:
      Nausea and vomiting
      Photophobia and phonophobia
   and
2) Other causes of headache have been ruled out

TABLE 3 Common Symptoms with Basilar Migraine

Vertigo	Weakness (usually bilateral)
Ataxia	Tinnitus
Paresthesias (usually bilateral)	Impaired hearing
	Double vision
Dysarthria	Loss of vision

The IHS criteria for the diagnosis of basilar migraine require an aura that contains two or more of the symptoms listed in Table 3. Patients with isolated episodes of vertigo do not meet the criteria for basilar migraine. Some have suggested that migraine-associated vertigo must be accompanied by other migraine symptoms such as headache, photophobia, and phonophobia (6), but this would exclude the common occurrence of isolated episodes of vertigo. Until the underlying genetic mutations are identified for the common migraine syndromes, it will be difficult to establish reliable clinical criteria for the wide range of symptoms associated with the syndrome.

TREATMENT

The treatment of migraine can be divided into three general categories: symptomatic, abortive, and prophylactic. Before embarking on drug treatment of migraine, it is important to recognize that there are many common triggers for migraine symptoms (Table 4). It is often helpful to have the patient keep a log of the migraine attacks, noting any possible triggers that might be regularly associated with the attacks. As a general rule, patients with migraine must live a regimented life, with regular sleep and eating patterns.

Symptomatic treatment of migraine includes analgesics, antiemetics, antivertiginous drugs, and sedatives. Antivertiginous and antiemetic medications are useful in patients in whom vertigo and nausea are prominent. Promethazine, 25 or 50 mg, orally or by suppository, is particularly effective for relief of both vertigo and nausea. Drugs in this class have a sedative effect that is usually acceptable in a patient who is eager to sleep. The decrease in gastric motility that occurs during migraine attacks can decrease the absorption of oral drugs, in addition to contributing to nausea and vomiting. Metoclopramide promotes normal gastric motility and may improve absorption of oral drugs. For many patients, aspirin or nonsteroidal anti-inflammatory drugs are adequate to relieve the headache.

To be effective, abortive drugs must be taken during the aura, if one is present, or at the earliest symptoms of headache onset. A wide range of drugs, including ergotamines, caffeine, serotonin receptor agonists, and sympathomimetics, has been effective in aborting migraine headaches. Currently, the most widely used abortive drugs are tryptans, agonists of the 5-hydroxytryptamine 1 receptor. These drugs will typically abort the headache in more than 70% of patients when taken at the earliest sign of onset, but a large percentage of

TABLE 4 Common Factors that Trigger Migraine Symptoms

Stress and emotional upset
Hormones: menstruation, use of oral contraceptives, and pregnancy
Sleep deprivation
Food: red wines, fermented cheeses, chocolate, and coffee
Eating disorders: fasting and binges

patients will have a recurrence within 24 hours, requiring remedicating. Although there have been anecdotal reports of tryptans aborting migraine-associated vertigo, there have been no placebo-controlled trials documenting efficacy.

Prophylactic treatment is necessary when migraine attacks are frequent and/or the severity cannot be ameliorated by symptomatic or abortive medicines. It is probably the most effective treatment for migraine equivalents, particularly episodic vertigo. Five major categories of drugs have been used: tricyclic amines, selective serotonin reuptake inhibitors, antiepileptic drugs, β blockers, and calcium channel blockers. In addition, many other drugs have been found effective according to small, controlled studies or uncontrolled observations. As a rule, the mechanism of action of these drugs in migraine is speculative. Most have been found to work on an empiric basis. In women whose migraine symptoms are periodic and premenstrual, nonsteroidal anti-inflammatory agents such as naproxen and ibuprofen or the carbonic anhydrase inhibitor, acetazolamide, can be taken for a few days each month when the migraine is expected, to prevent its appearance. In our experience, acetazolamide has been particularly effective in preventing episodes of vertigo in patients with migraine. A trial of migraine prophylaxis is warranted in any patient with episodic vertigo of unknown cause, who has a past history of migraine or a strong family history of migraine.

COMPLICATIONS AND PROGNOSIS

Rarely, patients with migraine can develop permanent damage to the brain, eye, or ear. It is unclear whether this damage results from the underlying genetic metabolic disorder or the associated vasospasm. Numerous studies have found that migraine is associated with an increased risk of stroke, particularly in young people. The IHS criteria for migrainous infarction include that (*i*) the incident occurs during a typical attack of MA; (*ii*) neurologic deficits are not completely reversible within seven days; and (*iii*) other causes of stroke have been excluded. With basilar migraine, infarction commonly occurs in the cerebellum, particularly in watershed areas between arterial supplies consistent with hypoperfusion due to vertebrobasilar vasospasm. In some cases, labyrinthine and brain infarction occur simultaneously, since the blood supply to the inner ears arises from the vertebrobasilar system (Fig. 2) (7). Whether sudden deafness unrelated to headache can be a migraine phenomenon is more difficult to prove, but we and others have noted a high incidence of migraine in patients presenting with sudden sensorineural hearing loss. Many of these patients will have other symptoms of vasospasm, including monocular visual loss, episodes of hemiparesis or hemianesthesia, and episodes of chest pain. A small percentage of patients with recurrent monocular visual loss will go on to infarct the retina, so prophylaxis with an antispasmodic agent such as Verapamil is recommended. Compared with controls, migraine patients have an increased incidence of unilateral caloric paresis and benign positional vertigo, presumably secondary to the recurrent vasospasm of the labyrinthine artery.

SUMMARY

Migraine is not a disease, but a syndrome with multiple causes. Several migraine syndromes have a clear autosomal-dominant pattern of inheritance, and recently, mutations have been identified in two different channel genes in families with the rare syndrome of hemiplegic migraine. Familial aggregation and twin studies in families with the more common migraine syndromes show that genetic factors are important, although the mode

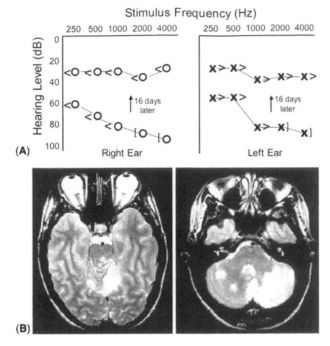

FIGURE 2 A 40-year-old man with known basilar migraine developed bilateral hearing loss associated with severe, throbbing occipital headaches, tinnitus, vertigo, ataxia, and right hemiparesis. **(A)** Audiometric testing showed a severe bilateral sensorineural hearing loss that largely recovered after 16 days. **(B)** MRI of the brain documented infarcts on the pons and cerebellum. *Abbreviation*: MRI, magnetic resonance imaging.

of inheritance is not always clear. Neurotologic symptoms are common with migraine, yet relatively little is known about the pathophysiology of such symptoms. Motion sensitivity with bouts of motion sickness occurs in approximately two-thirds of patients with migraine. Episodes of vertigo occur in about one-fourth of patients, and in some, vertigo is the only symptom (so-called migraine equivalent). Phonophobia is the most common auditory symptom, but fluctuating hearing loss and acute permanent hearing loss occur in a small percentage of patients. Migraine can mimic Ménière's disease, and so-called vestibular Ménière's disease is usually associated with migraine. Until the specific genetic causes are identified, however, diagnosis and treatment of these disorders will continue to be empiric.

REFERENCES

1. Baloh RW. Neurotology of migraine. Headache 1997; 37(10):615–621.
2. Haan J, Kors EE, Vanmolkot KR, et al. Migraine genetics: an update. Curr Pain Headache Rep 2005; 9(3):213–220.
3. von Brevern M, Zeise D, Neuhauser H, et al. Acute migrainous vertigo: clinical and oculographic findings. Brain 2005; 128(Pt 2):365–374.
4. Baloh RW, Andrews JC. Migraine and Meniere's disease. In: Harris JP, ed. Meniere's Disease. The Hague, The Netherlands: Kugler Publications, 1999:281–289.
5. Lee H, Lopez I, Ishiyama A, et al. Can migraine damage the inner ear? Arch Neurol 2000; 57(11): 1631–1634.
6. Neuhauser H, Lempert T. Vertigo and dizziness related to migraine: a diagnostic challenge. Cephalalgia 2004; 24(2):83–91.
7. Lee H, Whitman GT, Lim JG, et al. Hearing symptoms in migrainous infarction. Arch Neurol 2003; 60(1):113–116.

24

Pseudotumor Cerebri and Jugular Foramen Syndrome

Aristides Sismanis and David R. Salley
Department of Otolaryngology-Head and Neck Surgery, Virginia Commonwealth University Medical Center, Richmond, Virginia, U.S.A.

PSEUDOTUMOR CEREBRI SYNDROME

INTRODUCTION

Pseudotumor cerebri (PC) syndrome may present with otologic/neurotologic manifestations; therefore, otolaryngologists should be familiar with this entity, in order to establish early diagnosis and apply effective treatment.

DEFINITION

PC syndrome is a disorder characterized by increased intracranial pressure (ICP), normal cerebrospinal fluid (CSF) content, and absent neurologic signs, except for occasional V, VI, and VII cranial-nerve palsies. In the majority of cases, the etiology is unknown (1,2). Other synonyms of this disorder are idiopathic intracranial hypertension syndrome and benign intracranial hypertension syndrome, although the latter term is being used less often, because of the risk of visual loss.

EPIDEMIOLOGY

The annual incidence of PC syndrome has been estimated to be 0.9 per 100,000 people in the general population. This entity is more common in young African American females who are 20% or more above their ideal body weight (3–5). In males, this disorder is very rare. In 25% of patients, it may become chronic (2).

ETIOLOGY

The various etiologies of this entity are summarized in Table 1 (1,6–9).

PATHOGENESIS

Significant uncertainty exists regarding the pathophysiology of PC syndrome. Many studies have attempted to elucidate the underlying cause, often with conflicting results. Proposed theories include increased CSF production, cerebral edema, decreased CSF absorption, and elevated cerebral venous pressure (1,4,7,10,11). The latter theory is supported by the following studies: Anatomic obstruction of the venous transverse sinuses has recently been reported in PC patients; and direct retrograde cerebral venography with manometry has been recommended, in order to establish diagnosis (12,13). In another study, autotriggered elliptic-centric-ordered three-dimensional gadolinium-enhanced magnetic resonance venography (ATECO MRV) identified bilateral sinovenous stenosis in 27 of 29 patients with PC syndrome and in only 4 of 59 controls. It was not clear whether stenosis was a cause or effect of intracranial hypertension (14). There is evidence that in obese patients with PC syndrome, increased intracranial venous pressure most likely results from increased intra-abdominal, intrathoracic, and cardiac filling pressures (15). This pathophysiologic mechanism is further supported by an animal study demonstrating increased CSF pressure when intra-abdominal pressure was acutely raised (16).

Increased cerebral blood flow secondary to cerebrovascular resistance changes and CSF hypersecretion induced by elevated estrogen levels also have been reported as pathophysiologic mechanisms of PC syndrome (17).

TABLE 1 Etiologies of Idiopathic Intracranial Hypertension Syndrome

Medications
Amiodarone
Anabolic steroids
Chlordecone
Corticosteroids
Cyclosporine
Diphenylhydantoin
Divalproate
Growth hormone
Indomethacin
Leuprorelin acetate
Levothyroxine
Lithium carbonate
Minocycline
Nalidixic acid
Norplant
Penicillin
Sulfa antibiotics
Tetracyclines and related compounds
Vitamin A
All-trans retinoic acid

Endocrine disorders
Adrenal insufficiency
Hypoparathyroidism
Hyperthyroidism
Obesity
Menarche
Menstrual irregularities
Pregnancy
Polycystic ovary syndrome

Nutritional disorders
Hypervitaminosis A
Hypovitaminosis A
Hyperalimentation in nutritional deficiency

Obstruction of venous drainage
Cerebral venous thrombosis
Hypercoagulable states
Antiphospholipid antibody syndrome
Polycythemia
Mastoiditis
Superior vena cava syndrome
Increased right heart pressure
Bilateral radical neck dissection

Circulatory and hematologic
Iron-deficiency anemia
Sickle-cell anemia
Pernicious anemia
Gastrointestinal hemorrhage
Cryofibrinogenemia

Systemic disorders
Lupus erythematosus
Sickle-cell anemia
Sarcoidosis
Sleep apnea
Turner's syndrome
Human immunodeficiency virus infection
Paget's disease
Galactosemia
Head trauma
Nephrotic syndrome
Uremia
Infectious
Lyme disease
Infectious mononucleosis

Source: From Refs. 1,2,6–8.

The origin of pulsatile tinnitus (PT) in PC syndrome is secondary to the systolic pulsations of the CSF, which originate mainly from the arteries of the Circle of Willis. These pulsations, which are increased in magnitude in the presence of intracranial hypertension, are transmitted to the exposed medial aspect of the dural venous sinuses (transverse and sigmoid) and compress their walls synchronously with the arterial pulsations (3,18). The resulting periodic narrowing of the lumen converts the normal laminar blood flow to turbulent, which results in a low-frequency PT (3).

The low-frequency sensorineural hearing loss seen in many of these patients is secondary to the masking effect of the PT. This is supported by the fact that light digital compression over the ipsilateral internal jugular vein (IJV) results in cessation of the tinnitus and immediate improvement or normalization of hearing (3).

Stretching or compression of the cochlear nerve and brain stem, caused by the intracranial hypertension and/or possible edema, may also play a role in the hearing loss and dizziness encountered in these patients. This is supported by the abnormal auditory brainstem evoked responses (ABR) present in one-third of these patients (19).

CLINICAL MANIFESTATIONS

Although the classic presentation of PC syndrome consists of headaches and/or visual disturbances, PT alone or in association with hearing loss, dizziness, and aural fullness have been reported as the main manifestation(s) of this entity (3). Otolaryngologists, therefore, should be familiar with this syndrome, because these patients may present to them with the aforementioned symptomatology.

Headaches are described more often in the frontal region, are worse in a recumbent position and in the early morning hours, and may improve during the day.

Visual disturbances consist mainly of transient visual obscuration (short-duration episodes of visual clouding in one or both eyes). Visual obscurations are not a pathognomonic sign of PC syndrome, since they can occur with all etiologies of increased ICP with papilledema. They can also be present in patients without increased ICP, who have elevated optic discs from other causes.

DIAGNOSIS

Diagnosis of PC syndrome is made by exclusion of other causes of intracranial hypertension and is established by lumbar puncture (LP) and confirmation of CSF pressure of more than 200 mm of water with normal CSF constituents. Table 2 summarizes the modified Dandy criteria upon which diagnosis is based (20).

Consultation with a neuro-ophthalmologist or a neurologist is imperative for these patients.

Many of these patients are morbidly obese (body weight more than 100 lbs above ideal weight) and have an audible bruit in the ear canal and retroauricular area. Upon application of light digital pressure over the ipsilateral IJV, the bruit subsides (venous). Figure 1 depicts a typical PC syndrome patient who presented with PT. The remainder of the examination is usually normal.

Typically, PC syndrome patients have associated papilledema; however, absence of papilledema does not exclude this entity (21–23). In our experience, the majority of patients presenting with PT due to PC syndrome have no associated papilledema, and for this reason, some neurologists have been hesitant to perform LP and CSF measurement on these patients (24). It is therefore imperative for otolaryngologists to insist that this test be performed, in order to establish diagnosis.

Other serious comorbidities, such as diabetes mellitus, hyperlipidemia, hypertension, and obstructive sleep apnea, are common in patients with morbid obesity, and always deserve medical attention (25).

TABLE 2 Modified Dandy Criteria

An awake and alert patient
Presence of signs and symptoms of increased ICP
Absence of localized findings on the neurologic examination
    except paresis of abducens nerve
Normal cerebrospinal fluid findings except for increased pressure
Absence of deformity, displacement, and obstruction of the
    ventricular system on neuroimaging studies
No other cause of increased ICP identified

Abbreviation: ICP, intracranial pressure.
Source: From Ref. 3.

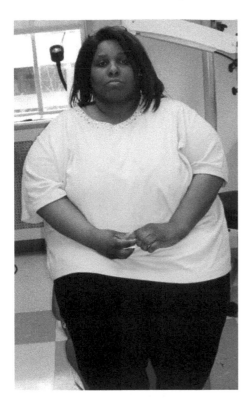

FIGURE 1 Pseudotumor cerebri patient.

Pure-tone (air and bone conduction) and speech audiometry should be performed in suspected cases. In cases with hearing loss in the low frequencies, something that can mimic Ménière's disease, a repeat audiogram should be obtained while the patient is applying light digital pressure over the ipsilateral IJV. This maneuver typically results in improvement or normalization of pure tones in patients with PT due to PC syndrome, because of elimination of the masking effect of the tinnitus (3). Discrimination is typically excellent in these patients. Figure 2A and B are representative audiograms of a patient with PT and PC syndrome.

Electronystagmography should be considered in cases with associated dizziness (3).

Neuroimaging is of utmost importance in the evaluation of these patients and always should precede LP. Patients suspicious for PC syndrome (young, obese females with PT) should undergo a brain magnetic resonance imaging (MRI) study combined with an MRV at their initial evaluation. Although in the literature, MRI findings of PC syndrome have been reported as normal in the majority of patients (26) (with the exception of an empty sella and/or small ventricles), a controlled study of 20 such patients disclosed flattening of the posterior sclera in 80% of patients, empty sella in 70%, distension of the perioptic subarachnoid space in 45%, enhancement of the prelaminar optic nerve in 50%, vertical tortuosity of the orbital optic nerve in 40%, and intraocular protrusion of the prelaminar optic nerve in 30% (27). Head MRV is obtained to eliminate stenosis/obstruction of the dural venous sinuses (12–14,28).

Serologic testing should be individualized and may include erythrocyte sedimentation rate, thyroid function tests, electrolytes, calcium, phosphorous, blood urea nitrogen (BUN), creatinine, serum cortisol, serum vitamin A level, and antinuclear antibodies (26).

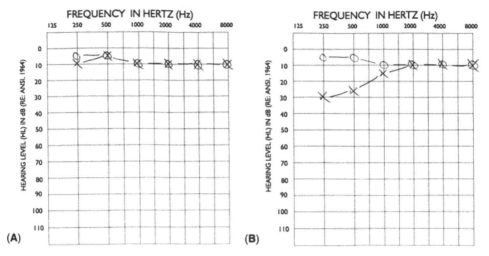

FIGURE 2 (A) Audiogram of a patient with PT and pseudotumor cerebri syndrome. Left low-frequency hearing loss is present. (B) Normalization of hearing loss while digital pressure is applied over the right internal jugular vein and the masking PT is eliminated. *Abbreviation*: PT, pulsatile tinnitus.

TREATMENT

The goals of management are to normalize ICP, prevent loss of vision, relieve PT and headache, and treat comorbidities.

Since the majority of these patients are obese females, some even morbidly obese, it is very important to make them aware of the relationship between their body weight and PC syndrome. Consultation with a dietician is essential; weight reduction results in decrease or resolution of symptoms (29).

Comorbidities, such as obstructive sleep apnea, gastroesophageal reflux, hypertension, diabetes mellitus, and hyperlipidemias, should be detected early on and addressed aggressively, as well.

Acetazolamide inhibits choroid plexus carbonic anhydrase and reduces CSF production by 50% to 60% (30). The recommended dose is 250 mg three times a day or 500 mg twice a day (31). PT may decrease with this treatment; however, it seldom subsides unless it is combined with weight loss.

Recently there has been some anecdotal evidence that the antiepileptic medication Topamax® (topiramate) is effective in PC syndrome. One of topirimate's mechanisms of action is inhibition of carbonic anhydrase, although this effect is weaker than that of acetazolamide. Furthermore, a potential side effect of Topamax is weight loss, which would be beneficial to many PC patients. Currently, we have no clinical experience with topiramate at our institution.

Furosemide (Lasix) has little effect on PC syndrome when given alone, but it has been used as an adjunct to acetazolamide (30).

Corticosteroids can rapidly lower ICP, but since their long-term use has the opposite effect (20), they are rarely indicated.

A lumbar peritoneal shunt should be considered for PC syndrome patients with progressive deterioration of vision, persistent headaches, and disabling PT (3,26,31,32). In morbidly obese patients, however, this procedure is often complicated by occlusion of the shunt secondary to increased intra-abdominal pressure (33).

Optic nerve sheath fenestration is helpful for progressive visual loss and headaches (31,34).

For morbidly obese patients who have failed to lose weight with dieting, effective weight loss can be achieved with bariatric surgery. Out of 16 patients who underwent this procedure, 13 experienced complete resolution of PT (35). A substantial majority of patients with obstructive sleep apnea, hyperlipidemia, hypertension, and diabetes mellitus experienced complete resolution or improvement following this type of surgery (25).

Recently, resolution of symptoms has been reported following retrograde venography and stenting of the transverse sinus in PC syndrome patients with associated stenosis/ obstruction of this structure (12,13,28).

The cooperation of an experienced neuro-ophthalmologist or neurologist, internist, ophthalmologist, dietician, and general surgeon is of utmost importance.

COMPLICATIONS

Visual problems are the most serious complications of PC syndrome and may include decreased visual acuity and visual field deficits. Loss of vision may precede the diagnosis or may occur after several years (20). Associated comorbidities such as diabetes mellitus, hyperlipidemia, hypertension, and obstructive sleep apnea may have disastrous results if left untreated.

PROGNOSIS

For patients with PC syndrome who lose weight, the prognosis is good. It has been reported that in 25% of patients, this entity may become chronic (2).

SUMMARY

Patients with PC syndrome may first present to an otolaryngologist with PT and other otologic/neurotologic symptoms. Associated comorbidities such as diabetes mellitus, hyperlipidemia, hypertension, and obstructive sleep apnea should be detected early and addressed aggressively. A team approach with a neuro-ophthalmologist or neurologist, ophthalmologist, internist, dietician, and general surgeon is of utmost importance.

JUGULAR FORAMEN SYNDROME

INTRODUCTION

Jugular foramen syndrome (JFS) is an uncommon clinical entity that often presents a diagnostic and management challenge to the otolaryngologist. The purpose of this section is to define this syndrome and elucidate the epidemiology, pathogenesis, clinical manifestations, diagnostic workup, and general treatment options for the syndrome.

DEFINITION

Various combinations of palsies of cranial nerves IX, X, and XI resulting from lesions in the area of the jugular foramen have been referred to as JFS. Eponyms include Vernet's and Collet-Sicard syndromes (36,37).

ETIOLOGY AND EPIDEMIOLOGY

Etiologies of JFS can be classified as neoplastic (primary and metastatic), traumatic, vascular, and infectious.

Primary lesions of the jugular foramen include glomus jugulare tumors, schwannomas, and meningiomas. Metastatic lesions to the jugular foramen are more common than primary neoplasms (36,38–42). Glomus jugulare tumors are the most common primary neoplasms of the jugular foramen. These are vascular tumors arising from neuroectodermally derived paraganglia present at the jugular fossa, the inferior tympanic canaliculus, the promontory, and within the vagus nerve. Paraganglia are very similar histologically and embryologically to the adrenal medulla. They, along with their derivative glomus tumors (jugulare and tympanicum), are typically supplied by the inferior tympanic branch of the ascending pharyngeal artery (43); however, the blood supply to glomus tumors may be very extensive, originating from the external carotid, the internal carotid, and the vertebral arteries (44). These tumors are more common in females (6:1 female-to-male ratio) and usually present in middle age. Functional tumors occur in 1% to 3% of cases with secretion of dopamine, serotonin, or norepinephrine. In such cases, patients may experience headache, labile blood pressure, sweating, and flushing (43). Approximately 3% of glomus jugulare tumors are malignant and develop metastases. Although hearing loss occurs in 80% and PT occurs in 60% of patients with glomus jugulare tumors, only 10% have cranial neuropathies.

Schwannomas are the second most common primary neoplasms. They most often involve the vagus nerve and originate from schwann cells. Malignant schwannomas are extremely rare. Sensorineural hearing loss may occur when schwannomas encroach on the cochlea and/or the internal auditory canal.

Meningiomas are the third most common primary neoplasms. They originate from arachnoid cap cells and may be associated with prior trauma, radiotherapy, or foreign body, although the nature of this association is not known. Like glomus jugulare, these tumors have a female predilection (2:1 female-to-male ratio). They also tend to present in middle age and can become metastatic in approximately 7% of the cases. These tumors may present with cerebellar signs, retrotympanic mass, and hearing loss, as well as lower cranial nerve palsies (45). Etiologies of JFS are summarized in Table 3.

PATHOGENESIS

Mass effect on neural contents of the jugular foramen from various neoplastic, vascular, infectious, and inflammatory processes is the main pathophysiologic mechanism of this syndrome. Trauma and direct injury to the nerves in the foramen is another etiology.

ANATOMY OF THE JUGULAR FORAMEN

The jugular foramen is limited anterolaterally by the temporal bone and posteromedially by the occipital bone. Anterior to the foramen lies the carotid artery, with the facial nerve coursing laterally. The foramen is divided by a fibrous or bony ridge connecting the jugular spine of the temporal bone to the jugular process of the occipital bone, to form the pars nervosa and the pars vascularis. Contrary to the suggestion of the names, the two segments each contain both vascular and nervous structures. Cranial nerves X and XI along with the jugular bulb usually occupy the pars vascularis, while cranial nerve IX and the inferior petrosal sinus traverse the pars nervosa. There are two openings in the dura medial to the sinus. These superior and inferior openings transmit cranial nerve IX and nerves X and XI, respectively. Exiting the skull base, nerve XI is posterior and nerve IX is anterior, with the vagus medial to the two in their caudad

TABLE 3   Etiologies of Jugular Foramen Syndrome

Neoplastic
   Benign
      Glomus jugulare tumor
      Schwannoma/neurilemmoma
      Meningioma
   Malignant
      Metastatic
        From head and neck primary tumors
      Kidney (39)
      Prostate (41)
      Skin (38)
   Primary
      Lymphoma (46)
      Myxoid chondrosarcoma (47)
      Chondroid chordoma (48)
      Malignant glomus tumors, schwannomas, and meningiomas
Infectious
   Neuroinflammatory disorders—varicella zoster (49)
   Parapharyngeal abscess (50)
Vascular
   Thrombosis/thrombophlebitis of the intraforaminal sigmoid sinus/jugular vein (36)
   Carotid dissection (51)
Traumatic
   Skull base fracture (52)
   Penetrating trauma (53,54)

extension. The vascular anatomy is variable but the inferior petrosal sinus usually enters the medial jugular bulb after passing medial to the internal carotid (44). The anatomical and functional innervation of cranial nerves IX–XI is outlined in Table 4.

CLINICAL MANIFESTATIONS

Hoarseness and dysphagia with aspiration are the cardinal manifestations of JFS. It has traditionally been thought that lesions involving the superior and recurrent laryngeal nerve lead to a lateral or cadaveric position of the paralyzed cord and associated breathy dysphonia. It has been reported, however, that site of nerve injury has no statistically significant relationship to vocal cord position (45).

    The combination of vocal cord and superior pharyngeal muscle paralysis along with decreased sensation of the pharynx makes these patients prone to aspiration pneumonia.

    Paralysis of the soft palate and superior constrictor muscles may lead to velopharyngeal insufficiency.

    Decreased taste sensation of the ipsilateral tongue and weakness of the ipsilateral trapezius and sternocleidomastoid muscles may be reported.

    Other manifestations such as PT and/or hearing loss are common in patients with glomus tumors.

DIAGNOSIS

A detailed history and a high index of suspicion are of paramount importance in making the diagnosis of JFS. Symptoms such as breathy voice, dysphagia, and aspiration should alert the astute physician to this syndrome. Subtle taste changes and neck and shoulder

TABLE 4 Anatomical and Functional Description of Cranial Nerves IX, X, and XI

IX (Glossopharyngeal)	X (Vagus)	XI (Spinal accessory)
Efferent	Efferent	Efferent
Special	*Special*	*Cranial root*
Stylopharyngeus	Voluntary muscles of pharynx and larynx, palatoglossus, palatopharyngus, levator veli palatini, salpingopharyngeus, and constrictors	Some fibers are accessory to vagus in innervation of pharynx and larynx and run primarily with the tenth nerve
General	*General*	*Spinal root*
Parasympathetics to smooth muscle and glands of pharynx, larynx, and some thoracoabdominal viscera	Parasympathetics to pharynx, larynx, and thoracoabdominal viscera	Trapezius and sterno-cleidomastoid muscles
Afferent	Afferent	Not afferent
Visceral	*Visceral*	
Carotid sinus and body	Baroreceptors, receptors from aortic arch, chemoreceptors from aortic body, sensory from larynx, esophagus, trachea and abdomino-thoracic viscera	
Somatic sensory	*Somatic sensory*	
External ear, medial surface of tympanic membrane, upper pharynx, and posterior third of tongue	Skin of posterior auricle and external auditory canal, parts of lateral tympanic membrane, and pharynx	
Special sensory	*Special sensory*	
Taste posterior third of tongue	Taste to epiglottic area	

weakness may also be noted. A history of unilateral hearing loss or PT may be associated with glomus tumors or other tumors that extend to the middle/inner ear.

Otoscopy may reveal a retrotympanic mass. Figure 3 depicts the otoscopic findings of a patient with a glomus jugulare tumor. Inspection of the oropharynx may reveal weakness of the ipsilateral soft palate with uvular deviation away from the lesion (curtain sign).

Examination of the upper aerodigestive tract is best accomplished with a fiberoptic nasopharyngoscope. Typically, there is ipsilateral hypesthesia of the pharynx as detected by lack of gag reflex, and the vocal fold may be immobilized. More directed examination of the supraglottis and lower pharynx can be done with flexible endoscopic evaluation of swallowing with sensory testing (55).

Laboratory testing should be individualized according to manifestations and clinical findings. For glomus jugulare tumors, serum should be screened for levels of epinephrine, norepinephrine, dopamine, and serotonin. Twenty-four-hour urinalysis should also be performed to assess for the presence of elevated metabolites of these substances, such as vanillylmandelic acid (VMA) and 5-hydroxyindole-acetic acid (5 HIAA) (43). Glomus tympanicum tumors do not require routine screening for these substances; however, these tests should be obtained if endocrine symptoms are present.

Audiological testing should be obtained in cases with hearing loss, PT, or retro-tympanic mass.

Imaging studies constitute the cornerstone of evaluation of these patients. Paragangliomas, meningiomas, schwannomas, and metastatic lesions have different

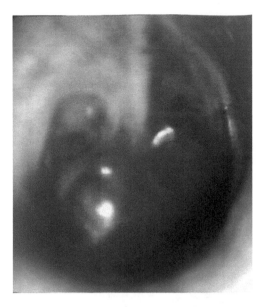

FIGURE 3 Otoscopic view of a glomus jugulare tumor.

radiographical characteristics. MRI and computed tomography (CT) are complementary to each other and are often used together to determine the nature and extent of the pathology under investigation. CT is superior to MRI for evaluating bone destruction; MRI is more useful for detection of dural invasion and intracranial extension (56–58).

For patients with a retrotympanic mass and/or PT, CT angiography (CTA) of the head is the preferable initial imaging study at our institution. This study can differentiate between a glomus tympanicum and a glomus jugulare tumor. It is also diagnostic of an ectopic carotid artery or a high jugular bulb. Figure 4 depicts a CTA of a patient with a glomus jugulare tumor. Since the upper neck is included in head CTA, a coexisting carotid body tumor can be detectable in patients with glomus tumors. For glomus jugulare cases, a head MRI should follow the CTA to better determine the size of the lesion and any possible intracranial extension. Carotid angiography is indicated only for prospective surgical cases to evaluate the collateral circulation of the brain (arterial and venous) in anticipation of possible vessel ligation and/or preoperative tumor embolization (59).

Bone scanning or positron emission tomography (PET) scanning is recommended if JFS occurs in a patient with a known or suspected history of malignancy.

Imaging characteristics of common jugular foramen tumors are depicted in Table 5.

TREATMENT

Treatment must be directed toward the primary etiology. An exhaustive discussion of treating the various etiologies of this syndrome is beyond the scope of this chapter, but modalities of choice for the most common causes will be addressed.

The three most common primary jugular foramen lesions, glomus jugulare, schwannoma, and meningioma, have traditionally been treated surgically through the lateral skull base approach (44,62). In an area so anatomically intricate, complete surgical resection can be difficult, and the risk of injury to cranial nerves VII–IX, as well as vascular and inner ear structures, can be considerable. However, recent advances in surgical techniques have allowed for thorough resection with acceptable morbidity. Another option for treatment is fractionated or Gamma knife radiation therapy (44,63). A recently published meta-analysis of surgery versus radiosurgery revealed that both are safe and efficacious

TABLE 5 Imaging Characteristics of Jugular Foramen Tumors

	Glomus jugulare	Schwannoma	Meningioma	Lymphoma/metastases
Computed tomography	Irregular shape Homogeneous Moth-eaten bony rim of destruction (20) Enhances with contrast	Smooth margin and smooth erosion of bone Less homogeneous than glomus Mild contrast enhancement	Osseous erosion with hyperostotic, sclerotic bone High contrast enhancement dural tails (60)	Osteolytic destruction with poorly demarcated borders (46)
Magnetic resonance	Small flow voids with "salt and pepper" appearance (61). Isointense with brain on T1 High T2 signal High contrast enhancement	Smooth contour Flow voids absent Low T1 signal similar to brainstem High T2 signal Marked contrast enhancement	Irregular lobulated borders Dural tails (60) Flow voids absent Low T1 signal similar to brainstem Variable T2 signal (44) Highest contrast enhancement	Signal characteristics similar to schwannoma
Angio	Intense contrast stain Vascular pedicle (46)	Not vascular	Not vascular Evaluation of venous drainage may determine need for sigmoid sinus occlusion prior to removal	Not typically useful

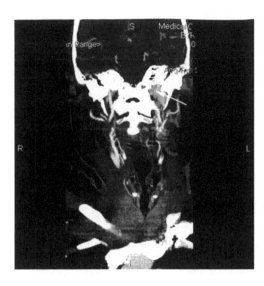

FIGURE 4 Computed tomography angiogram of patient with glomus jugulare (*arrow*).

modalities of treatment. Morbidity and recurrences were infrequent in both groups; however, the incidence of late recurrences (after 10–20 years) in the radiosurgery group is unknown (64). Gamma knife treatment has also been shown to be useful for meningiomas (63).

Since schwannomas and glomus jugulare tumors are typically benign and slow-growing lesions, observation should be considered in selected cases, particularly in older individuals and patients in poor general health.

Metastatic processes, of course, must be approached according to the specific pathology involved. In most cases, this will involve chemotherapy with or without radiotherapy.

In cases with uncompensated vocal cord paralysis, medialization should be considered. This can be accomplished by type I thyroplasty, vocal cord injection, or arytenoid adduction procedure. Vocal cord injection can be accomplished with micronized alloderm, calcium hydroxyapatite, and fat, among other substances. Vocal cord injection and type I thyroplasty are efficacious for medialization of the anterior vocal cord. If posterior medialization is also necessary, arytenoid adduction procedure is useful in conjunction with an anterior medialization procedure. Injection with gelfoam or collagen is the procedure of choice if recovery of function is expected.

COMPLICATIONS AND PROGNOSIS

Complications and prognosis vary widely and depend upon the underlying etiology and the type of treatment administered.

Regarding the main primary tumors of the jugular foramen, complications result from persistent paralysis of cranial nerves IX, X, and XI. Aspiration pneumonia is the most dangerous complication of this syndrome (65). Hoarseness and shoulder weakness are other complications.

For primary tumors, depending upon their extension, the inner ear, facial nerve, and eighth nerve are at risk. Other potential life-threatening complications include CSF leak and meningitis.

When preoperative embolization is used, stroke is another potential complication; however, this procedure is considered to be overall a safe and useful adjunct to surgery (66). Due to the benign nature of the common primary tumors, the overall prognosis is good if local control can be achieved.

SUMMARY

JFS can present a diagnostic and management challenge to the otolaryngologist. Glomus tumors and other primary tumors are common etiologies. A high index of suspicion, thorough examination, and proper imaging studies are necessary to establish diagnosis. For primary tumors, surgery and radiation therapy are the main modalities of treatment. Observation may be applied in selected cases.

R*EFERENCES*

1. Fishman RA. Benign intracranial hypertension. In: Fishman RA, ed. Cerebrospinal Fluid in Disease of the Nervous System. Philadelphia, PA: WB Saunders Co., 1980:128–139.
2. Sorensen PS, Krogsaa B, Gjerris F. Clinical course and prognosis of pseudotumor cerebri. A prospective study of 24 patients. Acta Neurol Scand 1988; 77(2):164–172.
3. Sismanis A. Otologic manifestations of benign intracranial hypertension syndrome: diagnosis and management. Laryngoscope 1987; 97(8 Pt 2 suppl 42):1–17.
4. Friedman DI. Pseudotumor cerebri. Neurosurg Clin N Am 1999; 10(4):609–621, Viii.
5. Galvin JA, Van Stavern GP. Clinical characterization of idiopathic intracranial hypertension at the Detroit Medical Center. J Neurol Sci 2004; 223(2):157–160.
6. Malm J, Kristensen B, Markgren P, et al. CSF hydrodynamics in idiopathic intracranial hypertension: a long-term study. Neurology 1992; 42(4):851–858.
7. Henry M, Driscoll MC, Miller M, et al. Pseudotumor cerebri in children with sickle cell disease: a case series. Pediatrics 2004; 113(3 Pt 1):E265–E269.
8. Oswald J, Meier K, Reinhart WH, et al. Pseudotumor cerebri in minocyline treatment. Schweiz Rundsch Med Prax 2001; 90(39):1691–1693.
9. Uddin AB. Drug-induced pseudotumor cerebri. Clin Neuropharmacol 2003; 26(5):236–238.
10. Karahalios DG, Rekate HL, Khayata MH, et al. Elevated intracranial venous pressure as a universal mechanism in pseudotumor cerebri of varying etiologies. Neurology 1996; 46(1):198–202.
11. King JO, Mitchell PJ, Thomson KR, et al. Cerebral venography and manometry in idiopathic intracranial hypertension. Neurology 1995; 45(12):2224–2228.
12. Higgins JN, Cousins C, Owler BK, et al. Idiopathic intracranial hypertension: 12 cases treated by venous sinus stenting. J Neurol Neurosurg Psychiatry 2003; 74(12):1662–1666.
13. Owler BK, Parker G, Halmagyi GM, et al. Pseudotumor cerebri syndrome: venous sinus obstruction and its treatment with stent placement. J Neurosurg 2003; 98(5):1045–1055.
14. Farb RI, Vanek I, Scott JN, et al. Idiopathic intracranial hypertension: the prevalence and morphology of sinovenous stenosis. Neurology 2003; 60(9):1418–1424.
15. Sugerman HJ, DeMaria EJ, Felton WL III, et al. Increased intra-abdominal pressure and cardiac filling pressures in obesity-associated pseudotumor cerebri. Neurology 1997; 49(2):507–511.
16. Josephs LG, Este-Mcdonald JR, Birkett DH, et al. Diagnostic laparoscopy increases intracranial pressure. J Trauma 1994; 36(6):815–818.
17. Gross CE, Tranmer BI, Adey G, et al. Increased cerebral blood flow in idiopathic pseudotumour cerebri. Neurol Res 1990; 12(4):226–230.
18. Langfitt TW. Clinical methods for monitoring intracranial pressure and measuring cerebral blood flow. Clin Neurosurg 1975; 22:302–320.
19. Sismanis A, Callari RH, Slomka WS, et al. Auditory-evoked responses in benign intracranial hypertension syndrome. Laryngoscope 1990; 100(11):1152–1155.
20. Wall M. Idiopathic intracranial hypertension. Neurol Clin 1991; 9(1):73–95.
21. Lipton HL, Michelson PE. Pseudotumor cerebri syndrome without papilledema. JAMA 1972; 220 (12):1591–1592.
22. Marcelis J, Silberstein SD. Idiopathic intracranial hypertension without papilledema. Arch Neurol 1991; 48(4):392–399.
23. Spence JD, Amacher AL, Willis NR. Benign intracranial hypertension without papilledema: role of 24-hour cerebrospinal fluid pressure monitoring in diagnosis and management. Neurosurgery 1980; 7 (4):326–336.
24. Sismanis A. Pulsatile tinnitus. A 15-year experience. Am J Otol 1998; 19(4):472–477.
25. Buchwald H, Avidor Y, Braunwald E, et al. Bariatric surgery: a systematic review and meta-analysis. JAMA 2004; 292(14):1724–1737. Erratum In: JAMA 2005; 293(14):1728.

26. Sismanis A, Smoker WR. Pulsatile tinnitus: recent advances in diagnosis. Laryngoscope 1994; 104(6 Pt 1):681–688.

27. Brodsky MC, Vaphiades M. Magnetic resonance imaging in pseudotumor cerebri. Ophthalmology 1998; 105(9):1686–1693.

28. Ogungbo B, Roy D, Gholkar A, et al. Endovascular stenting of the transverse sinus in a patient presenting with benign intracranial hypertension. Br J Neurosurg 2003; 17(6):565–568.

29. Kupersmith MJ, Gamell L, Turbin R, et al. Effects of weight loss on the course of idiopathic intracranial hypertension in women. Neurology 1998; 50(4):1094–1098.

30. McCarthy KD, Reed DJ. The effect of acetazolamide and furosemide on cerebrospinal fluid production and choroid plexus carbonic anhydrase activity. J Pharmacol Exp Ther 1974; 189(1):194–201.

31. Kesler A, Gadoth N. Pseudotumor cerebri (PTC—an update). Harefuah 2002; 141(3):297–300, 312.

32. Sismanis A, Butts FM, Hughes GB. Objective tinnitus in benign intracranial hypertension: an update. Laryngoscope 1990; 100(1):33–36.

33. Sugerman HJ, Felton WL III, Salvant JB Jr, et al. Effects of surgically induced weight loss on idiopathic intracranial hypertension in morbid obesity. Neurology 1995; 45(9):1655–1659.

34. Corbett JJ, Nerad JA, Tse DT, et al. Results of optic nerve sheath fenestration for pseudotumor cerebri. The lateral orbitotomy approach. Arch Ophthalmol 1988; 106(10):1391–1397.

35. Michaelides EM, Sismanis A, Sugerman HJ, et al. Pulsatile tinnitus in patients with morbid obesity: the effectiveness of weight reduction surgery. Am J Otolaryngology 2000; 21(5):682–685.

36. Lee KJ, Lee ME. Syndromes and eponyms. In: Lee KJ, ed. Essential Otolaryngology: Head and Neck Surgery. New York, NY: Mcgraw-Hill, 2003:207.

37. Robbins KT, Fenton RS. Jugular foramen syndrome. J Otolaryngol 1980; 9(6):505–516.

38. Schweinfurth JM, Johnson JT, Weissman J. Jugular foramen syndrome as a complication of metastatic melanoma. Am J Otolaryngol 1993; 14(3):168–174.

39. Boileau MA, Grotta JC, Borit A, et al. Metastatic renal cell carcinoma simulating glomus jugulare tumor. J Surg Oncol 1987; 35(3):201–203.

40. Watanabe H, Komiyama S, Soh N, et al. Metastases to the rouviere nodes and headache. Auris Nasus Larynx 1985; 12(1):53–56.

41. Wilson H, Johnson DH. Jugular foramen syndrome as a complication of metastatic cancer of the prostate. South Med J 1984; 77(1):92–93.

42. Greenberg HS, Deck MD, Vikram B, et al. Metastasis to the base of the skull: clinical findings in 43 patients. Neurology 1981; 31(5):530–537.

43. Gulya AJ. The glomus tumor and its biology. Laryngoscope 1993; 103(11 Pt 2 suppl 60):7–15.

44. Horn KL, Hankinson H. Tumors of the jugular foramen. In: Jackler RK, Brackmann DE, eds. Neurotology. Chicago, IL: Mosby, 1994:1059–1068.

45. Woodson GE. Configuration of the glottis in laryngeal paralysis. I: clinical study. Laryngoscope 1993; 103(11 Pt 1):1227–1234.

46. Eldevik OP, Gabrielsen TO, Jacobsen EA. Imaging findings in schwannomas of the jugular foramen. AJNR Am J Neuroradiol 2000; 21(6):1139–1144.

47. Slaba S, Haddad A, Zafatayeff S, et al. Imaging of an exceptional tumor: myxoid chondrosarcoma of the jugular foramen. J Med Liban 2001; 49(4):231–233.

48. Rupa V, Rajshekhar V, Bhanu TS, et al. Primary chondroid chordoma of the base of the petrous temporal bone. J Laryngol Otol 1989; 103(8):771–773.

49. Hayashi T, Murayama S, Sakurai M, et al. Jugular foramen syndrome caused by varicella zoster virus infection in a patient with ipsilateral hypoplasia of the jugular foramen. J Neurol Sci 2000; 172(1):70–72.

50. Thomasen I, Peitersen E, Peitersen B. Parapharyngeal abscess complicated by the jugular foramen syndrome. Report of a child aged 2. Ugeskr Laeger 1987; 149(30):2023.

51. Waespe W, Niesper J, Imhof HG, et al. Lower cranial nerve palsies due to internal carotid dissection. Stroke 1988; 19(12):1561–1564.

52. Hsu HP, Chen ST, Chen CJ, et al. A case of Collet-Sicard syndrome associated with traumatic atlas fractures and congenital basilar invagination. J Neurol Neurosurg Psychiatry 2004; 75(5):782–784.

53. Overholt EM, Dalley RW, Winn HR, et al. Penetrating trauma of the jugular foramen. Ann Otol Rhinol Laryngol 1992; 101(5):452–454.

54. Sacks AD. Penetrating trauma of the jugular foramen. Ann Otol Rhinol Laryngol 1993; 102(6):485.

55. Tabaee A, Murry T, Zschommler A, et al. Flexible endoscopic evaluation of swallowing with sensory testing in patients with unilateral vocal fold immobility: incidence and pathophysiology of aspiration. Laryngoscope 2005; 115(4):565–569.

56. Durden DD, Williams DW III. Radiology of skull base neoplasms. Otolaryngol Clin North Am 2001; 34(6):1043–1064, Vii.

57. Chong VF, Khoo JB, Fan YF. Imaging of the nasopharynx and skull base. Neuroimaging Clin N Am 2004; 14(4):695–719.

58. Ishida H, Mohri M, Amatsu M. Invasion of the skull base by carcinomas: histopathologically evidenced findings with CT and MRI. Eur Arch Otorhinolaryngol 2002; 259(10):535–539.

59. Remly KB, Coit WE, Harnsberger HR, et al. Pulsatile tinnitus and the vascular tympanic membrane: CT, MR, and angiographic findings. Radiology 1990; (174):383–389.

60. Macdonald AJ, Salzman KL, Harnsberger HR, et al. Primary jugular foramen meningioma: imaging appearance and differentiating features. AJR Am J Roentgenol 2004; 182(2):373–377.

61. Rao AB, Koeller KK, Adair CF. From the archives of the AFIP. Paragangliomas of the head and neck: radiologic-pathologic correlation. Armed Forces Institute of Pathology. Radiographics 1999; 19 (6):1605–1632.

62. Jackson CG, McGrew BM, Forest JA, et al. Lateral skull base surgery for glomus tumors: long-term control. Otol Neurotol 2001; 22(3):377–382.

63. Liscak R, Kollova A, Vladyka V, et al. Gamma knife radiosurgery of skull base meningiomas. Acta Neurochir Suppl 2004; 91:65–74.

64. Gottfried ON, Liu JK, Couldwell WT. Comparison of radiosurgery and conventional surgery for the treatment of glomus jugulare tumors. Neurosurg Focus 2004; 17(2):E4.

65. Ramina R, Maniglia JJ, Fernandes YB, et al. Jugular foramen tumors: diagnosis and treatment. Neurosurg Focus 2004; 17(2):E5.

66. Abud DG, Mounayer C, Benndorf G, et al. Intratumoral injection of cyanoacrylate glue in head and neck paragangliomas. AJNR Am J Neuroradiol 2004; 25(9):1457–1462.

Section 2

Differential Diagnosis and Treatment of Clinical Presentations in the Head and Neck

25

Otorrhea

Michael E. Hoffer, Ben J. Balough, and Darrell Hunsaker
*Department of Otolaryngology, Naval Medical Research Command,
Naval Medical Center, San Diego, California, U.S.A.*

INTRODUCTION

Ear drainage can represent a difficult problem for health-care professionals and the patients they treat. Drainage from the ear can be associated with a foul odor and can soil clothing, causing embarrassment to patients in social situations. In addition, individuals who wear hearing aids are often forced to keep the aids out of the ear during the period of drainage, which may further increase social isolation. In this chapter, we will begin by considering the infectious cause of otitis externa and otitis media as they relate to ear drainage; next, we will discuss allergic and inflammatory disorders; finally, we will examine systemic disorders that can produce otorrhea. After discussion of each disorder, we will examine therapeutic options.

DEFINITION

Drainage from the ear can originate from any of three sites—the external ear, the middle ear, or the brain. In analyzing otorrhea, several factors are important to consider, including the appearance of the discharge, the pattern of the discharge, and the chronicity of the discharge. The appearance of otorrhea can vary significantly. Otorrhea can take the form of purulent fluid as is the case in middle and external ear infections; clear, noninfected fluid as is seen in a cerebral spinal fluid (CSF) leak; or bloody as can be seen with infections or trauma. The pattern of the discharge is another important factor in diagnosing and treating this disorder. Discharge can be constant as is often seen with infectious etiologies or intermittent as can be seen with tympanostomy tube otorrhea. Additionally, the discharge can sometimes be observed to vary in intensity with pressure, as can be seen with CSF otorrhea. Finally, otorrhea can be described by the length of its course as acute or chronic. Arbitrarily, we label otorrhea lasting less than six weeks as acute and that lasting more than six weeks as chronic. While this time course may be a helpful diagnostic sign, intervention may affect time course as much as the etiology affects time course. A chronically draining ear may be from a middle-ear cholesteatoma or may simply be from untreated otitis externa. One etiology, otitis externa, may have resolved with antibiotic therapy, had it been treated, whereas the other, cholesteatoma, may have gotten better but not resolved with antibiotics. Therefore, knowledge of what treatment was applied and when it was applied is very important in using time course as a factor in determining etiology.

EPIDEMIOLOGY

The epidemiology of otorrhea is difficult to fully understand. Since the most common cause of this disorder worldwide is external and middle-ear infections, the rate of otorrhea will be higher in populations with a high rate of ear disease, such as Native Americans and Australian aborigines (1). The local environment also plays a role in the epidemiology of otorrhea. Increased rates of otitis externa are reported in individuals who swim in dirty water, such as lakes and ponds, as compared with those who spend more time in controlled aquatic environments. Increased rates of otitis media also are reported in those who have smokers in their household. An additional factor is the rate at which myringotomy tubes (PE tubes) are placed, since some studies indicate that over half of the individuals who receive PE tubes have drainage at some point while the tubes are in place (2).

PATHOGENESIS

Drainage from the ear can originate from a variety of sources. It is convenient to categorize the pathogenesis of this disorder according to the etiology. By far, the most common cause of otorrhea is infectious in etiology. In this category, acute bacterial infections of the external and middle ear are very common causes of ear drainage. Fungal infections of the external ear can also be common in certain environments or after aggressive treatment of a bacterial infection. While ear drainage most often is caused by common external and middle-ear bacteria, immunocompromised individuals can manifest otorrhea from infectious agents not commonly present in patients with healthy immune systems. In these individuals, a diligent search for the causative agent is critical in achieving a satisfactory outcome. Associated with the infectious causes is tympanostomy tube drainage, which can occur in a significant percentage of individuals who undergo the procedure (1,2). After bacterial infections, the next most common pathogenesis of otorrhea is a group of disorders that we categorize as allergic dermatitis. Once again, the frequency of these disorders is dependent on the environment and patient population. While allergy has been implicated as a major cause of ear drainage, the link may be difficult to prove in individual patients. Irritants, however, show a clear relationship and can range from hairspray to over-aggressive digitalization (or Q-tipping) of the ear. Finally, there is a group of "other disorders" that is largely composed of systemic disorders that may manifest with otorrhea. The most well known, but certainly not the only disorder in this class, is Wegener's granulomatosis (Chapter 8). Diagnosis of these disorders is critical, since systemic complications may be associated and the ear drainage may be the first sign of a more serious systemic disorder.

DIAGNOSIS AND TREATMENT

The Infectious Etiologies

Acute Bacterial Otitis Externa.   Both the external ear and the middle ear are susceptible to infection and both can present with otorrhea. External-ear infections (acute otitis externa) are most often caused by irritation to the ear, either from manipulation (fingers, Q-tips, etc.) or from environmental factors (water, debris, etc.). External-ear infections will present with ear pain and drainage. In bacterial otitis externa, the discharge is typically purulent. The main pathogens are Pseudomonas and Staphylococcal species, with a variable amount of anaerobes, as well (3). Typically, the ear will appear red and inflamed and be extremely sensitive to touch. In some cases, the ear can swell to the point where the tympanic membrane cannot be seen through the ear canal. Less commonly, the ear will demonstrate vesicles and pustules. Generally, this appearance is driven by pathology, since the vesicular lesions that tend to drain a clear, watery fluid, are usually viral in origin. In most cases, acute otitis externa can be controlled, but if the disease is allowed to progress, complications, including a true canal stenosis, can occur (4).

In the treatment of the draining ear, the first priority is to diagnose the cause and location of the drainage. Often, this is impossible to accomplish without the use of a microscope and a set of equipment (suction, cerumen loops, etc.) capable of cleaning debris out of the ear. When the disorder is recognized as an acute otitis externa, antimicrobial ear drops should be utilized. The best eardrop is controversial. Clearly, if an eardrum perforation is seen or a tube is in place, a nonototoxic medicine should be utilized. In fact, even when the eardrum is intact, there is mounting evidence that both non–antibiotic-containing and aminoglycoside-containing eardrops are becoming less effective over time (5,6). We utilize a quinolone antibiotic drop containing steroids. This gives increased effectiveness and is safe if the eardrum becomes ruptured or opened during the disease process (6). Our standard regimen is four to five drops b.i.d., pumped in by depressing the tragus (7). If the ear canal is narrow, we will place a wick and saturate it with antibiotics twice a day. We are careful to change the wick every two to three days. Finally, if there is no response or a severe infection, systemic antibiotics may be necessary.

Noninvasive Fungal Otitis Externa. Fungal otitis externa most often presents with a clear or white discharge and may be apparent by the presence of fungal elements in the external canal. Usually, the ear has minimal pain but significant itching. In rare cases, noninvasive fungal infections can also present with granulation tissue and pain (8). Fungal otitis externa can present primarily but often is a secondary complication due to the elimination of the normal aural flora when eardrops are used for otorrhea. Although noninvasive fungal infection is usually limited to the external ear canal, a recent study discovered fungal DNA in the middle ear of individuals with otorrhea (9). The significance of this finding has not yet been fully defined.

Fungal drainage can be a difficult condition to treat. Again, good aural care is crucial in treating these infections. With a mild fungal infection, acidification of the ear canal with an acid-based eardrop can be effective, but the drop can cause pain in the patient. Filling the ear canal with an antifungal cream, such as clotrimizole, often can be effective. Due to the need to completely fill the canal with the cream, reapplication should be done in the clinic, and patients often will require several applications over a two-week period to gain control over the fungal infection.

Infectious Otitis Media. Otorrhea can also present with otitis media. Several patterns of middle-ear pathology can produce drainage. Middle-ear fluid in acute otitis media can spontaneously rupture the eardrum and spill into the external auditory canal, or a middle ear with cholesteatoma can drain. Additionally, fluid can drain from the middle ear through tympanostomy tubes that were placed to ventilate the middle ear.

Tympanostomy tube drainage is not uncommon, and typically occurs in two patterns. It has been estimated that 10% of all tubes drain during the first week after surgery. The fact that antibiotic eardrops and nonantibiotic eardrops are equally effective at controlling this drainage suggests that most of this early drainage is sterile fluid or treated acute otitis media fluid that has been sterilized (10). As for latter drainage, that fluid has been cultured and the most common pathogens found have been *Streptococcus pneumonia* and *Haemophilus influenza* (11). Antibiotic-containing eardrops approved for middle-ear use are the most effective treatment option for this drainage. In cases that are refractory to antibiotic eardrops, we add oral antibiotics and, if these fail, we consider changing the tubes. As new vaccination patterns emerge, the predominant microorganisms found in middle-ear secretions may change over time. Finally, in chronic otitis media with cholesteatoma, the middle ear is, by definition, infected and will drain into the external ear.

Infections in Immunocompromised Individuals. A special type of external otitis is termed malignant otitis externa. This is a bacterial otitis externa present in diabetic or immunocompromised patients in whom there is osteomyelitis of the skull base. The disorder is caused by *Pseudomonas aeruginosa* infection and may be recognized by granulation tissue in the external ear. The ear also may present with significant inflammation and erythema (12). A culture of the ear positive for Pseudomonas does not make the diagnosis, since Pseudomonas is part of the flora of a normal ear and can also be positive in simple otitis externa. The best diagnostic test is a bone scan looking for evidence of the osteomyelitis. It is important for clinicians to keep a high index of suspicion for this disorder, since, if not treated appropriately, the disorder can progress to lateral sinus thrombosis, involvement of the temporal mandibular joint (TMJ), multiple cranial nerve involvement, and meningitis (13,14).

Treatment of malignant otitis externa can be complex. Antibiotic therapy is the mainstay of treatment and must continue until there are clear signs of resolution of the osteomyelitis. The fluoroquinolone class of antibiotics represents a convenient oral group of medicines that could achieve adequate tissue levels to treat malignant otitis externa; however, resistance is possible. We recommend consultation with an infectious disease specialist in some cases. There has been significant debate over the years as to the role of debridement of granulation tissue. Some argue for limited and relatively gentle cleaning of the external ear, whereas others argue for aggressive debridement, to include an operative procedure. Perhaps the most rational approach is early debridement concomitant with appropriate antibiotic therapy, allowing the disease progression to guide treatment.

Malignant otitis externa is not the only disorder unique to immunocompromised patients such as those infected with HIV or those receiving chemotherapy. These individuals are especially likely to manifest aural discharge from a host of common and noncommon infectious agents. In this group of individuals, the practitioner must be especially vigilant to discover the pathologic agent, as well as to rule out the possibility of a malignant otitis externa. In HIV patients in particular, *Pneumocystis carinii*–infected aural polyps can occur and drain in the external canal (15). Fungal disease can be particularly aggressive in this group of patients. Invasive fungal disorders, while much more common in the sinuses, can also affect the ear and mastoid (16). Aggressive surgical treatment combined with systemic antifungal therapy is necessary in this group of individuals.

Allergy and Dermatitis

There is clear evidence that otitis media with effusion is highly related to an allergic diathesis. When this converts to chronic draining otitis media, the allergic component would seem to still be relevant, although direct evidence is scant (17–19). Therefore, the surgeon must consider allergy evaluation, based on a patient history of other allergic diatheses, especially of the unified respiratory epithelium. Patients with chronic draining ear and allergic rhinitis, chronic rhinosinusitis, and asthma are strong candidates for allergy workup before contemplating surgical treatment.

Contact allergy to chemicals used in ear drops is the most common type of dermatologic otitis externa. Hairsprays, dyes, and cosmetics can also result in an eczematoid and draining otorrhea. If the source of external canal weeping is not obvious, routine patch testing is strongly suggested (20). The "autoeczematization" (ID) reaction, which is an autoimmune reaction that may involve only the external auditory canal, has been recorded for over 70 years in the otolaryngology literature. Recent studies confirm that this is due to a local reaction to distant fungus infections, most commonly dermatophytid in the feet and inguinal area. Control of the primary fungal infection with prolonged antifungal systemic treatment will nearly always control the ear reaction (21,22). There are other less-common dermatologic conditions that may focus on the ear. Atopic dermatitis, which has recently been found to result from a superantigen reaction to *Staphylococcus aureus* exotoxin, has been implicated in otitis externa (23). A special cause of contact dermatitis is the overuse of some ear drops in which the preservative or a component of the drop itself irritates the ear. In these individuals, the drops have often been administered to clear up an infectious etiology of otorrhea. In the case of contact dermatitis, the infectious otorrhea will stop as the drops become effective and then will begin again with a slightly different character as the drops become noxious.

Most autoimmune and contact allergy reactions of the external auditory canal and pinna skin are treated primarily by eliminating the source and controlling the local reaction with topical steroids. Care must be taken to avoid skin atrophy caused by prolonged topical steroid use. Necrosis of external auditory canal skin and temporal bone exposure may occur.

Other Etiologies

While the vast majority of otorrhea is infectious in etiology, there are a number of other important causes. Trauma can cause otorrhea in several different fashions. Head injury or surgery can create a CSF leak from the middle fossa or posterior fossa into the mastoid. The CSF can then pass into the middle ear and escape through the tympanic memberane (TM), if it, too, is damaged or opened by the traumatic event or surgery. More commonly, trauma will be associated with bloody otorrhea due to damage to the eardrum or external auditory canal. This type of otorrhea is often associated with head injury, digital manipulation of the external canal, or removal of cerumen from the ear.

A number of systemic diseases have been associated with otorrhea. The classic systemic etiology associated with otorrhea is Wegener's. Approximately 20% of individuals with Wegener's granulomatosis will have otologic involvement. Wegener's can cause inflammation and granulation tissue in the external ear and/or the middle ear, and both sites will be associated with a discharge. In addition to Wegener's disease, aural discharge has been associated with Churg–Strauss syndrome (Chapter 8) and Behçet's syndrome (Chapter 3) (24,25). Churg–Strauss syndrome produces otorrhea in much the same fashion as Wegener's by forming granulation tissue. In Behçet's disease, the evidence suggests that aural discharge occurs as a result of opportunistic infections.

Tuberculosis (TB), although technically infectious in etiology, can often be associated with an aural form. Although the classic description of TB otitis media is a single central perforation with profuse, painless discharge (26,27), the disorder can cause a host of otologic complications, many of which will also present with otorrhea. A more detailed discussion of TB can be found in Chapter 12.

COMPLICATIONS AND PROGNOSIS

In the treatment of the draining ear, the first priority is to diagnose the cause and location of the drainage. Often, this is impossible to accomplish without the use of a microscope and equipment (suction, cerumen loops, etc.) capable of cleaning debris out of the ear. If there is a systemic condition causing the disorder, it must be treated. After making the appropriate diagnosis, good local care is imperative. The ear must be cleaned of all debris, but in so doing, the practitioner must avoid causing additional trauma to the already irritated ear canal.

In treating individuals with otorrhea, a number of issues should be kept in mind. Whereas drainage does not always completely stop five to seven days after treatment, there should be some effect by that time. If there is no effect within one week, or if the condition gets better and then returns within two weeks, an alternate diagnosis and treatment plan should be considered. In particular, this group of patients is at risk for serious complications and should be followed closely until the symptoms resolve and an adequate search for other disorders can be performed.

SUMMARY

Otorrhea is a common otologic condition that can be caused by a variety of disorders. While in many cases the drainage is secondary to a "simple swimmer's ear" which can be cured in a matter of a few days, in other cases, the cause of the drainage is much more significant and difficult to treat. Making the proper diagnosis, understanding how to gently clean the ear, and utilizing the appropriate treatment regimen are essential in treating this disorder. Persistent drainage that is difficult to control may signify a more significant condition and will require vigilance by the treating practitioner.

REFERENCES

1. Bluestone CD. Studies in otitis media: Children's Hospital of Pittsburgh-University of Pittsburgh progress report—2004. Laryngoscope 2004; 114(11 Pt 3 suppl 105):1–26.
2. Kacmarynski DS, Levine SC, Pearson SE, et al. Complications of otitis media before placement of tympanostomy tubes in children. Arch Otolaryngol Head Neck Surg 2004; 130(3):289–292.
3. Roland PS, Stroman DW. Microbiology of acute otitis externa. Laryngoscope 2002; 112(7 Pt 1):1166–1177.
4. Luong A, Roland PS. Acquired external auditory canal stenosis: assessment and management. Curr Opin Otolaryngol Head Neck Surg 2005; 13(5):273–276.
5. van Balen FA, Smit WM, Zuithoff NP, et al. Clinical efficacy of three common treatments in acute otitis externa in primary care: randomised controlled trial. BMJ 2003; 327(7425):1201–1205.
6. Cantrell HF, Lombardy EE, Duncanson FP, et al. Declining susceptibility to neomycin and polymyxin B of pathogens recovered in otitis externa clinical trials. South Med J 2004; 97(5):465–471.
7. Roland PS, Anon JB, Moe RD, et al. Topical ciprofloxacin/dexamethasone is superior to ciprofloxacin alone in pediatric patients with acute otitis media and otorrhea through tympanostomy tubes. Laryngoscope 2003; 113(12):2116–2122.
8. Marzo SJ, Leonetti JP. Invasive fungal and bacterial infections of the temporal bone. Laryngoscope 2003; 113(9):1503–1507.
9. Kim EJ, Catten MD, Lalwani AK. Detection of fungal DNA in effusion associated with acute and serous otitis media. Laryngoscope 2002; 112(11):2037–2041.
10. Kumar VV, Gaughan J, Isaacson G, et al. Oxymetazoline is equivalent to ciprofloxacin in preventing postoperative otorrhea or tympanostomy tube obstruction. Laryngoscope 2005; 115(2):363–365.
11. Mandel EM, Casselbrant ML, Kurs-Lasky M. Acute otorrhea: bacteriology of a common complication of tympanostomy tubes. Ann Otol Rhinol Laryngol 1994; 103(9):713–718.
12. Antonelli PJ, Schultz G, Cantwell JS, et al. Inflammatory proteases in chronic otitis externa. Laryngoscope 2005; 115(4):651–654.
13. Nadol JB Jr. Histopathology of Pseudomonas osteomyelitis of the temporal bone starting as malignant external otitis. Am J Otolaryngol 1980; 1(5):359–371.
14. Mardinger O, Rosen D, Minkow B, et al. Temporomandibular joint involvement in malignant external otitis. Oral Surg Oral Med Oral Pathol Oral Radiol Endod 2003; 96(4):398–403.
15. Lucente FE. Acquired immunodeficiency syndrome (AIDS). In: Lucente FE, Lawson W, Novick N, eds. The External Ear. Philadelphia, PA: WB Saunders, 1995:95.
16. Pelton SI, Klein JO. The promise of immunoprophylaxis for prevention of acute otitis media. Pediatr Infect Dis J 1999; 18(10):926–935.
17. Smirnova MG, Birchall JP, Pearson JP. The immunoregulatory and allergy-associated cytokines in the aetiology of the otitis media with effusion. Mediators Inflamm 2004; 13(2):75–88.
18. Bernstein JM. Role of allergy in eustachian tube blockage and otitis media with effusion: a review. Otolaryngol Head Neck Surg 1996; 114(4):562–568.
19. Doyle WJ. The link between allergic rhinitis and otitis media. Curr Opin Allergy Clin Immunol 2002; 2(1):21–25.
20. Millard TP, Orton DI. Changing patterns of contact allergy in chronic inflammatory ear disease. Contact Dermatitis 2004; 50(2):83–86.
21. Atzori L, Pau M, Aste M. Erythema multiforme ID reaction in atypical dermatophytosis: a case report. J Eur Acad Dermatol Venereol 2003; 17(6):699–701.
22. Derebery J, Berliner KI. Foot and ear disease–the dermatophytid reaction in otology. Laryngoscope 1996; 106(2 Pt 1):181–186.
23. Skov L, Baadsgaard O. Bacterial superantigens and inflammatory skin diseases. Clin Exp Dermatol 2000; 25(1):57–61.
24. Ishiyama A, Canalis RF. Otological manifestations of Churg-Strauss syndrome. Laryngoscope 2001; 111(9):1619–1624.
25. Venzor J, Hua Q, Bressler RB, et al. Behçet's-like syndrome associated with idiopathic CD4$^+$ T-lymphocytopenia, opportunistic infections, and a large population of TCR [α][β]$^+$ CD4$^-$ CD8$^-$ T cells. Am J Med Sci 1997; 313(4):236–238.
26. Greenfield BJ, Selesknick SH, Fisher L, et al. Aural tuberculosis. Am J Otol 1995; 16(2):175–182.
27. Linstrom CJ, Lucente FE, Joseph EM. Infections of the external ear. In: Bailey BJ, Calhoun KH, eds. Head and Neck Surgery-Otolaryngology. Vol. 2. Philadelphia, PA: Lippincott-Raven, 1998:1965–1980.

26

Vertigo, Disequilibrium, and Dizziness

Joel A. Goebel
Department of Otolaryngology-Head and Neck Surgery, Washington University School of Medicine, St. Louis, Missouri, U.S.A.

Timothy E. Hullar
Department of Otolaryngology-Head and Neck Surgery and Department of Anatomy and Neurobiology, Washington University School of Medicine, St. Louis, Missouri, U.S.A.

INTRODUCTION

Due to the complexity of the balance mechanism in the human body, a variety of systemic diseases can create a sense of dizziness or imbalance. In order to maintain postural control and gaze stability, the body employs *sensory input, central integration, and motor output* to create appropriate responses to changes in the visual world and support surface. Accordingly, diseases that alter or destroy one or more sensory inputs to the brain, interfere with brainstem and cortical integration and formulation of motor commands, or interrupt motor responses will result in postural or visual instability. The critical feature for localizing the site of lesion in such patients is a thorough history of the nature of the problem and a comprehensive balance examination.

In general, most patients who suffer from *vertigo*—a false sensation of movement in their visual world—will have dysfunction of the vestibular labyrinth or eighth nerve, with a minority having lesions in the cerebellum, brainstem, or cerebral cortex. In contrast, patients with *disequilibrium*—a sense of poor coordination with the surrounding environment—can have lesions affecting visual, vestibular, and somatosensory input, central integration, or motor output. Finally, patients complaining of *lightheadedness or near syncope* usually have a cardiovascular or cerebrovascular etiology.

With these distinctions in mind, this chapter is devoted to defining systemic processes that can cause vertigo, disequilibrium, or lightheadedness, and the optimal strategies for treatment of these symptoms.

DEFINITION

As mentioned in the introduction, patients with balance complaints can be divided into three general categories, based on the nature of their symptoms. Patients who present with *vertigo* as their chief complaint will describe a strong sense of motion in their visual world such as spinning, tumbling, or rocking from side to side. In the majority of cases, the problem originates from an imbalance of signals from the vestibular periphery, a situation perceived by the brain as a sense of self-motion relative to the visual surroundings. Vertigo tends to come in attacks lasting minutes to hours with minimal symptoms between spells. Accompanying complaints such as hearing loss, tinnitus, aural fullness, phonophobia, and blurry vision with head movement are common and underscore the peripheral nature of the process. In less common cases of central nervous system (CNS) involvement, complaints such as dysarthria, dysphagia, altered sensorium, photophobia, or seizure activity may accompany the vertigo that may last minutes to hours but can persist even longer.

In contrast to vertigo, *disequilibrium* tends to be a less well-defined sensation of abnormal interaction with the environment, particularly when the patient is moving. Disequilibrium tends to be more troubling while the patient is upright and lessen while in the seated or supine position. Patients with disequilibrium can suffer from a variety of sensory input, central integration, and motor output problems.

Finally, *lightheadedness* is a sensation of "floating" or "nearly passing out" and can usually be seen in two main conditions: poor blood flow to the brain due to cardiovascular or cerebrovascular disease or anxiety and hyperventilation syndromes. In its most severe manifestation, syncopal episodes occur and a cardiovascular, cerebrovascular, or epileptic source is identified.

EPIDEMIOLOGY

Although dizziness can be seen in almost any age group, the probability of suffering some form of vertigo, disequilibrium, and/or lightheadedness increases with age. Roughly 30%

of patients over the age of 65 complain of dizziness (1), and dizziness accounts for 2% of all chief complaints of elderly patients (2). In a review of several studies of patients with dizziness, just under half of the patients had peripheral vestibulopathy, while cerebrovascular disease was responsible for 6%, cardiac disease for 1.5%, and brain tumor for less than 1% (3). Due to the complexity of postural control, many systemic diseases that affect cerebral blood flow cause disequilibrium or lightheadedness, and therefore, the incidence of these problems increases sharply with age.

PATHOGENESIS

As mentioned in the previous sections, dizziness can be broken down into three main categories—vertigo, disequilibrium, and lightheadedness—and the pathogenesis of these three symptoms will vary. In most cases, vertigo occurs whenever the normal inputs from the semicircular canals or the eighth cranial nerve become disturbed and the brain is fooled into thinking that the head is in motion when in fact it is not. This can occur by a variety of mechanisms. Hair-cell function can be affected by infection (bacterial labyrinthitis secondary to otitis media), localized inflammatory disease (i.e., cholesteatoma or cholesterol granuloma) with otic capsule erosion, metastatic disease, chronic granulomatous disease (i.e., Wegener's granulomatosis, sarcoidosis, and histiocytosis), or autoimmune disease (i.e., Cogan's syndrome). The latter two of these are discussed in Chapters 6 and 8, respectively. Likewise, eighth nerve function is susceptible to injury from granulomatous and metastatic lesions of the petrous apex, viral inflammation, and leukemic or lymphomatous infiltrate. Diseases that cause microangiopathic changes such as diabetes, hypertension, and renal failure can also lead to asymmetric labyrinthine damage and vertigo. Vascular, primary neoplastic, metastatic, and degenerative processes within the brainstem, vestibulocerebellum, and insular cortex can generate a sense of vertigo by interrupting the central connections and cortical representations of the vestibulo-ocular reflex (VOR). Finally, bilateral loss of vestibular function may present with vertigo at its onset but usually progresses to gait instability and oscillopsia with head movement.

In contrast, patients presenting with disequilibrium as their primary complaint could have diffuse interruption of central brainstem pathways used to integrate sensory input (i.e., demyelination) or generate motor output (cerebellar atrophy, extensive internal capsule small vessel disease, basal ganglia disease, and normal pressure hydrocephalus), or they may suffer from musculoskeletal or somatosensory dysfunction (osteoarthritis, rheumatoid arthritis, lower motor neuron disease, and peripheral neuropathy). Depending on the etiology and site of dysfunction, patient complaints may range from mild instability while standing to inability to ambulate without assistance.

The pathogenesis of lightheadedness is a decrease in blood flow and hence oxygen to the brainstem and cerebral and cerebellar cortices that generates a gradual decline in function. In its mildest form, hyperventilation creates a sense of floating or giddiness. In more severe cases, cerebral blood pressure drops due to cardiac arrhythmia, dehydration, lower extremity venous pooling, or dysautonomia and can actually lead to syncope, which is almost never due to labyrinthine disease. In these patients, movement against gravity (getting out of a bed or chair and going up in an elevator) creates more symptoms than movement with gravity (lying or sitting down). Finally, lightheadedness due to primary psychiatric disease can present with a constellation of other symptoms (globus sensation, sense of impending doom, and unexplained anxiety) that usually makes it possible to diagnose these cases.

CLINICAL MANIFESTATIONS

Vertigo

Systemic diseases that affect the labyrinth or eighth nerve to cause vertigo can be infectious, inflammatory, primary neoplastic, paraneoplastic, metastatic, autoimmune, or degenerative.

Infectious causes for vertigo include suppurative or toxic labyrinthitis secondary to otitis media, viral labyrinthitis or neuritis (frequently from the herpes virus family), otosyphilis, Lyme disease, and bacterial and viral meningitis. In such cases, accompanying signs of middle ear or meningeal involvement will be seen, which helps facilitate the diagnosis.

Inflammatory diseases include chronic granulomatous disease such as eosinophilic granuloma or histiocytosis, Wegener's granulomatosis, sarcoidosis, amyloidosis, cholesterol granuloma, and invasive cholesteatoma. Characteristic lesions within the middle ear or temporal bone on examination or imaging are aided with serologic testing (i.e., sedimentation rate, anti-neutrophile cytoplasmic antibody (c-ANCA)) and tissue biopsy for diagnosis. In cases of suspected systemic involvement, pulmonary, renal, and CNS function tests and imaging may be useful.

Autoimmune causes for vertigo include Cogan's syndrome (consisting of dizziness, progressive sensorineural hearing loss, and uveitis), systemic lupus erythematosus (Chapter 1) rheumatoid arthritis (Chapter 1) and steroid-responsive autoimmune hearing loss (Chapter 5). Characteristic ocular, cutaneous, and extremity findings in addition to serology are crucial to making the correct diagnosis.

Sometimes, a *neoplasm* may present with vertigo or cause vertigo as a primary symptom. In most cases, the neoplasm is likely to be primary to the temporal bone or eighth nerve, such as with vestibular schwannoma, but neoplasms causing vertigo may also be a part of a systemic disease. Paraneoplastic cerebellar degeneration is the most common paraneoplastic syndrome affecting the brain. In this syndrome, anti-Yo antibodies target the Purkinje cells of the cerebellum, leaving the patient with symptoms of ataxia, headache, dysarthria, nystagmus, and vertigo. This syndrome is most commonly associated with cancer of the breast, ovary, and lung (4), and often the paraneoplastic symptoms are those that bring the patient to medical attention (5). Treatment of the primary tumor has been reported to improve the paraneoplastic symptoms (6).

Primary neoplasms related to systemic disease that may present with vertigo include neurofibromatosis (NF)-2 and endolymphatic sac tumor. NF-2 is a genetic condition caused by errors in the structure of the tumor suppressor gene *merlin*, normally responsible for regulating the cell's actin cytoskeleton (7). The condition is characterized by vestibular schwannomas (Fig. 1). Although hearing loss is by far the most common presenting symptom, almost 10% of patients with NF-2 come to medical attention due to vertigo. Over half of patients with NF-2 have been reported to have skin tumors and over one-third have cafe-au-lait spots, more commonly associated with NF-1. In addition, over one-third have ocular manifestations, including juvenile posterior subcapsular lenticular opacities or juvenile cortical cataract (8).

Endolymphatic sac tumors that may present with vertigo (9) are sometimes part of the clinical spectrum of von Hippel-Lindau disease, which is also characterized by hemangioblastomas of the CNS and retinal hemangioblastomas, renal-cell carcinoma, and pancreatic neuroendocrine tumors and pheochromocytomas, and is caused by a mutation of the *VHL* tumor suppressor gene. Proteins transcribed in response to hypoxia, including vascular endothelial growth factor, may be upregulated in patients with the disorder (10).

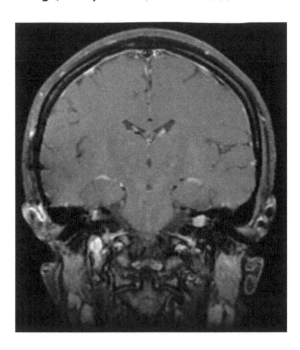

FIGURE 1 Magnetic resonance image of a patient with bilateral vestibular neuromas consistent with neurofibromatosis-2.

Some distant neoplasms are known to metastasize to the temporal bone, where they may cause vertigo. Tumors with primary sites in the breast, lung, stomach, kidney, prostate, and larynx have been found in the middle and inner ear (11). Such tumors have been reported to cause sudden cranial neuropathy, including eighth-nerve dysfunction (12,13), although it has not been shown that rapidly worsening cochlear or vestibular symptoms require a full metastatic workup. In addition, leukemic infiltrates can invade the temporal bone and otic capsule, causing a combination of unilateral hearing loss, vertigo, and facial nerve weakness.

Degenerative causes for vertigo include idiopathic bilateral vestibular loss and central brainstem degenerative syndromes. In many cases, the presence or absence of CNS signs and symptoms alerts the clinician to the source of the problem.

In all of the above-mentioned cases, the neurotologic examination will reveal nystagmus that usually beats in the direction of the uninvolved side, in addition to a variety of auditory, facial, and brainstem abnormalities, depending upon the site and extent of the lesion.

Disequilibrium

Any of the abovementioned disease processes may cause disequilibrium rather than vertigo if they do not involve the labyrinth itself but instead cause dysfunction with brainstem integration, cortical perception, or musculoskeletal function. In such cases, other cranial nerve or somatic deficits point toward the etiology of the problem. Common examples include loss of vibration sensation and joint proprioception in diabetic and hypertensive patients, poor muscle strength, and joint deformity in cases of severe osteoarthritis or rheumatoid arthritis and the wide-based ataxic gait of patients with cerebellar cortical disease.

Medications are common causes of imbalance and disequilibrium, especially in the elderly (14). Gentamicin toxicity may cause vertigo in the acute setting, but a patient's compensatory ability and symmetric vestibular loss may prevent this symptom from persisting. A patient may first manifest this after recovering from an acute illness enough to begin ambulating, sometimes with the most prominent long-term sequela consisting of difficulty walking in the dark (15). Furosemide is another medication that may be given in the context of systemic disease that can cause imbalance. Cisplatin is a common cause of disequilibrium in patients receiving chemotherapy. Amiodarone was once a common cause for vertigo or imbalance in patients with cardiac disease (16), but lowered doses now favored by cardiologists seem to have decreased the rate of this complication somewhat. Antipsychotics and anticonvulsants can cause instability and disequilibrium, symptoms that are often accompanied by eye findings such as spontaneous nystagmus.

Deficiency of vitamin B12 can be related to imbalance but only rarely to true vertigo. Subacute combined degeneration related to deficiency of the vitamin may be found in those with gastric disease or in vegetarians (17).

Migraine-associated dizziness is a common disease that manifests itself as headaches with nausea, photophobia, and dizziness of variable intensity, duration, and quality in young to middle-aged patients, manifesting more commonly in women than in men. A key to making this diagnosis is a high level of suspicion in younger, otherwise healthy patients with a personal or familial migraine history and light sensitivity during their dizziness (18).

Lightheadedness

The primary systemic conditions causing lightheadedness affecting the heart and cerebrovascular circulation are related to anxiety or other psychiatric disorders. Sometimes, reproduction of a patient's symptoms during hyperventilation is indicative of anxiety-related dizziness; these patients will often admit to generalized anxiety or even panic attack. When accompanied by horizontal nystagmus, however, the presence of cerebellopontine angle tumor must also be considered (19). A positive hyperventilation test, along with a history of cardiac arrhythmias, orthostasis, and carotid bruit, are all common manifestations of altered cerebral flow due to cardiac disease, cerebrovascular compromise, or vasoconstriction. Most commonly, extensive small vessel cerebrovascular disease is found on imaging in elderly patients with additional risk factors such as hypertension, diabetes, and hypercholesterolemia. Occasionally, dysautonomia associated with diabetes or hypoadrenalism can be identified. In many cases, medication effects need to be considered, especially with aggressive antihypertensive therapy and sedative medications in the elderly.

DIAGNOSIS

Diagnosis of vestibular disorders depends in large part on the history taken from the patient. Patients may benefit initially by localizing the source of symptoms to the vestibular periphery or CNS, a distinction that may also help determine what systemic diseases may be involved. Peripheral disorders tend to manifest more episodically, with signs attributed to movement in certain directions (such as extending the head or turning the head while lying down) or with sensations of intense spinning vertigo. Central disorders may be more constant and feature a more general sensation of imbalance or disequilibrium and may be related to certain postures such as lying down or attempting to ambulate. These divisions are not precise, however, and a strong clinical suspicion must be maintained for pathology in either area. In addition to patient history, the bedside examination is critically useful for determining the source of a patient's symptoms. A positive reaction to the Dix-Hallpike examination, indicative of benign positional vertigo, reflects disease almost certainly limited to the vestibular periphery. Nystagmus following headshaking or a lag of the VOR during rapid head thrusts is each indicative of peripheral disease, with the latter able to distinguish disease from individual canals. Abnormal loss of visual ability during dynamic visual acuity testing is indicative of a loss of VOR function, but it is not particularly localizing.

Laboratory testing may be useful in detecting systemic disease in patients with vertigo. Vestibular function tests include caloric exams, rotary chair exams, and platform posturography. Abnormal caloric and rotary chair examinations may indicate peripheral vestibular loss, while patterns of sway during platform posturography may indicate difficulties with sensory integration or motor control. An audiogram may help detect subclinical hearing loss in patients suspected of having peripheral vestibular loss, while magnetic resonance imaging (MRI) may give evidence of cerebellar degeneration, small vessel disease, or tumor.

An attempt to distinguish between peripheral and central processes is important in helping determine the systemic diseases that may be related to symptoms of vertigo. Disequilibrium falls more into the category of central disorders, because it usually manifests with a general sense of imbalance and lack of coordination, and rarely, spinning vertigo. On the other hand, lightheadedness may be associated with assuming a position, commonly that involves going from a lying or sitting to a standing position, where orthostatic symptoms are prominent. These patients require evaluation of blood pressure changes throughout the day (including medication effects) and a workup of the autonomic system, including tilt-table testing, and will often need carotid studies including Doppler or magnetic resonance angiography (MRA). MRA has the advantage of being able to image the vertebral arteries and the circle of Willis during the same examination.

Only a small number of patients suffering from a systemic disease will initially present with dizziness. In these patients it is crucial to consider other, more commonly encountered causes before planning expensive, time-consuming, and, often frustrating, tests for undiagnosed systemic disease. Conditions with other otologic signs point to causes limited to the ear, such as Ménière's disease. In some cases, particular infectious diseases may be suspected. A clinical history of sexually transmitted diseases may lead to a diagnosis of otosyphilis using rapid plasma reagin (RPR) or veneral disease research laboratory (VDRL) tests, and, if positive, a follow-up fluorescent antitreponemal [fluorescent treponemal antibody absorption test (FTA–ABS)] confirmatory study (20). Lyme disease is well known to present with cranial nerve findings; a patient with a history of tick exposure or spreading rash should have immunologic testing for Lyme disease and therapy initiated promptly (21).

Patients presenting with ocular symptoms deserve prompt referral to an ophthalmologist, with the consideration that an inflammatory condition such as Cogan's syndrome is responsible. Similarly, in patients with mucosal lesions, unexplained skin rashes, or joint pain, the possibility must be considered that an autoimmune disease is responsible and appropriate laboratory tests performed. These include erythrocyte sedimentation rate, rheumatoid factor, antinuclear antibody, and anticytoplasmic antibody studies.

Patients presenting with disequilibrium should be carefully examined for other neurologic signs. Problems noted on neurologic examination, such as cerebellar ataxia, may be indicative of spinocerebellar degenerative disease or a cause such as West Nile virus infection (22). Serum titers as well as MRI are appropriate in these cases.

TREATMENT AND PROGNOSIS

Patients with symptoms of imbalance often require symptomatic relief as well as treatment of the underlying systemic disorder. Benzodiazepines such as clonazepam are particularly useful in controlling symptoms of vertigo, and to a lesser extent, disequilibrium, and offer a degree of anxiety reduction that meclizine does not. Essential to the treatment of imbalance is management of the underlying systemic condition. This may be relatively simple in cases where the symptoms are related to overmedication or a relatively treatable condition such as migraine, but much of the time, the balance function that has been lost cannot be regained and therapy must be directed toward vestibular rehabilitation (23). Prognosis for patients with severe bilateral peripheral vestibular loss is poorer than for unilateral dysfunction, while patients with disruption of central pathways may be able to compensate significantly if the systemic disease process is controlled. Ongoing efforts to develop sensory substitution protocols may provide patients with severe vestibular loss increased rehabilitative potential (24).

REFERENCES

1. Kwong EC, Pimlott NJ. Assessment of dizziness among older patients at a family practice clinic: a chart audit study. BMC Fam Pract 2005; 6(1):2.
2. Sloane PD. Dizziness in primary care. Results from the National Ambulatory Medical Care Survey. J Fam Pract 1989; 29(1):33–38.
3. Kroenke K, Hoffman RM, Einstadter D. How common are various causes of dizziness? A critical review. South Med J 2000; 93(2):160–167.
4. Liu S, Tunkel R, Lachmann E, et al. Paraneoplastic cerebellar degeneration as the first evidence of cancer: a case report. Arch Phys Med Rehabil 2000; 81(6):834–836.
5. McLellan R, Currie JL, Royal W, et al. Ovarian carcinoma and paraneoplastic cerebellar degeneration. Obstet Gynecol 1988; 72(6):922–925.
6. Kearsley JH, Johnson P, Halmagyi GM. Paraneoplastic cerebellar disease. Remission with excision of the primary tumor. Arch Neurol 1985; 42(12):1208–1210.
7. Neff BA, Welling DB. Current concepts in the evaluation and treatment of neurofibromatosis type II. Otolaryngol Clin North Am 2005; 38(4):671–684, ix.
8. Evans DG, Huson SM, Donnai D, et al. A clinical study of type 2 neurofibromatosis. Q J Med 1992; 84(304):603–618.
9. Silveira RL, Gusmao SS, Pittella JE, et al. Endolymphatic sac adenocarcinoma: case report. Arq Neuropsiquiatr 2002; 60(3-B):847–851.
10. Zatyka M, da Silva NF, Clifford SC, et al. Identification of cyclin D1 and other novel targets for the von Hippel-Lindau tumor suppressor gene by expression array analysis and investigation of cyclin D1 genotype as a modifier in von Hippel-Lindau disease. Cancer Res 2002; 62(13):3803–3811.
11. Cureoglu S, Tulunay O, Ferlito A, et al. Otologic manifestations of metastatic tumors to the temporal bone. Acta Otolaryngol 2004; 124(10):1117–1123.
12. Hill BA, Kohut RI. Metastatic adenocarcinoma of the temporal bone. Arch Otolaryngol 1976; 102 (9):568–571.
13. Ingelaere PP, Simpson RH, Garth RJ. Metastatic renal cell carcinoma presenting as an aural polyp. J Laryngol Otol 1997; 111(11):1066–1068.
14. Tinetti ME, Williams CS, Gill TM. Dizziness among older adults: a possible geriatric syndrome. Ann Intern Med 2000; 132(5):337–344.
15. Rinne T, Bronstein AM, Rudge P, et al. Bilateral loss of vestibular function: clinical findings in 53 patients. J Neurol 1998; 245(6–7):314–321.
16. Arbusow V, Strupp M, Brandt T. Amiodarone-induced severe prolonged head-positional vertigo and vomiting. Neurology 1998; 51(3):917.
17. Hemmer B, Glocker FX, Schumacher M, et al. Subacute combined degeneration: clinical, electrophysiological, and magnetic resonance imaging findings. J Neurol Neurosurg Psychiatry 1998; 65(6):822–827.
18. Reploeg MD, Goebel JA. Migraine-associated dizziness: patient characteristics and management options. Otol Neurotol 2002; 23(3):364–371.
19. Minor LB, Haslwanter T, Straumann D, et al. Hyperventilation-induced nystagmus in patients with vestibular schwannoma. Neurology 1999; 53(9):2158–2168.
20. Linstrom CJ, Gleich LL. Otosyphilis: diagnostic and therapeutic update. J Otolaryngol 1993; 22 (6):401–408.
21. Lorenzi MC, Bittar RS, Pedalini ME, et al. Sudden deafness and Lyme disease. Laryngoscope 2003; 113(2):312–315.

22. Burton JM, Kern RZ, Halliday W, et al. Neurological manifestations of West Nile virus infection. Can J Neurol Sci 2004; 31(2):185–193.
23. Cowand JL, Wrisley DM, Walker M, et al. Efficacy of vestibular rehabilitation. Otolaryngol Head Neck Surg 1998; 118(1):49–54.
24. Tyler M, Danilov Y, Bach-Y-Rita P. Closing an open-loop control system: vestibular substitution through the tongue. J Integr Neurosci 2003; 2(2):159–164.

27

Tinnitus

Erik S. Viirre and Quyen Nguyen
Department of Surgery, Division of Otolaryngology-Head and Neck Surgery and School of Medicine, University of California, San Diego, California, U.S.A.

INTRODUCTION

Almost all people periodically experience sound sensations that they ultimately realize are coming from inside their ears or inside their head. These sensations are called tinnitus. Most often the cause of tinnitus is related to the hearing system itself, such as the tinnitus that occurs with hearing loss. However, there are a variety of systemic diseases that are associated with tinnitus. To discuss the etiologies underlying the tinnitus types that are associated with systemic conditions, we will use the categories of tinnitus labeled "objective" and "subjective". For an overview of disease and tinnitus, we will first examine some epidemiologic links to tinnitus.

EPIDEMIOLOGY OF TINNITUS

It has been found through epidemiologic studies that although chronic tinnitus is quite common and is found in both men and women, young and old, it is typically the elderly male who has spent a lifetime working in an industrial job who is most commonly diagnosed with tinnitus [(1), pp. 16–41]. Interestingly, across multiple epidemiologic studies from different countries, the prevalence of tinnitus shows a strong correlation with level of hearing loss. The more severe the hearing loss, the stronger is the perception of tinnitus. Although there is also a direct correlation with increasing age, male sex, lower income, lower education, and poor overall health status [(1), pp. 16–41], surveys of the available literature suggest that once hearing level is accounted for, the above correlations are no longer as strong.

OBJECTIVE TINNITUS

Objective tinnitus is a physical sound that emanates from the body, such as pulsing blood flow through the great vessels in the neck or tetanic contractions of the stapedius muscle on the tympanic membrane. With a stethoscope, microphone, or just the unaided ear, an observer can sometimes hear an objective tinnitus. Objective sounds in the head are relatively rare. In objective tinnitus, etiologies can be separated in terms of whether the tinnitus is pulsatile or nonpulsatile. Pulsatile tinnitus has a rhythmic/repeating periodicity. Pulsatile tinnitus can have a musculoskeletal, vascular, or respiratory etiology. Most of the cases of objective tinnitus are local in origin, such as musculoskeletal activity from the stapedius muscle, tensor tympani muscle spasms in the middle ear, or myoclonus of the palate (Table 1). Vascular causes such as arteriovenous shunts, glomus tumors, high-riding dehiscent jugular bulbs, aberrant carotid arteries, persistent stapedial arteries, and microvascular compression can cause pulsatile tinnitus through a structural mechanism. Another rare condition that results in pulsating noises in the head is pseudotumor cerebri, which results from intracranial hypertension; this is discussed in detail in Chapter 24. However, systemic disorders can present with a pulsing sound through generation of high-speed vascular flow with audible turbulence. Hyperdynamic states such as pregnancy (2), anemia [(1), p. 257], hypertension, and hyperthyroidism [(3), p. 13] cause tinnitus. Another local cause of pulsatile tinnitus may be airflow through a patulous eustachian tube (Table 1). Objective nonpulsatile tinnitus may be recordable but may not necessarily have a rhythmic/repeating periodicity. Etiologies of objective nonpulsatile tinnitus include temporomandibular joint dysfunction, spontaneous otoacoustic emissions, and superior/posterior canal dehiscence syndrome (Table 2). These are all local causes of an objective sound.

TABLE 1 Etiologies of Objective Pulsatile Tinnitus

Musculoskeletal	Arteriovenous shunts
Stapedial muscle spasm	Congenital AVM
Tensor tympani muscle spasm	Posttraumatic AVM
Palatal myoclonus	Glomus tumors
Vascular	*Hyperdynamic cardiovascular system*
Arterial	**Pseudotumor cerebri**
Aberrant carotid artery	**Pregnancy**
Carotid stenosis	**Anemia**
Persistent stapedial artery	**Hyperthyroidism**
Venous	**Hypertension**
High-riding dehiscent jugular bulb	**Respiratory**
Sigmoid/transverse sinus obstruction	Patulous eustachian tube

Note: Systemic disorders are highlighted in bold type.
Abbreviation: AVM, arteriovenous malformations.
Source: From Ref. 1.

SUBJECTIVE TINNITUS

In contrast to objective tinnitus, subjective tinnitus appears to be an inappropriate activation of the auditory system. At some point in the multilink pathway of translation of sound pressure waves in the air to neural code in the brain, there is activity that is not normally present. The higher centers in the brain interpret this inappropriate activity as a sound, despite the absence of a true sound stimulus. It appears that there can be triggers for the inappropriate activity anywhere along the chain of structures in the auditory system. Perhaps the most common cause of tinnitus is not a systemic disease, but a local one: hearing loss. It is theorized (4) that autoregulatory mechanisms in the auditory system trying to compensate for the hearing loss are overactive resulting in generation of signals that the higher cortical auditory centers interpret as sound. The sound sensations in subjective tinnitus are quite varied but are commonly described as "buzzing," "ringing," "hissing," or similar sounds. The phenomenon of tinnitus with hearing loss is analogous to the "phantom limb pain" phenomenon, where cortical stimulation is perceived in the absence of external input. Our understanding of tinnitus causes is still rudimentary, however, as a large number of people with tinnitus appear to have no known auditory or systemic pathology.

Through understanding that there can be inappropriate activations of the auditory system presenting as tinnitus, we can determine possible pathogenic links from systemic diseases that result in the generation of inappropriate sound sensations. In our review of systemic diseases that can cause tinnitus, we will go by body systems and their known pathologies.

Neurologic System

Interestingly, most tumors of the nervous system are silent with respect to the auditory system. However, tumors located on the eighth nerve can cause an insidious compression of the nerve and progressive loss of hearing, and result in the appearance of tinnitus. These

TABLE 2 Etiologies of Objective Nonpulsatile Tinnitus

Temporomandibular joint dysfunction
Superior canal dehiscence syndrome
Posterior canal dehiscence syndrome

acoustic neuromas are well described elsewhere (5). The very common condition of migraine can present with tinnitus. Migraine may be a genetic calcium channel defect of neurons and can present with multiple unusual manifestations (see Chapter 23 for detailed discussion of migraines). Cure (6) gives a report of multiple sclerosis (MS) patients presenting with tinnitus. MS lesions can appear throughout the brain and spinal cord and thus could be expected to affect locations in the auditory system, reduce signal transmission, and activate the compensatory mechanisms that result in tinnitus.

Psychological Disorders

There is an increased incidence of depression and anxiety in people with tinnitus, and the converse also appears to be true. There are direct limbic inputs to a variety of locations in the auditory system and these inputs can make the auditory system more sensitive. Thus, an abnormal percept of sound from activation of the auditory system could also be activated or enhanced from the limbic system. High levels of stress or anxiety, therefore, could present as tinnitus [(1), p. 278].

Musculoskeletal System

The auditory nerve passes through the auditory canal of the temporal bone on its way to the brainstem. The auditory canal may be very narrow, and as described above with acoustic neuromas, impingement of the nerve can result in hearing loss and tinnitus. Systemic bony diseases, such as osteogenesis imperfecta or Paget's disease (Chapter 21), can result in bony overgrowth. Thus, the canal can become narrowed, impinge on the nerve, and present as tinnitus (7).

Endocrine System

Disorders of the endocrine system can appear with tinnitus, although the mechanism is sometimes unclear. Addison's disease can present with hyperacusis, a condition closely related to tinnitus (8). Hyperacusis is a subjective sensitivity to sound where people find sounds of intensities typical in the world to be uncomfortable. Approximately 50% of people with tinnitus have hyperacusis. Hypothyroidism can present with tinnitus [(3), p. 32]. There may be a link between subclinical depression, hypothyroidism, and tinnitus. As described above, the hyperdynamic cardiac state that appears in pregnancy can result in a pulsatile objective tinnitus; however, the hormonal changes that occur with pregnancy and premenstrually also appear to have an influence on the auditory system and can trigger the common subjective tinnitus sensations.

Paraneoplastic syndrome was first described by Moersch (9). In this syndrome, malignant tumors manifest antibody sites against which immune responses are developed. The immune responses can cross-react with neural tissues, typically cerebellar or brainstem. Thus, unusually, tinnitus may be the first manifestation of a remote pulmonary or renal tumor (10). Soon after the appearance of tinnitus, more severe brainstem or cerebellar symptoms appear, including ataxia, hearing loss, diplopia, and uncontrollable nystagmus.

Immune System

Immune activation against tissues in the auditory system can damage auditory function and result in a secondary tinnitus. Generalized autoimmune disorders such as systemic lupus erythematosus and rheumatoid arthritis are associated with tinnitus; these are discussed in detail in Chapter 1. Further, the autoimmune diseases of the ear, such as Cogan's syndrome (Chapter 6), can result in bilateral hearing loss and the appearance of tinnitus [(1), p. 56].

Other Causes

Infectious. Although infections of the various structures of the ear might well be expected to affect hearing and thus trigger tinnitus, infections of locations remote to the ear can do the same. Meningitides can cause tinnitus, as can Bell's palsy. Syphilis (Chapter 15) can affect the labyrinth as well as the rest of the nervous system. Finally, it is curious that Lyme disease can have a hearing manifestation. As described above under endocrine disorders with Addison's disease, hyperacusis is associated with tinnitus and with Lyme disease. Fallon (11) reports that 48% of their cohort of Lyme disease had hyperacusis.

Genetic. There are familial hearing loss disorders that can have associated tinnitus. Williams syndrome, which has manifestations throughout multiple body systems, has a 95% incidence of hyperacusis (12). There has been one report of a familial objective tinnitus that is presumably genetic in nature [(1), p. 350]. As described above, tumors on the eighth nerve can present with tinnitus. The condition of neurofibroma type II is familial and results in multiple fibromas on nerves throughout the body. Unfortunately, both auditory nerves are common sites for these fibromas and they may first appear as tinnitus (13).

Iatrogenic. Treatments that result in cases of tinnitus are obviously indirect manifestations of a systemic disease. There have been many thorough reviews of pharmaceuticals that cause tinnitus. Table 3 is adapted from Snow [(1), p. 273]. The prototypical pharmaceutical that has tinnitus as an adverse effect is acetylsalicylic acid (ASA). ASA was first described to result in tinnitus in the 1850s when it was developed for clinical use (14). Indeed, today "ringing in the ears" is used as a clinical sign of ASA overdose. Thus systemic diseases such as headache, arthritis, and other causes of pain, when treated with ASA, "cause" tinnitus. Further, it may well be that successful treatment of a systemic disease "causes" tinnitus to be relieved by obviating the need for symptomatic management that indirectly causes tinnitus. It is suggested that successful management of temporomandibular joint disorders might relieve tinnitus by reducing the need for ASA or non-steroidal anti-inflammatory (NSAIDs) [(3), p. 228].

Returning to the two types of tinnitus, there are two general mechanisms by which drugs can cause tinnitus: increasing activity that causes objective tinnitus and increasing activity that causes subjective tinnitus. For example, taking an angiotensin-converting enzyme inhibitor could cause a hyperdynamic cardiac state. The increased blood flow can be just enough for the vibration sensors in the auditory system to activate, and a pulsatile tinnitus could appear after taking the drug. In contrast, ASA is apparently toxic to the outer hair cells in the cochlea. Thus, direct stimulation of these cells by ASA gives rise to the ringing. In Table 3, the mechanism of tinnitus production by a drug is given, where understood.

TABLE 3 Pharmacologic Causes of Tinnitus

Pharmaceutical	Possible mechanism
Acetylsalicylic acid	Hair-cell toxicity
NSAIDs	Hair-cell toxicity
Cis-platinum	Hair-cell toxicity
Caffeine	Central nervous system stimulant
ACE inhibitors	Cardiac hyperdynamic state
α-adrenergic blockers	Cardiac hyperdynamic state
Benzimidazole inhibitors	Unknown

Abbreviations: NSAIDs, non steroidal anti-inflammatory; ACE. angiotensin-converting enzyme.

FURTHER READING

For complete reviews of tinnitus including epidemiology, experimental research, and clinical management, the reader is referred to the excellent monographs by Tyler (3) and Snow (1). For a briefer outline that emphasizes clinical approaches to tinnitus, Baloh (15) is recommended.

REFERENCES

1. Snow JB Jr. Tinnitus: Theory and Management. Lewiston, NY: BC Decker, 2004.
2. Gurr P, Owen G, Reid A, et al. Tinnitus in pregnancy. Clin Otolaryngol Allied Sci 1993; 18(4): 294–297.
3. Tyler R. Tinnitus Handbook. San Diego, CA: Singular: [South] Africa, 2000.
4. Jastreboff PJ, Gray WC, Gold SL. Neurophysiological approach to tinnitus patients. Am J Otol 1996; 17(2):236–240.
5. Raut VV, Walsh RM, Bath AP, et al. Conservative management of vestibular schwannomas—second review of a prospective longitudinal study. Clin Otolaryngol Allied Sci 2004; 29(5):505–514.
6. Cure JK, Cromwell LD, Case JL, et al. Auditory dysfunction caused by multiple sclerosis: detection with MR imaging. AJNR Am J Neuroradiol 1990; 11(4):817–820.
7. Nager GT. Paget's disease of the temporal bone. Ann Otol Rhinol Laryngol 1975; 84(4 Pt 3 suppl 22):1–32.
8. Henkin RI, Daly RL. Auditory detection and perception in normal man and in patients with adrenal cortical insufficiency: effect of adrenal cortical steroids. J Clin Invest 1968; 47(6):1269–1280.
9. Moersch FP, Woltman HW. Progressive fluctuating muscular rigidity and spasm ("stiff-man" syndrome); report of a case and some observations in 13 other cases. Mayo Clin Proc 1956; 31(15):421–427.
10. Savastano M, Bottin R, Andreoli C, et al. Tinnitus as a presenting symptom in secondary neuropathy: a case report. Int Tinnitus J 1995; 1(2):153–154.
11. Fallon BA, Nields JA, Burrascano JJ, et al. The neuropsychiatric manifestations of Lyme borreliosis. Psychiatr Q 1992; 63(1):95–117.
12. Nigam A, Samuel PR. Hyperacusis and Williams syndrome. J Laryngol Otol 1994; 108(6):494–496.
13. Drsata J, Celakovsky P, Vokurka J, et al. Neurofibromatosis 2: two case reports. Int Tinnitus J 2003; 9 (2):116–118.
14. McCabe PA, Dey FL. The effect of aspirin upon auditory sensitivity. Ann Otol Rhinol Laryngol 1965; 74:312–325.
15. Baloh RW. Dizziness, Hearing Loss, and Tinnitus. New York, NY: FA Davis Co., 1998.

28

Sensorineural Hearing Loss

Joel Guss and Michael J. Ruckenstein
Department of Otorhinolaryngology: Head and Neck Surgery, University of Pennsylvania School of Medicine, Philadelphia, Pennsylvania, U.S.A.

INTRODUCTION

Hearing loss resulting from dysfunction of the inner ear or the eighth cranial nerve is a common patient complaint, particularly in the aging population. Most commonly, sensorineural hearing loss results from a disease process that is specific to the ear; common examples include presbycusis (hearing loss associated with aging) and hearing loss secondary to noise exposure. However, there are multisystemic diseases associated with inner ear or vestibulocochlear nerve pathology. In addition, certain treatments of systemic diseases may be ototoxic. This chapter will review those systemic disease processes that can cause sensorineural hearing loss.

DEFINITION

Sensorineural hearing loss is defined as an increase in the sound reception threshold secondary to dysfunction of the inner ear or the cochlear branch of the eighth cranial nerve. In contrast, conductive hearing loss results from pathology within the external, or, more commonly, the middle ear. In mixed hearing loss, there are both conductive and sensorineural components. The vast majority of systemic diseases are associated with sensorineural hearing loss. One notable exception is Wegener's granulomatosis, which commonly manifests with middle-ear pathology; this is discussed in detail in Chapter 8.

PATHOGENESIS

There are a variety of sites within the auditory apparatus that may be affected by multisystemic diseases. The external and middle ear serve primarily to amplify the sound stimulus. Particularly critical to this function are the tympanic membrane and middle ear bones (ossicles). The inner ear functions to convert the acoustic energy transmitted to the cochlea into an electrical signal that is transmitted to the central nervous system (CNS) via the eighth cranial nerve afferent fibers. This task falls specifically to the sensory receptors within the cochlea known as the inner hair cells. The adjacent outer hair cells participate in this process by maintaining the precise tuning of the cochlea (i.e., the ability of the cochlea to transmit the precise pitch characteristics of the stimulus that ultimately correspond to stimulus clarity). The bipolar cell bodies of the cochlear nerve fibers reside in the spiral ganglion. Axons from these cells form the cochlear nerve and terminate in the ipsilateral cochlear nucleus, from which projections are sent bilaterally to ultimately terminate in the auditory cortex.

Hair-cell function is dependent on the cochlea maintaining precise electrolyte concentrations within its fluid-containing compartments. These fluid compartments, known as the cochlear ducts (scalae), contain either a solution analogous to intracellular (endolymph) or an extracellular (perilymph) fluid. The endolymphatic compartment (scala media), with its high potassium concentrations, is tightly isolated from the sodium-rich perilymphatic compartments (scala vestibuli and scala tympani). The maintenance of these gradients creates an electrochemical gradient of 80 to 100 mV that drives hair-cell depolarization—the key process in auditory stimulus transmission to afferent nerve fibers. These electrolyte concentrations in the scala media are maintained by Na^+-K^+-ATPase enzyme on the surface of cells in the stria vascularis, a highly vascular and metabolic tissue. Gap junctions are intercellular channels formed by proteins called connexins and are thought to be important in electrolyte metabolism in the stria vascularis and other inner ear supporting cells. Mutations in a gene (*GJB2*) coding for connexin 26 are an important cause of genetic hearing loss. Blood supply to the cochlea is exclusively from the labyrinthine artery, which is usually a branch of the anterior inferior cerebellar artery.

Sensorineural hearing loss results when one or more components of the inner ear or cochlear nerve are damaged. For example, hearing loss associated with aging (presbycusis) is associated with hair-cell, stria vascularis, and neural pathologies. Noise and most ototoxins primarily affect hair cells, although other cochlear structures may also be involved. The following discussion pertains to systemic diseases that may result in auditory pathology.

CLINICAL MANIFESTATIONS

Genetic Diseases

Congenital hearing loss is common, and about one-half of cases are thought to be genetic. Genetic hearing loss is typically classified as syndromic or nonsyndromic. When hearing loss consistently coexists with other pathologic findings, it is considered part of a syndrome; when it exists in isolation, it is nonsyndromic. As our focus is on systemic diseases, nonsyndromic hearing loss, which accounts for two-thirds of hereditary hearing loss, will not be discussed extensively. Mutations in the *GJB2* gene coding for connexin 26 are now thought to account for over half of the cases of nonsyndromic genetic hearing loss (1). Nearly 100 mutations have been identified, some being quite specific to individual ethnic groups. Hearing loss tends to be moderate to severe, symmetric, and nonprogressive. There are no associated temporal bone malformations, and patients tend to do well after cochlear implantation.

There are more than 400 syndromes associated with sensorineural hearing loss. It is important not to confuse genetic hearing loss with congenital hearing loss. While genetic hearing loss may be present at birth, it may also appear later in life. The pattern of inheritance may be autosomal dominant or recessive, X-linked, or mitochondrial. A complete list of syndromes is the subject of complete textbooks; as such, several prominent syndromes with multisystemic manifestations are reviewed below.

Pendred Syndrome. Pendred syndrome is an autosomal-recessive mutation of the *PDS* gene, thought to encode a chloride–iodide transporting enzyme (2). Manifestations include a euthyroid, multinodular goiter by the second decade, congenital deafness, and an abnormal perchlorate discharge test. Temporal bone imaging typically demonstrates a Mondini-type cochlear malformation in which the cochlea is incompletely formed.

Jervell and Lange-Nielsen Syndrome. Jervell and Lange-Nielsen syndrome is marked by bilateral severe sensorineural hearing loss in association with electrocardiographic evidence of a prolonged QT interval and syncopal attacks during childhood (3). Sudden death may occur. Inheritance is autosomal recessive.

Alport Syndrome. Alport syndrome is predominantly X-linked, although some cases are autosomal recessive. It is the most common cause of hereditary nephritis in the United States and is marked by progressive high-frequency sensorineural hearing loss, hematuria, and ocular malformations. Symptoms appear during the first decade, and all males progress to end-stage renal failure. The mutation involves genes encoding type IV collagen (4).

Branchio-Oto-Renal Syndrome. Also affecting the kidneys is the branchio-oto-renal (BOR) syndrome with renal anomalies, multiple branchial cleft cysts, fistulae and sinuses, and hearing loss that may be purely sensorineural but is typically mixed. External-, middle-, and inner-ear malformations are common. BOR is autosomal dominant and caused by mutations in the *EYA1* gene (5).

Neurofibromatosis Type 2. Neurofibromatosis (NF) type 2 is a multisystemic disease resulting from mutation of the *NF2* gene (6). Inheritance is autosomal dominant, although half of the cases represent de novo mutations. Bilateral vestibular schwannomas are the best-known feature of the disease. Patients most commonly present with unilateral sensorineural hearing loss, but bilateral deafness eventually develops. Dumbbell-shaped spinal cord schwannomas, intracranial meningiomas, other CNS tumors, and "juvenile cataracts" are also associated with this syndrome. Notably absent are the cutaneous manifestations of NF1 (i.e., café au lait spots, axillary freckling, and cutaneous neurofibromas). Rarely, NF1 can involve the eighth cranial nerve.

Mitochondrial Syndromes. The mitochondrial syndromes are a fascinating set of diseases, and sensorineural hearing loss is a common component. Mitochondrial DNA forms a closed circular molecule similar to that seen in prokaryotes and codes for 13 proteins, mostly involved in oxidative metabolism. All the mitochondrial DNA in an individual is inherited from the mother, because the oocyte contributes all of the cytoplasm and organelles to the embryo. Male and female offspring are affected equally. Penetrance of mutations is complex, because there are about 100,000 copies of the mitochondrial chromosome in each cell (as opposed to only two copies of each nuclear chromosome).

The A1555G mitochondrial DNA mutation is associated with nonsyndromic hearing loss and an increased sensitivity to aminoglycoside toxicity. Hearing loss may develop several months after administration of the antibiotic and is thought to account for up to one-third of aminoglycoside-induced hearing loss (7). Mitochondrial encephalopathy, lactic acidosis, and stroke-like (MELAS) syndrome is characterized by strokes and encephalopathy at an early age, myopathy and metabolic acidosis, recurrent headaches and vomiting, as well as other systemic manifestations (8). A bilateral symmetric, progressive, high-frequency sensorineural hearing loss is seen in 70% of the patients. In maternally inherited diabetes and deafness, hearing loss precedes glucose intolerance and both tend to occur in adulthood (8). Kearns–Sayre syndrome is characterized by progressive external ophthalmoplegia, cardiac conduction abnormalities, retinitis pigmentosa, and ataxia. Onset is before the age of 20 and sensorineural hearing loss is seen in 60% of the cases (8).

Infectious Diseases

Hearing loss is an uncommon presenting symptom of a systemic infectious disease but may develop during the course of several viral and bacterial infections. Pathogens may infect the inner ear and auditory pathways in utero, resulting in congenital syndromes that often include deafness, or infection may be acquired after birth. As the fluids of the inner ear are not easily accessible for sampling, the implication of viral pathogens as the causes of sensorineural hearing loss has often depended on circumstantial evidence, including an associated viral illness—for example, an upper respiratory infection—or demonstration of seroconversion during the time of hearing loss.

Cytomegalovirus. Cytomegalovirus (CMV) is a large, double-stranded DNA virus belonging to the herpesvirus family. Its name is derived from the typical appearance of infected tissues, containing massively enlarged cytomegalic inclusion cells. CMV is the most common congenital infection in the world. Of babies born in the United States, 1% are infected; the likely route of infection is transplacental. Of these babies, 10% will exhibit symptomatic infection or cytomegalic inclusion disease, almost exclusively when primary maternal infection occurs during pregnancy. Of those babies that survive the neonatal period, the majority will have severe neurologic deficits and severe bilateral sensorineural hearing loss. Possibly more significant, from an epidemiologic point of view, is hearing loss that develops in those children with apparently asymptomatic congenital CMV infection (9).

Between 6% and 23% of these infants will go on to develop sensorineural hearing loss. Most cases will be mild, but up to one-quarter will be severe. Hearing loss may be unilateral or bilateral and may develop months or years after birth and be missed on routine audiometric screening. It is thought that asymptomatic CMV infection causes 20% to 30% of congenital hearing loss. In the healthy adult, CMV infection is usually asymptomatic or may cause a mononucleosis-like syndrome. In human immunodeficiency virus (HIV)-infected or transplant patients, severe multisystemic disease may ensue, but hearing loss is not common.

Rubella. Rubella is a member of the *Togaviridae* family. The significance of this virus is that primary maternal infection during the first trimester of pregnancy may result in the congenital rubella syndrome. Sensorineural hearing loss is the most common manifestation, seen in up to 60% of affected infants. Hearing loss may be bilateral or unilateral, may manifest as late as the second year of life, and may be the only sign of infection (10). Other features are ocular malformations including cataracts and retinopathy, cardiac malformations, and CNS disease. Postnatal infection produces German measles, a mild viral illness.

Varicella-Zoster Virus. Varicella-zoster virus (VZV) is also a herpes virus. Primary VZV infection results in varicella, or chickenpox. Once primary infection is cleared, VZV remains dormant in the dorsal root ganglia. Reactivation of the virus, often during periods of suppressed cellular immunity, results in shingles, or a dermatomal vesicular eruption. Reactivation of VZV in the geniculate ganglion results in a painful vesicular eruption in the external ear, known as herpes zoster oticus. When facial paralysis accompanies these other symptoms, the disorder is known as Ramsay Hunt syndrome. Extension of the inflammatory process to involve the vestibulocochlear nerve may result in sensorineural hearing loss and vertigo.

Mumps and Measles Viruses. Mumps and measles viruses are members of the paramyxoviridae family; infection is rare in the developed world since vaccination began, although it is common worldwide. Mumps infection commonly presents with unilateral or bilateral parotitis and orchitis in males. Sensorineural hearing loss is uncommon, affecting less than 0.05% of patients, and tends to be unilateral. Similarly, hearing loss is uncommon in measles infection, seen in approximately 0.1% of patients (10). The classic presentation of measles involves cough, coryza, conjunctivitis, white oral mucosal lesions known as Koplik spots, and a maculopapular rash.

Human Immunodeficiency Virus. HIV infection is associated with a significant incidence of sensorineural hearing loss, although this relationship is not fully understood. The etiology is likely variable and includes a high incidence of middle-ear disease, opportunistic infections and malignancies of the CNS, viral labyrinthitis and neuritis, meningitis, and ototoxicity from medications used to treat HIV infection and its complications (11). HIV is discussed in detail in Chapter 16.

Meningitis. Most bacterial infections involving the inner ear represent extension of inflammation or infection from the CNS, or, less commonly, the middle ear. Meningitis may result in bacterial invasion of the labyrinth via the internal auditory canal or the cochlear aqueduct. Sensorineural hearing loss is a common complication of meningitis, particularly in children. Up to one-third of patients with bacterial meningitis sustain some loss of hearing (12). The hearing loss is typically bilateral and stable, though it may be unilateral and progressive or fluctuating. Male sex, computed tomography (CT) scan evidence of elevated intracranial pressure, nuchal rigidity, low cerebrospinal fluid (CSF) glucose levels, and *Streptococcus pneumoniae* as the infective agent are all associated with an increased incidence of postmeningitic sensorineural hearing loss (13).

Otitis Media. Acute otitis media can produce a sterile serous labyrinthitis secondary to the passage of bacterial toxins and inflammatory mediators into the inner ear fluids, likely through the round window or a dehiscent lateral semicircular canal in patients with chronic middle-ear disease and cholesteatoma. This typically causes a mild high-frequency hearing loss. Entrance of bacteria into the inner ear will lead to a suppurative labyrinthitis, which is heralded by severe hearing loss and vertigo (14).

Syphilis. Syphilis may cause sensorineural hearing loss in its congenital or acquired form. The disease is caused by a spirochete, *Treponema pallidum*. Infection may be sexually transmitted or may be acquired in utero. Congenital infection usually spreads through the placenta, although it may be acquired during delivery, and most commonly occurs with maternal primary or secondary infection during pregnancy. There is a high incidence of stillbirth in fetuses infected with syphilis; of those that are born alive, one of two syndromes may result. Early congenital syphilis refers to manifestations within the first two years of life and is usually fatal. It occurs as a result of active systemic infection. Symptoms of early congenital syphilis include skeletal malformations, organomegaly, rash, CNS disease, and syphilitic rhinitis (snuffles) productive of purulent secretions rich in spirochetes. Late congenital syphilis presents after the age of two and results from residual scarring and inflammation from earlier infection; it may present with hearing loss in childhood but also as late as the third or fourth decade of life (15). The hearing loss can present suddenly and may be associated with vestibular symptoms (16). Hutchinson's triad of late congenital syphilis includes Hutchinson's teeth (notched central incisors), interstitial keratitis of the eye, and sensorineural hearing loss.

Acquired syphilis is sexually transmitted in almost all cases. The course and pathogenesis of the disease is elaborate. The spirochete penetrates intact mucous membranes and spreads systemically long before the primary lesion appears. The primary lesion is the chancre, a painless ulcerative lesion at the site of inoculation associated with regional lymphadenopathy; it heals in four to six weeks. Secondary syphilis represents disseminated infection and appears 6 to 12 weeks after the primary lesion. Constitutional symptoms, a maculopapular rash involving the palms and soles, condyloma lata, and mucous patches are the most common manifestations. With resolution of untreated secondary disease, a period of latency begins. The late or tertiary manifestations of syphilis appear years after the primary infection, although they probably represent the end-stage of a pathologic process that began with inoculation. The major categories of tertiary syphilis include neurosyphilis, cardiovascular syphilis that may result in aortic aneurysms, and gummas, which are benign granulomatous lesions that may occur anywhere in the body (17).

Hearing loss can be associated with early or late acquired syphilis. Sensorineural hearing loss arising during the secondary stage of syphilis is thought to result from a basilar meningitis affecting the cochlear nerve. This appears as a sudden, rapidly deteriorating, bilateral hearing loss. Luetic labyrinthitis may develop as part of late acquired syphilis and presents in a variable manner with asymmetric involvement being common. Vestibular symptoms may be more prominent than hearing loss. Gummas may form along the brainstem, the eighth nerve, and the temporal bone and vestibule and result in sensorineural hearing loss (16). Syphilis is discussed in greater detail in Chapter 15.

Lyme Disease. Sensorineural hearing loss has also been reported in association with infection with another spirochete, *Borrelia burgdorferi*, the causative organism of Lyme disease. The organism is introduced into the skin by the bite of an infected tick of the genus Ixodes. The spirochete has particular tropism to the skin, CNS, heart, joints, and eyes. It is not fully clear which features are a result of disseminated infection and which result from the systemic inflammatory response. In the head and neck, Lyme disease is most commonly associated with facial paresis, particularly in children. There have been reports of sudden sensorineural hearing loss or a Ménière's-like syndrome in Europe (Selmanzi Z), although there has yet to be an association between Lyme disease and inner-ear pathology in North America (18,19).

Autoimmune Diseases

Autoimmune inflammation of the inner ear may occur in isolation as an organ-specific process or may be part of a systemic autoimmune syndrome (20). Evidence is mounting to support the existence of an organ-specific cochlear autoimmune disease. The presence of antibodies to cochlear antigens, such as the 68 kD inner-ear antigen, as well as an impressive response to immunosuppressive medications, implicate autoimmunity as the underlying pathologic process in some patients with "idiopathic" sensorineural hearing loss. These patients with autoimmune inner-ear disease (more accurately termed immune-mediated inner-ear disease, since proof for autoimmunity is still lacking) have a fluctuating progressive sensorineural hearing loss, often associated with vertigo and tinnitus. Generally, hearing loss progresses rapidly, within a period of weeks and months, to an irreversible end-stage disease. While at any given moment, one ear may be more significantly affected, the process eventually affects both ears.

Cogan's syndrome (Chapter 6) is a rare disease characterized by nonsyphilitic interstitial keratitis associated with vertigo, tinnitus, and hearing loss (21). If the same labyrinthine complaints are associated with other forms of ocular inflammation (e.g., uveitis and episcleritis), the condition is known as atypical Cogan's disease. The auditory and vestibular dysfunction resembles that seen in Ménière's disease and, untreated, progresses to profound deafness within weeks or months. The interval between ocular and otologic disease varies from a few weeks to a year; either organ may be affected first. The etiology of Cogan's syndrome is unknown. While the relatively focal inflammation suggests organ-specific autoimmunity, this has not been proven. Like other vasculitides, the disease may represent a hypersensitive immune reaction to a viral infection.

The systemic vasculitides may involve the labyrinth. Wegener's granulomatosis (Chapter 8) is a systemic vasculitis of medium and small blood vessels resulting in a triad of necrotizing granulomas of the upper airway, necrotizing glomeruloncphritis, and systemic necrotizing angiitis. Chronic otitis media is the most common otologic manifestation of Wegener's, but sensorineural hearing loss will occur in a significant number of patients. Immune-mediated inner-ear disease can also be a component of polyarteritis nodosa (PAN). Postmortem temporal bone histopathologic studies on patients with PAN have demonstrated vasculitic changes within the labyrinth. Systemic lupus erythematosus, rheumatoid arthritis, Sjögren's syndrome, and relapsing polychondritis have also been associated with cases of sudden hearing loss and histopathologic evidence of labyrinthitis.

Ototoxicity

The major ototoxic agents in use remain cisplatin and aminoglycosides. Cisplatin ototoxicity manifests as hearing loss, while aminoglycosides may cause auditory and/or vestibular complaints. Gentamicin and streptomycin are much more likely to present with vestibular complaints, specifically imbalance. In contrast, amikacin, kanamycin, and dihydrostreptomycin are more toxic to the cochlea. Tobramycin carries an approximately equivalent risk of toxicity to the cochlea and vestibular labyrinth.

Loop diuretics and vancomycin are rarely ototoxic on their own; more commonly, they potentiate the ototoxic effects of the aminoglycosides or cisplatin. High-dose intravenous erythromycin may cause a reversible sensorineural hearing loss. Quinine derivatives and salicylates can cause reversible tinnitus.

DIAGNOSIS

The vast majority of patients with hearing loss need only an audiogram to confirm the diagnosis. As stated earlier, most of these patients will be diagnosed with diseases limited to the inner ear such as presbycusis, noise-induced hearing loss, and ototoxicity. Asymmetry in hearing loss warrants the performance of magnetic resonance imaging (MRI) scan with paramagnetic enhancement to rule out a retrocochlear etiology.

In the pediatric patient with unilateral sensorineural hearing loss, a CT scan is warranted to rule out a bony malformation of the inner ear. A young patient with bilateral hearing loss should undergo genetic testing for Connexin 26 (*GJB2*) mutations. Other tests that have been advocated in the workup of pediatric patients for sensorineural hearing loss include urinalysis (Alport), electrocardiogram (EKG) (Jervell and Lange-Nielsen), thyroid function tests (Pendred), and electroretinography (Usher). Newer studies question the cost-effectiveness of ordering these tests in the absence of other history or physical findings implicating these syndromes.

A small fraction of adult patients will present with symptoms of hearing loss that warrant further investigation. Unfortunately, our testing options remain limited and often rely on circumstantial evidence. Patients with sudden unilateral sensorineural hearing loss require an audiogram and an MRI scan. Further testing is usually not warranted.

Patients with rapidly progressive sensorineural hearing loss (evolving over weeks to months), be it unilateral or bilateral, require a workup for autoimmune disease and syphilis. The screening tests have not been standardized and vary somewhat between sites. Our screening evaluation typically involved obtaining complete blood count (CBC), sedimentation rate, electrolytes, blood urea nitrogen (BUN), creatinine, urinalysis, antinuclear antibody (ANA) screen, rheumatoid factor, anti-Sjögren's antibodies, C3 & C4 levels, antinuclear cytoplasmic antibody (c-ANCA), antiphospholipid antibody screen, Lyme titers, and fluorescent treponemal antibody-absorption test (microhemagglutination assay for antibodies to *T. pallidum*) (FTA-ABS [MHA-TP]). Western blot for heat-shock protein 70 (HSP-70) may be supportive of a diagnosis of "autoimmune" steroid-responsive sensorineural hearing loss. In our screening of over 300 patients with progressive, idiopathic sensorineural hearing loss, only ANA levels (in bilateral disease) and antiphospholipid antibodies have shown any significant elevations. Patients with very rapidly progressive bilateral sensorineural hearing loss (evolving over days to weeks) should also undergo a lumbar puncture, for analysis of CSF for infection and malignancy.

TREATMENT

Medications

Many treatments have been advocated for sudden sensorineural hearing loss, which is presumed to be of viral (or rarely vascular) origin. The diagnosis of "autoimmune" inner-ear disease is still predicated by a documented response to corticosteroid administration (20). Treatment strategies have varied between reports, but, in general, a dose of prednisone, 40 to 60 mg in the adult for two weeks, is an appropriate therapeutic trial. Substantial improvement on this dosage regimen would then warrant a slow taper of steroids over several months with close observation for recurrence. Even prompt administration of these doses results in a significant improvement in only approximately 40% to 50% of cases. Antiviral agents, vasodilators, antiplatelet agents, and anticoagulants have no proven role in the management of this entity.

There are several circumstances that warrant special mention. Patients with Ménière's disease and certain forms of genetic hearing loss may manifest spontaneous fluctuations in hearing. In these situations, the administration of steroids at the onset of the hearing loss may result in a false impression that the subsequent spontaneous improvement in hearing was actually the result of steroid administration. Thus, in patients in whom there is question of whether the hearing is actually responding to steroids, it is often prudent to withhold the administration of prednisone for two weeks, to see if there is spontaneous resolution of the hearing loss. If the hearing loss does not resolve during that time frame, then administration of steroids would be warranted and a positive therapeutic response would support the diagnosis of "autoimmune" inner-ear disease.

Patients who show a definite therapeutic response to steroids, but relapse when weaned from these drugs, pose another therapeutic dilemma. To date, an efficacious prednisone-sparing regimen has not been developed. Numerous drugs including methotrexate, azothiaprine, and etanercept have been shown to be ineffective in maintaining patients' hearing. While cyclophosphamide, given as an oral regimen or in monthly intravenous boluses, has traditionally been used in this patient group, its efficacy has not been definitively established. In addition, it carries specific, undesirable complications. In patients who cannot be maintained in remission without chronic use of prednisone, a reasonable alternative is to discontinue treatment, allow the disease to take a natural course, and then utilize a cochlear implant. These patients typically perform extremely well with cochlear implants and can avoid the complications of prolonged use of potentially toxic medications.

Ototoxicity Prophylaxis

Most forms of ototoxicity ultimately result from the generation of free radicals in the affected portions of the inner ear. A considerable amount of basic science literature has accumulated investigating the systemic and transtympanic (through the middle ear) administration of agents that counteract free radical formation. A variety of promising candidates have been identified. Thus, within the coming years, it is reasonable to anticipate the development of an agent or agents that will be administered prophylactically to patients at risk for ototoxic reactions (e.g., patients undergoing chemotherapy with cisplatin).

Prosthetics

Hearing-aid amplification remains the mainstay of rehabilitation for patients with sensorineural hearing loss. Unfortunately, hearings aids are amplifiers, not clarifiers, and, as such, leave patients less than satisfied.

Cochlear implants have revolutionized the management of patients with severe sensorineural hearing loss or deafness. They are the only prosthesis that successfully replaces sensory function. Many objective studies have proven their value in the treatment of pediatric patients' prelingual and postlingual severe-to-profound sensorineural hearing loss, and in adults with postlingual sensorineural hearing loss. Implant devices and surgical techniques have been refined since their introduction and surgical complications are rare. This remains a rapidly expanding and exciting field as software and hardware become more sophisticated and indications for use of these devices broaden.

SUMMARY

The vast majority of cases of sensorineural hearing loss involve processes, be they genetic, aging, or due to noise or ototoxicity, which are specific to the inner ear and/or cochlear nerve and do not require any evaluation for systemic disease. In selected cases, however, an evaluation for systemic infectious or inflammatory disease is warranted. A variety of agents are currently being developed that may allow for the prevention of ototoxicity via the transtympanic administration of these drugs. Hearing aids remain the main form of rehabilitation for patients with hearing loss. Cochlear implants already offer excellent rehabilitation for those patients with severe-to-profound hearing loss, and this technology continues to evolve at a rapid pace.

REFERENCES

1. Kenneson A, Van Naarden Braun K, Boyle C. GJB2 (connexin 26) variants and nonsyndromic sensorineural hearing loss: a HuGE review. Genet Med 2002; 4(4):258–274.
2. Kopp P. Pendred's syndrome: identification of the genetic defect a century after its recognition. Thyroid 1999; 9(1):65–69.
3. Cusimano F, Martines E, Rizzo C. The Jervell and Lange-Nielsen syndrome. Int J Pediatr Otorhinolaryngol 1991; 22(1):49–58.
4. Kashtan CE. Familial hematuria due to type IV collagen mutations: Alport syndrome and thin basement membrane nephropathy. Curr Opin Pediatr 2004; 16(2):177–181.
5. Rodriguez Soriano J. Branchio-oto-renal syndrome. J Nephrol 2003; 16(4):603–605.
6. Uppal S, Coatesworth AP. Neurofibromatosis type 2. Int J Clin Pract 2003; 57(8):698–703.
7. Usami S, Abe S, Shinkawa H, et al. Sensorineural hearing loss caused by mitochondrial DNA mutations: special reference to the A1555G mutation. J Commun Disord 1998; 31(5):423–434.
8. Fischel-Ghodsian N. Mitochondrial deafness. Ear Hear 2003; 24(4):303–313.
9. Fowler KB, Boppana SB. Congenital cytomegalovirus (CMV) infection and hearing deficit. J Clin Virol 2006; 35(2):226–231.
10. Davis LE, Johnsson LG. Viral infections of the inner ear: clinical, virologic, and pathologic studies in humans and animals. Am J Otolaryngol 1983; 4(5):347–362.
11. Gurney TA, Murr AH. Otolaryngologic manifestations of human immunodeficiency virus infection. Otolaryngol Clin North Am 2003; 36(4):607–624.
12. Wellman MB, Sommer DD, McKenna J. Sensorineural hearing loss in postmeningitic children. Otol Neurotol 2003; 24(6):907–912.
13. Woolley AL, Kirk KA, Neumann AM Jr, et al. Risk factors for hearing loss from meningitis in children: the Children's Hospital experience. Arch Otolaryngol Head Neck Surg 1999; 125(5):509–514.
14. Goldstein NA, Casselbrant ML, Bluestone CD, et al. Intratemporal complications of acute otitis media in infants and children. Otolaryngol Head Neck Surg 1998; 119(5):444–454.
15. Azimi P. Syphilis. In: Behrman RE, Kliegman R, Jenson HB, eds. Nelson Textbook of Pediatrics. 17th ed. Philadelphia, PA: WB Saunders Co., 2000:978–982.
16. Zoller M, Wilson WR, Nadol JB Jr, et al. Detection of syphilitic hearing loss. Arch Otolaryngol 1978; 104(2):63–65.
17. Lukehart SA. Syphilis. In: Braunwald E, Fauci AS, Kasper DL, et al., eds. Harrison's Principles of Internal Medicine. 15th ed. New York, NY: McGraw-Hill, 2001:1044–1052.
18. Quinn SJ, Boucher BJ, Booth JB. Reversible sensorineural hearing loss in Lyme disease. J Laryngol Otol 1997; 111(6):562–564.
19. Peltomaa M, Pyykko I, Sappala I, et al. Lyme borreliosis, an etiological factor in sensorineural hearing loss? Eur Arch Otorhinolaryngol 2000; 257(6):317–322.
20. Ruckenstein MJ. Autoimmune inner ear disease. Curr Opin Otolaryngol Head Neck Surg 2004; 12:426–430.
21. St. Clair EW, McCallum RM. Cogan's syndrome. Curr Opin Rheumatol 1999; 11(1):47–52.

29

Facial Nerve Paralysis

Quinton Gopen
Department of Otology and Laryngology, Harvard Medical School, Boston, Massachusetts, U.S.A.

Jeffrey P. Harris
Department of Surgery, Division of Otolaryngology-Head and Neck Surgery, University of California and VA San Diego Healthcare System, San Diego, California, U.S.A.

ANATOMY

The facial nerve is one of 12 cranial nerves. It contains motor nerve fibers responsible for facial expression as well as other nerve fibers involved in sensation, taste, and secretory function. The motor pathway begins within the premotor and motor cortex. Upper motor neurons then connect the premotor and motor cortex to the facial nucleus located within the pons. Lower motor neurons exit from the facial nucleus and continue on to innervate the various mimetic muscles of facial expression. It is important to note that the forehead receives bilateral innervation from the facial nucleus, whereas the remaining facial musculature receives only ipsilateral innervation from the facial nucleus. Along with the muscles of facial expression, the facial nerve innervates the auricular, posterior digastric, stylohyoid, platysma, buccinator, and stapedial muscles.

The facial nerve also contains parasympathetic nerve fibers in charge of the secretory function of the lacrimal gland, submandibular gland, and sublingual gland. This parasympathetic innervation is derived from the superior salivatory nucleus within the pons. These parasympathetic fibers synapse within the sphenopalatine ganglion, stimulating lacrimal gland secretion, and within the submandibular ganglion, stimulating submandibular gland and sublingual gland secretion.

In addition to the motor and autonomic functions of the facial nerve listed above, the facial nerve contains sensory nerve fibers subserving taste from the anterior two-thirds of the tongue via the chordae tympani nerve. These fibers synapse within the geniculate ganglion and continue on to the solitary nucleus within the pons. The facial nerve also innervates cutaneous sensation to the postauricular area, conchae, and a small portion of the superior tympanic membrane. These fibers synapse within the geniculate ganglion and continue on to the spinal nucleus of the trigeminal nerve within the pons.

The course of the facial nerve can be divided into intracranial, intratemporal, and extratemporal segments. The intracranial segment, known as the pontine or cisternal segment, spans roughly 25 mm and connects the facial nerve from its origin in the brainstem to the entrance of the internal auditory canal (IAC), where the intratemporal course of the nerve then begins.

The intratemporal portion can be divided into four segments: meatal, labyrinthine, horizontal, and vertical. The meatal segment courses from the beginning of the medial portion of the IAC, termed the porus acousticus, to the lateral end of the IAC, termed the fundus. The facial nerve lies within the anterosuperior quadrant of the IAC, demarcated by the falciform crest horizontally and Bill's bar vertically. The facial nerve is still ensheathed by an extension of the meninges at this point. The next segment, termed the labyrinthine or petrous segment, is only 5 mm in length and runs from the fundus of the IAC to the geniculate ganglion. It is here that the bony channel through which the nerve runs, the fallopian canal, is at its narrowest dimension of 0.7 mm, leaving the nerve particularly vulnerable to traumatic or compressive forces. The labyrinthine segment contains the geniculate ganglion housing cell bodies for sensation as well as taste. The greater superficial petrosal nerve branches off from the facial nerve here and continues on to supply parasympathetic innervation to the lacrimal gland. At this point, the facial nerve turns abruptly and runs in an anterior-to-posterior plane. This point or turn is termed the first genu of the facial nerve. The next segment, the tympanic or horizontal segment, spans 10 mm in length and continues from the geniculate ganglion to the second genu of the facial nerve. This is the most common site of facial nerve dehiscence, found in half of the population. Once again, the facial nerve has a change in course and at the second genu turns to run in a superior-to-inferior direction. The ensuing mastoid or vertical segment is 15 mm in length and runs from the second genu to the stylomastoid foramen.

Branches to the stapedius muscle and the chordae tympani nerve exit from this segment of the facial nerve. This ends the intratemporal course of the facial nerve.

Once the nerve has left the stylomastoid foramen, it becomes extratemporal and quickly branches at the pes anserinus into the temporozygomatic and cervicofacial divisions. Most often, the facial nerve divides further into five branches: temporal, zygomatic, buccal, marginal mandibular, and cervical. However, numerous branching patterns have been described and the extratemporal nerve course is known to be highly variable.

The arterial supply to the facial nerve is from both the carotid and the vertebrobasilar systems. The meatal segment is supplied by labyrinthine branches of the anterior inferior cerebellar artery (AICA). The labyrinthine segment is supplied by the petrosal artery, a branch of middle meningeal artery coming from the internal maxillary artery. The stylomastoid artery supplies the mastoid and tympanic segments (Fig. 1).

*T*REATMENT

The management of a facial nerve injury is largely dependent on its anticipated return of function. Electrophysiologic testing, such as electroneurography (ENoG), can be helpful in predicting the ultimate prognosis for facial nerve recovery. Electrophysiologic testing is never relevant for paresis, but if the nerve is paralyzed it can be a valuable tool for predicting prognosis for recovery. Care must be taken to time the evaluation appropriately, as a test before Wallerian degeneration has occurred (approximately 72 hours after injury) will be erroneous. Optimal timing is approximately one week after the injury and must be completed within two to three weeks of the injury. The ENoG test uses a stimulating electric current over the peripheral facial nerve branches with the response measured by an electrode placed within the muscles of facial expression. The normal side is evaluated and a comparison between the responses of the two sides is reported. The amplitude of the response measured by the electrode is directly proportional to the number of intact motor

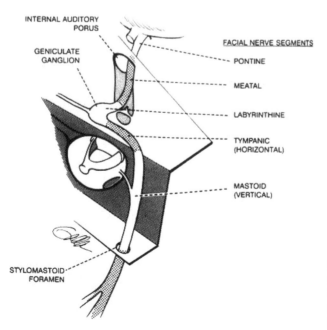

FIGURE 1 Facial nerve segments. *Source:* Courtesy of W. R. Wilson, Parthenon Publishing Group, Boca Raton, FL, U.S.A.

axons. Greater than 90% degeneration within 10 days of paralysis is associated with a 50% chance of poor prognosis (1).

Whether or not recovery is anticipated, management should focus on eye protection. Taping the eye closed at night in addition to frequent eye lubrication is critical to avoiding exposure keratitis and visual loss. Patients often experience increased tearing with facial paralysis, a result of the loss of the pumping action afforded by eyelid closure into the lacrimal canaliculus. If a longer or indefinite period of facial nerve dysfunction is anticipated, reversible therapy such as a gold weight will aid the patient in achieving complete lid closure for as long as needed.

Specific therapy depends on the mechanism of facial nerve injury. If the nerve remains in continuity and the injury is secondary to compression from traumatic, neoplastic, or infectious etiologies, anti-inflammatory medications such as corticosteroids or decompressive surgery may be employed. Antiviral medications are often dispensed in treating Bell's palsy but remain controversial in their efficacy. Decompression of the entire facial nerve can be accomplished with a combined transmastoid and middle cranial fossa approach. If the patient has no usable hearing, a translabyrinthine approach could also be used for complete nerve decompression.

If the nerve has been severed, the first treatment should be direct anastomosis. This is often difficult, given the bony course of the nerve, and defects greater than 1 cm cannot usually be reapproximated even with rerouting maneuvers. If direct anastomosis cannot be completed, cable grafting is the next appropriate step. The greater auricular nerve is an excellent donor nerve, providing up to 10 cm of length. Alternatively, if a longer segment is required, the sural nerve provides up to 25 cm of available length. Occasionally, the proximal end of the nerve is no longer viable or usable; this precludes any attempts at anastomotic reconstruction. In this scenario, the patient may benefit from a hypoglossal to facial nerve anastomosis. Facial crossover grafts from the uninvolved facial nerve to the contralateral involved facial nerve have also been described.

The above techniques all attempt to regain dynamic facial nerve function, but static rehabilitation is also used in facial nerve rehabilitation. Static surgical therapy usually involves rehabilitating the lower face (mouth) or rehabilitating the upper face (eye). Techniques used for lower facial rehabilitation include facial slings, temporalis or masseter muscle transfer, and lip wedge resections. Eyelid rehabilitation is usually focused on eyelid closure and can be accomplished with a gold weight placement or a palpebral spring. Any ectropion that forms due to loss of innervation to the periorbital musculature can be addressed with a canthopexy or lateral canthotomy.

*S*YSTEMIC DISEASE WITH FACIAL NERVE DYSFUNCTION

An overview of the systemic diseases discussed is given in Table 1.

INFECTIOUS DISEASES

Lyme Disease

Lyme disease, also termed Bannwarth's syndrome, is caused by an infection with the spirochete *Borrelia burgdorferi* transmitted by tick bites. It is a systemic disease affecting the skin, nervous system, heart, and joints. Symptoms may be mild and can include fever, fatigue, migratory arthritis, myalgia, headache, meningismus, lymphadenopathy, and skin lesions. Erythema migrans, a characteristic skin lesion found in Lyme disease, is defined as an enlarging, annular erythematous skin lesion seen in half of infected patients (2).

TABLE 1 Systemic Disease Overview

Infectious	Idiopathic	Metabolic	Systemic neoplasms
Lyme disease	Sarcoidosis	Paget's disease	Leukemia
Syphilis	Melkersson-Rosenthal	Fibrous dysplasia	Lymphoma
Leprosy	Guillain-Barre	Osteopetroses	Multiple myeloma
Mumps	Histiocytosis X	Porphyria	
Tuberculosis	Sjögren's syndrome	Myasthenia gravis	
Varicella-Zoster	Multiple sclerosis	Hypothyroidism	
Bell's palsy	Lupus	Diabetes mellitus	
Mycoplasma	Amyotrophic lateral sclerosis	Malignant hypertension	
Polio	Mixed connective tissue disease	Pregnancy	
Mononucleosis	Polyarteritis nodosum	Vaccinations	
Cytomegalovirus	Wegener's granulomatosis	Toxicity	
AIDS	Pseudotumor cerebri	Embolization	
Cat scratch	Kawasaki syndrome		
Tetanus	Amyloidosis		
Otic			

Neurologic involvement may present as meningitis, encephalitis, peripheral neuropathy, myelitis, or cranial neuropathy. Cranial neuropathies are quite common and found in 60% of patients (3). Facial paralysis is the most common neurologic manifestation affecting 10% to 31% of patients (4,5). Recent studies have demonstrated 2.2% of all patients with facial paralysis have serologic evidence of Lyme disease (3). In Western Europe, Lyme disease is now the leading cause of acute facial nerve paralysis in children and represents the most common etiology for facial paralysis in endemic areas (2). Bilateral facial nerve involvement is also common in Lyme disease and is present in 13% to 25% of cases (3,5). Children with Lyme disease have a higher incidence of facial paralysis than adults. Studies cite up to 55% involvement of the facial nerve in children (3), with an increased incidence of bilateral facial nerve involvement (2).

The mechanism of injury to the facial nerve results from direct axonal damage by the spirochetes (2). Diagnosis is made by measuring IgM and IgG titers for antibodies against *B. burgdorferi*. Although the IgM titers are present first, patients may not seroconvert for three to four weeks. Furthermore, the IgM response quickly dissipates. IgG antibody titers develop in patients around six to eight weeks after infection and remain elevated until the infection resolves. Unfortunately, facial nerve involvement typically occurs early in Lyme disease before seroconversion can occur (2). Additional laboratory findings can include cerebrospinal fluid (CSF) pleocytosis, elevated CSF protein, and increased erythrocyte sedimentation rate (ESR), but these are all nonspecific findings.

Treatment involves prolonged antibiotic therapy to eradicate the causative spirochetes. *B. burgdorferi* is highly sensitive to tetracycline but only moderately sensitive to penicillin. A standard treatment is 2 g or 100 mg/kg ceftriaxone daily for 14 days or doxycycline 100 mg b.i.d. for four weeks. Other antibiotics used include erythromycin and imipenem. Corticosteroids are given to treat severe carditis and arthritis. It is important to note that patients can be reinfected after curative treatment.

The prognosis for facial nerve recovery is quite good, even in the absence of antibiotic therapy. One investigation demonstrated 78% of cases with facial involvement recovered completely within three months; the remaining 22% had some residual weakness with grade I–II House–Brachmann paresis (5).

Syphilis

Syphilis is a systemic infection caused by the spirochete *Treponema pallidum*, a facultative anaerobic bacterium. Syphilis infections are extremely diverse in their presentation and are known for their ability to mimic almost any disease. Syphilis can be classified into one of five stages: primary, secondary, congenital, latent, and tertiary (6). Primary syphilis is seen with the initial infection and usually shows a chancre at the site of inoculation. Patients are typically asymptomatic. Secondary syphilis is a systemic infection with patients exhibiting fever, headache, chills, arthralgias, malaise, and photophobia. Congenital syphilis involves vertical transmission of the infection to the fetus. The spectrum of afflictions in congenital syphilis is extremely diverse and can be delayed in its presentation until adulthood. In the latent phase, patients have serologic evidence of the infection but are otherwise free of any clinical signs or symptoms. Some patients progress to tertiary syphilis marked by destructive lesions involving any organ system. Tertiary syphilis has three types: cardiovascular, mucocutaneous, and neurosyphilis. Neurosyphilis ultimately affects approximately 10% of untreated patients, with the central nervous system directly damaged by the spirochetes (7). Common sequelae of neurosyphilis include injury to the dorsal columns, so-called tabes dorsalis, as well as interstitial keratitis and cranial neuropathies. Cranial neuropathies most commonly affect the facial and cochleovestibular nerves. Facial paresis or paralysis is often found with unilateral or bilateral involvement (7). Facial paralysis almost always occurs within one year of primary infection and is usually a complete paralysis. The likely cause of damage to the facial nerve is an obliterative endarteritis of the terminal nutrient arterioles. This causes ischemia, inflammation, and ultimately, necrosis of the facial nerve (8).

Diagnosis is confirmed by various serologic tests. The venereal disease research laboratory (VDRL) or rapid plasma reagin (RPR) tests are used for screening, but both tests have a high false-positive rate. The fluorescent treponemal antibody absorption (FTA-ABS) test is a more reliable test that has high sensitivity but remains positive even after the spirochetes have been eradicated. Demonstration of the spirochetes in CSF or a positive VDRL CSF test may be required for definitive diagnosis in some cases. Treatment of neurosyphilis involves long-term penicillin (six weeks) as well as prednisone for months (30–60 mg q.d.). The prognosis for facial nerve recovery is variable but usually good with early antibiotic therapy. A direct relation between duration of paralysis and recovery was observed in a literature review of all cases of facial involvement since 1945 (9). A more detailed discussion of syphilis can be found in Chapter 15.

Leprosy

Leprosy, also known as Hansen's disease, is caused by an infection with the bacillus *Mycobacterium leprae*. It is most common in warm, wet areas in the tropics and subtropics. This chronic infectious disease usually affects the skin, peripheral nerves, and mucous membranes of the aerodigestive tract and eyes. In 2002, the number of new cases detected worldwide was 763,917, with the majority occurring in the endemic areas of Brazil, India, Madagascar, Mozambique, Tanzania, and Nepal. The number of new cases detected in the United States for 2002 was 96 (10). *M. leprae* is usually spread from person to person in close contact by respiratory droplets. As the bacterium has a propensity to invade peripheral nerves, cranial neuropathies including the facial nerve are not uncommon. Leprosy remains one of the most common causes of peripheral neuropathy worldwide, with some degree of nerve involvement in every case (11). Estimates of 3% to 5% involvement of the facial nerve in leprosy infections have been reported, with facial nerve involvement typically occurring after prolonged infection, on average 12.1 years (12). Both paresis and paralysis can occur, and several investigators have reported that the upper facial nerve branches, particularly the zygomatic branch, are more likely to be affected (13).

Diagnosis is suggested by clinical presentation in endemic areas but can only be confirmed by biopsy. The pathogenesis of nerve damage is from direct injury by the mycobacterium with early invasion of the dermal nerve twigs. As the invasion progresses, Schwann cells and endothelial cells swell from direct infiltration by the organisms. One study demonstrated greater involvement of the distal portions of the nerve, suggesting retrograde spread of infection (11). Treatment of leprosy is with dapsone as well as clofazamine and rifampin. Due to the low likelihood of recovery of nerve function, aggressive surgical rehabilitation and eye protection have been advocated. As the trigeminal nerve is also commonly involved, eye damage from exposure keratitis is a particularly important concern and further advocates for early and aggressive surgical therapy toward eye protection. Facial nerve decompression is not indicated, as involvement of the nerve appears to be along the peripheral portion and not within the enclosed bony segments (11). The mycobacteria are discussed in greater detail in Chapter 12.

Mumps

Mumps is caused by infection with an RNA paramyxovirus. The most common presentation is parotid gland swelling and pain; the testicles, pancreas, kidneys, eyes, and ovaries are also often involved. As mumps has a predilection for neural tissue, neurologic involvement is present in 5% to 30% of cases and may manifest as meningitis, encephalitis, or cranial neuropathies (14). Among cranial nerve involvement, the facial and cochleovestibular nerves are most commonly affected. Some investigators report facial paralysis as a rare sequelae of mumps (15) while others report a higher incidence, as high as 15% (14).

The pathogenesis of neural involvement has not been investigated in the literature. It remains unclear whether facial nerve involvement is related to parotitis, aseptic meningitis, direct viral injury, or swelling along the intracanalicular course of the nerve (14).

Diagnosis is made clinically and can be confirmed with serologic titers. Up to 30% of cases demonstrate lymphocytosis of the CSF, but this is a nonspecific finding (14). Treatment remains symptomatic for this viral infection. Prevention using mumps vaccinations remains the most effective measure for control. Since the introduction of vaccination against the virus, there has been a dramatic decrease in the incidence of infection. Facial paralysis in mumps appears to have a poor prognosis, with a small review of the literature showing only 25% of patients with complete recovery (16).

Tuberculosis

Tuberculosis is caused by an infection with the bacterium *Mycobacterium tuberculae*. In 2004, 14,517 cases of tuberculosis were reported in the United States (17). The infection is spread via respiratory droplets. Pulmonary symptoms predominate, but any organ system can be affected. Spread to the ear can be via direct extension through the nasopharynx, from hematogenous spread, or on rare occasions, via direct implantation through a preexisting tympanic perforation. Tubercular otitis media occurs in 1% of all tuberculosis cases and currently accounts for roughly 0.1% of all cases of otitis media (18–20). Presentation of tubercular otitis is variable but classically is a painless, copious otorrhea with multiple or total tympanic membrane perforations and granulation tissue. Tubercular otitis media has a higher incidence of postauricular fistulae, preauricular lymphadenopathy, and facial nerve involvement when compared to other bacterial causes of otitis media. It is important to note that only 42% of patients with tubercular otitis media have evidence of pulmonary tuberculosis (19).

Facial paralysis is sometimes present in tuberculosis infections and has been estimated at 40% in patients with tubercular otitis (21). The incidence of facial nerve involvement in tuberculosis otitis media seems to be decreasing, with a 30% incidence before 1953 versus a 16% incidence after 1953 (19). The incidence of facial nerve involvement is increased in pediatric patients, with the highest elevation in children less than 10 years of age. Although infections are often bilateral, facial nerve involvement is almost always unilateral (22). In fact, clinicians should have a high index of suspicion for tuberculosis in any child with facial paralysis and otorrhea (21). Damage to the facial nerve is from direct involvement with the mycobacterium on the nerve itself or through nerve impingement from a sequestrum or subperiosteal abscess.

Diagnosis can be made through cell culture, but mycobacterium is difficult to isolate and often takes a prolonged incubation before identification can be made. The purified protein derivative (PPD) test, a skin test for tuberculosis, can be used as a screening tool and often identifies patients with previous exposure to tuberculosis. Chest X rays along with sputum cultures are used to identify patients with active pulmonary disease. Histopathology demonstrates the classic finding of caseating granulomas and acid fast bacilli. The treatment of tuberculosis entails multiple concurrent antibiotics over extended periods. Isonazid, rifampin, pyrazinamide, ethambutol, and streptomycin all have activity against the mycobacterium.

The treatment of facial palsy in active tubercular otitis media or mastoiditis is controversial. Singh published a review of 43 patients to assess the role of surgery in tuberculous mastoiditis. Of the patients, 17 had facial paralysis in this study. He found that 92% of patients treated with antituberculosis medical therapy without surgery had recovery of the facial nerve, with only 80% of patients undergoing surgery (cortical mastoidectomy and removal of sequestrum) obtaining recovery. In the surgical patients, facial nerve decompression was not performed as a part of the operation. These results may reflect more severe cases being selected into the surgical group. The authors concluded that the only role for surgery is incision and drainage of a postauricular abscess or removal of sequestrum, if present; and chemotherapeutic management is the treatment of choice for tubercular mastoiditis (22). Harbert in 1964 had a similar conclusion and felt that surgical intervention was contraindicated as a treatment for facial paralysis in tuberculosis infections (23). However, many other investigators have advocated strongly for decompressive surgery. These investigators cite complete facial nerve recovery, without hearing loss or other complications, as the expected outcome of decompressive surgery (20,24–26).

The prognosis of facial nerve recovery depends heavily on early diagnosis and treatment with antitubercular drugs. In a review by Singh, when treatment was initiated within five days of developing facial palsy, nearly all patients had complete nerve recovery. When therapy was delayed more than two months after developing facial palsy, patients rarely demonstrated a favorable outcome (22). See Chapter 12 for further discussion of tuberculosis.

Herpes Zoster Oticus (Varicella-Zoster, Chicken Pox)

The varicella-zoster virus is a neurotropic DNA virus. Initial infection with the varicella-zoster virus is commonly known as chicken pox and displays a very characteristic vesicular cutaneous eruption. The virus can remain dormant in ganglion cells for many years, with subsequent reactivation of the dormant virus resulting in shingles. Neurologic involvement has been found in chicken pox and includes encephalitis, myelitis, and cerebellar ataxia. Chicken pox has very rarely been associated with facial nerve involvement. As of 1999, only 12 cases of facial palsy in association with an initial varicella-zoster infection were reported in the English literature (27). In contrast, reactivation of the latent virus has a high incidence of facial nerve involvement. Herpes zoster oticus, also termed Ramsay Hunt syndrome, is a specific subset of varicella-zoster reactivation. Patients with herpes zoster oticus present with the classic triad of otalgia, auricular vesicles, and facial paralysis. Patients may also develop other cranial neuropathies, as well as hyperacusis and sensorineural hearing loss. In fact, facial nerve involvement is so common with varicella-zoster reactivation that it remains second only to Bell's palsy as the most common cause of acute peripheral facial paralysis in the United States.

The mechanism of neuropathy appears to be from the neurotropic virus, which causes a diffuse lymphocytic and plasma cell infiltrate of the neural tissue with perivascular and perilymphatic cuffing. This has been demonstrated along the entire length of the facial nerve with some cases undergoing substantial demyelination (28). Alternatively, the viral infection could lead to compressive ischemia as the nerve swells along its tight bony canal.

Diagnosis is often clinical but can be confirmed by direct fluorescence antibody staining for varicella-zoster virus using Tzank preparations as well as serum titers. Magnetic resonance imaging demonstrates facial nerve enhancement with gadolinium in roughly 50% of patients (29).

Treatment is with valacyclovir 1000 mg t.i.d. for seven days, as well as prednisone 1 mg/kg/day (divided) tapered over 7 to 10 days. Sensorineural hearing loss and vertigo may be present with herpes zoster oticus but not with Bell's palsy. The prognosis is poorer than for Bell's palsy, with only 50% demonstrating satisfactory improvement. The course of facial nerve paralysis evolves more slowly, over three weeks. Surgical decompression has remained an extremely controversial issue. Investigators arguing against decompression claim that facial paralysis is unaltered by surgical intervention (30,31). Others have been strong advocates for decompression of the facial nerve, although a lack of consensus as to the areas of decompression remains. May performed a prospective study and concluded that transmastoid decompression of the facial nerve to the labyrinthine segment favorably alters the natural history in patients with herpes zoster oticus when they have a poor prognosis for spontaneous recovery based on electrophysiologic testing (32). Herpes and related viral diseases are discussed in detail in Chapter 10.

Bell's Palsy

Bell's palsy is characterized by a sudden onset of facial paresis or paralysis. Bell's palsy is the most common cause of facial paralysis worldwide, with an incidence of up to 30 cases per 100,000 individuals (33). It may be associated with facial numbness, otalgia, hyperacusis, decreased tearing, or taste changes. Other neurologic symptoms should be absent because Bell's palsy remains a diagnosis of exclusion.

In some patients, the inflammation along the nerve can be detected by an enhancing signal using magnetic resonance imaging with gadolinium contrast agent.

Herpes simplex virus has been implicated using polymerase chain reaction (PCR) techniques as the likely causative agent in Bell's palsy (33). The mechanism of injury appears to be viral insult with direct injury to ganglion cells as well as Schwann cells, resulting in secondary edema and inflammatory demyelination (34). Fisch, using intraoperative-evoked electromyography (EMG), determined that the pathologic constriction of the facial nerve is at the meatal foramen of the intralabyrinthine segment in 94% of patients (1).

Prognosis is good, with 85% of patients achieving complete recovery. A study of over 1000 patients followed for at least 15 years demonstrated that all patients had some recovery within six months: 71% achieved normal function, 13% had slight dysfunction, 12% had mild dysfunction, and 4% had severe dysfunction (35). Treatment is controversial, but recent studies advocate corticosteroid and antiviral therapy over corticosteroid therapy alone. A double blind prospective trial of prednisone versus prednisone and acyclovir in Bell's palsy patients demonstrated that acyclovir 500 mg 5 times a day for 10 days with prednisone did produce a statistically significant improvement in outcome. This included improved return of volitional muscle motion and prevention of nerve degeneration on ENoG over prednisone therapy alone (36). Prednisone dosing is a 1 mg/kg/day (divided) taper over 7 to 10 days, and acyclovir dosing is 1000 mg/day (5 times/day) for seven days. Surgical therapy remains an extremely controversial topic, with strong advocates both for and against its use. All agree that for patients with incomplete paralysis, the prognosis is excellent and surgical therapy should not be considered. ENoG has been shown to predict which patients are most likely to have a poor prognosis. It is in those patients where some would advocate surgical decompression of the nerve. Gantz et al. have advocated that for patients with more than 90% degeneration of ENoG after two weeks along, with no voluntary motor unit EMG potentials, the overall outcome is poor enough (58% chance of a poor outcome of House-Brackmann grade III or IV) to warrant surgical decompression using a middle fossa approach. Using this protocol, the outcome improved to a 91% chance of achieving a House-Brackmann grade I or II in the same patient population. Decompression medial to the geniculate ganglion appears to be most critical, with many studies demonstrating that decompression of the vertical segment alone has dubious efficacy. Late decompression beyond two weeks was also of no clinical benefit (37).

Mycoplasma

Mycoplasma pneumoniae is a small bacterium that lacks a cell wall and commonly causes upper respiratory tract infections and pneumoniae. The overall incidence of infection in the United States has been estimated at 1.7 cases/1000 people/year (38) with 6.8% of all pneumonia caused by this pathogen (39). Symptoms include fever, cough, malaise, and headache, but as many as 25% of patients are asymptomatic. Extrapulmonary manifestations do occur, with neurologic sequelae estimated in 0.1% of all cases (39). Neurologic findings are variable and include psychosis, meningitis, transverse myelitis, ataxia, peripheral neuropathies, and cranial neuropathies. Facial nerve involvement, alone or in conjunction with other neurologic sequelae, is considered rare but has been reported by several authors (40–42). Bilateral facial paralysis has also been associated with mycoplasm infections (43,44).

The mechanism of neurologic injury is uncertain, but many theories have been put forward; these include antigen–antibody reactions, microembolisms, thrombus formation, neurotoxins, and direct viral invasion of the tissue (43).

Diagnosis is often difficult and made clinically. Viral serum titers are difficult to perform, expensive, and time consuming. A fourfold rise in the specific antimycoplasma antibody is considered definitive, with titers of 1:64 or greater highly suggestive of infection. Isolation of *M. pneumoniae* from the sputum is also considered diagnostic. Cold agglutinins have been used but have a low sensitivity, at only 66%, with frequent false positives from other viral infections (43). Recent advances with PCR may allow for more definitive diagnosis.

Treatment is with tetracycline or erythromycin, as the organism is entirely resistant to penicillin since it lacks a cell wall. Facial nerve decompression has not been studied or discussed in the current world literature.

The prognosis is usually good, with most patients demonstrating return of the affected neurologic function within five months (43). The prognosis and time course of facial nerve involvement is thought to be similar to that of Bell's palsy.

Polio

Polio, also termed poliomyelitis, is a small RNA enterovirus transmitted by fecal-oral contamination. It is highly contagious and often remains asymptomatic. When patients are symptomatic, presentation varies but typically includes mild flu-like symptoms of fever, odynophagia, and diarrhea. A minority of cases progress to aseptic meningitis with paralysis of the extremities and respiratory musculature.

Facial paralysis is commonly associated with polio and can be an isolated finding in the disease. Large series have estimated 11% to 18% involvement of facial paralysis in polio infection (44–46). Agius in 1945 reported 426 cases of poliomyelitis in the Malta epidemic of the early 1940s and found 47 cases of facial paralysis (11%) (47). Neuropathy results from direct damage by the neurotropic polio virus. Injury to the facial nerve occurs peripherally rather than at the level of the facial nucleus.

Treatment of the systemic disease is primarily preventative. Salk developed the first vaccine against the polio virus, which was introduced in the early 1950s. The disease is now eradicated in North America, with only 250 cases reported worldwide in the first half of 2005 (17). Only physiotherapy has been studied as a treatment for facial paralysis due to polio virus and was not found to be beneficial (48).

The prognosis for facial nerve recovery is variable. Winters found roughly one-third of the patients with facial involvement had incomplete paralysis, one-third had complete paralysis but recovered to only slight weakness, and one-third had little recovery with moderate or severe facial weakness during long-term (>two years) followup (48). Moore found seven of eight patients presenting with complete facial paralysis from polio virus had some residual weakness one year or longer after illness (49). Agius found only 10 patients of 47 with facial paralysis from polio virus demonstrated persistent facial weakness on two-year followup (47).

Mononucleosis

Mononucleosis is caused by an infection with the Epstein-Barr virus (EBV), a DNA virus in the Herpes virus family. It typically presents with fever, sore throat, malaise, lymphadenopathy, and hepatosplenomegaly. It is estimated that 90% of adults have serologic evidence of prior EBV infection. Diagnosis is confirmed by the clinical picture, characteristic hematologic changes, and immunologic findings. Hematologic changes include atypical lymphocytosis of peripheral monocyte cells. Immunologic findings are an elevated heterophil antibody test, the most specific test used for mononucleosis. The heterophile antibody is an IgM antibody produced by infected B lymphocytes. It is not directed against EBV infected cells but rather is a result of the viral transformation of the B cell into a plasmacytoid state induced by the virus. It is present in 90% of cases by the third week of infection. Immunofluorescence techniques are also available to detect antibodies to EBV (50).

Neurologic involvement has been documented in 5.5% of cases with EBV infection (51). Neurologic sequelae are variable and include encephalopathy, meningoencephalitis, seizures, Guillain–Barre syndrome, and cranial neuropathy. Isolated involvement of all 12 cranial nerves has been reported. Facial nerve involvement is a well-recognized sequelae of the infection and was first recognized in 1937 by Gsell (52). The paralysis can be either unilateral (53–55) or bilateral (56), usually presenting as a rapid onset of complete paralysis with typical full recovery of function over the ensuing several weeks (57). Theories of nerve involvement include direct neural cytotoxic injury by the virus, local pressure from viral lymphadenopathy, edema of the facial nerve course, autoimmune response to the antibody–antigen complexes, and vasculitis. Treatment is supportive only and the infection is self-limited with full recovery anticipated. Please refer to Chapter 10 for detailed discussion of EBV.

Cytomegalovirus

Cytomegalovirus (CMV) is a large DNA virus of the Herpes virus group. It is estimated that 50% to 80% of adults have prior evidence of CMV infection (58). The infection is usually subclinical when contracted by immunocompetent infants and adults and infrequently may lead to a mononucleosis-type syndrome. However, significant sequelae exist from in-utero infections as well as infections in immunocompromised patients.

Neurologic involvement almost always is associated with immunosuppression or in-utero infections. Neurologic sequelae include encephalitis, myelitis, polyneuritis, and cranial nerve involvement (59). Facial nerve involvement has been implicated in CMV infections, but the true incidence of facial nerve involvement is difficult to quantify, given the ubiquitous nature of the virus and its relatively asymptomatic state in immunocompetent patients. However, one study documented significant levels of CMV-specific antibodies of IgM and/or IgG in 64 of 88 patients (73%) presenting with idiopathic acute peripheral facial palsy (60). Importantly, though, CMV replication of the dormant virus and acute facial palsy may be only coincidental and not pathologically linked (60).

The pathogenesis of neurologic involvement is likely due to direct injury by the virus, which results in cell lysis after infection. The diagnosis is made by histopathologic identification of inclusion bodies and enlarged cells as well as elevated titers of antibodies to CMV. Treatment is with gangcyclovir, only used in immunosuppressed patients. Treatment for immunocompetent patients is symptomatic, but infectious patients should avoid exposure to pregnant women. The prognosis for facial recovery is good, with most reported cases recovering full function within weeks to months (58).

AIDS/Human Immunodeficiency Virus

Human immunodeficiency virus (HIV) is a retrovirus that is transmitted through blood or other body fluids. As the HIV destroys the CD4+ helper T-cells, the patient inevitably becomes immunodeficient, at which point the patient is considered to have acquired immunodeficiency syndrome, better known as AIDS. The conversion to the diagnosis of AIDS is met when the CD4+ count drops below 200 or when the patient exhibits any immunodeficient-defining symptom such as Kaposi's sarcoma, candidiasis, CMV disease, toxoplasmosis, or *Pneumocystis carinii* pneumonia. Initial symptoms are mild, most often fever, night sweats, fatigue, and mild lymphadenopathy. As the virus progresses and the patient becomes immunodeficient, opportunistic infections predominate. Immunosuppression also predisposes patients to neoplasms, particularly Kaposi's sarcoma and lymphoma. Diagnosis is usually made using an enzyme-linked immunosorbent assay (ELISA) test. If the ELISA test is positive, a Western blot test is performed for confirmation. Together, these two tests result in a sensitivity of over 99.9% in detecting HIV.

Central nervous system disease is present in 69% of cases, with the peripheral nervous system affected in 8% of HIV cases. Of the peripheral nervous system dysfunctions, the facial nerve is most common, found in approximately 5% of patients (61). A similar study of 170 AIDS patients found a 4.1% incidence of facial paralysis (62). Facial paralysis is abrupt in onset and usually unilateral (63). The mechanism of facial nerve injury may be a direct effect of the neurotropic virus, secondary involvement due to parotid or other neoplastic processes, or immunosuppression leading to reactivation of herpes zoster or other viruses. Multidrug therapy is the current standard therapy for HIV infection. Reverse transcriptase and protease inhibitors are effective and block HIV replication; fusion inhibitors are also used and block HIV entry into the cell. The prognosis for facial paralysis is good, with the majority of patients having complete or near-complete recovery of facial function (64).

A detailed discussion of HIV and AIDS can be found in Chapter 16.

Cat-Scratch Disease

Cat-scratch disease is caused by a systemic infection with *Bartonella henselae*, a bacteria colonizing cat saliva. The infection typically presents as a skin lesion at the site of a cat scratch with ensuing local lymphadenopathy. Infection is manifested by lymphadenopathy, but infected individuals may display fever, fatigue, anorexia, or headaches. It is most commonly a pediatric disorder, affecting individuals usually younger than 21 years of age. Neurologic involvement is estimated to affect 2% to 3% of patients, presenting as encephalopathy, seizures, cerebellar ataxia, hemiparesis, myelitis, or cranial neuropathies. Curiously, neurologic involvement has an increased incidence in adult patients. Facial nerve involvement is considered rare (65).

The mechanism of facial nerve involvement remains unclear. Parotid enlargement is found in 3% of cases and may cause direct involvement of the peripheral branches of the facial nerve (66). Other authors have theorized direct invasion due to the granulomatous lesions around the facial nerve (67). Alternatively, the bacteria could have a direct effect on the facial nerve or cause injury to the nerve secondary to edema along its course within the temporal bone.

Diagnosis is made clinically and confirmed using serologic titers for antibodies to *B. henselae*. Histopathologic findings are not diagnostic but typically demonstrate micro-abscesses with necrotic centers surrounded by epithelioid cells. Warthin–Starry staining can identify the causative bacterium. Treatment of the infection is symptomatic. Suppurative lymphadenopathy is treated by aspiration. The prognosis for facial nerve recovery is considered good, but too few cases exist for meaningful data to be extrapolated.

Chapter 11 contains a detailed discussion of cat-scratch disease.

Tetanus

Tetanus results from the neurotoxin secreted by the bacterium *Clostridium tetani*. On average, the Centers for Disease Control (CDC) has reported 90 cases per year in the United States since vaccinations were implemented to prevent the infection (68). The most consistent early symptom is trismus. Without treatment, the infection is lethal in 30% of patients. A rare localized form of tetanus, termed cephalic tetanus, causes facial paralysis and usually results from an ipsilateral facial wound.

Cephalic tetanus refers to tetanus with paresis or paralysis of any muscle supplied by the cranial nerves. This flaccid paralytic involvement is differentiated from the more common spastic muscle involvement usually seen in tetanus infections. Cephalic tetanus remains a rare variant of tetanus infections, with one review finding cephalic tetanus in 23 cases out of a total of 1025 cases with diagnosed tetanus infections (2.2%) (69).

Various mechanisms have been proposed. One difficulty has been explaining how the toxin or bacteria causes a flaccid paralysis instead of the more typical spastic paralysis. Rose theorized a compressive theory of facial injury (70). Russel favored neuritis due to the tetanus toxin (71). Binet thought that the neurotoxin may behave in a dose-dependent fashion, causing flaccid paralysis at lower concentrations and spastic paralysis at higher concentrations (72). Brunner theorized that selected subtypes of tetanus toxin having different effects might provide the answer (73). Vakil proposed a central etiology of dysfunction, citing an EMG study that did not demonstrate any denervation potentials as evidence (69).

The treatment for cephalic tetanus is the same as for generalized tetanus. Elimination of the toxin by wound debridement and killing active bacteria with penicillin as well as administration of the antitoxin and initiation of immunization are crucial. Patients may also require varying degrees of supportive therapy. The facial paralysis often persists despite resolution of muscle spasm in other parts of the body (69).

Otic Diseases

Acute Otitis Media.   Acute otitis media is a suppurative infection of the middle-ear cavity. Facial nerve involvement is considered a complication of the infection and often occurs from direct pathogen invasion of a dehiscent portion of the facial nerve course, most commonly in the horizontal segment of the facial nerve. Treatment consists of systemic antibiotic therapy against the most common pathogens: *Haemophilus influenzae, Moraxella catarrhalis*, and *Streptococcus pneumoniae*. Drainage of the infected fluid from the middle-ear space with a wide myringotomy is mandatory. If mastoiditis is present, a cortical mastoidectomy for drainage is indicated. Any sequestrum must be removed. Most physicians do not advocate facial nerve decompression in this setting.

Chronic Otitis Media.   Chronic otitis media is an infection lasting more than six weeks with persistent otorrhea. Facial nerve involvement in this setting requires decompression of the facial nerve in addition to long-term antibiotics.

Cholesteatoma.   Cholesteatoma is caused by squamous epithelium present within the middle-ear space. Cholesteatoma commonly causes bony erosion of the ossicles and can lead to serious complications such as fistulas, CSF otorrhea, meningitis, and facial paralysis. When facial paralysis occurs, urgent removal of the cholesteatoma and decompression of the facial nerve is indicated, much akin to cases of chronic otitis media.

Malignant Otitis Externa.   Malignant otitis externa, also termed necrotizing otitis externa, is a skull-based osteomyelitis of otogenic origin. Patients present with severe otalgia, otorrhea, and cranial neuropathies. The facial nerve is the most common cranial nerve involved with studies ranging from 24% to 43% (74). The usual pathogen is *Pseudomonas aeruginosa* and often occurs in immunocompromised patients, typically with diabetes mellitus. Diagnosis is clinical, with an elevated sedimentation rate characteristic on serum evaluation (75). Patients also display increased tracer uptake on technetium or gallium nuclear medicine scans. Treatment requires aggressive blood sugar control and long-term antibiotic therapy directed toward *P. aeruginosa*. Hyperbaric oxygen has also proven beneficial in treating the chronic osteomyelitis. Prognosis is guarded, with mortality near 20% (74). Facial nerve recovery is also reported as quite poor in the literature, with little or no recovery of function, the rule. Surgical therapy is conservative with only minor debridement when necessary.

IDIOPATHIC DISEASES

Sarcoidosis

Sarcoidosis is a chronic, idiopathic, granulomatous disease with a strong predilection for African American and Puerto Rican women in their third or fourth decades of life. Patients most often present with pulmonary symptoms, including shortness of breath, hemoptysis, nonproductive cough, and dyspnea on exertion; however, the spectrum of patient presentation can range from asymptomatic to involvement of any organ system. When neurologic involvement is present, the term neurosarcoidosis has been used.

Neurologic involvement can be central or peripheral. Diabetes insipidus, basal leptomeningitis, and peripheral neuropathy are frequent manifestations (76). An estimated 12% of all patients with sarcoidosis and 50% of patients with neurosarcoidosis have facial paralysis, which remains the most frequent neurological presentation of the disorder. The paralysis can be either unilateral or bilateral in up to 33%

of patients. Any case of bilateral facial paralysis deserves consideration of sarcoidosis as a possible etiology (77).

The association of uveitis, parotid gland enlargement, facial paralysis, and fever was first identified by Heerfordt in 1909 and bears his name to this day as Heerfordt's syndrome. Facial nerve involvement was thought to be from direct involvement of facial nerve branches within the parotid gland (78). Recent evidence, however, implicates a more proximal involvement. Serial examinations of the facial nerve and electrical stimulation at different sites along the entire motor path have suggested that the involvement is characterized by a demyelination process that starts in the cerebellopontine angle and spreads distally into the facial nerve canal (79). The mechanism of injury may be toxic factors, direct invasion by granulomas, or a disturbance in calcium metabolism. Pathologic studies reveal inflammatory changes with the nerve fibers uninjured, suggesting the injury may be to the vasa nervorium (76).

Sarcoidosis remains a diagnosis of exclusion. The Kveim-Siltzbach skin test involves injection of antigen extracted from the spleens of sarcoid patients. The injected area is then biopsied four to eight weeks later, with a positive test demonstrating a nodule with the characteristic histopathologic findings seen in the disorder: a noncaseating granuloma with Schaumann's bodies (laminated concretions composed of calcium and proteins). Asteroid bodies can also be found and are stellate inclusions enclosed within giant cells and centrospheres. Serologic evaluation reveals elevation of many nonspecific markers: elevated ESR (83%), angiotensin converting enzyme (ACE) (73%), liver function tests (LFTs) (65%), EBV (80%), gammaglobulinemia (66%), anergic skin testing (85%), hypercalcemia (5%), or hypercalciuria (25%). Bilateral hilar adenopathy demonstrated on chest X-ray (CXR) is the typical and most common radiologic finding.

Treatment of the systemic disease depends largely on the patient's symptoms. Patients demonstrating spontaneous remission require no further treatment. Immunosuppressive therapy is reserved for cardiac, neurologic, hypercalcemia, or more severe sequelae. Typical treatment of severe sequelae consists of high-dose systemic corticosteroids and topical corticosteroids for nasal disease.

Treatment of facial paralysis is with immunosuppressive therapy. Over 80% of patients respond to corticosteroid therapy with complete recovery of facial nerve function (77). Recurrent paralysis is rare. Some authors have recommended facial nerve decompression if facial nerve recovery does not occur, but reports are only anecdotal and no consensus on indications or timing is currently available (80).

Please refer to Chapter 6 for further discussion of sarcoidosis.

Melkersson-Rosenthal Syndrome

Melkersson-Rosenthal syndrome is characterized by a triad of recurrent episodes of facial paralysis and facial edema along with a fissured tongue. Other neurologic sequelae have been documented, including headache, trigeminal neuralgia, cranial nerve dysfunction, and autonomic dysfunction. Although the etiology is unknown, recent investigation points toward a granulomatous disease leading to recurrent attacks of edema and inflammation of the face and oral cavity with a predilection for facial nerve involvement. Facial nerve involvement may be unilateral or bilateral, with varying frequencies of attacks and progression. No confirmatory blood test, histopathology, or radiographic evaluation is available, as the diagnosis is entirely clinical.

Treatment for the intermittent attacks of facial edema consists of topical, intralesional, or systemic corticosteroid therapy. Mixed results have also been found with various other therapies, including dapsone, clofazimine, sulfasalazine, and antihistamines (81). Recurrent attacks of facial paralysis may result in synkinesis or residual paralysis. For such cases, many investigators now propose surgical decompression as the treatment of choice. Initial surgical procedures decompressing only the horizontal and vertical segments of the facial nerve left patients with continued attacks of facial paralysis (82). Evidence has mounted that the likely site of involvement is within the labyrinthine segment, and current recommendations are for patients with an increasing frequency, duration, and severity of facial paralysis attacks to undergo a combined middle-fossa transmastoid decompression of the entire course of the intratemporal facial nerve and opening of the nerve sheath (81). This procedure has been shown in several series to prevent further attacks of facial paralysis (83).

Guillain-Barre Syndrome

Guillain-Barre syndrome, also known as Landry's ascending paralysis or acute inflammatory demyelinating polyneuropathy, is characterized by rapidly progressive ascending paralysis following a viral or bacterial infection. The incidence is approximately one per 50,000 individuals in the United States (84). Initially, patients exhibit weakness or abnormal sensations in the extremities. Paralysis often ensues, with progression of the extremity weakness involving the muscles of respiration and often facial paralysis or other cranial neuropathies.

Current theories of the pathogenesis of Guillain-Barre syndrome postulate a postviral autoimmune demyelination of the nervous system. Guillain-Barre disorder should always be considered in any patient presenting with bilateral facial nerve involvement. In a study of 43 patients with bilateral facial involvement, six patients were diagnosed with Guillain-Barre syndrome or a variant thereof (85). Many variations of Guillain-Barre syndrome have been described, some with particular predilection for cranial nerve involvement. In fact, a syndrome of multiple cranial nerve palsies as a variant of Guillain-Barre syndrome was first described by Guillain himself in 1937 and included bilateral facial paralysis (86). Another variant known as Miller-Fisher syndrome consists of ataxia, areflexia and ophthalmoplegia and has been strongly associated with facial diplegia (87).

Diagnosis of Guillain-Barre syndrome and its variants is largely based on clinical symptoms, but lumbar puncture and nerve conduction testing can be confirmatory. Treatment with intravenous immunoglobulins or plasmapheresis can hasten the course and dampen the severity of the paralysis. Corticosteroid therapy, sometimes prolonged, has also been found beneficial in randomized trials. During the acute stages of the disease, patients often require extensive support, including artificial respiration. Despite the dramatic progression, the prognosis is quite good, with over 80% of patients achieving a full recovery.

Histiocytosis X

Histiocytosis X, also known as Langerhan's cell histiocytosis (LCH), is a granulomatous disease of idiopathic etiology. There are three subtypes: localized LCH, chronic disseminated LCH, and acute disseminated LCH.

Localized LCH, also called eosinophilic granuloma, occurs primarily in older children and young adults. There is a male predilection with the typical presentation as an osteolytic bone lesion usually in the frontal or temporal areas. Other areas affected include the skull, long bones, ribs, vertebrae, pelvis, maxilla, or mandible. Presentation is variable and based on local symptoms depending on the location of the osteolytic bony lesion. Typically, lesions present with dull pain as well as a soft-tissue mass over the involved site. Treatment is with surgical excision and low-dose radiation therapy, usually 6 Gy. The prognosis is excellent.

Chronic disseminated LCH, also termed Hand-Schuller-Christian disease, affects children and young adults. An osteolytic bone lesion, usually within the mandible, combined with multiorgan involvement, is characteristic. Patients may also have gingival swelling, pain, and premature tooth loss. The triad of a skull lesion, exopthalmos, and diabetes insipidus from sphenoid roof erosion into the sella turcia is present in 10% of cases. Treatment is with multimodal therapy: surgical excision of the lesion combined with chemotherapy and radiation therapy. Despite aggressive therapy, a 30% mortality rate exists.

Finally, acute disseminated LCH, also termed Letterer-Siwe disease, occurs in infants less than three years old. Presentation is with extraskeletal involvement including fever, proptosis, hepatosplenomegaly, adenopathy, multiple bony lesions, bone marrow invasion, anemia, thrombocytopenia, and exfoliative dermatitis. Chemotherapy using vinblastine and steroids has been purported, but the prognosis has been uniformly dismal.

The histopathology of these three forms of LCH demonstrates sheets of polygonal histiocytes, termed Langerhan's cells, present in a varying background of inflammatory cells. Frequently, characteristic "Birbeck granules" or "X bodies" are seen as trilaminar rod-shaped organelles within the nuclear cytoplasm on electron microscopy. Radiographic findings are usually scalloped lytic bony lesions that can often mimic malignant cancers.

Facial nerve involvement occurs in 3% of LCH cases (14 of 500 in the literature) and can occur intracranially at the level of the facial nucleus, along the intratemporal course or less commonly along the peripheral extent of the nerve. Injury to the nerve results from interruption of the vascular supply of the nerve rather than from direct invasion of the neural tissue or compression by the disease (88).

Treatment is primarily directed toward eradicating the disease, usually with low-dose radiation therapy. As the disease improves, facial nerve recovery is expected. Facial nerve decompression is contraindicated, as the granulomas are quite soft and unlikely to cause compressive injury to the nerve. Furthermore, identification of the nerve is quite difficult due to the granulomatous involvement, and risk of iatrogenic injury to the nerve is considered substantial; in fact, the incidence of iatrogenic injury in such cases is as high as 12% (88).

Histiocytosis is discussed further in Chapter 19.

Sjögren's Syndrome

Sjögren's syndrome is an autoimmune disorder of unknown etiology. It occurs in isolation, known as primary Sjögren's syndrome, or secondary to a connective tissue disease. It primarily affects women over 50 years of age. Typical presentation involves dryness of the eyes, termed xeropthalmia, along with dryness of the mouth, termed xerostomia. The pathogenesis of the disorder involves a monocytic infiltration and damage to the salivary and lacrimal glands. Typical symptoms include dysphagia, pancreatitis, parotid enlargement, vasculitis, epistaxis, nasal crusting, corneal ulceration, dental caries, oral ulcers, and neurologic dysfunction. There is an increased risk of other malignancies associated with this disorder, particularly lymphoma.

Laboratory evaluation may demonstrate mild anemia, leukopenia, eosinophilia, elevated ESR, hypergammaglobulinemia, elevated rheumatic factor, SSA/Ro, or SSB/La. Diagnosis can be confirmed with a biopsy of the salivary glands, with the most typical site being a minor salivary gland within the lip. Schirmer's test can help with the diagnosis and is abnormal if less than 5 mm of the filter paper is moistened in five minutes when draped over the lower eyelid.

Neurologic involvement is observed in approximately 20% to 25% of patients with primary Sjögren's syndrome and can involve either the peripheral or the central nervous system (89). Focal neurologic deficits, diffuse neurologic dysfunction, and psychiatric as well as cognitive impairment have all been reported. Although episodes of neurologic impairment are typically transient, they often recur and are multifocal. Over time, patients typically sustain recurrent attacks and develop progressive neurologic impairment. Of those patients with neurologic involvement, the cranial nerves are involved in 19.5% of this subset. Cranial nerve involvements were distributed as follows: cochlear nerve (7.3%), trigeminal nerve (6.1%), facial nerve (4.9%), and olfactory nerve (2.5%) (90). Treatment is primarily supportive, but when neuropathy develops, several investigators have advocated cyclophosphamide therapy. Corticosteroid treatment may be less efficacious. Intravenous immunoglobulins and plasmapheresis have also been anecdotally reported to have benefit.

See Chapter 2 for detailed discussion of Sjögren's syndrome.

Multiple Sclerosis

Multiple sclerosis is an autoimmune disorder characterized by patches of demyelination throughout the nervous system. Presentation is highly variable but typically involves a neurologic deficit such as paresthesia, visual disturbance, motor weakness, or autonomic dysfunction. The disease has a highly variable clinical spectrum, with some patients entering into remission and others deteriorating with recurrent and unremitting exacerbations of neurologic dysfunction. Diagnosis is confirmed by characteristic sclerotic patches on fluid attenuated inversion recovery (FLAIR) sequence using magnetic resonance imaging as well as lumbar puncture demonstrating oligoclonal bands. Facial palsy is considered a common feature of multiple sclerosis and has a reported prevalence of 20% (91).

Facial nerve involvement is from demyelination of the facial nerve along its course and within its nucleus at the pons. Although it typically occurs years after initial diagnosis, a literature review revealed a range of 1% to 5% of patients with facial paralysis as the initial presenting symptom (91).

Preventative medications used for multiple sclerosis are Copaxone and β-interferon injections. Treatment is with high-dose corticosteroids for exacerbations. In a recent study, 22 patients with multiple sclerosis and facial palsy were treated with corticosteroids at the onset of facial palsy, with 12 of the 22 demonstrating complete recovery. The remaining 10 patients had variable facial nerve function ranging from mild abnormality of mobility to asymmetry at rest in the most severe cases. Of four untreated multiple sclerosis patients with facial palsy, one had full recovery with persisting facial nerve dysfunction in the other three (91).

Systemic Lupus Erythematosus

Systemic lupus erythematosus is a chronic autoimmune inflammatory disorder caused by abnormal deposition of antigen–antibody complexes. Kaposi is credited with the first description of the disorder in 1872 and noted "disturbed neurologic function" in his report (92). Although any organ system in the body can be affected, patients most often have arthritis (88%), butterfly rash (79%), pericarditis (64%), and kidney dysfunction (48%). Neurologic sequelae of lupus are common and have been estimated at 37% of patients (93). Neurologic manifestations are quite diverse and can include motor deficits, seizures, cranial nerve dysfunction, headaches, cerebral hemorrhages, and myelitis. Cranial neuropathy has been estimated in 11% of cases (93). The facial nerve is the most common cranial nerve involved, with a roughly 5% prevalence. Bilateral facial involvement has also been described (94).

The underlying pathogenesis of neurologic involvement is unknown, but many autopsy studies have implicated microvascular injury as the mechanism. Some investigators have noted deposition of antibody–antigen complex within the choroid plexus with ensuing damage and dysfunction of CSF production. The facial nerve, in particular, appears to be vulnerable, with pathologic lesions demonstrated along its course from the facial nucleus to the neuromuscular junction (92).

Diagnosis is confirmed with specific blood tests including elevated ESR, antinuclear antibodies (ANA), anti-Sm, anti-DNA, anti-ribonuclear protein (anti-RNP), anti-Ro (SSA), anti-La (SSB), and anticardiolipin antibody. A urinalysis commonly identifies elevated protein consistent with nephrotic syndrome characteristic of the kidney damage caused by the antigen–antibody deposition in lupus.

Treatment of lupus involves immunosuppressive therapy, usually high doses of corticosteroids for exacerbations. Immuran and cytoxan have also been used. Nonsteroidal anti-inflammatory drugs can be used for mild symptom control. Antimalarials such as hydroxyquinine have been shown to reduce the severity and frequency of exacerbations. Plasmapheresis, monoclonal antibodies, and total lymphoid irradiation have also shown some benefit but are considered experimental. The prognosis is variable, with 84% of patients demonstrating partial or complete improvement in their neurologic dysfunction with corticosteroid treatment (93).

See Chapter 1 for detailed discussion of systemic lupus emythemetosus (SLE).

Amyotrophic Lateral Sclerosis

Amyotrophic lateral sclerosis, or Lou Gehrig's disease, is a progressive degeneration of selected upper and lower motor neurons, of unknown etiology. Patients present with dysfunction of the voluntary muscles, most often having problems with ambulation as well as difficulties with tongue movements, causing dysphagia and dysarthria. This dysfunction inevitably progresses to respiratory difficulties as the disease worsens, but cognitive, sensory, and autonomic nerve functions are spared. Eye movements are usually not involved with this disorder. Diagnosis is made by demonstrating upper motor neuron disease on exam (spasticity with exaggerated reflexes), fasciculations, and EMG findings. Although the hypoglossal nerve is by far the most common cranial nerve affected in the disorder (66%), the facial nerve can also be affected (23%) (95).

The mechanism of injury is unknown, but pathologic examination has demonstrated symmetric demyelination of the pyramidal column with loss of anterior horn cells and motor nuclei. Diagnosis is based on history and clinical examination as well as EMG. Treatment is supportive and often involves physical therapy as well as respiratory support. Tracheostomy and gastrostomy tubes are often required. Chronic aspiration can complicate the course and may require additional procedures such as epiglottic oversew or laryngectomy in refractory cases. Only 50% of patients survive for three years after diagnosis, with only 20% of patients surviving for greater than five years after the diagnosis (95).

Mixed Connective Tissue Disease

Mixed connective tissue disease is characterized by a combination of overlapping features of systemic lupus erythematous, scleroderma, and polymyositis. Typical presentation is with Raynaud's phenomenon, arthralgias, inflammatory myopathy, lymphadenitis, skin or mucosal lesions, and serositis. A key distinguishing factor of the disorder is a high titer of antibody to ribonucleoprotein, a finding absent in any of these three disorders (SLE, scleroderma, and polymyositis). Neurologic dysfunction is present in approximately 10% to 15% of cases, usually presenting with facial pain, facial paresthesias, or aseptic meningitis (96,97). Facial nerve involvement, although far less common than trigeminal nerve involvement, has been described and is felt to be an early manifestation of the disorder (98). Although CSF analysis has suggested an inflammatory involvement of the cranial nerves at the meningeal level, there remains an absence of direct evidence for the neurologic dysfunction found in these patients. Current theories implicate a vasculitis as the mechanism of neural injury (99). The prognosis for the disease is quite poor without treatment, but immunosuppressive therapy such as corticosteroids has a dramatic efficacy. Case reports have shown complete facial nerve recovery after corticosteroid treatment (99).

Polyarteritis Nodosum

Polyarteritis nodosum is a vasculitis involving medium-sized arteries, most commonly at their bifurcations. Presentation usually involves the gastrointestinal tract as postprandial abdominal pain with nausea. Patients may also demonstrate kidney dysfunction, subcutaneous palpable nodules, fevers, livedo reticularis, and mononeuritis multiplex. Unlike Wegener's granulomatosis, lung involvement is not typically seen. Nervous system involvement is most often a peripheral neuropathy. Although cranial nerve palsies are uncommon, the facial nerve is the most frequently involved nerve and has been reported by several investigators (100–102). Diagnosis is confirmed with biopsy demonstrating granulomatous vasculitis as well as an elevated serum perinuclear anti-neutrophil cytoplasmic antibody (p-ANCA) and an elevated ESR with anemia. Without treatment, the overall prognosis is dismal. Treatment involves high-dose corticosteroids. Dudley and Goodman performed decompression surgery on a patient with bilateral facial paralysis from polyarteritis nodosum and found no effect (102).

Wegener's Granulomatosis

Wegener's granulomatosis is an idiopathic vasculitis of small arteries, arterioles, and capillaries primarily affecting the upper aerodigestive tract, lungs, and kidneys. Typical presentation is in middle-aged patients with a slight male predominance. Otologic manifestations are common and range from 19% to 45% of cases (103). They include conductive hearing loss, sensorineural hearing loss, otalgia, otorrhea, and serous otitis media. Neurologic involvement is frequent with nearly half of patients demonstrating either peripheral or central neuropathy (104). Cranial nerve involvement was reported in 6.5% of patients (105). When the ear is affected by the disorder, facial nerve involvement has been estimated at 5% (103,106). Injury to the facial nerve may be from destructive granulomatous lesions involving the skull base, necrotizing vasculitis, or compressive effect due to granuloma in the middle ear (107). Pathologically, the disorder is characterized by noncaseating granulomas with necrotizing vasculitis. Diagnosis can be facilitated using a sensitive serum marker, c-ANCA.

   Treatment consists of immunosuppressive therapy, including methotrexate, cyclophosphamide, and prednisone; Septra may help keep patients in remission. Immunosuppressive therapy now offers a 70% to 85% remission rate, which is remarkable, considering the invariably fatal outcome within one year without treatment. Several studies have demonstrated almost universal resolution of neuropathy with institution of systemic immunosuppressive therapy (108). In rare cases where facial nerve involvement persists after systemic therapy has been instituted, many have advocated against facial nerve decompression, citing concerns of increased risk of nerve injury due to granulation tissue surrounding the nerve (103,109,110). Dagum, in a literature review, reported six cases of facial paralysis in Wegener's granulomatosis, all of whom had resolution of the paralysis with treatment of the disease (107).

   Chapter 8 discusses Wegener's granulomatosis is further detail.

Pseudotumor Cerebri

Pseudotumor cerebri is a condition of unknown etiology characterized by elevated intracranial pressure without hydrocephalus occurring in the absence of intracranial masses or CSF outflow obstruction. It was first recognized by Quiricke in 1897 (111). Typically, middle-aged women are affected and present with headache, visual disturbances, and pulsatile tinnitus. Cranial nerve palsies are common, with the abducens nerve most often affected, in as many as 60% of cases (111). An association between pseudotumor cerebri and facial nerve paralysis, either unilateral or bilateral, has also been reported in the literature. In a 1996 review, 14 cases of facial palsy in patients with pseudotumor cerebri were identified. Of the 14 cases, three were bilateral and 11 were unilateral. In 13 of the 14 cases, facial paralysis resolved with correction of the elevated intracranial pressure (112). The likely mechanism of facial involvement is traction on the extra axial facial nerve. Treatment is centered on addressing the elevated intracranial pressures, with diamox, serial lumbar punctures, or lumboperitoneal shunts.

See Chapter 24 for a detailed discussion of pseudotumor cerebri.

Kawasaki Disease

Kawasaki disease, also known as acute infantile febrile mucocutaneous lymph-node syndrome, is a syndrome of unknown etiology affecting children. Children typically present with fever, irritability, strawberry tongue, conjunctival congestion, cervical lymphadenopathy, and desquamating rash on the palms and soles. In the United States, approximately 3000 cases are diagnosed annually. Neurologic manifestations of the syndrome include aseptic meningitis, irritability, meningeal signs, seizures, and encephalopathy (113).

Facial nerve paralysis was first noted in 1974 by Murayama, with 28 cases documented by the year 2000 (114). Facial palsy is usually transient, ranging from two days to three months. Complete recovery was the rule for all infants who survived the syndrome. Facial nerve palsy is likely due to a vasculitis involving the facial nerve. Vasculitis typically involves the coronary arteries in Kawasaki's syndrome and is a significant determinant of morbidity and mortality occurring in 25% of untreated cases. When facial nerve involvement is present, the incidence of coronary artery aneurysms is increased to 54%. Aggressive treatment for the systemic syndrome is warranted to prevent coronary aneurysms. Intravenous immunoglobulin and aspirin therapy are the current treatments employed (115).

Kawasaki disease is discussed in further detail in Chapter 9.

Amyloidosis

Amyloidosis is a disease resulting from abnormal protein deposits in extracellular tissue. The disease can be localized or systemic and can be further subclassified as primary, secondary, and familial. In primary amyloidosis, the protein fibrils form without a known cause. Secondary amyloidosis results from multiple myeloma or other chronic diseases that generate an abnormal amount of protein breakdown. Familial amyloidosis refers to a hereditary version of the disorder. Presentation is initially asym-ptomatic but proteinuria may be an early finding. Cardiac, dermatologic, gastrointestinal, and other organ systems show dysfunction depending on the location of the abnormal protein deposition. Any organ system in the body can be involved.

Neurologic involvement is usually of the peripheral nerves, the spinal nerve roots, and the autonomic ganglia, with the brain usually spared (116). Peripheral neuropathy in amyloidosis is found in 17% of patients. Cranial nerve involvement is rare in amyloidosis. Although cranial neuropathies are more common in familial amyloidosis, recent reviews have demonstrated cranial nerve involvement in primary amyloidosis (117). The facial nerve is rarely involved in cases of primary, secondary, and familial amyloidosis.

Although the mechanism of damage remains unknown, electromyographic studies have shown evidence of chronic partial denervation with amyloid deposits demonstrated in the perineurium (116). Some hypothesize that a progressive buildup of amyloid fibrils around cells results in injury. Amyloid deposits have been demonstrated to involve the facial nerve directly, with nearly complete replacement of the nerve (118).

Diagnosis is confirmed with biopsy demonstrating green birefringence of the abnormal protein using Congo red staining when viewed with a polarizing light. Serologic or urinary identification of homogeneous protein fibrils is also possible. Treatment with alkylating agent–based chemotherapy has had some success in amyloidosis. Clinical trials are underway for corticosteroid and α-interferon treatment. Colchicine may be beneficial in some forms of familial amyloidosis.

METABOLIC DISORDERS

Paget's Disease

Paget's disease is a common osteodystrophy characterized by abnormal bone metabolism where focal areas of bone are resorbed, then replaced in excess. It is estimated to affect 7% of males and 4% of females over the age of 55 (119). Although 85% of cases of Paget's disease are asymptomatic, typical presentations of pain, arthritis, fractures, and high-output cardiac failure are characteristic (120). Skull enlargement with bony impingement of neural foramina can lead to neuropathy, but this appears to be an uncommon occurrence. Of the cranial nerves involved, the auditory and olfactory nerves are the most commonly affected. When involvement of the facial nerve occurs, it usually presents as hemifacial spasm occurring in 7% of patients with Paget's disease. Facial paresis or paralysis has also been found in roughly 2% of Paget's patients. Diagnosis is confirmed by characteristic radiographic findings with demineralized areas giving a washed out or blurry appearance. Laboratory abnormalities showing an elevated alkaline phosphatase level are consistent with increased bone metabolism. Treatment is with antiosteoclastic agents including calcitonin, plicamycin (mithramycin), and etidronate (etidronic acid). The prognosis is considered good with the exception of sarcomatous transformation, which occurs in roughly 10% of the cases (120).

Paget's disease is discussed in detail in Chapter 21.

Fibrous Dysplasia

Fibrous dysplasia is another osteodystrophy or developmental disturbance of bone formation and is also discussed in Chapter 21. In fibrous dysplasia, bone is resorbed and then replaced with haphazardly arranged fibrous tissue. Fibrous dysplasia is classified as monostotic, polyostotic, or McCune–Albright syndrome. McCune–Albright syndrome is a polyostotic fibrous dysplasia along with endocrine abnormalities consisting of skin changes over the neck and trunk, precocious puberty, accelerated skeletal growth, hyperparathyroidism, acromegaly, hyperthyroidism, Cushing's disease, and diabetes mellitus.

The etiology of fibrous dysplasia is unknown and there is a small incidence of malignant transformation into osteosarcoma. Usually, the disease starts within the first decade of life and stabilizes after puberty. The disorder typically presents as a painless bony growth involving the face or skull. Facial asymmetry may be present with variable progression to gross deformation commonly seen.

Neuropathy has been well described and is due to direct compressive effects of the abnormal bony remodeling. When the temporal bone is involved, the most common clinical manifestations are external auditory canal stenosis and conductive hearing loss. Although optic neuropathy is more frequent, facial paralysis has also been associated with fibrous dysplasia. Facial palsy has been reported in 9% of patients with temporal bone involvement (121).

Diagnosis is confirmed by characteristic bony lesions on radiographs that appear as "ground glass" with a cortex that is always intact. Histopathologic features consist of immature woven bone arranged in "Chinese character" appearance from the fibrocolla-genous cellular spindly stroma and is considered pathognomonic for the disease. There is no known medical treatment for this disorder and patients typically undergo conservative surgical bony remodeling procedures. Facial paralysis from mechanical compression of the nerve by abnormal bony remodeling is treated by surgical decompression of the nerve.

Osteopetroses

Osteopetroses are rare genetic osseous dysplasias characterized by bony sclerosis and abnormal bone metabolism with increased bone density. The skull is frequently involved and various cranial neuropathies have been described secondary to bony impingement of the skull foramina. The incidence of cranial neuropathies in osteopetroses has been estimated at 16%. Although the facial nerve is the most common cranial nerve involved, the optic and vestibulocochlear nerves are also affected (122).

One subtype of osteopetroses, termed sclerosteosis, has a proclivity for facial nerve involvement. It is characterized by syndactyly, conductive hearing loss, and sclerosis, and almost always has progressive recurrent facial nerve palsy (123). Attacks of facial paralysis commonly begin in childhood, are recurrent, and often alternate sides of the face. Total nerve degeneration is the rule and recovery with significant synkinesis at three to five months is the usual outcome (124).

There has been speculation regarding the mechanism of injury. As the fallopian canal is narrowed, the nerve may become more susceptible to edematous involvement with viral reactivation as the culprit. As the bony impingement worsens, the delicate vascular supply to the nerve may be interrupted. Finally, as the bony growth progresses, there may be direct crush injury to the nerve itself (125). Dort, in a temporal bone study, found significant narrowing along the course of the facial nerve, particularly within the labyrinthine segment, but also in the distal temporal and mastoid segments, supporting this notion. However, he also demonstrated bony obliteration of the stylomastoid artery and proposed ischemia as another etiology for facial nerve injury (123).

Treatment of the disorder is difficult, because no known medication has been demonstrated to halt the progression of the disease. Surgical decompression of the facial nerve has been efficacious and favorable outcomes have been reported by various investigators. Current recommendations are to decompress the facial nerve early in the course of the disease using a combined transmastoid-middle fossa approach along the entirety of the nerve's course (123).

Porphyrias

Porphyrias are a group of metabolic disorders characterized by defects in the synthesis of heme, a metalloporphyrin that is the product of porphyrin metabolism. Presentation of the disorder typically involves abdominal pain, vomiting, constipation, hypertension, tachycardia, photosensitivity, psychosis, and neuropathy. Neuropathy is estimated to affect 10% to 40% of patients and is primarily motor (126). Cranial neuropathies have been described but facial paralysis is rare (127). Although the mechanism of neuropathy is unknown, several autopsy as well as biopsy studies have implicated a distal axonal lesion (128). Investigators have hypothesized that some of the abnormally elevated heme byproducts, such as delta-aminolevulinic acid, may have a direct neurotoxic effect. Alternatively, heme deficiency in neural tissue may be cytotoxic or may lead to neurotransmitter dysfunction. Diagnosis is confirmed by identifying a markedly increased urinary porphobilinogen level. Treatment of an acute attack involves intravenous hemin therapy started as soon as possible. Intravenous glucose alone is appropriate only for mild attacks or until hemin is available. The prognosis for recovery of facial neuropathy is variable, but typically, recovery is slow over many months and often with incomplete return of function or residual synkinesis. Repeated attacks usually lead to progressive dysfunction with the ultimate long-term prognosis dependent on the ability to adequately prophylax against recurrence of the attacks (126).

Myasthenia Gravis

Myasthenia gravis is an autoimmune disorder with antibodies directed at the postsynaptic receptors for the neurotransmitter acetylcholine. As the receptors are destroyed, the axonal nerve signals cannot be communicated to the muscles, resulting in progressive muscle fatigue and paralysis. Typical presentation is ocular weakness including ptosis and ophthalmoplegia and is present in 90% of the cases. The facial nerve can be involved with myasthenia gravis and can be unilateral or bilateral of varying severity (129,130). In rare cases, the facial nerve can even be involved without any ocular weakness (131). Diagnosis can be made by giving a test dose of edrophonium, because patients with myasthenia gravis show dramatic improvement in muscle weakness after intravenous infusion. Finding antibodies to the acetylcholine receptor in the serum is diagnostic. Treatment consists of anticholinesterase inhibitors that prevent the breakdown of acetylcholine at the neurosynaptic junction providing more availability of this neurotransmitter to function on the reduced numbers of receptors available. As with other muscle weakness found in this disorder, the facial nerve function dramatically improves with neostigmine or other anticholinesterase inhibitors.

Hypothyroidism

Thyroid hormone plays a critical role in regulating metabolism. In hypothyroidism, the basal metabolic rate is decreased due to a lack of thyroid hormone, resulting in bradycardia, cold intolerance, alopecia, and weight gain. Neurologic symptoms are relatively common in hypothyroidism and include paresthesias in up to 80% of patients as well as ataxia, coma, headache, seizure, cerebellar signs, and psychosis (132,133). Cranial nerve involvement has also been reported, with the vestibulocochlear nerve most commonly affected in 15% to 31% of patients with hypothyroidism (132). Involvement of the facial nerve is considered rare. Its mechanism is thought to be a compressive phenomenon. In hypothyroidism, myxedematous infiltration and swelling of the soft tissue are hypothesized to have a compressive effect on the facial nerve through the tight confines of the fallopian canal. Anecdotal reports of facial nerve decompression in hypothyroidism have been described (134), but additional reports state that the facial paralysis resolves as the thyroid abnormality is corrected (133). Treatment involves thyroid hormone supplementation.

Diabetes Mellitus

Diabetes mellitus results from a lack of insulin production causing an elevated level of serum glucose. The presentation ranges from asymptomatic to ketotic coma. Neurologic

TABLE 2 Malignant Hypertension and Facial Paralysis Review

Investigator	Year	Patients with malignant HTN	Patients with facial involvement (percentage)
Clark (140)	1956	79	7 (8.9%),
Lloyd (141)	1966	35	6 (17.1%)
Amberg (142)	1929	25	2 (8%)
Rance (143)	1974	70	2 (2.9%)
Trompeter (144)	1982	45	2 (4.4%)
Totals	1929–1982	254	19 (7.5%)

Abbreviation: HTN, hypertension.

sequelae are quite common and most often are seen as a peripheral neuropathy in the lower legs. The incidence of facial neuropathy in diabetic patients has been estimated between 0.5% and 2.5% without a clear link to blood glucose control (135,136). This incidence of facial involvement is elevated when compared to the incidence of facial paralysis in the general population of 0.1%. In fact, Korzyn reported that among 130 cases studied of facial palsy, 20% had diabetes with as many as 66% demonstrating impaired glucose tolerance (137).

The primary systemic effects are caused by injury to the microvascular blood supply from the elevated serum glucose levels that result in impaired microvascular circulation. The blood supply to the facial nerve can be affected by diabetes resulting in facial paralysis that can be temporary or permanent. The most susceptible area of the facial nerve to vascular compromise is the labyrinthine segment, a watershed area where the carotid and vertebrobasilar systems connect. Treatment involves aggressive control of blood sugars with frequent monitoring of glucose levels. Corticosteroid therapy for facial nerve dysfunction is contraindicated, as glucocorticoids result in a substantial elevation of serum glucose.

Malignant Hypertension

Moxon first reported hypertension as a cause of facial paralysis in 1869 (138). Since that time, an association between peripheral facial paralysis and hypertension has been confirmed. Paine reported on 80 pediatric cases presenting with facial palsy over a seven-year period at Boston's Children's Hospital and found two cases (2.5%) resulted from malignant hypertension (139). This link is substantiated by a review of the literature on pediatric malignant hypertension, which reveals a consistent incidence of facial nerve involvement ranging from 3% to 17% (Table 2).

An association between malignant hypertension and peripheral facial paralysis in adults has also been found. In a review by Clarke of 190 patients with malignant hypertension, 38% were found to have various neurologic sequelae including focal brain ischemia, cerebral hemorrhage, subarachnoid hemorrhage, hypertensive encephalopathy, mental disturbances, convulsions, and cranial neuropathies. The facial nerve was the most common cranial nerve involved with an incidence of 10% for isolated facial nerve involvement in adults with malignant hypertension (140).

The pathogenesis of the lower motor nerve involvement of the facial nerve may be from recurrent hemorrhage within the facial canal. This theory has been supported by two autopsies where blood clots were identified within the facial canal (138,141). Alternatively, edema of the nerve with compression of the blood supply could cause the paralysis.

The prognosis for facial nerve recovery is quite good with treatment aimed at correcting the hypertensive state (145). An anecdotal report of facial nerve decompression in a patient with hypertension as the etiology resulted in complete return of facial nerve function (146). However, given the excellent outcome without surgery, many advocate a more conservative approach. Glucocorticoid therapy is contraindicated as this may exacerbate the hypertensive state (147). Investigators now stress the need to measure blood pressure in any child presenting with facial paralysis (148).

Pregnancy

An increased risk of acute facial paralysis has been noted in pregnancy dating as far back as Sir Charles Bell in his 1830 publication (149). Pregnant women have a 3.3-fold increased risk for facial paralysis when compared to age-matched nonpregnant women (149). Timing of the facial paralysis during pregnancy is as follows: 5% in the first trimester, 6% in the second trimester, 71% in the third trimester, and 18% within one week postpartum (150). Of the cases, 35% had incomplete paralysis with 65% of cases demonstrating complete paralysis within 10 days of its onset. An increased risk for facial paralysis was also correlated with preeclampsia with a sixfold increased risk identified (151).

There are many possible mechanisms for facial nerve involvement in pregnancy. Elevated progesterone levels are known to cause an increase in extracellular fluid content, which could result in edema and injury to the facial nerve along its tight bony course within the temporal bone (152). This might explain the increased incidence of facial paralysis in the third trimester, when progesterone levels are at their highest.

Viral inflammation or immunosuppression during pregnancy is the alternative explanation (153). Naib demonstrated that the incidence of herpes simplex in pregnant women is higher than in nonpregnant women. Gestational immunosuppression from rising cortisol levels is well known and may then lead to viral reactivation. In terms of prognosis, no effect or correlation of facial involvement was identified on neonatal outcome (151). For incomplete paralysis, all patients demonstrated complete recovery. For the pregnant women demonstrating complete facial paralysis, only 52% achieved satisfactory outcome. This is statistically significant when compared to aged-matched nonpregnant women as well as men with Bell's palsy, who achieved 77% to 88% incidence of satisfactory outcome (House Brackman I or II). Corticosteroid therapy did not appear to alter the outcome. One author has advocated induction of delivery early in the last week of pregnancy followed by facial nerve decompression (154).

Vaccinations

In 1999, a review of 1526 patients in Switzerland, who were given the intranasal influenzae vaccine, found 11 cases of facial paralysis ranging from 3 to 43 days after the vaccination was administered, yielding an incidence of 0.7%. The intranasal influenzae vaccine is a virosomal vaccine that also contains adjuvant heat-labile *Escherichia coli* toxin. The facial paralysis resolved in 10 of 11 patients. When compared to the spontaneous incidence of 0.02% in this patient population, this was considered a significant increase in the incidence of facial paralysis and the intranasal influenzae vaccine was removed from the market. Since that time, a second intranasal influenzae vaccination has been introduced based on live attenuated cold-adapted influenzae virus, without any cases of facial paralysis (155).

Additional investigations have been performed for parenteral influenza vaccines. Using the vaccine adverse event reporting system in the United States for the years 1991–2001, a total of 197 reports of facial paralysis were documented after injection of influenza vaccines. The study compared the incidence of facial paralysis with influenza vaccine to the incidence of facial paralysis to other vaccines and concluded a "possible association between influenza vaccines and increased risk of Bell's palsy" (156).

A study of the incidence of facial paralysis after hepatitis B vaccination revealed 10 cases over a three-year period with 850,000 vaccines administered. Analysis found that this was not an increase over the expected incidence of Bell's palsy but did find an association with Guillain–Barre syndrome, with five cases documented over the same three-year time period (157).

Toxicity

Toxic exposures have, on rare occasions, resulted in facial paralysis. Ethylene glycol, or antifreeze, has resulted in unilateral and bilateral facial paralysis when ingested. Patients who have ingested glycol also have ataxia, dysarthria, and visual changes (158). Arsenic intoxication has also been linked with facial paralysis. A single case report of neurologic and gastrointestinal disturbances presenting as facial paralysis and pancreatitis following arsenic intoxication was described in a literature review (159). Chronic arsenic toxicity is known to cause a symmetric polyneuropathy of sensory and motor nerves, but cranial nerve involvement is rare. Lithium toxicity has also been reported to cause facial nerve involvement (160). Chronic alcohol intoxication was hypothesized as the cause of bilateral facial paralysis in a patient with Wernicke–Korsakoff syndrome (158).

Some chemotherapeutic agents have been linked with facial nerve involvement. Paclitaxel has been reported to cause bilateral facial paralysis after only a single cycle (161).

Embolization for Epistaxis

Arterial embolization has been used to treat recalcitrant epistaxis since 1974 (162). Since that time, a literature review reveals 13 cases of facial paralysis after embolization of branches of the external carotid artery. The majority occurred immediately after embolization, with most of the others occurring within the first hour after embolization (163). In one case after bilateral middle meningeal artery ligation, a patient developed bilateral facial paralysis within 36 hours of embolization, which lasted five months before the patient demonstrated full recovery (164).

Facial nerve paralysis occurred using both absorbable and nonabsorbable materials for the embolization (163). Complete recovery of the facial nerve occurred in only 40% of the cases.

Theories about the pathogenesis of injury are related to the major blood vessels that supply the facial nerve along its course. The internal auditory artery is a branch of the AICA coming from the basilar artery and supplies the portion of the nerve running within the IAC. The petrosal artery is a branch of the middle meningeal artery coming from the internal maxillary artery and supplies the labyrinthine and horizontal segments of the facial nerve. Finally, the stylomastoid artery is a branch of either the occipital artery or the posterior auricular artery and supplies the vertical portion of the facial nerve.

A detailed discussion of epistaxis can be found in Chapter 31.

SYSTEMIC NEOPLASMS

Leukemia

Leukemia represents a hematogenous malignancy of the white blood cells. Four different subtypes exist: acute myelogenous leukemia (AML), chronic myelogenous leukemia, acute lymphomatoic leukemia, and chronic lymphomatoid leukemia. These diseases are discussed in detail in Chapter 17.

Presentation varies dramatically depending on the subtype, but patients usually suffer from inadequate hematopoietic production of precursor cells due to leukemic infiltration of the bone marrow. Infections, bleeding, pallor, lethargy, malaise, and fever are frequent symptoms (165). Diagnosis is confirmed with characteristic elevation of the white-blood cell count and diagnostic finding on bone marrow biopsy. Extramedullary disease occurs, most often involving the central nervous system and testes (165). An uncommon manifestation of myelogenous leukemias is the chloroma, also known as a granulocytic sarcoma or myeloblastoma, occurring in roughly 5% of patients with AML (166). Chloromas represent a focal deposition, or mass, comprised of immature myeloid cells. Chloromas can be found in any location.

Temporal bone involvement has been found in 36% of temporal bones evaluated in leukemic patients (167). Facial nerve paralysis has been associated with leukemia but is considered unusual (168). Facial nerve involvement is most often seen with meningeal leukemia with involvement of the facial motor nucleus (167). Less commonly, direct invasion of leukemic cells, such as a chloroma along any portion of the course of the facial nerve, including the parotid gland, can lead to facial nerve dysfunction (169,170). The leukemic invasion involves the perineurium, and to a lesser extent, the endoneurium (167). Treatment involves chemotherapy with focal radiation therapy at the site of the chloroma. When the chloroma involves the mastoid bone, surgical treatment is restricted to obtaining a biopsy for diagnosis, and recovery occurs without decompression of the facial nerve (171).

Lymphoma

Lymphoma represents a malignancy of the lymphoreticular epithelial system. It is generally divided into Hodgkin's and non-Hodgkin's lymphoma. This is discussed further in Chapter 17. Although the presenting systems are quite variable, lymphadenopathy is usually a prominent feature. Patients may also develop fatigue and night sweats. Non-Hodgkin's lymphoma more commonly involves extranodal sites. Lymphoma can involve the temporal bone either primarily or from metastatic disease.

When facial nerve involvement occurs, it is usually from direct involvement of the lymphoma along the course of the facial nerve. It is considered an exceptionally rare complication of lymphoma (172) but is well described (173–176). Tucci reports two cases of primary lymphoma of the temporal bone which presented with facial paresis (174). In both cases, the facial paresis recovered completely after chemotherapeutic treatment was given. Metastatic involvement of the temporal bone is much more common than primary lymphoma involvement. Treatment depends on the type of lymphoma but is primarily multidrug chemotherapy. Facial paralysis involved with temporal bone lymphoma usually follows the course of the disease (175).

Multiple Myeloma

Multiple myeloma, also known as myeloma or plasma cell myeloma, is a hematogenous malignancy of the plasma cells. It is the second most common hematogenous malignancy behind non-Hodgkin's lymphoma. Patients early in the disease are often asymptomatic but later can develop lower back and rib pain as well as anemia and kidney dysfunction. Diagnosis is confirmed by the presence of excess protein (so-called M protein) in the blood or urine and an increased number of plasma cells on bone marrow biopsy.

The first case of multiple myeloma of the temporal bone was published in 1979 by Lavine. Shone documented the first case of facial involvement with multiple myeloma in 1985 (177), with other investigators presenting similar cases (178–180). Temporal bone histopathology in multiple myeloma patients has shown a high percentage of involvement, with 87% of bones examined at autopsy of patients succumbing to the disease demonstrating evidence of multiple myeloma. When alive, only 12% of these same patients demonstrated otologic symptoms (181). Although the temporal bone is commonly involved in the terminal stages of the disease, symptoms related to temporal bone involvement are often outweighed by the overwhelming skeletal disease (182). Treatment regimens include radiation therapy, bisphosphonates, and stem-cell transplants.

See Chapter 17 for further discussion of this topic.

*R*EFERENCES

1. Fisch U. Surgery for Bell's palsy. Arch Otolaryngol 1981; 107(1):1–11.
2. Cook SP, Macartney KK, Rose CD, et al. Lyme disease and seventh nerve paralysis in children. Am J Otolaryngol 1997; 18(5):320–323.
3. Peltomaa M, Pyykko I, Seppala I, et al. Lyme borreliosis and facial paralysis—a prospective analysis of risk factors and outcome. Am J Otolaryngol 2002; 23(3):125–132.
4. Bingham PM, Galetta SL, Athreya B, et al. Neurologic manifestations in children with Lyme disease. Pediatrics 1995; 96(6):1053–1056.
5. Angerer M, Pfadenhauer K, Stohr M. Prognosis of facial palsy in Borrelia burgdorferi meningopolyradiculoneuritis. J Neurol 1993; 240(5):319–321.
6. http://www.cdc.gov/epo/dphsi/casedef/syphiliscurrent.htm (accessed October 2005).
7. Johnson RA, White M. Syphilis in the 1990s: cutaneous and neurologic manifestations. Semin Neurol 1992; 12(4):287–298.
8. Cintron R, Pachner AR. Spirochetal diseases of the nervous system. Curr Opin Neurol 1994; 7(3):217–222.
9. Verduijn PG, Bleeker JD. Secondary syphilis of the facial nerve. Arch Otolaryngol 1982; 108(6):382–384.
10. http://www.cdc.gov/ncidod/dbmd/diseaseinfo/hansens_t.htm (accessed October 2005).
11. Selby RC. Neurosurgical aspects of leprosy. Surg Neurol 1974; 2(3):165–177.
12. Antia NH, Divekar SC, Dastur DK. The facial nerve in leprosy. I. Clinical and operative aspects. Int J Lepr Other Mycobact Dis 1966; 34(2):103–117.
13. Reichart PA, Srisuwan S, Metah D. Lesions of the facial and trigeminal nerve in leprosy. An evaluation of 43 cases. Int J Oral Surg 1982; 11(1):14–20.
14. Beardwell A. Facial palsy due to the mumps virus. Br J Clin Pract 1969; 23(1):37–38.
15. Manning JJ, Adour KK. Facial paralysis in children. Pediatrics 1972; 49(1):102–109.
16. Endo A, Izumi H, Miyashita M, et al. Facial palsy associated with mumps parotitis. Pediatr Infect Dis J 2001; 20(8):815–816.
17. http://www.mass.gov/dph/cdc/tb/ (accessed October 2005).
18. Stone JW. Tuberculosis of the middle ear. Arch Otolaryngol 1967; 86(4):407–411.
19. Skolnik PR, Nadol JB Jr, Bake AS. Tuberculosis of the middle ear: review of the literature with an instructive case report. Rev Infect Dis 1986; 8(3):403–410.
20. Lucente FE, Tobias GW, Parisier SC, et al. Tuberculosis otitis media. Laryngoscope 1978; 88(7 pt 1):1107–1116.
21. Samuel J, Fernandes CM. Tuberculous mastoiditis. Ann Otol Rhinol Laryngol 1986; 95(3 pt 1):264–266.
22. Singh B. Role of surgery in tuberculous mastoiditis. J Laryngol Otol 1991; 105(11):907–915.
23. Harbert F, Riordan D. Tuberculosis of the middle ear. Laryngoscope 1964; 74:198–204.
24. Windle-Taylor PC, Bailey CM. Tuberculosis otitis media: a series of 22 patients. Laryngoscope 1980; 90(6 pt 1):1039–1044.
25. Plester D, Pusalkar A, Steinbach E. Middle ear tuberculosis. J Laryngol Otol 1980;94(12): 1415–1421.
26. Legent F, Baron F. Facial paralysis and tuberculosis otitis. Significance of early neural decompression. Ann Otolaryngol Chir Cervicofac 1975; 92(4–5):235–240.
27. van der Flier M, van Koppenhagen C, Disch FJ, et al. Bilateral sequential facial palsy during chickenpox. Eur J Pediatr 1999; 158(10):807–808.
28. Guldberg-Moller J, Olsen S, Kettel K. Histopathology of the facial nerve in herpes zoster oticus. AMA Arch Otolaryngol 1959; 69(3):266–275.

29. Muecke M, Amedee RG. Herpes zoster oticus: diagnosis and management. J La State Med Soc 1993; 145(8):333–335.
30. Dickins JR, Smith JT, Graham SS. Herpes zoster oticus: treatment with intravenous acyclovir. Laryngoscope 1988; 98(7):776–779.
31. Uri N, Greenberg E, Meyer W, et al. Herpes zoster oticus: treatment with acyclovir. Ann Otol Rhinol Laryngol 1992; 101(2 pt 1):161–162.
32. May M, Blumenthal F. Herpes zoster oticus: surgery based upon prognostic indicators and results. Laryngoscope 1982; 92(1):65–67.
33. Murakami S, Mizobuchi M, Nakashiro Y, et al. Bell palsy and herpes simplex virus: identification of viral DNA in endoneurial fluid and muscle. Ann Intern Med 1996; 124(1 pt 1):27–30.
34. Friedman RA. The surgical management of Bell's palsy: a review. Am J Otol 2000; 21(1):139–144.
35. May M, Hughes GB. Facial nerve disorders: update 1987. Am J Otol 1987; 8(2):167–180.
36. Adour KK, Ruboyianes JM, Von Doersten PG, et al. Bell's palsy treatment with acyclovir and prednisone compared with prednisone alone: a double-blind, randomized, controlled trial. Ann Otol Rhinol Laryngol 1996; 105(5):371–378.
37. Gantz BJ, Rubinstein JT, Gidley P, et al. Surgical management of Bell's palsy. Laryngoscope 1999; 109(8):1177–1188.
38. Foy HM, Kenny GE, McMahan R, et al. Mycoplasma pneumoniae pneumonia in an urban area. Five years of surveillance. JAMA 1970; 214(9):1666–1672.
39. Levine DP, Lerner AM. The clinical spectrum of Mycoplasma pneumoniae infections. Med Clin North Am 1978; 62(5):961–978.
40. Murray HW, Masur H, Senterfit LB, et al. The protean manifestations of Mycoplasma pneumoniae infection in adults. Am J Med 1975; 58(2):229–242.
41. Yesnick L. Central nervous system complications of primary atypical pneumonia. AMA Arch Intern Med 1956; 97(1):93–98.
42. Endtz LJ, Hers JF. Mycoplasma pneumoniae polyradiculitis. Lancet 1970; 1(7642):358.
43. Ernster JA. Bilateral facial nerve paralysis associated with Mycoplasma pneumonia infection. Ear Nose Throat J 1984; 63(12):585–590.
44. Klar A, Gross-Kieselstein E, Hurvitz H, et al. Bilateral Bell's palsy due to Mycoplasma pneumoniae infection. Isr J Med Sci 1985; 21(8):692–694.
45. Falk W. The 1950 Poliomyelitis Epidemic. Acta Med Orient 1951; 10:105.
46. Marberg K. Observations on poliomyelitis during the 1950 epidemic in Israel. Acta Med Orient 1952; 11(4):61–77.
47. Agius T, Bartolo AE, Coleiro C, et al. Clinical Features of Poliomyelitis Epidemic in Malta, 1942–1943. Br Med J 1945; 1:759.
48. Winter ST. Facial paralysis in poliomyelitis; a follow-up of 58 patients. Pediatrics 1957; 19(5):876–880.
49. Moore EW. The fate of the face in poliomyelitis. Lancet 1952; 1(22):1092–1093.
50. Carpenter CCJ. Fever and febrile syndromes. In: Andreoli TE, Bennett JC, Carpenter CCJ, Plum F, eds. Cecil Essentials of Medicine. 4th ed. Philadelphia, Pennsylvania: W. B. Saunders Company, 1997:671–672.
51. Silverstein A, Steinberg G, Nathanson M. Nervous system involvement as the heralding and-or major manifestation of infectious mononucleosis. Trans Am Neurol Assoc 1971; 96:16–20.
52. Gsell O. Meningitis serosa bei pfeiffer—schem drusenfieber (mononucleosis infectiosa). Dtsch Med Wochenschr 1937; 63:1759–1762.
53. Grose C, Feorino PM, Dye LA, et al. Bell's palsy and infectious mononucleosis. Lancet 1973; 2(7823):231–232.
54. Michel RG, Pope TH Jr, Patterson CN. Infectious mononucleosis, mastoiditis, and facial paralysis. Arch Otolaryngol 1975; 101(8):486–489.
55. Snyderman NL. Otorhinolaryngologic presentations of infectious mononucleosis. Pediatr Clin North Am 1981; 28(4):1011–1016.
56. Weintraub MI. Bilateral facial palsy. A rare presentation of infectious mononucleosis. Clin Pediatr (Phila) 1977; 16(12):1158–1159.
57. Johnson PA, Avery C. Infectious mononucleosis presenting as a parotid mass with associated facial nerve palsy. Int J Oral Maxillofac Surg 1991; 20(4):193–195.
58. Strauss M. Cytomegalovirus and the otolaryngologist. Laryngoscope 1981; 91(12):1995–2006.
59. Leonard J, Tobin J. Polyneuritis associated with CMV infections. Q J Med 1971; 40:435–442.
60. Mair IW, Traavik T. Peripheral facial palsy and viral replication. Acta Otolaryngol 1983; 95(5–6):528–531.

61. Sene-Diouf F, Ndiaye M, Diop AG, et al. Epidemiological, clinical and progressive aspects of neurological manifestations associated with retroviral infections: eleven year retrospective study. Dakar Med 2000; 45(2):162–166.

62. Schielke E, Pfister HW, Einhaupl KM. Peripheral facial nerve palsy associated with HIV infection. Lancet 1989; 1(8637):553–554.

63. Belec L, Georges AJ, Vuillecard E, et al. Peripheral facial paralysis indicating HIV infection. Lancet 1988; 2(8625):1421–1422.

64. Murr AH, Benecke JE Jr. Association of facial paralysis with HIV positivity. Am J Otol 1991; 12 (6):450–451.

65. Walter RS, Eppes SC. Cat scratch disease presenting with peripheral facial nerve paralysis. Pediatrics 1998; 101(5):E13.

66. Premachandra DJ, Milton CM. Cat scratch disease in the parotid gland presenting with facial paralysis. Br J Oral Maxillofac Surg 1990; 28(6):413–415.

67. Yose M, Nishihira O, Inoue S, et al. Facial nerve palsy due to cat scratch disease. Facial Nerve Res 1985; 5:167–169.

68. Jagoda A, Riggio S, Burguieres T. Cephalic tetanus: a case report and review of the literature. Am J Emerg Med 1988; 6(2):128–130.

69. Vakil B.J, Singhal BS, Pandya SS, et al. Cephalic tetanus. Neurology 1973; 23(10):1091–1096.

70. Rose E. Der starrkrampf beim menschen. Deutsche Chirurgie 1897; 3:358–374.

71. Russel BW. Diseases of the Nervous System. 3rd ed. London: Oxford University Press, 1948:783.

72. Binet T. Sur le tetanus cephalique. Rev Chir (Paris) 1909; 50:427–439.

73. Brunner C. Experimentelle und klinische studien uber den kopftetanus. Zuricher Chirurgishchen Klinik 1894; 11:307–348.

74. Rubin J, Yu VL. Malignant external otitis: insights into pathogenesis, clinical manifestations, diagnosis, and therapy. Am J Med 1988; 85(3):391–398.

75. al Dousary S, Attallh M, al Rabah A, et al. Otitis externa malignant. A case report and review of literature. Otolaryngol Pol 1998; 52(1):19–22.

76. Hybels RL, Rice DH. Neuro-otologic manifestations of sarcoidosis. Laryngoscope 1976; 86(12):1873–1878.

77. James DG. Differential diagnosis of facial nerve palsy. Sarcoidosis Vasc Diffuse Lung Dis 1997; 14 (2):115–120.

78. Lower EE, Broderick JP, Brott TG, et al. Diagnosis and management of neurological sarcoidosis. Arch Intern Med 1997; 157(16):1864–1868.

79. Glocker FX, Seifert C, Lucking CH. Facial palsy in Heerfordt's syndrome: electrophysiological localization of the lesion. Muscle Nerve 1999; 22(9):1279–1282.

80. Bopp FP, Cheney ML, Donzis PB, et al. Heerfordt syndrome: a cause of facial paralysis. J La State Med Soc 1990; 142(2):13–15.

81. Dutt SN, Mirza S, Irving RM, et al. Total decompression of facial nerve for Melkersson-Rosenthal syndrome. J Laryngol Otol 2000; 114(11):870–873.

82. Tamaki H, Ogino S, Miyaguchi M. Recurrent facial palsy. In: Graham M, House W, eds. Disorders of the Facial Nerve. New York, New York: Raven Press, 1982:243–248.

83. Graham MD, Kemink JL. Total facial nerve decompression in recurrent facial paralysis and the Melkersson-Rosenthal syndrome: a preliminary report. Am J Otol 1986; 7(1):34–37.

84. http://www.guillain-barre.com/overview.html (accessed October 2005).

85. Keane JR. Bilateral seventh nerve palsy: analysis of 43 cases and review of the literature. Neurology 1994; 44(7):1198–1202.

86. Guillain G. Les Polyradiculonevrites avec dissociation albumino cytologique et a evolution favorable (syndrome de Guillain et Barre). J Belge Neurol Psychiatr 1938; 38:323–329.

87. Shuaib A, Becker WJ. Variants of Guillain-Barre syndrome: Miller Fisher syndrome, facial diplegia and multiple cranial nerve palsies. Can J Neurol Sci 1987; 14(4):611–616.

88. Tos M. Facial palsy in Hand-Schuller-Christian's disease. Arch Otolaryngol 1969; 90(5):563–567.

89. Alexander EL. Central nervous system (CNS) manifestations of primary Sjogren's syndrome: an overview. Scand J Rheumatol Suppl 1986; 61:161–165.

90. Delalande S, de Seze J, Fauchais AL, et al. Neurologic manifestations in primary Sjogren syndrome: a study of 82 patients. Medicine (Baltimore) 2004; 83(5):280–291.

91. Fukazawa T. Facial palsy in multiple sclerosis. J Neurol 1997; 244(10):631–633.

92. Adelman DC, Saltiel E, Klinenberg JR. The neuropsychiatric manifestations of systemic lupus erythematosus: an overview. Semin Arthritis Rheum 1986; 15(3):185–199.

93. Feinglass EJ, Arnett FC, Dorsch CA, et al. Neuropsychiatric manifestations of systemic lupus erythematosus: diagnosis, clinical spectrum, and relationship to other features of the disease. Medicine (Baltimore) 1976; 55(4):323–339.

94. Blaustein DA, Blaustein SA. Antinuclear antibody negative systemic lupus erythematosus presenting as bilateral facial paralysis. J Rheumatol 1998; 25(4):798–800.

95. Carpenter RJ III, McDonald TJ, Howard FM Jr. The otolaryngologic presentation of amyotrophic lateral sclerosis. Otolaryngology 1978; 86(3 pt 1):479–484.

96. Sharp G. Mixed connective tissue disease. Bull Rheum Dis 1975; 25:828–831.

97. Nitsche A, Leiguarda RC, Maldonado Cocco JA, et al. Neurological features in overlap syndrome. Clin Rheumatol 1991; 10(1):5–9.

98. Alfaro-Giner A, Penarrocha-Diago M, Bagan-Sebastian JV. Orofacial manifestations of mixed connective tissue disease with an uncommon serologic evolution. Oral Surg Oral Med Oral Pathol 1992; 73(4):441–444.

99. Hamza M, Annabi A, Ayed K, et al. Mixed connective tissue disease (Sharp syndrome) with involvement of the trigeminal nerve and facial paralysis. Sem Hop 1983; 59(36):2555–2556.

100. Per-Lee JH, Parsons RC. Vasculitis presenting as otitis media. South Med J 1969; 62(2):161–165.

101. Rose GA, Spencer H. Polyarteritis nodosa. Q J Med 1957; 26(101):43–81.

102. Dudley JP, Goodman M. Periarteritis nodosa and bilateral facial paralysis. Arch Otolarygnol 1969; 90(2):139–146.

103. Drinias V, Florentzson R. Facial palsy and Wegener's granulomatosis. Am J Otolaryngol 2004; 25 (3):208–212.

104. de Groot K, Schmidt DK, Arlt AC, et al. Standardized neurologic evaluations of 128 patients with Wegener granulomatosis. Arch Neurol 2001; 58(8):1215–1221.

105. Nishino H, Rubino FA, DeRemee RA, et al. Neurologic involvement in Wegener's granulomatosis: an analysis of 324 consecutive patients at the Mayo Clinic. Ann Neurol 1993; 33(1):4–9.

106. McCaffrey TV, McDonald TJ, Facer GW, et al. Otologic manifestations of Wegener's granulomatosis. Otolaryngol Head Neck Surg 1980; 88(5):586–593.

107. Dagum P, Roberson JB Jr. Otologic Wegener's granulomatosis with facial nerve palsy. Ann Otol Rhinol Laryngol 1998; 10(7):555–559.

108. Kornblut AD, Wolff SM, Fauci AS. Ear disease in patients with Wegener's granulomatosis. Laryngoscope 1982; 92(7 pt 1):713–717.

109. Calonius IH, Christensen CK. Hearing impairment and facial palsy as initial signs of Wegener's granulomatosis. J Laryngol Otol 1980; 94(6):649–657.

110. Bibas A, Fahy C, Sneddon L, et al. Facial paralysis in Wegener's granulomatosis of the middle ear. J Laryngol Otol 2001; 115(4):304–306.

111. Bakshi SH, Oak JL, Chawla KP, et al. Facial nerve involvement in pseudotumor cerebri. J Postgrad Med 1992; 38(3):144–145.

112. Capobianco DJ, Brazis PW, Cheshire WP. Idiopathic intracranial hypertension and seventh nerve palsy. Headache 1997; 37(5):286–288.

113. Amano S, Hazama F. Neural involvement in Kawasaki disease. Acta Pathol Jpn 1980; 30(3):365–373.

114. Poon LK, Lun KS, Ng YM. Facial nerve palsy and Kawasaki disease. Hong Kong Med J 2000; 6 (2):224–226.

115. Park MS, Lee HY, Kim HM, et al. Facial nerve paralysis associated with Kawasaki disease. Yonsei Med J 1991; 32(3):279–282.

116. Little KH, Lee EL, Frenkel EP. Cranial nerve deficits due to amyloidosis associated with plasma cell dyscrasia. South Med J 1986; 79(6):677–681.

117. Traynor AE, Gertz MA, Kyle RA. Cranial neuropathy associated with primary amyloidosis. Ann Neurol 1991; 29(4):451–454.

118. Braganza RA, Tien R, Hoffman HT, et al. Amyloid of the facial nerve. Laryngoscope 1992; 102(12 pt 1):1372–1376.

119. Barker DJ, Clough PW, Guyer PB, et al. Paget's disease of bone in 14 British towns. Br Med J 1977; 1(6070):1181–1183.

120. Hullar TE, Lustig LR. Paget's disease and fibrous dysplasia. Otolaryngol Clin North Am 2003; 36 (4):707–732.

121. Megerian CA, Sofferman RA, McKenna MJ, et al. Fibrous dysplasia of the temporal bone: ten new cases demonstrating the spectrum of otologic sequelae. Am J Otol 1995; 16(4):408–419.

122. Johnston CC Jr, Lavy N, Lord T, et al. Osteopetrosis. A clinical, genetic, metabolic, and morphologic study of the dominantly inherited, benign form. Medicine (Baltimore) 1968; 47(2):149–167.

123. Dort JC, Pollak AC, Fisch U. The fallopian canal and facial nerve in sclerosteosis of the temporal bone: a histopathologic study. Am J Otol 1990; 11(5):320–325.

124. Hofmeyr LM, Hamersma H. Sclerosing bone dysplasias: neurologic assessment and management. Curr Opin Otolaryngol Head Neck Surg 2004; 12(5):393–397.

125. Miyamoto RT, House WF, Brackmann DE. Neurotologic manifestations of the osteopetroses. Arch Otolaryngol 1980; 106(4):210–214.

126. Albers JW, Fink JK. Porphyric neuropathy. Muscle Nerve 2004; 30(4):410–422.

127. Meyer UA, Schuurmans MM, Lindberg RL. Acute porphyrias: pathogenesis of neurological manifestations. Semin Liver Dis 1998; 18(1):43–52.

128. Cavanagh JB, Mellick RS. On the nature of peripheral nerve lesions associated with acute intermittent porphyria. J Neurol Neurosurg Psychiatry 1965; 28:320–327.

129. Weintraub MI. Facial diplegia. Arch Otolaryngol 1976; 102(5):311–312.

130. Spillane JA. The face in neurological diagnosis. Br J Hosp Med 1983; 30(5):321–322, 324–325.

131. Chia LG. Facial weakness without ocular weakness in myasthenia gravis. Muscle Nerve 1988; 11 (2):185–186.

132. Sanders V. Neurologic manifestations of myxoedema. N Engl J Med 1962; 266:599–603.

133. Cox NH, Chew D, Williams JG, et al. Bell's Palsy associated with hypothyroidism. Br J Clin Pract 1985; 39(4):158–159.

134. Earll JM, Kolb FO. Facial paralysis occurring with hypothyroidism. A report of two cases. Calif Med 1967; 106(1):56–58.

135. Watanabe K, Hagura R, Akanuma Y, et al. Characteristics of cranial nerve palsies in diabetic patients. Diabetes Res Clin Pract 1990; 10(1):19–27.

136. Takasu T. A study of the disorder of the nervous system in diabetes mellitus. Adv Neurol Sci 1964; 8:1.

137. Korczyn AD. Bell's palsy and diabetes mellitus. Lancet 1971; 1(7690):108–109.

138. Moxon M. Apoplexy into canal of Fallopius in a case of Bright's disease, causing facial paralysis. Trans Pathol Soc London 1869; 20:420–422.

139. Paine RS. Facial paralysis in children; review of the differential diagnosis and report of ten cases treated with cortisone. Pediatrics 1957; 19(2):303–316.

140. Clarke E, Murphy EA. Neurological manifestations of malignant hypertension. Br Med J 1956; 44 (5005):1319–1326.

141. Lloyd AV, Jewitt DE, Still JD. Facial paralysis in children with hypertension. Arch Dis Child 1966; 41(217):292–294.

142. Amberg S. Hypertension in the young. Am J Dis Child 1929; 37:335–350.

143. Rance CP, Arbus GS, Balfe JW, et al. Persistent systemic hypertension in infants and children. Pediatr Clin North Am 1974; 21(4):801–824.

144. Trompeter RS, Smith RL, Hoare RD, et al. Neurological complications of arterial hypertension. Arch Dis Child 1982; 57(12):913–917.

145. Tirodker UH, Dabbagh S. Facial paralysis in childhood hypertension. J Paediatr Child Health 2001; 37(2):193–194.

146. Voorhees RL, Zeitzer LD, Ross M. Hypertension and associated peripheral facial paralysis. Laryngoscope 1972; 82(5):899–902.

147. Siegler RL, Brewer ED, Corneli HM, et al. Hypertension first seen as facial paralysis: case reports and review of the literature. Pediatrics 1991; 87(3):387–389.

148. Harms MM, Rotteveel JJ, Kar NC, et al. Recurrent alternating facial paralysis and malignant hypertension. Neuropediatrics 2000; 31(6):318–320.

149. Hilsinger RL Jr, Adour KK, Doty HE. Idiopathic facial paralysis, pregnancy, and the menstrual cycle. Ann Otol Rhinol Laryngol 1975; 84(4 pt 1):433–442.

150. Gillman GS, Schaitkin BM, May M, et al. Bell's palsy in pregnancy: a study of recovery outcomes. Otolaryngol Head Neck Surg 2002; 126(1):26–30.

151. Falco NA, Eriksson E. Idiopathic facial palsy in pregnancy and the puerperium. Surg Gynecol Obstet 1989; 169(4):337–340.

152. Rosenbaum RB, Donaldson JO. Peripheral nerve and neuromuscular disorders. Neurol Clin 1994; 12(3):461–478.

153. Cohen Y, Lavie O, Granovsky-Grisaru S, et al. Bell palsy complicating pregnancy: a review. Obstet Gynecol Surv 2000; 55(3):184–188.
154. Pulec JL. Collected letter. Int Corresp Soc Opthalmol Otolaryngol 1974; 19:42–43.
155. Sendi P, Locher R, Bucheli B, et al. Intranasal influenza vaccine in a working population. Clin Infect Dis 2004; 38:974–980.
156. Zhou W, Pool V, DeStefano F, et al. A potential signal of Bell's palsy after parenteral inactivated influenza vaccines: reports to the Vaccine Adverse Event Reporting System (VAERS) – United States, 1991–2001. Pharmacoepidemiol Drug Saf 2004; 13(8):505–510.
157. Shaw FE Jr, Graham DJ, Guess HA, et al. Postmarketing surveillance for neurologic adverse events reported after hepatitis B vaccination. Am J Epidemiol 1988; 127(2):337–352.
158. Rice JP, Horowitz M, Chin D. Wernicke-Korsakoff syndrome with bilateral facial nerve palsies. J Neurol Neurosurg Psychiatry 1984; 47(12):1356–1357.
159. Zaloga GP, Deal J, Spurling T, et al. Unusual manifestations of arsenic intoxication. Am J Med Sci 1985; 289(5):210–214.
160. McCall WV, Coffey CE. Transient facial palsy during lithium toxicity. J Clin Psychopharmacol 1987; 7(4):280–281.
161. Lee RT, Oster MW, Balmaceda C, et al. Bilateral facial nerve palsy secondary to the administration of high-dose paclitaxel. Ann Oncol 1999; 10(10):1245–1247.
162. Sokoloff J, Wickbom I, McDonald D, et al. Therapeutic percutaneous embolization in intractable epistaxis. Radiology 1974; 111(2):285–287.
163. de Vries N, Versluis RJ, Valk J, et al. Facial nerve paralysis following embolization for severe epistaxis (case report and review of the literature). J Laryngol Otol 1986; 100(2):207–210.
164. Metson R, Hanson DG. Bilateral facial nerve paralysis following arterial embolization for epistaxis. Otolaryngol Head Neck Surg 1983; 91(3):299–303.
165. Rhee D, Myssiorek D, Zahtz G, et al. Recurrent attacks of facial nerve palsy as the presenting sign of leukemic relapse. Laryngoscope 2002; 112(2):235–237.
166. Sood BR, Sharma B, Kumar S, et al. Facial palsy as first presentation of acute myeloid leukemia. Am J Hematol 2003; 74(3):200–201.
167. Paparella MM, Berlinge NT, Oda M. Otological manifestations of leukemia. Laryngoscope 1973; 83(9):1510–1526.
168. Zappia JJ, Bunge FA, Koopmann CF Jr, et al. Facial nerve paralysis as the presenting symptom of leukemia. Int J Pediatr Otorhinolaryngol 1990; 19(3):259–264.
169. Gotay V. Unusual otologic manifestations of chronic lymphocytic leukemia. Laryngoscope 1976; 86(12):1856–1863.
170. Schattner A, Kozack N, Sandler A, et al. Facial diplegia as the presenting manifestation of acute lymphoblastic leukemia. Mt. Sinai J Med 2001; 68(6):406–409.
171. Chapman P, Johnson SA. Mastoid chloroma as relapse in acute myeloid leukemia. J Laryngol Otol 1980; 94(12):1423–1427.
172. Ho TP, Carrie S, Meikle D, et al. T-cell lymphoma presenting as acute mastoiditis with a facial palsy. Int J Pediatr Otorhinolaryngol 2004; 68(9):1199–1201.
173. Bockmuhl U, Bruchhage KL, Enzmann H. Primary non-Hodgkin's lymphoma of the temporal bone. Eur Arch Otorhinolaryngol 1995; 252(6):376–378.
174. Tucci DL, Lambert PR, Innes DJ Jr. Primary lymphoma of the temporal bone. Arch Otolaryngol Head Neck Surg 1992; 118(1):83–85.
175. Lang EE, Walsh RM, Leader M. Primary middle-ear lymphoma in a child. J Laryngol Otol 2003; 117(3):205–207.
176. Laubert A, Mausolf A, Bernhards J, et al. Non-Hodgkin's lymphoma: a differential diagnosis of otogenic facial paralysis. HNO 1991; 39(3):98–101.
177. Shone GR. Facial palsy due to myeloma of the temporal bone. J Laryngol Otol 1985; 99(9):907–908.
178. Marks PV, Brookes GB. Myelomatosis presenting as an isolated lesion in the mastoid. J Laryngol Otol 1985; 99(9):903–906.
179. Funakubo T, Kikuchi A. A case of myeloma with facial palsy. Acta Otolaryngol Suppl 1994; 511:200–203.
180. Quinodoz D, Dulguerov P, Kurt AM, et al. Multiple myeloma presenting with external ear canal mass. J Laryngol Otol 1998; 112(5):469–471.
181. Li W, Schachern PA, Morizono T, et al. The temporal bone in multiple myeloma. Laryngoscope 1994; 104(6 pt 1):675–680.
182. Schuuknecht HF. Neoplastic growth. In: Schuknecht HF, ed. Pathology of the Ear. 2nd ed. Philadelphia, Pennsylvania: Lea and Febiger, 1993:492–498.

30

Headache

Christy M. Jackson
Department of Neurosciences and School of Medicine, University of California, San Diego, California, U.S.A.

INTRODUCTION

With the development of more effective headache therapy, headache sufferers are becoming more educated and are seeking physician advice for pain control. The magnitude of headache and its impact on quality of life and work productivity is significant.

With the introduction of subcutaneous sumatriptan in 1993, physicians entered a new era of headache management. In 2003, the International Headache Society (IHS) formulated a revised classification scheme for headaches (1). This classification scheme serves to standardize research and treatment protocols. A complete listing of the individual headache classifications may be found in this encompassing publication.

In this chapter, the evaluation, workup, and treatment of primary and secondary headache presenting to the otolaryngologist's office will be reviewed.

CLASSIFICATION

Headache syndromes are classified as primary or secondary. Primary headache syndromes are those in which no underlying organic pathology exists. The most common primary headache syndromes include migraine with and without aura, cluster, tension-type, and analgesic rebound or medication overuse headache (MOH).

Secondary headaches account for 2% to 3% of headache complaints received by physicians. These disorders arise from an underlying organic etiology such as systemic disease, vascular malformations, or structural causes. One popular patient complaint is of "sinus" headache. A recent article reviews the literature on sinus headache and finds that patients presenting with a complaint of "sinus" headache actually have a 58% to 88% incidence of migraine-type headache (2). Recognizing the diagnosis of migraine in these cases increasingly falls on the otolaryngologist. Multiple over-the-counter sinus remedies effectively relieve migraine symptoms by providing vasoconstriction of medium bore arterioles, thus reinforcing to the patient the idea of sinus pathology. As migraine often presents with nasal congestion, a systematic approach to the diagnosis and treatment of migraine is necessary. This approach is discussed elsewhere in this text.

PATIENT HISTORY

A systematic approach focusing on a complete history is recommended initially. At the University of California San Diego (UCSD) Headache Clinic, a patient's first contact is devoted to an in-depth review of the history. A headache questionnaire (Appendix 1) is utilized to elicit historical features of the headache and to help guide the examiner in the determination of whether the headache is of primary or secondary etiology. The 10-page questionnaire elicits such information as age of onset, characteristics of pain, associated features, triggers, and whether the pain has changed in character or intensity.

Important historical information includes family history of headaches and whether the headaches are progressively worsening. Sudden onset of severe pain with change in mentation or otherwise focal neurologic exam would lead the examiner to consider secondary headache etiologies such as subarachnoid hemorrhage, meningitis, or mass lesion. However, the patient who presents with recurrence of severe headaches that have occurred intermittently for years would point the examiner to a primary headache syndrome such as migraine, cluster, or tension-type.

Most commonly, the headaches will be of intermediate severity and have developed subacutely. A complete history of prior headache experience is necessary to identify whether the patient has, in fact, suffered from a primary headache disorder in the past, and whether this presentation may be a recurrence of the same. Examples include the resurgence of migraine in a woman in her perimenopausal years, which has features of tinnitus and vertigo, but no true pain. This is termed acephalgic migraine and responds to migraine therapies, often including a low-dose estrogen patch for a few months.

PRIMARY HEADACHES

By far, in most instances of a patient presenting with a complaint of headache, the underlying etiology will be nonorganic (primary). The most common primary headaches a physician will see are migraine with or without aura, cluster, tension-type, and analgesic rebound headache (MOH).

Migraine Headache

Migraine without Aura. These headache episodes, formerly known as common migraine, are defined by specific criteria set forth by the IHS (1). Patients must fulfill two of the four characteristics of Group A listed below and fulfill one of the two characteristics of Group B to satisfy diagnostic criteria.

Group A. Two of the following criteria must be met:

Pain is unilateral
Pain is pulsatile or throbbing
Pain is moderate to severe and may inhibit or restrict ability to function
Pain is aggravated by routine physical activity such as bending over or climbing stairs

Group B. One of the two following criteria must be met:

Presence of nausea *and/or* vomiting
Presence of photophobia *and* phonophobia

Migraine with Aura. Migraine with aura, formerly known as classic migraine, is defined as headache that meets the criteria listed above and is preceded by a 15- to 20-minute episode of visual or sensory aura. These auras represent a cortical spreading depression and may be of several types. Teichopsia are described as brightly colored flashes of light or rippling images that begin in the corner of the visual field and spread, often in a crescent pattern. Fortification spectra are sharply angled lines coalescing to resemble the architectural ground plan of a fort. Sensory auras are described by patients as parasthesias that classically involve the arm and face. Other symptoms that comprise aura may include unilateral weakness, aphasia, and mental slowing.

Treatment. Treatment of migraine begins with determining whether a preventative medicine should be utilized. If a patient will be using abortive medications more than two to three days per week, a preventative medicine is recommended in order to lessen the chance of MOH. β blockers, tricyclic antidepressants (TCAs), valproate and topiramate, as well as calcium channel blockers are the most widely used prophylactic medications. Counseling the patient to maintain good sleep hygiene, exercise aerobically regularly, and avoid food triggers is another effective strategy to decrease headache frequency. Abortive medications include NSAIDs, tramadol, ergots, and triptans. Avoidance of narcotic use as a routine abortive medication is recommended.

Tension-Type Headaches

Tension-type headaches are commonly seen in clinical practice and are often difficult to differentiate from the milder forms of migraine. They may occur episodically with a frequency of less than 15 days monthly or chronically with a frequency of 15 or more days monthly.

The IHS criteria for tension-type headaches include two of the following features (1):

It is a band-like pressure that is nonpulsatile
It is not aggravated by routine physical activity
It is of mild or moderate intensity, not preventive of daily activities
It is of bilateral distribution

Sensitivity to light or sound is not found in tension-type headaches and is used in clinic to differentiate this form of headache from migraine.

Treatment.   Episodic tension-type headaches are common and often respond to physiological approaches to correct imbalances in refractive error, dental alignment, or cervical alignment. Pharmacologic treatment with nonsteroidal anti-inflammatory agents and muscle relaxants are often of benefit in treatment of episodic pain. For chronic tension-type sufferers, prophylaxis with TCAs is effective. Increasingly, the use of biofeedback, acupuncture, and physiotherapy are being utilized for both episodic and chronic tension-type headache control. Trials of Botox® for treatment of tension-type headaches have proved unsuccessful (3).

Cluster Headaches

Cluster headaches are severe, unilateral, retro-orbital, and invariably described by patients as a searing, burning pain behind one eye. The headache pain lasts from 15 to 180 minutes and recurs in clusters, often at the same time each day. Cluster patients present very differently from migraineurs. They may pace in an agitated fashion in anticipation of the next episode. The patient often tries to relieve pain by putting pressure on the orbit or even striking the side of the face to provide distraction from the pain. The migraineur, on the other hand, is very sensitive to movement and stimuli.

Treatment.   Episodic cluster can be treated effectively with a variety of abortive agents. Ergotamine tartrate or sumatriptan injection, with or without inhalation of 100% oxygen (7 L/min), is highly effective. Intranasal lidocaine (4% solution) may abort a cluster episode, and steroid pulses have been effective in suppressing bouts of cluster attacks. Chronic cluster headaches (regularly occurring attacks) may respond well to prophylaxis with methysergide, verapamil, lithium, or high-dose NSAIDs such as indomethacin.

ANALGESIC REBOUND (MEDICATION OVERUSE) HEADACHES

Increasingly, patients are presenting for medical attention with symptoms of vague, diffuse headache that is present upon waking and lasts throughout the day. Often the patient will state that the pain may worsen at times into pain that has migrainous or tension-type features. When analgesic medications are taken more than two to three days weekly, a superimposed headache may develop that will be responsive only to the medication that is, unfortunately, now causing it. Medications thought to cause analgesic rebound if used too frequently include the triptans, ergotamines, narcotics, vasoconstrictors such as pseudoephedrine, and caffeine-containing medications (4).

Treatment

The treatment in these cases is to withdraw the patient from the offending medication for a period of time while beginning a preventative medication. Although rebound headaches are active, preventative medications will be ineffective. The most difficult issue is to find pain relief for the patient while removing the offending medication. Some patients respond to prednisone tapers of 10 days, while a newer approach is to use a naratriptan taper for 90 days (5). Preventative medications may then be initiated either for migraine (most commonly) or for tension-type headache. The primary effort is to prevent the headache frequency from increasing once again, as nearly all analgesics, if used too frequently, have been implicated in this type of headache.

SECONDARY HEADACHES

Table 1 describes common secondary headache syndromes and the recommended evaluation for each.

A summary statement from The American Academy of Neurology in 1994 supports neuroimaging in patients with atypical headache patterns and a history of seizures or focal neurologic signs or symptoms (6). Neuroimaging is not thought to be warranted in adults with a prior diagnosis of migraine, no recent change in headache pattern, and a normal neurologic exam.

Under most circumstances, a computed tomography (CT) of the brain will suffice to rule out acute causes of headache as well as to locate mass lesions and increased intracranial pressure. If the focus of pain is thought to lie in the posterior fossa, however, magnetic resonance imaging (MRI) will be the most helpful imaging tool. For example, cases of Arnold-Chiari 1 malformation will often be missed on routine CT of the brain, because the sagittal image of the posterior fossa is needed to adequately evaluate this. The Arnold-Chiari malformations are characterized by extension of posterior fossa contents through the foramen magnum. Chiari 1 malformation is currently defined as extension of the cerebellar tonsils more than 5 mm below the foramen magnum (7). Extension of the cerebellar tonsils up to 3 mm may be found in the normal population (8). Figure 1 demonstrates mild cerebellar tonsillar herniation that would be considered within normal limits.

Although Chiari malformations are congenital, symptoms often do not manifest until the third and fourth decades of life, or even later. Patients may present with headache, lower cranial nerve palsies, central vertigo, ataxia, or dissociated anesthesia of the trunk and extremities (7). Definitive diagnosis is made by MRI that shows the compressed tonsils extending through the foramen magnum into the cervical subarachnoid space (9). In this author's experience, the MRI of a mild Arnold-Chiari 1 malformation may be read as normal. When a cerebrospinal fluid (CSF)-gated flow study is employed to evaluate pressure in the CSF space at the base of the brain, one may often find an increase in the local pressure that results in recurrent headache and posterior fossa symptoms.

The following case is that of a 40-year-old white male presenting with intractable headaches, diagnosed as tension-type headache at the age of seven. This diagnosis should raise concern, as tension-type headache is not typically diagnosed at an early age unless ocular strabismus is the cause. Additionally, these headaches would not remain persistent despite multiple standard therapies. The patient had undergone numerous CT scans of the brain to identify the etiology; these had returned read as normal. When an MRI of the brain was ordered, the diagnosis of mild Arnold-Chiari 1 malformation was made. Figure 2 demonstrates extension of the cerebellar tonsils into the foramen magnum at the length of approximately 5 to 6 mm. The headaches were treated with high-dose indomethacin and a prophylactic of valproic acid. No lower cranial nerve findings have arisen, nor has any significant hydrocephalus. The patient is seen on a routine basis with an MRI scan every two years to evaluate for hydrocephalus and/or syrinx formation. He has continued to do well.

TABLE 1 Secondary Headache Syndromes

Syndrome	Presenting features	Evaluation
Infectious		
Meningitis		
Acute	Nuchal rigidity, fever	Exam, CT brain, LP
Chronic	Nuchal rigidity, fever, mental status changes	Exam, CT or MRI, LP
Sinusitis	Sinus tenderness, nasal drainage, congestion	Exam, plain films
Vascular		
Temporal arteritis	Scalp tenderness, jaw claudication, tender, poorly pulsatile artery	Exam, ESR
Stroke	Sudden in onset with focal neurologic features	Exam, CT brain
SAH	Sudden in onset with nausea, vomiting, LOC or focal exam HTN, tachycardia	Exam, CT brain, LP
Mass lesions		
Tumor	Progressive in onset, postural worsening, possible focal exam	Exam, CT/MRI brain*
Abscess	Fever, focal exam	Exam, CT with and without contrast
Hematoma	HTN, tachycardia, N/V, focal neuro exam	Exam, CT brain
Toxin		
Decongestant rebound	Headache only responsive to med	Exam, taper from med
Analgesic rebound	Headache only responsive to med	Exam, taper from med
Lead encephalopathy	Chronic progressive headache Peripheral limb weakness	CBC, heavy metal screen exam
Oral estrogens	Temporal relationship, progressive worsening	Exam, removal of med
Nitrates	Temporal relationship, pulsatile quality	Exam, removal of med
Autoimmune		
SLE, Sjögren's, Behcet's, ulcerative colitis		
Metabolic		
Hypothyroidism	Fatigue, constant pain frontal location	Exam, delayed reflexes, thyroid-stimulating hormone
Uremia	Constant ill-defined pain	Chemistries, exam
Hypoxia	Pain often present upon waking	Sleep study, exam
Hypercarbia	Constant pain, worse with exertion	Sleep study, exam
Abnormal CSF circulation		
Pseudotumor cerebri	Visual obscurations, disc edema worse upon wakening	Exam, CT brain, LP
CSF obstruction	Neck stiffness, N/V, visual obscuration, disc edema, worse upon wakening	Exam, MRI brain for posterior fossa
Low CSF pressure	Worse with upright positions, relieved with recumbency, rhinorrhea, otorrhea	Exam, CT brain, LP
Arnold-Chiari	Neck stiffness, vertigo, lower cranial nerve findings, hydrocephalus	Exam, MRI, CSF flow study

*MRI of the brain is suggested when lesions of the cerebellum or brainstem are suspected.
Abbreviations: SAH; SLE; CSF, cerebrospinal fluid; LOC; HTN; N/V; CT, computed tomography; MRI, magnetic resonance imaging; LP; ESR; CBC.

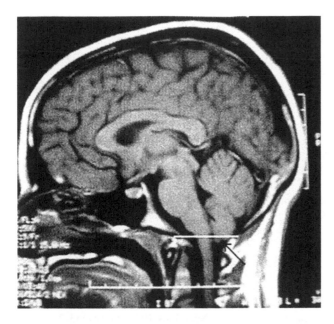

FIGURE 1 Tonsillar herniation within normal limits. Sagittal T1-weighted magnetic resonance image showing tonsillar herniation of 3 to 4mm.

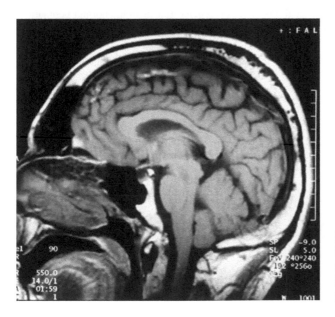

FIGURE 2 Arnold-Chiari I Malformation. Sagittal T1-weighted magnetic resonance image showing tonsillar herniation of 6 to 7 mm.

SUMMARY

The goal of the first physician–patient encounter in the evaluation of headache is to rule out the 2% to 3% of cases that represent secondary or organic headaches. The most common organic headaches in otolaryngology practice have been summarized, with emphasis on analgesic rebound headache presenting as sinus headache, and Arnold-Chiari 1 malformation presenting as headache with vertigo and ataxia. Primary headaches have been described with an overview of diagnostic and treatment strategies. At UCSD, a close referral relationship with the Headache Clinic has helped in efficiently identifying the infrequent organic headache as well as identifying and treating the more common primary headaches that may present atypically.

REFERENCES

1. Headache Classification Subcommittee of the International Headache Society. The international classification of headache disorders. 2nd ed. Cephalalgia 2004, 24(suppl 1):9–160.
2. Mehle ME, Schreiber CP. Sinus headache, migraine, and the otolaryngologist. Head Neck Surg 2005; 133(4):489–496.
3. Boudreau G. Treatment of chronic tension-type headache with botulinum toxin: a double-blind, placebo-controlled clinical trial. Cephalalgia 2005; 25(11):1101; author reply 1101–1102.
4. Couch JR. Rebound-withdrawal headache (medication overuse headache). Curr Treat Options Neurol 2006; 8(1):11–19.
5. Sheftell FD, Rapoport AM, Tepper SJ, et al. Naratriptan in the preventive treatment of refractory transformed migraine: a prospective pilot study. Headache 2005; 45(10):1400–1406.
6. Practice parameter: the utility of neuroimaging in the evaluation of headache in patients with normal neurologic examinations (summary statement). Report of the Quality Standards Subcommittee of the American Academy of Neurology. Neurology 1994; 44(7):1353–1354.
7. Solomon D. Distinguishing and treating causes of central vertigo. Otolaryngol Clin North Am 2000; 33(3):579–601.
8. Aboulezz AO, Sartor K, Geyer CA, et al. Position of cerebellar tonsils in the normal population and in patients with Chiari malformation: a quantitative approach with MR imaging. J Comput Assist Tomogr 1985; 9(6):1033–1036.
9. Pokharel D, Siatkowski RM. Progressive cerebellar tonsillar herniation with recurrent divergence insufficiency esotropia. J AAPOS 2004; 8(3):286–287.

*A*PPENDIX I

UCSD HEADACHE CENTER
HEADACHE QUESTIONNAIRE

DATE:

TO ALL HEADACHE CLINIC PATIENTS:

We would appreciate your cooperation in filling out this form. In our evaluation of headache, your history is typically our most valuable tool for diagnosis and subsequent treatment. If you have any questions regarding this form, please ask.

PATIENT PORTION

A. Identification

Name:_____

Age:_____

Sex:_____

Date of birth:_____

Address:_____

_____

_____

Phone #:_____

  How were you referred to the UCSD Headache Clinic?_____

  _____

  _____

  _____

  Who is your primary physician? _____

  _____

B. Headache History

How old were you when you had your first significant headache? _____

Over the past 2 months, how many individual headache attacks have you averaged per month?_____

How long does a typical headache attack last?_____

a) 0–1 hr_____   b) > 1–6 hr_____   c) > 6–12 hr_____

d) > 12–24 hr_____   e) > 24–48 hr_____   f) > 48–72 hr_____

g) > 72 hr_____   h) constant_____   i) too variable_____

j) unknown_____

Has there been any recent change in the character or frequency of your headaches? No_____Yes_____

If yes, please specify what type of change:_____

Check any of the following factors which seem to trigger a headache attack in you:

☐ alcohol (specify types:_____)

☐ menstruation

☐ emotional stress

☐ odors (please list:_____)

☐ fatigue

☐ missing meals

☐ caffeine

☐ changes in weather

☐ other (please specify:_____)

Are your headaches ever incapacitating (e.g., have to leave work or school or lie down undisturbed)? No_____Yes_____

How many days per month are you incapacitated by headache?_____

Where on this line does your typical (average) headache fall?

|———|

no pain   unbearable pain

Overall, how disabled do you feel you have been by headaches over the past 2 months?

|———|

no problem with headaches   totally disabled by frequent/severe headache

Is your headache pain ever throbbing? No_____Yes_____Unknown_____

(If yes, what percent of your headache attacks involve "throbbing" pain?_____%
_____ unknown

Is your headache ever localized to one side?_____% _____
_____ unknown

Does your headache typically occur at a certain time of day or on certain days of the week or month? No____Yes_____(If yes, please describe_____)

Do you have any warning symptoms which alert you that you are going to have a headache attack? No___Yes____(If yes, what type of warning do you have?_____
_____)

Do you ever experience any of the following symptoms in association with your headache attacks (before, during, or after)? Please check the appropriate boxes:

□ nasal congestion
□ nausea (with what % of attacks do you experience nausea?_____%
    _____unknown
□ vomiting (with what % of attacks do you experience vomiting?_____%
    _____unknown
□ diarrhea
□ visual changes (e.g., visual distortion, "flash cubes," "zig-zags," "blind spots," "sparkles"). (Please describe:_____).
□ inability to tolerate bright light (photophobia)
□ inability to tolerate loud noise (phonophobia)
□ numbness and/or tingling in face, arm, or leg (Please describe: _____).
□ speech disturbance (Please describe:_____).
□ loss of balance
□ vertigo (i.e., a spinning/"merry-go-around" sensation)
□ extreme thirst, food cravings (Please describe:_____).

What makes your headache worse?_____
_____.

What seems to help your headache?_____
_____.

C. Medical and Social History

Are you currently having difficulties with your sleeping (insomnia, early morning awakening, "always sleepy," etc.)? No____Yes____

Do you consider yourself to be currently under a significant amount of stress? No_____
Yes _____

Do you adhere to a regular exercise program? No____ Yes____

Do you eat at regular intervals? No____ Yes_____

Do you sleep at regular intervals? No_____ Yes_____

Are you currently receiving formal treatment (counseling and/or medications) for anxiety or depression? No_____ Yes_____

Please check the appropriate boxes:

☐ history of snoring

☐ history of lung disease

☐ anemia

☐ hypertension (high blood pressure)

☐ arthritis

☐ history of thyroid disease

☐ treated for depression in past

☐ recent weight loss

☐ past or present problems with significant motion sickness

☐ do you smoke cigarettes now? (Number of cigarettes per day_____)

☐ any significant head injury? (If yes, within the past six months? No___Yes_____)

☐ history of seizures

☐ any other significant medical or psychiatric problem or conditions for which you are under medical care? If yes, please explain:_____

_____

_____

What medications are you presently taking? (Please include over-the-counter medications, herbs, and birth control pills):_____

_____

_____

Have you taken oral contraceptives or estrogen replacement therapy in the past? No___Yes_____ (If yes, effect on your headaches? Better _____ worse _____ no change _____ can't recall _____)

Have you been pregnant? No____Yes_____ (If yes, effect on your headaches? Better_____ worse_____no change_____ can't recall_____

Have you seen a doctor in the past for your headaches? No_____ Yes_____ His/Her diagnosis (if known):_____

Have you had a CAT scan in the past? No_____ Yes_____ Unknown_____

Have you had a brain MRI scan in the past? No____Yes____Unknown____

What medications have you tried in the past for your headaches (e.g., Inderal, Cafergot, Elavil)?_____

D. Family History

Has anyone in your family had a significant problem with headaches or been diagnosed as having migraine or "sick" headaches? No____Yes_____(If yes, who?_____) unknown_____

E. Other

Is there anything else you think is pertinent for your doctor to know?_____

_____

_____

31

Epistaxis

Mark J. Shikowitz
Albert Einstein School of Medicine and Department of Otolaryngology and Communicative Disorders, Long Island Jewish Medical Center, New Hyde Park, New York, U.S.A.

- Vascular Anatomy **442**
- Physiology of the Nose and the Nasal Lining **443**
- Etiology of Epistaxis **444**
  - Local Factors **445**
  - Systemic Factors **446**
- Epistaxis Management **447**
  - Control of Epistaxis in the Outpatient Setting **447**
  - Nasal Packing **448**
  - Maxillary Artery Ligation **452**
  - Endoscopic Management of Epistaxis **452**
  - Endoscopic Ligation of the Sphenopalatine Artery **453**
  - Septal Dermatoplasty **453**
  - Ethmoid Artery Ligation **454**
  - Selective Embolization **454**
- Juvenile Angiofibromas **456**
- References **457**

VASCULAR ANATOMY

A clear understanding and knowledge of nasovascular anatomy is essential for expediency and safety in controlling nasal hemorrhage. Regardless of the type of technology, new or old, utilized to control nasal hemorrhage, it is the clear understanding of the various potential sources of the blood supply that is important. Whether control of the problem is via more traditional anterior or posterior packing of the nose, open surgical approach, or endoscopic approach followed by selective angiography and embolization, one premise still holds true: the offending source of blood supply to the region must clearly be defined and controlled to prevent potential unwarranted side effects and complications.

The internal and the external carotid artery systems are the primary vascular supply to the nose. The external carotid artery serves as the major contributor. The internal carotid artery supplies blood to the anterior and posterior ethmoid arteries. The larger anterior and smaller posterior ethmoid arteries branch off the ophthalmic artery within the orbit itself. Both of these vessels pass through the periorbital fascia through the shared wall of the medial orbit and lateral fovea ethmoidalis bone along the frontoethmoidal suture line. The frontoethmoidal suture line is approximately at the level of the cribriform plate. The posterior ethmoid artery enters its foramen within 4 to 7 mm of the optic nerve greater than 80% of the time. The anterior ethmoidal artery enters its foramen 14 to 22 mm posterior to the maxillolacrimal suture greater than 80% of the time (1). It has been noted that the anterior ethmoid artery may be absent 7% to 14% of the time (2,3). It has also been demonstrated that the posterior ethmoid artery may be absent 31% of the time (3). The anterior and the posterior ethmoid arteries pass through the ethmoid air cells and give rise to the medial and lateral branches. Of these, the medial branches of the ethmoid arteries supply the superior septum in the Little's area. The lateral branches of the ethmoid arteries supply the superior and the middle turbinates (Fig. 1).

The external carotid artery supplies blood to the nose through two different branches. The primary branch is the maxillary artery; the secondary supply is via the facial artery. The maxillary artery is the terminal branch of the external carotid artery. The facial artery supplies the superior labial artery, which then gives rise to the nasal arterial branches medial to the septum and lateral to the nasal ala. The maxillary artery then passes into the infratemporal fossa, either lateral to the superior and inferior heads of the lateral pterygoid muscle or between the superior and inferior heads. From here, the artery enters the pterygopalatine fossa through the pterygomaxillary fissure. The maxillary artery passes through the pterygopalatine fossa within the fat pad. The maxillary artery and its branches are usually anteroinferior to the maxillary and vidian nerves.

This is an important anatomical point to remember when undertaking a maxillary artery ligation for control of epistaxis. Although the maxillary artery gives rise to several branches, four primary vessels are relevant in the control of epistaxis. These include the descending greater palatine artery, the pharyngeal artery, the posterior nasal artery, and the sphenopalatine artery. The descending palatine artery may give rise to two or three branches. The largest is the greater palatine artery of the greater palatine canal. The lesser palatine artery passes through the lesser palatine canal and foramen, and supplies blood to the soft palate. The greater palatine artery has a varied course to the nose by first passing inferiorly through the greater palatine canal and foramen and then traveling within the lateral hard palatal mucosa. These bilateral paired arteries meet in the anterior portion of the nose in the midline and pass superiorly through the single midline incisor foramen. The greater palatine artery also supplies blood to the septum and floor of the nose. The maxillary artery bifurcates into the sphenopalatine and posterior nasal arteries at or distal to the sphenopalatine foramen. The sphenopalatine artery supplies the septal mucosa in the

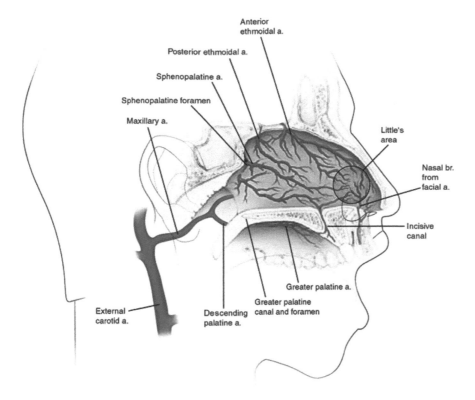

FIGURE 1 A sagittal view demonstrating the arterial branches of the internal carotid artery. The nasal septum is supplied via branches from the facial artery and maxillary artery. "Little's area" is comprised of anastomosis from the sphenopalatine, anterior ethmoid, greater palatine, and nasal branches of the facial artery.

region of the anterior inferior septum anastomosis with the greater palatine artery, the anterior ethmoidal artery, and the nasal branches of the facial artery forming Kiesselbach's plexus or Little's area (1,4). It is this complex meeting or net of vessels in the anterior portion of the septum that make this region play such a prominent role in epistaxis. The posterior nasal artery supplies the turbinates and the lateral nasal wall. Superiorly, it often anastomoses with the ethmoid arteries (5). Inferiorly, it anastomoses with the pharyngeal arterial branch of the maxillary artery, forming Woodruff's naso-nasopharyngeal plexus (6).

It can be seen that the nose and its surrounding structures have an extremely complex and often variable blood supply. It is for this reason that treatment of epistaxis is often a complicated process requiring both skill and superior knowledge of the anatomical vascular supply. With the development of newer and less invasive techniques such as nasal endoscopy, the exact location becomes even more important for selective control of bleeding. The use of angiographic techniques, both for identifying the offending vessel and for therapeutic control with embolization, is another means of utilizing and understanding anatomy to our and the patient's benefit.

PHYSIOLOGY OF THE NOSE AND THE NASAL LINING

The functional design of the internal nose provides a streamlined passage for a laminar airflow and exchange. This laminar airflow may be considered similar to air passing over an airfoil or airplane wing. Any disruption of this airflow creates turbulence and will alter its physiology. The lining of the nose is comprised of pseudostratified ciliated columnar epithelium.

As air passes over this layer, particulate matter is filtered and the air is humidified. In addition to this, the nose has the capability of temperature control, from warming air from the subzero temperatures of the North and South Poles to cooling air from the high temperatures of the earth's deserts, to help the lungs function properly. In effect, it acts as the body's radiator to help in this process. The many convolutions within the nasal cavity itself increase its surface area, much as the fins do on a car's radiator. All of these factors help the nose to work more effectively. The lining of the nose along the inferior and middle turbinates contains a highly vascular lamina propria. The arterioles in the turbinates pass within the conchal bone and are surrounded by a venous plexus. Arterial dilatation will effectively block the venous outflow and result in mucosal congestion. This submucosal plexus of veins, also known as the cavernous nasal plexus, is similar to erectile tissue found in other parts of the body and provides for rapid engorgement under parasympathetic control. Stimulation of this parasympathetic process can occur from a variety of sources, including thermal, psychogenic, mechanical, sexual, or chemical (7). A crucial physiological point is that the nasoseptal cartilage does not have its own intrinsic blood supply and must depend on the vessels within the mucoperichondrial layer that covers it. A significant disruption of the mucoperichondrium may cause a loss of cartilage, resulting in either perforation of the nasal septum, or, when significant enough, nasal collapse. This point must always be taken into consideration when treating epistaxis. The nasal lining contains multiple mucous and serous glands, especially along the turbinates, which are responsible for maintaining the secretions and protective blanket for the mucosa. Any loss of these secretions may result in the loss of cilia or ciliary activity and prevent the normal passage of secretions and debris through the nose.

ETIOLOGY OF EPISTAXIS

The etiology of epistaxis may be divided into two major categories, local and systemic. The most common local factors seen by the otolaryngologist include trauma related to digital manipulation or sports injury. Relatively cold temperatures with low humidity will also result in increased epistaxis. This is common in the cooler northern climates during the winter, due to the relatively low humidity of the ambient air, complicated by the use of central heating systems without humidification. The chronic use of nasal decongestant sprays will also alter the nasal lining, in addition to chronically decreasing the blood supply to the nasal septum. In cases of prolonged use of nasal decongestants, septal perforation has been seen to occur. This will alter the change of nasal airflow from its usual laminar state to one of turbulence, thus increasing the drying and crusting of the remaining nasal mucosa, especially at the edges of the perforation. Anatomic deformities including deviated nasal septum may also alter the state of the nasal lining (8,9).

In children, foreign bodies may play a role. Intranasal tumors, both malignant and benign, can be heralded by recurrent and often significant epistaxis. The use of nasal prongs and oxygen in the hospital or home setting is another frequently seen cause. With the recognition of obstructive sleep apnea as a significant medical condition and the use of continuous positive airway pressure (CPAP) with its continuous flow of positive pressure through the nasal passages, there has been a rise in the number of patients with recurrent epistaxis (9). Any medication inhaled nasally, which can alter the pseudostratified columnar epithelium or effectiveness of the ciliary blanket, can cause epistaxis (8).

Systemic factors contributing to epistaxis include vascular disorders, blood dyscrasias, alcohol consumption, hypertension, various infectious diseases, vitamin deficiencies, inflammatory diseases, and granulomatous diseases.

Local Factors

By far, one of the most common causes of epistaxis, especially in children and participants in sporting activities, is trauma. It is for this reason that epistaxis occurs along the anterior nasal region in 90% to 95% of cases. It is often seen in children who suck their thumbs and in adolescents and adults as a result of chronic digital manipulation of the nose. Individuals who participate in sports with a high rate of contact with the nasal and facial structures also run the risk of recurrent epistaxis and complications related to its treatment (1). Basketball players, boxers, soccer players, and other athletes who do not wear headgear or facial protection have an increased incidence of recurrent problems: along with the risk of epistaxis, a septal hematoma secondary to repeat trauma can accelerate the risk of complications if not treated appropriately. Continuous trauma to the nasal structures may result in devitalization of the mucoperichondrium, with loss of the vascular supply to the cartilage and/or exposure of the cartilage with subsequent perforation. Septal perforations result in loss of laminar airflow, increase in turbulence, and increase in the drying, scab formation, and continued bleeding (10). Trauma to the nasal skeleton and surrounding facial structures may result in a simple nasal fracture or severe and often life-threatening midface and base-of-skull fractures. Motor vehicle accidents, especially in the days before the common use of seat belts and air bags, often resulted in exsanguinating arterial hemorrhage.

Trauma to structures adjacent to the nose, such as the orbit, sinuses, or middle ear, may result in nasal hemorrhage, without being primary nasal epistaxis. Recurrent and often massive epistaxis in a young adolescent male, with or without nasal obstruction, may be the initial symptoms of juvenile angiofibroma (JA) (11–13).

Massive epistaxis in a patient who presents with the classic triad of prior monocular blindness, ipsilateral orbital fractures, and delayed epistaxis with a recent history of head and neck trauma, should always make one suspicious of a post-traumatic pseudoaneurysm of the internal carotid artery. Delayed epistaxis is often seen following cosmetic and post-traumatic maxillofacial reconstructive surgery. Local irritation and inflammation of the nasal and sinus lining due to upper respiratory tract infections, sinusitis, allergic rhinitis, or environmental irritants such as tobacco, smoke, or chemical exposure, may alter the normal protective mucosal blanket, allowing drying, crusting, exposure, and hemorrhage. With the increasing use of nasal steroid sprays for the control of allergic rhinitis, there has been an increase in epistaxis secondary to their drying effects on the mucosa. Several companies have placed their steroids in an aqueous carrying agent, in an attempt to decrease some of these drying side effects. Persistent unilateral rhinorrhea, foul-smelling nasal discharge, and recurrent bleeding are cause for strong suspicion of foreign body or a tumor in the nose. It is often surprising upon questioning that a child remembers sticking something up his or her nose but was afraid to tell the parents. The foreign body often induces an intense inflammatory response, with the formation of granulation tissue. This granulation tissue often makes it difficult at first to differentiate the foreign body from some other possible source, such as a nasal tumor. Careful removal of the offending foreign body will often result in resolution of all of the nasal symptoms (1).

Any form of intranasal surgery including septoplasty, traditional sinus surgery, or endoscopic sinus surgery, can cause epistaxis as a postoperative complication. Epistaxis following surgery can be immediate or can occur up to several weeks after the surgical procedure.

Systemic Factors

The control of bleeding after blood-vessel injury involves a complex interaction among three systems: the blood vessel wall, the platelets, and the plasma coagulation protein. The three phases of hemostasis consist of (*i*) formation of a hemostatic plug, (*ii*) formation of fibrin, and (*iii*) stability of fibrin and fibrolytic activity (14,15). The interaction of these systems results in normal hemostasis, but if any portion is deficient, bleeding can occur.

The patient with hemostasis disorders may be identified early in life. A history of bruising without significant trauma, prolonged bleeding after dental work or minor cuts, and unusually heavy menorrhea, all are indicators. The most common hereditary bleeding disorder associated with epistaxis is Von Willebrand's disease (VWD). This disease is an autosomal-dominant inherited disorder that presents clinically with mucocutaneous hemorrhage, excessive bleeding after surgery or trauma, and epistaxis. Approximately 60% of patients with VWD complain of recurrent epistaxis. During the course of normal hemostasis, the subendothelium is exposed during injury to the vessel wall, causing platelet aggregation. This is induced by Von Willebrand factor (VWF). When this factor is deficient, there is an increased bleeding time. Unless the bleeding time is specifically performed as a part of the preoperative evaluation, the problem may be missed. The diagnosis is most commonly made with quantitative immunoelectrophoresis or enzyme-linked immunoassay.

Presurgical prophylaxis in patients with Von Willebrand's is with desmopressin. Desmopressin increases VWF and factor VIII level. This non–blood-product therapy has been recommended over cryoprecipitate.

Functional defects often associated with epistaxis include hemophilia A. This is the most common hemophilia and is secondary to a functional defect of the procoagulant portion of factor VIII. Factor VIII is a complex of two molecules: VWF and procoagulant factor VIII. Hemophilia B is less common, and is secondary to factor IX deficiency. This is also known as Christmas disease. Both hemophilia A and B are sex linked, male inherited, and detected by a prolonged partial thromboplastin time. The difficulty with epistaxis may be variable and can be associated with the severity of the disease (1).

Factor XIII deficiency is a rare autosomal-recessive disorder in which only a homozygote shows the bleeding tendency. Factor XIII, also known as "fibrin-stabilizing factor," is essential in fibrin stabilization and in protection from proteolytic degradation. This may result in delayed bleeding after trauma or surgery as well as impaired wound healing (14). There may be an increase in mortality due to uncontrolled bleeding and intracranial hemorrhage. Acquired factor XIII deficiency can result from inflammatory bowel diseases and acute leukemia (15). Replacement therapy with fresh frozen plasma or factor XIII concentrates has been utilized to control postoperative hemorrhage (14,16,17).

Hereditary hemorrhagic telangiectasia, also known as Osler–Weber–Rendu disease, was first described by Babington in 1865. It is an autosomal-dominant inherited disorder characterized by a strong family history, multiple telangiectasias, arteriovenous malformations that may rupture and bleed, and epistaxis. Symptoms vary according to the location of the lesion; skin, nasal mucosa, gastrointestinal tract mucosa, and pulmonary, cerebral, and hepatic circulation are commonly affected (1,18,19).

Pathological examination reveals thin-walled vessels without smooth muscles and increased angiogenesis resulting in vascular proliferation (arteriovenous fistula and mucosal fragility). Even minor trauma such as nose blowing can cause epistaxis. Epistaxis is the presenting symptom in 90% of patients. Of the patients, 62% become symptomatic by age 16, and almost all patients by 40 years of age. Conservative methods of hemostasis without the use of cautery and cartilage sparing have been recommended as the initial means of treatment. More detailed and advanced forms of treatment will be discussed later in this chapter (20,21).

EPISTAXIS MANAGEMENT

Epistaxis is a common disorder treated by emergency department (ED) staff and otolaryngologists worldwide (22,23). It is the most common emergency in otorhinolaryngology (24). The annual incidence of epistaxis is 11% (23), with 15 patients per 10,000 requiring physician care and 1.6 per 10,000 requiring hospital admission (22,25–27). Epistaxis is rarely life threatening; however, the complications and outcome of uncontrolled nasal bleeding can be serious and may include significant blood loss, myocardial infarction, stroke, and airway compromise (22). Uncontrolled or unrecognized epistaxis is more common from a posterior bleeding point. Fortunately, most cases of epistaxis originate in the anterior portion of the nasal septum in Kiesselbach's plexus (22,28).

Exsanguinating epistaxis is an uncommon condition but may be life threatening. This condition is more commonly seen in trauma patients with injury to the midface, resulting in maxillary artery laceration. These patients require immediate triage, evaluation, and control of the airway.

Control of the bleeding is essential, along with replacement of fluid loss to prevent hypovolemia and shock. Hypovolemia may be recognized by the effects of inadequate tissue perfusion, cool clammy skin, decreased urinary output, central nervous system symptoms, anxiety, depression, tachypnea, tachycardia, and weak pulses (1). The study reported by Beer et al. (28) on blood loss estimation in epistaxis found that once the measured volume was above 100 mL, visual estimation became grossly inaccurate, and staff tended to grossly underestimate larger blood volume loss. In many severely injured patients, the midfacial skeleton is unstable, making it difficult to adequately place packing and control epistaxis. These patients may require anterior and posterior nasal packs and additional nasopharyngeal packs, once the airway is controlled by intubation or tracheotomy. If packing fails to control the hemorrhage, then external carotid artery ligation and/or ethmoid artery ligation may be performed under local anesthesia (1,24,29–31). If the patient can be stabilized, angiography with embolization may be the treatment of choice prior to carotid artery ligation. Patients with a prior history of sphenoid sinus surgery and recurrent epistaxis may have developed a carotid cavernous sinus fistula. Recurrent epistaxis in patients who have suffered head trauma may have also developed a pseudoaneurysm of the intracavernous internal carotid artery. This can occur weeks to years after the trauma and may be associated with monocular blindness and orbital fracture (32). Angiography with embolization has become the primary mode of diagnosis and treatment in these cases. The physician performing this procedure must have a high index of suspicion based on a good medical history and intimate knowledge of the anatomy and surrounding vascular structures.

Control of Epistaxis in the Outpatient Setting

Unlike the massive life-threatening epistaxis seen following trauma or surgical procedures, most patients seeking help for epistaxis in the ED or physician's office are hemodynamically stable and able to respond to questions. After initial resuscitation, a careful medical history is vital. The relevant points to be covered should include frequency and duration of the epistaxis; length of time of each occurrence; recent traumas and surgeries; history of finger manipulation; conditions of the living environment, e.g., dry heat, air conditioning, or low moisture content; coronary or vascular disease; hypertension; connective-tissue disorder; coagulopathies; and hematologic disorders. Medications are import, particularly anticoagulants such as warfarin, aspirin, Plavix, Coumadin, and the like.

Identification of the bleeding point is essential in controlling the epistaxis with localized therapy. The majority of patients will present with anterior or posterior epistaxis. Anterior epistaxis most commonly arises in Little's area and is often venous in origin. Posterior epistaxis most commonly arises in the posterior septum, followed by the lateral nasal wall and Woodruff's naso-nasopharyngeal plexus. This is often arterial in nature (1,26,33). Identifying a specific bleeding point will often take a great deal of time, patience, understanding, and skill. Studies have shown that ED training is often deficient in this respect, and increased levels of training are required in order for the ED to be an effective first line (24). Where possible, the patient should be in a sitting position and as comfortable as possible. Proper equipment should include protective clothing and eye protection, appropriate head light or head mirror, nasal speculum, Bayonet forceps, Frazier and Yankauer suction, and a selection of topical vasoconstrictive and anesthetic agents. Commonly available vasoconstrictive agents for topical use include oxymetazoline hydrochloride 0.05%, phenylephrine hydrochloride 0.25%, and cocaine solution 4% or 10%. For anesthesia, topical lidocaine hydrochloride 4% is useful, as is cocaine in either concentration. These agents may be applied by spray or dropper, or on pledgets. Proper preparation of the nasal lining may be even more important in posterior epistaxis.

The increasingly widespread availability of rigid or flexible fiberoptic nasopharyngoscopes in both EDs and otolaryngologist offices has dramatically improved visualization. After application of one of the vasoconstrictive agents and anesthetic agents, the nose can be more easily examined. Although these agents often may stop the bleeding before identification is made, every effort should be made to identify the offending vessel, since epistaxis may reoccur once their effect has worn off.

Other methods of controlling or decreasing epistaxis include local submucosal injection of 1% lidocaine plus 1:100,000 parts epinephrine.

An injection of local anesthetic with epinephrine into the pterygopalatine canal may be helpful in controlling a posterior nasal bleed. This may be effective by itself, or it may slow the bleeding substantially, allowing cauterization or packing under a more controlled situation. The ability to identify the greater palatine foramen is essential to this technique. It is located in the hard palate just anterior to the soft palate junction. It may be palpated as a slight depression in the mucosa just medial to the last molar tooth and in front of the hamulus process. Practicing palpating this point during routine surgical procedures, such as tonsillectomy, may be beneficial when an emergency with active bleeding arises.

Approximately 3 mL of local anesthesia 1% lidocaine (Xylocaine) with 1:100,000 epinephrine (adrenaline) should be injected into the pterygopalatine canal and then into the pterygopalatine fossa to block the sphenopalatine branch of the internal maxillary artery. A slight bend in the needle may help with accurate placement. The needle should only be advanced to 28 mm; at a depth of 40 mm, the needle may enter the orbit. As always, aspiration before injection is important (20).

Nasal Packing

Over the years, nasal packing techniques and materials have continued to evolve; however, the basic principle is not new. Nasal packing for epistaxis was first documented by Hippocrates in the fifth century BC (27). The nose is a complex and convoluted passageway. All packing works by one essential principle: maintaining pressure on the walls of damaged blood vessels and allowing an organized clot to form. The placement of nasal packing is uncomfortable and often traumatic for the patient. The use of topical vasoconstrictive agents and local anesthesia may help but not eliminate the discomfort. The removal of packing may also be uncomfortable and result in recurrent bleeding (22). Packing may remain in place for three to five days, resulting in additional complications.

Anterior Nasal Packing. Traditional anterior nasal packing consists of careful placement of Vaseline gauze (0.5 × 72 inch) coated with an antibiotic ointment in a layered fashion (Fig. 2). The use of local anesthesia not only decreases the pain, allowing the physician or ED staff better control, but may also reduce the risk of a vasovagal response by blocking the nasal–vagal reflex (11). This technique requires certain equipment and training for proper placement. The very end of the gauze should not be placed posterior in the nose, but the pack should be grasped several centimeters beyond the end, leaving the end near the anterior choana or nostril. This will help prevent aspiration or displacement of the pack. Care must be taken to place each ensuing section back toward the posterior choana, to be fully effective. Molding the finished pack with slight digital pressure will help to fill the convolutions of the nasal cavity. The technique is demonstrated in Figure 2. Removal of this gauze can often roughen the already friable mucosa, resulting in recurrent bleeding. If possible, a protective layer of Telfa or absorbable hemostatic material such as Surgicel or Oxycel (oxidized regenerated cellulose) may be placed over the bleeding site prior to traditional packing. This may help to prevent recurrent epistaxis upon removal. In significant bouts of epistaxis, this may not be feasible.

Because of the time involved, special training, and discomfort to the patient with traditional packing, new types of nasal packing material have been developed. One such innovation is compressed hydroxylated polyvinyl acetal (Merocel) or polyvinyl alcohol (PVA) (Expandacell® Rhino Rocket®). Rhino Rockets are hydrophilic and expand to many times their original size when wet. Often, newly developed packs are comprised of expandable preshaped balloons with a softer coating, e.g., Rapid Rhino Nasal Pack with Gel Knit (Shippert Medical Technologies, Englewood, New Jersey, U.S.A.) (Fig. 3). These new packs are more easily inserted by ED staff. Prospective studies examining these newer packs have shown that packing with coated expandable balloons may be easier to insert for some physicians. Both types of nasal packs, those with a coating and those without, were found to be equally effective in controlling epistaxis (1,22).

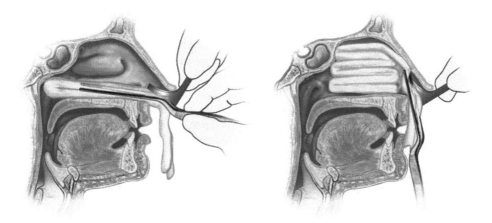

FIGURE 2 The proper technique is demonstrated for the placement of a traditional Vaseline gauze anterior nasal pack.

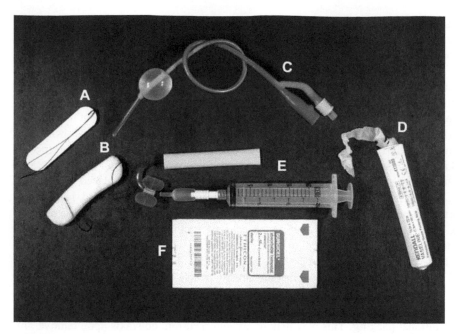

FIGURE 3 Various packing material and packs use to control epistaxis. (A) Merocel 2000 Laminated Nasal Dressing. 8 cm with drawstring (Medtronic XOMED, Jacksonville, FL, U.S.A.). (B) Ultracell Classic Nasal Pack (Ultracell Medical Technologies Inc., North Stonington, CT, U.S.A.). (C) 30 cc Foley Catheter. (D) 1/2" × 72" Vaseline Gauze Packing Strip. (The Kendall Co., Mansfield, MA, U.S.A.) (E) Rapid Rhino 7.5 cm Anterior-Posterior Nasal Pack (Applied Therapeutics Ltd., Glenfield Leicestershire, U.K.). (F) Surgicel Absorbable Hemostat (Oxidized Regenerated Cellulose) (Ethicon Inc., Somerville, NJ, U.S.A.).

Even anterior nasal packing is not without risk. Toxic shock syndrome (TSS), diagnosed with the use of vaginal packing, can also occur with nasal packing. *Staphylococcus aureus* can colonize the nasal packages and produce TSS toxin I. The majority of TSS cases follow nasal or sinus surgery where the mucosal barrier is disrupted, but it also can occur after packing for epistaxis. Infection is accompanied by sudden onset of fever, vomiting, diarrhea, hypotension, rash, desquamation, and eventual shock. Early recognition and intervention is essential to prevent a potentially fatal outcome. Appropriate use of prophylactic oral antibiotics is recommended with nasal packing (1,34).

Special cases of anterior epistaxis that may require a less aggressive form of packing include those patients with chronic disorders that may lead to coagulopathies or mucosal vascular fragility. These disorders may include leukemia, collagen vascular diseases, septal perforations, or coagulopathies (35). Control of hemorrhage initially with Surgicel or Oxycel or Avitene® (microfibrillar cross-linked bovine tropocollagen) has been successful in many patients (36). This minimally invasive method has avoided further destruction of nasal mucosa and decreased rebleeding upon removal (1).

Posterior Nasal Packing. If a patient continues to bleed despite a well-placed deep anterior pack, a posterior nasal pack may be indicated. The placement of a posterior pack is not without potential complications and should be carefully evaluated. The traditional posterior pack is often constructed from cylindrical dental rolls (rolled gauze sponges, umbilical tape, and silk tie). Red rubber catheters are useful for pulling the umbilical tape or silk tie through the nose. Because of the cumbersome method of application, the patient must be well informed of the method, risks, and techniques utilized for placement. Intravenous access for fluid resuscitation and possible sedation is advised. If this is not feasible, then placement in the operating room under anesthesia may be considered. One technique is as follows:

Rolling a surgical sponge tightly or placing three long cylindrical dental rolls together may form the posterior nasopharyngeal pack. These may be tied together tightly with two #1-0 silk sutures. The silk suture should be left long enough that it can be brought out through the nose. An alternative is to tie two umbilical tapes to the nasopharyngeal roll once it is formed. Two red rubber catheters are passed to the already decongested nasal cavities, into the oral cavity, and withdrawn through the mouth. The ends of the silk sutures or umbilical tapes are tied to the red rubber catheters. The red rubber catheters are pulled through the nose, taking the sutures or umbilical tapes with them, and eventually the posterior pack. This is simultaneously passed into the oral cavity and advanced behind the soft palate. Once the posterior pack is in place, a good anterior pack is now placed. Finally, the posterior pack is secured by tying the sutures or umbilical tapes over a second bolster in front of the columella (Fig. 4).

All patients with a posterior pack should be admitted to the hospital, to be monitored in an appropriate setting. Pulse oximetry is highly recommended, since these patients may have decreased oxygen saturation or hypoventilation. IV hydration, antibiotics, and judicial analgesia are important. If not well protected, columellar necrosis or alar necrosis

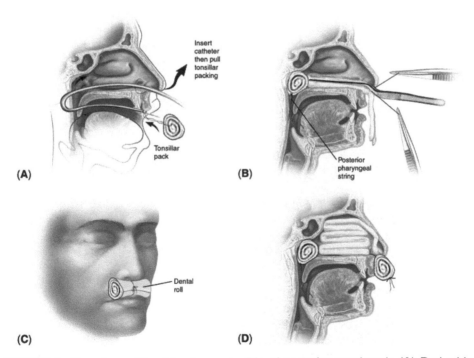

(A)

(B)

(C)

(D)

FIGURE 4 The steps utilized to place a traditional posterior nasal pack. (**A**) Red rubber catheters are passed through the nose until visible in the oropharynx. The catheters are then tied with silk sutures or umbilical tape. (**B**) The catheters are pulled out through the nose. The silk sutures or the umbilical tapes are secured to the posterior pack. The posterior pack is pulled and manually pushed into place. An anterior pack is then placed. (**C**) The silk sutures or umbilical tape is secured over dental rolls to maintain forward pressure and protect the columella. (**D**) Finished view of posterior pack.

may occur. This has been seen to develop several days after the pack is removed, secondary to vascular tissue compromise. The external nose should be checked routinely for any signs of vascular compromise. Posterior packs are routinely left in place for three to five days. The pressure may be slowly released and the pharynx observed for any signs of rebleeding. The patient who fails anterior and posterior packing may be a candidate for further intervention; this will be discussed later.

An alternative to the traditional posterior pack is the balloon pack. Initially, a 30 cc Foley catheter balloon was utilized. Passing the Foley catheter through the nose was easier, faster, and could be done in the ED without sedation or a trip to the operating room. Once the balloon was appropriately inflated, usually with saline, the catheter was held tightly in position with a clamp. It is imperative that the caudal structures of the nose be well padded with multiple surgical sponges. Even with this, necrosis was not uncommon. This concept was further improved with the development of specifically designed epistaxis balloon packs. Some are a combination of balloons with Merocel packing, with or without integrated breathing tubes. Like all other packs, these are placed blindly, and pressure on the specific bleeding site cannot be guaranteed.

Maxillary Artery Ligation

Transantral ligation of the maxillary artery has become a standard for the control of epistaxis. Hirsh reported this procedure in 1936 (36), and the names Caldwell and Luc have become synonymous with this approach (5,37,38). The Caldwell–Luc antrostomy can be performed under local anesthesia. The incision extends from the root of the canine tooth to the malar eminence over the first molar tooth. It should be located about 1 cm above the gingival margin to decrease bleeding and allow adequate tissue for suturing the incision closed. The upper lip flap is freed in the subperiosteal plane, being careful to preserve the infraorbital nerve. The antrum is entered with a fine osteotome or rotating cutting burr (37). The posterior maxillary sinus wall is identified and a laterally based U-shaped mucosal incision is made. The posterior maxillary wall is then removed. The remainder of the procedure is best performed under magnification with either surgical loops or operating microscope. The fat is carefully teased away, and the vessels, maxillary artery, and distal branches within the pterygopalatine fossa are clipped. Several studies have recommended that anterior ethmoid artery ligation be performed at the time of maxillary artery ligation (5,39); however, the overall benefit and long-term results are uncertain. Ligation of the sphenopalatine artery by a microsurgical approach was introduced in the 1970s (5,40–43). Selective sphenopalatine artery ligation where it exited the sphenopalatine foramen, using the transantral approach, was described by Simpson. The advantage of this technique was that it avoided the pterygomaxillary fossa. This was thought to avoid the complication from collateral circulation (44).

Endoscopic Management of Epistaxis

The nasal cavities have often been an area of uncertainty in the identification of bleeding sites. Limited visual access, even with a strong headlamp light, has often resulted in a less-than-satisfactory outcome. The advent of fiberoptic technology for illumination has made visualization of the deep recesses of the nose a reality. Surgical rigid endoscopes are available with various angles, making the visualization easier. They also allow cauterization of specific bleeding sites. Monopolar suction cautery has proven particularly well suited to this application (1). Bipolar cautery also has been utilized. Several reports have demonstrated lower complication rates, higher success rates, and shorter hospitalization times (41,42). Temporary palatal numbness is the major adverse effect of this procedure.

Endoscopic Ligation of the Sphenopalatine Artery

The transantral approach has been the gold standard for control of severe epistaxis, with a success rate of 80% to 95%. It has been considered to have a low complication rate; however, hypesthesia or neuralgia of the infraorbital nerve, scarring of the gingivolabial sulcus, painful sublabial incision, and oroantral fistula may occur. There is also the risk of collateral blood flow and continued or recurrent epistaxis. In order to prevent these complications, endoscopic ligation of the sphenopalatine artery via a transnasal approach has been described (43). If necessary, temporary control of bleeding is obtained with packing. This procedure can be performed under local anesthesia, but general anesthesia may be preferable. The anterior pack is removed, and the nose is decongested with oxymetazoline 0.05% solution on cottonoids or neurosurgical patties. The posterior pack may be led down to allow drainage of accumulated blood and reinflated if necessary to temporarily control bleeding. The nose is examined with a 30° 4 mm endoscope. Visibly bleeding vessels can be cauterized with a monopolar suction cautery or bipolar cautery. As in any surgery, adequate visualization is necessary; therefore, an endoscopic anterior ethmoidectomy or septoplasty may be indicated.

An uncinectomy is performed, followed by a large middle meatal antrostomy. Care should be taken not to injure the nasolacrimal duct. The antrostomy is enlarged in a posterior direction until level with the posterior wall of the maxillary sinus. A Cottle elevator is utilized to elevate the lateral nasal wall in a subperiosteal plane. This sphenopalatine foramen is located in the superomedial corner of the maxillary sinus. The surrounding bone is removed, with a Kerrison rongeur confirming the sphenopalatine artery. If the patient's nose permits entry of an endoscope with necessary instruments, the endoscope can be placed into the antrum with a trocar. The sphenopalatine artery may be coagulated or ligated with a hemoclip (43).

Some authors have reported that advantages of endoscopic ligation of the sphenopalatine artery have included decreased surgical time, decreased morbidity, and a shorter recovery (43). Other studies, however, have shown that inpatient treatment with nasal packing was associated with a lower overall hospital charge. It was thought that all three methods (packing, arterial ligation, and embolization) had similar complication rates (45). Further evaluation is necessary before a statement can be made for one method over the others.

Septal Dermatoplasty

The objective of dermatoplasty is to replace the fragile respiratory epithelium with a tougher epithelium such as skin. The procedure is most commonly described in the treatment of epistaxis in patients with Osler-Weber-Rendu disease. Saunders described the operation in 1960 (46). The best donor site is the anterior thigh wall above the knee. A split-thickness skin graft of about 0.014" is harvested with a dermatome. A ring curette is utilized to remove all of the mucosa from the anterior half of the nasal septum, floor, and lateral walls of the nose. Laterally, the mucosa of the inferior turbinate is also removed. A narrow strip of skin is resected from the mucocutaneous junction of the vestibule to act as a sewing edge to attach the graft with a #4-0 absorbable suture. The grafts are placed in the nose like a sleeve. Careful packing is very important. Packing should be coated with antibiotic ointment and left in place for five days. After several weeks, the interior of the nose can be cleaned daily with oil, soap, and water. Even after septal dermatoplasty, recurrent epistaxis can occur, but it is usually not as severe as it was preoperatively.

Ethmoid Artery Ligation

The anterior and posterior ethmoid arteries supply blood to the upper portion of the nose from the internal carotid artery system. Ligation of these arteries can decrease blood flow to decrease epistaxis. This is often performed conjointly with maxillary artery ligation. Knowledge of the anatomy of the region is extremely important to prevent complications. The anterior ethmoid artery foramen lies 14 to 22 mm posterior along the frontoethmoidal suture line. The posterior ethmoid artery is further back at a very variable location. Of significance is the location of the optic nerve, which lies 4 to 7 mm more posterior than the posterior ethmoidal artery.

The procedure to ligate these arteries has been extensively described. In brief, a Lynch incision is made in a curvilinear manner between the inner canthus and the middle of the nose. The area is first infiltrated with local anesthesia (1% lidocaine and 1:100,000 epinephrine) down to the level of the periosteum. The eye can be protected with a corneal shield or a #5-0 silk tarsorrhaphy stitch, after placement of ophthalmic antibiotic ointment. Dissection is carried down to the level of the periosteum. The periosteum is incised and elevated posteriorly down to the frontoethmoid suture line. Malleable retractors are very useful during this dissection. The artery can be ligated with bipolar cautery or vascular clips (Fig. 5). Ethmoid artery ligation is still an important surgical procedure, even with newer methods such as angiography and embolization. In specific cases, the artery may need to be ligated prior to angiography and embolization to prevent the embolization particles from entering the ophthalmic circulation.

Selective Embolization

Epistaxis is generally widespread, with 60% of the adult population having an episode during their life, while only 6% of patients require treatment (31,47). The conservative methods to control epistaxis have included pressure, vasoconstriction, and anterior and posterior packing. When these conservative methods have failed, surgical ligation has been undertaken. In 1974, Sokoloff et al. (48) described the embolization techniques to stop

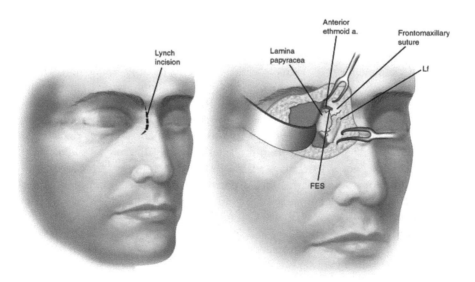

FIGURE 5   The technique of anterior ethmoid artery ligation via a Lynch incision.

intractable epistaxis. Since that time, multiple reports utilizing this basic technique with various catheters and embolic materials have been reported.

The use of this technique is seen in many areas including arteriovenous malformations, pseudoaneurysms, bleeding varices, shrinking of fibroids, and vascular tumors of the head and neck. Diagnostic angiography with embolization is commonly performed under local anesthesia via the femoral approach. A variety of catheters and microcatheters have been developed to get to the different sources of epistaxis. Once in the proper location, an embolic material is injected via the catheter to occlude the offending vessel. The type of embolic utilized depends on the desired level of occlusion, desired duration of occlusion, and catheter system compatibility (Table 1).

The technique most commonly used at our institution is as follows:

Prior to embolization, complete diagnostic arteriography of the internal and external carotid circulations is performed bilaterally, and, if indicated, the vertebral arteries' circulation is studied, as well. This is usually performed from a femoral artery approach, utilizing a 4- or 5-French diagnostic catheter. If embolization is to be performed, an open-ended guiding catheter usually is used. The catheter is advanced through a groin sheath and positioned in either the common carotid artery or the external carotid artery trunk. A microcatheter of under 2.8-French in diameter, in conjunction with micro-guidewires, is then utilized for selective catheterization of the appropriate vessel(s).

Embolization is then performed with an appropriate agent. In the case of epistaxis or preoperative tumor embolization, particulate agents are generally employed. Following embolization, which is performed during observation with real-time fluoroscopy, completion arteriography is generally performed through the microcatheter and/or guiding

TABLE 1 Embolic Agents

Absorbable material
    Gelfoam
    Autologous blood clot
    Avitene
    Ethibloc
Nonabsorbable material
    Particulate agents
    Autologous fat and muscles
    PVA
    Spherical PVA
    Acrylics
Injectable agents
    NBCA [Onyx (not currently available in United States), silicone]
Sclerosing agents
    Boiling contrast
    ETOH (absolute alcohol)
    Sodium morrhuate
    Sotradecol
Occlusion devices
    Detachable balloons
    Coils, microcoils
    Detachable coils
    Spider, clamp shells
    Amplatzer

Abbreviations: PVA, polyvinyl alcohol; NBCA, N-butyl cyanoacrylate; ETOH, ethyl alcohol.

catheter, and, depending on the vascular territory and level of embolization, collateral circulation might be evaluated with respect to the need for further embolization.

This technique, even in the best hands, is not without the risk of complication. The major complications reported in the literature have included stroke, blindness, facial paralysis, *grand mal* seizure, trismus, soft-tissue necrosis, and swelling of the cheek. Most of these cases occurred when utilizing permanent embolic agents such as PVA. Minor complications have been reported to range from 2.2% to 25% (31,49–51). These may include mild-to-moderate temporal pain, headache, and temporofacial pain.

JUVENILE ANGIOFIBROMAS

JA is a benign, highly vascular tumor that almost exclusively occurs in the nasopharynx of adolescent males. The average age of onset is 15 years. JA typically originates in the superior margin of the sphenopalatine foramen. It accounts for only 0.5% of all head and neck tumors (11,12,52). The most common presenting symptoms are severe recurrent epistaxis with nasal obstruction. The histologic origin of these tumors is uncertain, but they

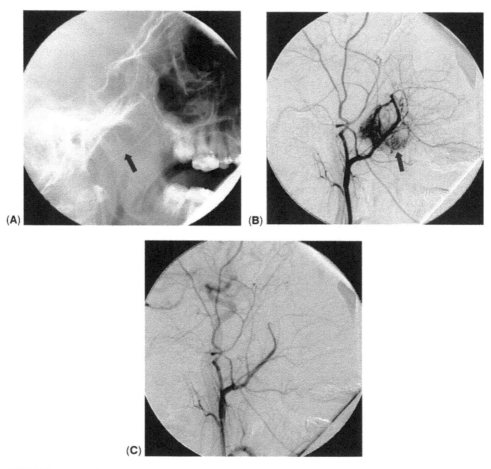

FIGURE 6 (**A**) Catheter in internal maxillary artery (*arrow*). (**B**) Right ECA preembolization. The tumor mass can be seen (*arrow*) (**C**) Right ECA postembolization. The tumor blush is gone. *Abbreviation*: ECA, external carotid artery.

have a highly vascularized and proliferative nature (12,53). Bone erosion may occur in the region of the orbit and the skull base. If the disease process is allowed to progress, facial deformity, proptosis, blindness, and cranial nerve palsy may occur. Fisch classified JAs into four types. The stages may help plan the correction (54).

Removal of the tumor depends on its extent and the training of the surgeon. Previously, the majority of these tumors were removed through an open approach, commonly via a lateral rhinotomy (11). Craniofacial resections have been utilized in advanced JAs (52,55,56). More recently, endoscopic removal has been popularized for lower-stage lesions (57). With the increase in interventional radiology and selective embolization, removal of these tumors can be accomplished without major blood loss. Effective preoperative embolization is most important when one wants to attempt endoscopic removal of these tumors (Fig. 6A–C).

REFERENCES

1. Santos PM, Lepore ML. Epistaxis in head and neck surgery. In: Bailey BJ, ed. Otolaryngology. Vol. 1. 2nd ed. Philadelphia, PA: Lippincott-Raven, 1998:513–529.
2. Shaheen OH. Arterial epistaxis. J Laryngol Otol 1975; 89(1):17–34.
3. Kirchner JA, Yanagisawa E, Crelin ES Jr. Surgical anatomy of the ethmoidal arteries. A laboratory study of 150 orbits. Arch Otolaryngol 1961; 74:382–386.
4. Hollinshead WH. Anatomy for Surgeons. Vol. 1: The Head and Neck. 3rd ed. Philadelphia, PA: Harper & Row, 1982.
5. Pearson BW, MacKenzie RG, Goodman WS. The anatomical basis of transantral ligation of the maxillary artery in severe epistaxis. Laryngoscope 1969; 79(5):969–984.
6. Woodruff GH. Cardiovascular epistaxis and the naso-nasopharyngeal plexus. Laryngoscope 1949; 59 (11):1238–1247.
7. Lang J. Clinical Anatomy of the Nose, Nasal Cavity and Paranasal Sinuses. Stell PM, trans. New York, NY: Thieme Medical Publishers, 1989.
8. Howard BK, Rohrich RJ. Understanding the nasal airway: principles and practice. Plast Reconstr Surg 2002; 109(3):1128–1146.
9. Rappai M, Collop N, Kemp S, et al. The nose and sleep-disordered breathing: what we know and what we do not know. Chest 2003; 124(6):2309–2323.
10. Diamantopoulos II, Jones NS. The investigation of nasal septal perforations and ulcers. J Laryngol Otol 2001; 115(7):541–544.
11. Mann WJ, Jecker P, Amedee RG. Juvenile angiofibromas: changing surgical concept over the last 20 years. Laryngoscope 2004; 114(2):291–293.
12. Bales C, Kotapka M, Loevner LA, et al. Craniofacial resection of advanced juvenile nasopharyngeal angiofibroma. Arch Otolaryngol Head Neck Surg 2002; 128(9):1071–1078.
13. Scholtz AW, Appenroth E, Kammen-Jolly K, et al. Juvenile nasopharyngeal angiofibroma: management and therapy. Laryngoscope 2001; 111(4 Pt 1):681–687.
14. Karabulut AB, Aydin H, Mezdegi A, et al. Recurrent bleeding following rhinoplasty due to Factor XIII deficiency. Plast Reconstr Surg 2001; 108(3):806–807.
15. Andreoli TE, Bennet JC, Carpenter CC. Cecil Essentials of Medicine. 3rd ed. Philadelphia, PA: Saunders, 1993:400–416.
16. Burrows RF, Ray JG, Burrows EA. Bleeding risk and reproductive capacity among patients with factor XIII deficiency: a case presentation and review of literature. Obstet Gynecol Surv 2000; 55 (2):103–108.
17. Gerlach R, Raabe A, Zimmermann M, et al. Factor XIII deficiency and postoperative hemorrhage after neurosurgical procedures. Surg Neurol 2000; 54(3):260–265.
18. Klepfish A, Berrebi A, Schattner A. Intranasal tranexamic acid treatment for severe epistaxis in hereditary hemorrhagic telangiectasia. Arch Intern Med 2001; 161(5):767.
19. Peery WH. Clinical spectrum of hereditary hemorrhagic telangiectasia (Osler-Weber-Rendu disease). Am J Med 1987;82(5):989–997.
20. Bowie EJW, Owen CA Jr. Primary vascular disorders. In: Colman RW, Hirsch J, Marder VI, et al., eds. Hemostasis and Thrombosis: Basic Principles and Clinical Practice. Philadelphia, PA: JB Lippincott Co., 1994:134–168.

21. Porteous ME, Burn J, Proctor SJ. Hereditary haemorrhagic telangiectasia: a clinical analysis. J Med Genet 1992; 29(8):527–530.
22. Singer AJ, Blanda M, Cronin K, et al. Comparison of nasal tampons for the treatment of epistaxis in the emergency department: a randomized controlled trial. Ann Emerg Med 2005; 45(2):134–139.
23. Wurman LH, Sack JG, Flannery JV Jr, et al. The management of epistaxis. Am J Otolaryngol 1992; 13(4):193–209.
24. Wild DC, Spraggs PD. Treatment of epistaxis in accident and emergency departments in the UK. J Laryngol Otol 2002; 116(8):597–600.
25. Josephson GD, Godley FA, Stierna P. Practical management of epistaxis. Med Clin North Am 1991; 75(6):1311–1320.
26. Viducich RA, Blanda MP, Gerson LW. Posterior epistaxis: clinical features and acute complications. Ann Emerg Med 1995; 25(5):592–596.
27. Perretta LJ, Denslow BL, Brown CG. Emergency evaluation and management of epistaxis. Emerg Med Clin North Am 1987; 5(2):265–277.
28. Beer HL, Duvvi S, Webb CJ, et al. Blood loss estimation in epistaxis scenarios. J Laryngol Otol 2005; 119(1):16–18.
29. Hassard AD, Kirkpatrick DA, Wong FS. Ligation of the external carotid and anterior ethmoidal arteries for severe or unusual epistaxis resulting from facial fractures. Can J Surg 1986; 29(6): 447–449.
30. Kurata A, Kitahara T, Miyasaka Y, et al. Superselective embolization for severe traumatic epistaxis caused by fracture of the skull base. AJNR Am J Neuroradiol 1993; 14(2):343–345.
31. Oguni T, Korogi Y, Yasunaga T, et al. Superselective embolisation for intractable idiopathic epistaxis. Br J Radiol 2000; 73(875):1148–1153.
32. Chambers EF, Rosenbaum AE, Norman D, et al. Traumatic aneurysms of cavernous internal carotid artery with secondary epistaxis. Am J Neuroradiol 1981; 2(5):405–409.
33. Jackson KR, Jackson RT. Factors associated with active, refractory epistaxis. Arch Otolaryngol Head Neck Surg 1988; 114(8):862–865.
34. Fairbanks DN. Complications of nasal packing. Otolaryngol Head Neck Surg 1986; 94(3): 412–415.
35. Montgomery RR, Coller BS. Von Willebrand disease. In: Colman RW, Hirsch J. Marder VJ, et al., eds. Hemostasis and Thrombosis: Basic Principles and Clinical Practice. 3rd ed. Philadelphia, PA: JB Lippincott Co., 1994:134–168.
36. Hirsch C. Ligation of the internal maxillary artery in patients with nasal hemorrhage. Arch Otolaryngol 1936; 24:589–596.
37. Bernstein L. The Caldwell-Luc operation. Otolaryngol Clin North Am 1971; 4(1):69–77.
38. Macbeth R. Caldwell-Luc operation 1952–1966. Arch Otolaryngol 1968; 87(6):630–636.
39. Metson R, Lane R. Internal maxillary artery ligation for epistaxis: an analysis of failures. Laryngoscope 1988; 98(7):760–764.
40. Prades J. Abord endonasal de la fosse pterygo-maxillaire. LXXIII Cong Franc Compt. Rendus des Seanc 1976; 290–296.
41. Prades J, Bosch J, Tolasa A. Garsi DLM, ed. Microcirugia Endonasal. Madrid, Espana, 1977.
42. Prades J. Salvat, ed. Microcirugia Endonasal de la Fosa Pterigomaxilar y del Meato Medio. Barcelona, Espana, 1980.
43. Snyderman CH, Carrau RL. Endoscopic ligation of the sphenopalatine artery for epistaxis. Operative techniques in Otolaryngology—Head and Neck Surgery 1997; 8(2):85–89.
44. Simpson GT II, Janfaza P, Becker GD. Transantral sphenopalatine artery ligation. Laryngoscope 1982; 92(9 Pt 1):1001–1005.
45. Goddard JC, Reiter ER. Inpatient management of epistaxis. Outcomes and cost. Otolaryngol Head Neck Surg 2005; 132(5):707–712.
46. Saunders WH. Epistaxis. In: Paparella MM, Shumrick DA, Glusckman JL, eds. Otolaryngology. Vol. 3. 2nd ed. Philadelphia, PA: WB Saunders Company, 1980:1994–2000.
47. Small M, Murray JA, Maran AG. A study of patients with epistaxis requiring admission to hospital. Health Bull (Edinb) 1982; 40(1):20–29.
48. Sokoloff J, Wickbom I, McDonald D, et al. Therapeutic percutaneous embolization in intractable epistaxis. Radiology 1974; 111(2):285–287.
49. Vitek J. Idiopathic intractable epistaxis: endovascular therapy. Radiology 1991; 181(1): 113–116.
50. Tseng EY, Narducci CA, Willing SJ, et al. Angiographic embolization for epistaxis: a review of 114 cases. Laryngoscope 1998; 108(4 Pt 1):615–619.

51. Moreau S, De Rugy MG, Babin E, et al. Supraselective embolization in intractable epistaxis: review of 45 cases. Laryngoscope 1998; 108(6):887–888.

52. Wormald PJ, Van Hasselt A. Endoscopic removal of juvenile angiofibromas. Otolaryngol Head Neck Surg 2003; 129(6):684–691.

53. Schiff M, Gonzalez AM, Ong M, et al. Juvenile nasopharyngeal angiofibroma contain an angiogenic growth factor: basic FGF. Laryngoscope 1992; 102(8):940–945.

54. Fisch U. The infratemporal fossa approach for nasopharyngeal tumors. Laryngoscope 1983; 93(1): 36–44.

55. Mishra SC, Shukla GK, Bhatia N, et al. Angiofibromas of the postnasal space: a critical appraisal of various therapeutic modalities. J Laryngol Otol 1991; 105(7):547–552.

56. Herman P, Lot A, Chapot R, et al. Long-term follow-up of juvenile nasopharyngeal angiofibromas: analysis of recurrences. Laryngoscope 1999; 109(1):140–147.

57. Tseng HZ, Chao WY. Transnasal endoscopic approach for juvenile nasopharyngeal angiofibroma. Am J Otolaryngol 1997; 18(2):151–154.

32

Oral Lesions: Stomatitis and Glossitis

Joseph C. Whitt

Oral and Maxillofacial Pathology, School of Dentistry, University of Missouri, Kansas City, Kansas, U.S.A.

Stomatitis

INTRODUCTION

Stomatitis refers to an inflammatory process involving the mucous membrane of the mouth that may manifest itself through a variety of signs and symptoms including erythema, vesiculation, bulla formation, desquamation, sloughing, ulceration, pseudomembrane formation, and associated discomfort. Stomatitis may arise due to factors that may be of either local, isolated conditions or of systemic origin. For example, a solitary oral ulcer with a history of a recurrent pattern may be classified as recurrent aphthous stomatitis, a purely local phenomenon. Another clinically-similar-appearing lesion, on the other hand, may represent an oral mucosal manifestation of a more generalized disease process such as Crohn's disease. Stomatitis may involve any site in the oral cavity, including the vermillion of the lips, labial/buccal mucosa, dorsal/ventral tongue, floor of mouth and hard/soft palate, and gingivae.

DIFFERENTIAL DIAGNOSIS

The differential diagnosis of stomatitis is challenging because the inflammatory response of the oral mucous membrane is nonspecific. The signs and symptoms of stomatitis (e.g., erythema, erosion, ulceration, pain, and discomfort) are the final common pathway for a wide variety of disease processes. For example, recurrent aphthous stomatitis, herpes simplex, and mucous membrane pemphigoid (MMP) all evolve to an ulcer even though early lesions may or may not be ulcerated.

Differential diagnosis of stomatitis is an art and skill that must be practiced. It begins with a thorough understanding of the signs and symptoms of a wide variety of local and systemic disease processes that might be responsible for the patient's condition (1–4). One uses this knowledge to eliminate unlikely candidates and to identify particular entities as likely candidates (5–8). Knowledge of the relative incidence of each potential cause is important to make a realistic ordering of the list of possible diagnoses, since common things tend to happen commonly. Additional factors such as the patient's age, gender, and the anatomic location of the lesions are usually helpful in ordering the differential diagnosis.

The goal in establishing a differential diagnosis should not be to develop a long laundry list of possibilities but to develop a short list of two to three conditions that might explain the patient's condition and serve as the basis to guide additional investigations to further refine the list. With a sound working diagnosis in hand, the appropriate initial management of the patient may begin. On occasion, a definitive diagnosis may not be reached and the patient's response to treatment and disease progression may provide the additional knowledge to classify the disease process.

When approaching a patient with a chief complaint suggesting stomatitis, one must first seek to understand the individual's current health status and drug history, as a number of disease processes that present as stomatitis may be manifestations of a systemic disease or related to the patient's use of systemic medications. Determine the historical aspects of the particular complaint. There are a number of clinical features that are important to observe while gathering the clinical information to make a differential diagnosis for a patient presenting with stomatitis. If the patient is wearing a dental prosthesis, have him/her remove it, in order to perform a thorough examination. What is the clinical appearance of the lesions? If ulcers are present, determine whether they were preceded by blisters. Where are the lesions located? Are they predominately anterior or posterior in the oral cavity? Are the gingivae involved? The specific site and extent of involvement of the lesions may provide key clues, as some disease processes preferentially involve certain sites over other sites. Does it appear to be a generalized or localized process? The presence or absence of associated constitutional symptoms or other skin and mucosal lesions are useful pieces of information to narrow the considerations. Did the condition arise acutely or are the lesions part of a chronic process? The type of onset and the duration of the condition are critical to establish. Establishing or excluding a history of a chronic, recurring disease process with exacerbation and remission also helps to narrow the differential. Determine if there are local modifying factors present. Learn whether prior attempts at managing the condition have been successful.

Adjunctive Aids to Diagnosis

In addition to physical examination and clinical laboratory investigations, a number of adjunctive procedures are available including culture, exfoliative cytology, brush biopsy (Oral CDx), and incisional or excisional surgical biopsy. Appropriate planning is important, since additional laboratory studies may require special handling of specimens for proper submission. For example, direct immunofluorescence (DIF) studies require the biopsy specimen be submitted fresh and immediately frozen as the immunofluorescent reagents are applied to frozen sections. Alternatively, the specimen may be submitted in specific immunofluorescence transport media. Biopsy may not always provide a definitive answer since many conditions exhibit a nonspecific histopathologic appearance and cannot be differentiated on the basis of the microscopic changes. While biopsy may not provide a definitive diagnosis on all occasions, it may nevertheless be useful in excluding some conditions from the differential diagnosis. It is important to carefully consider the site of biopsy. In most cases, perilesional tissue provides the best features for pathologic interpretation. Gentle handling of the specimen, including avoidance of pinching with tissue forceps, anesthetic injection into the specimen, and tight knotting of suture material around the specimen, is important to avoid disruption of fragile tissue relations in inflammatory disease processes.

HERPETIC STOMATITIS

Herpes simplex virus (HSV) infection of the oral mucous membrane may present as a generalized or localized stomatitis and is typically caused by herpes simplex virus type I (HSV-I), although an increasing number of oral infections are caused by type II virus due to creative sexual practices (9). The virus is transmitted by direct contact with infected saliva or secretions. Virus may be shed in the absence of active lesions. The majority of individuals in the population are seropositive, although few are able to recall a primary infection, indicating that the majority of primary infections are subclinical. Primary infection of the oral mucosa is followed by latency in the trigeminal ganglion. A percentage of those infected experience reactivation of the virus and subsequent secondary herpetic lesions.

Primary Herpetic Gingivostomatitis

Primary herpetic gingivostomatitis represents the primary infection of the HSV in an individual without prior exposure to the virus, and is accompanied by constitutional symptoms of fever, malaise, and cervical lymphadenopathy. Symptomatic primary infection usually occurs in childhood and is frequently accompanied by painful gingivitis with red, swollen gingiva (Fig. 1). The lesions may affect any mucosal surface, including

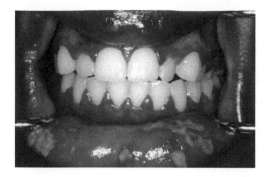

FIGURE 1 Primary herpetic gingivosto-matitis. This 18-year-old female presented with constitutional symptoms, painful, ten-der, swollen, red gingiva and multiple oral ulcers covered by yellowish fibrinous mem-branes. The ulcers were preceded by vesicles that rapidly ruptured, producing confluent ulcers, which take on a geo-graphic pattern. *Source*: Courtesy of Charles Dunlap, DDS.

both the keratinized masticatory mucosa and the nonkeratinized mucosa. Lesions begin as vesicles and rapidly ulcerate to form confluent ulcers. The lesions generally heal without scarring in 10 to 14 days.

Recurrent (Secondary) Herpetic Infections

When triggered, the latent virus in the trigeminal ganglion travels down a sensory nerve axon to the respective dermatome, where it infects epithelial cells and produces vesicles at the affected site. Prior to the appearance of the vesicles, patients typically report prodromal symptoms of tingling. The vermillion border of the lip (herpes labialis) and adjacent skin is the most commonly affected site (Fig. 2). Common synonyms for herpes labialis include cold sores and fever blisters. Intraoral lesions of secondary herpes may be seen on the keratinized mucosa over bone (Fig. 3), typically on the palate or gingiva.

Differential Diagnosis

Both primary herpes simplex and erythema multiforme (EM) exhibit a sudden onset of disease. The lip lesions of primary herpetic gingivostomatitis may bear a resemblance to the crusted lip lesions of EM (Fig. 4). Exfoliative cytology may be useful to differentiate the two by demonstrating the characteristic viral cytopathic effect produced as the epitheliotropic herpes virus replicates within the keratinocytes. Viral culture may also be useful. Lesions of herpangina, caused by the Coxsackie virus, may clinically resemble oral herpes virus infections but typically affect the more posterior areas of the oral cavity. Oral mucosal involvement in herpes zoster may be difficult to distinguish from a zosteriform presentation of recurrent intraoral herpes simplex. Recurrent aphthous stomatitis can be readily differentiated from herpetic infections since it is neither preceded by vesicles nor accompanied by fever or gingivitis. Recurrent aphthous stomatitis generally involves the

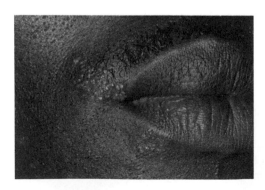

FIGURE 2 Secondary herpes (herpes labialis). Young adult with a long history of recurrent lesions of lip that appear several times a year and heal in 10 to 14 days. Ulcers are preceded by small vesicles that rupture and crust.

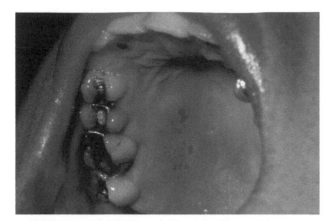

FIGURE 3 Recurrent intraoral herpes. This 30-year-old female experienced prodromal symptoms of itching and burning of palatal mucosa for less than one day followed by the appearance of multiple 1- to 2-mm painful vesicles. Note the slightly edematous, erythematous base. The lesions are now ulcerated, as the vesicles ruptured when a diagnostic exfoliative cytologic smear was harvested several minutes previously. The smear was diagnostic for herpes virus cytopathic effect. The patient did not recall an episode of primary infection.

nonkeratinized mucosa. Recurrent intraoral herpes simplex is limited to involvement of the heavily keratinized masticatory mucosa of the gingiva and palate—areas that are located over bone and are fixed and nonmovable (Fig. 5).

Treatment, Complications, and Prognosis

Mild cases of primary herpetic gingivostomatitis generally require supportive care with proper hydration. Compromised oral function in more severe cases may require

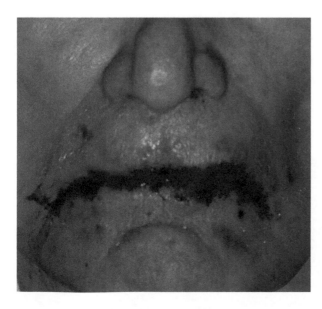

FIGURE 4 Herpetic gingivostomatitis. The crusted appearance of this elderly male's lips suggested the possibility of erythema multiforme. An exfoliative cytologic smear demonstrated the characteristic viral cytopathic effect of herpes simplex virus.

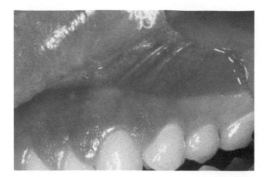

FIGURE 5 Mucogingival junction. Observing the location of ulcers relative to the mucogingival junction is important in differentiating recurrent aphthous stomatitis from recurrent intraoral herpes simplex. Recurrent aphthous stomatitis generally involves the nonkeratinized, freely movable mucosa. Recurrent intraoral herpes simplex is limited to involvement of the heavily keratinized masticatory mucosa of the gingiva and palate—areas that are located over bone and are fixed and nonmovable.

intravenous hydration. Systemic antiviral therapy may be effective if administered early in the course of the disease. Most cases of herpes labialis require only supportive care. Recent studies have shown modest benefit from topical pencyclovir 1%, if applied at the onset of prodromal symptoms. Avoidance of initiating factors such as ultraviolet light by using sunscreen is effective. Active herpetic lesions are sources of infectious virus that can be transmitted to other skin sites (herpes whitlow and herpes gladiatorum). The virus may also be autoinnoculated by transferring the organism from perioral lesions to the ocular mucosa. Herpetic encephalitis is a rare complication of herpetic infection. The clinical appearance of herpetic lesions may be atypical in the immunocompromised host, typically producing more chronic, painful lesions that are not limited to keratinized mucosa in distribution (10). In such situations, systemic acyclovir is effective in limiting the morbidity associated with the lesions. Refer to section on Herpetic glossitis later in this chapter. A number of cases of recurrent EM are preceded by recurrent herpes simplex (Fig. 6).

The herpes viruses are discussed in more detail in Chapter 10.

RECURRENT APHTHOUS STOMATITIS

Recurrent aphthous stomatitis (canker sore) is one of the most common forms of stomatitis. The majority of the population will experience some manifestation of this disease process

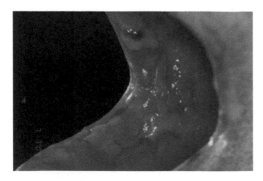

FIGURE 6 Erythema multiforme. Young male with explosive onset of widespread oral ulceration. Note the lack of peripheral keratotic striae.

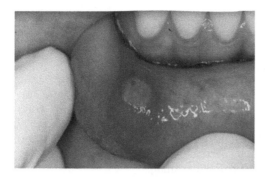

FIGURE 7 Solitary minor aphthous lesion. This solitary ulcer began as a red macule that subsequently ulcerated. A yellowish fibrinous membrane covers the surface. Note the erythematous halo at the periphery of the ulcer. The intensity of the erythematous flare may be related to the degree of secondary infection. On a dry skin surface this fibrinopurulent membrane would appear as a crust.

during their lifetime. The etiology of recurrent aphthous stomatitis is poorly understood. It may not even be a single disease entity since the associated factors seem to be different in different individuals. The infiltrate of T-lymphocytes present in these lesions points to some type of immunologic process (11–15). Aphthae arise as erythematous macules that soon ulcerate and are covered by a fibrinous membrane. Aphthae are ulcerated lesions from their inception. They are not preceded by vesicles. There are several clinical forms of aphthae: minor, major, and herpetiform.

Minor Aphthae
Smaller, shallow aphthae less than 0.5 cm are termed minor aphthae and may be solitary (Fig. 7) or multiple (Fig. 8). An erythematous halo frequently surrounds the ulcerated area. They are relatively superficial and heal without scarring in 7 to 10 days.

Major Aphthae
Larger, deeper aphthae greater than 0.5 cm are termed major aphthae (Fig. 9). As with minor apthae, major aphthae may be solitary or multiple. Due to the depth and extent of tissue destruction, they are slower to heal and often heal with scarring.

Herpetiform Aphthae
Multiple, small aphthae (usually less than 1 mm each) are termed herpetiform aphthae (Fig. 10). Patients with herpetiform aphthae tend to have shorter periods of remission. The

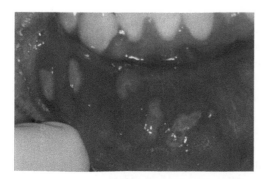

FIGURE 8 Multiple minor aphthae. This individual relates a history of recurring multiple aphthae. These five lesions of the lower lip arose several days previously. Involvement of the process is limited to this site. Aphthae located on highly movable structures such as the lower lip may produce a high degree of discomfort.

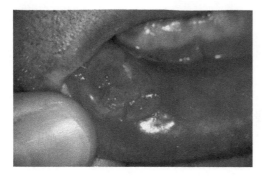

FIGURE 9 Solitary major aphtha. Adult male with a large, deep lesion of lower lip present for two weeks. Borders are rolled and indurated. Because they are associated with deeper destruction and healing by secondary intention, major aphthae may heal with scarring.

term "herpetiform" refers to the clinical appearance of the ulcers that resemble the ulcers produced by the HSV. The herpes virus is not the cause.

Differential Diagnosis
Patients will generally relate a history of recurrence of similar lesions. One of the considerations in the differential diagnosis of aphthous stomatitis is herpetic stomatitis. Recurrent intraoral herpes occurs on the keratinized mucosa of the palate and gingiva, whereas aphthous stomatitis occurs almost exclusively on the nonkeratinized mucosa (Fig. 5). Aphthous stomatitis should not be confused with primary herpetic gingivostomatitis due to the lack of both constitutional symptoms and of gingival involvement in the former. EM exhibits an acute onset, where aphthous stomatitis is a chronic disease. Traumatic ulcers may resemble aphthae; however, the clinical history is helpful in distinguishing them (Figs. 11 and 12). Other conditions such as Crohn's disease (Fig. 13), celiac disease, ulcerative colitis, neutropenia, Behçet's disease, and Reiter syndrome may be associated with oral mucosal ulcers indistinguishable from aphthous stomatitis (16). Crohn's disease and ulcerative colitis are discussed in detail in Chapter 20 and Behçet's disease in Chapter 3.

Treatment, Complications, and Prognosis
Aphthae located on highly movable structures such as the tongue and soft palate produce a high degree of discomfort. Topical analgesics may be used to reduce local discomfort. Topical steroids are also effective in reducing symptoms, as is Amlexanox (17). Short-term systemic steroid therapy is effective for lesions failing topical treatment. The treatment goal should generally be not to achieve a cure but to palliate and reduce the frequency of recurrence. Major aphthae may heal with scarring. In HIV-positive individuals, aphthous lesions follow a different course than in immunocompetent persons. In HIV-infected individuals, aphthae tend to occur more frequently, heal more slowly, and cause more discomfort (18). Intralesional steroid injections may be required to resolve severe aphthous lesions in HIV-infected individuals.

VARICELLA ZOSTER STOMATITIS

Like all viruses of the herpes family, the varicella zoster virus (human herpes virus-3) exhibits a pattern of primary infection followed by latency, and possibly, secondary

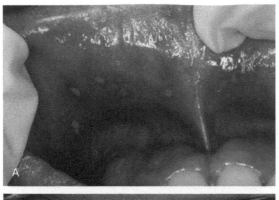

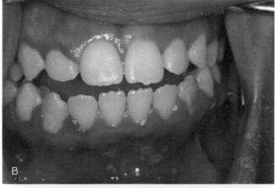

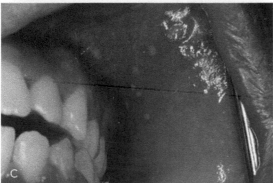

FIGURE 10 Herpetiform aphthae. Herpetiform aphthae are so named because the clinical appearance resembles that of herpes simplex. The lesions of recurrent intraoral herpes simplex arise on the keratinized masticatory mucosa, which is fixed and immobile and located over the bone. These aphthae involve the freely movable nonkeratinized mucosa. Based on the clinical appearance, pseudomembraneous candidiasis could be included in the differential diagnosis; however, these lesions do not wipe off and are quite painful. *Source*: Courtesy of Charles Dunlap, DDS.

reactivation. In contrast to HSV, in which the primary infection is usually subclinical, the primary infection of varicella zoster virus commonly produces symptomatic disease as varicella (chicken pox). Reactivation of the latent virus in the trigeminal ganglion due to a compromise in immunity produces a prodrome of pain in the distribution of the involved trigeminal nerve division that precedes the skin/mucosal lesions of herpes zoster (shingles).

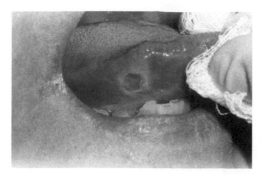

FIGURE 11 Traumatic ulcer. This is a chronic ulcer associated with several broken-down sharp teeth in the mandibular dental arch. The white periphery, slightly rolled border, and clinical history of nonrecurrence and chronicity help differentiate it from recurrent aphthous stomatitis. Since this is a high-risk site for oral cancer, this lesion should be submitted for microscopic examination, should it not regress after elimination of the suspected etiologic agent.

Differential Diagnosis

Although vesicles that rupture to form shallow ulcers may involve any oral mucosal site in varicella, the differential diagnosis is not usually problematic due to the constitutional symptoms and cutaneous lesions that dominate the clinical picture. In the early phase of zoster, the clinical picture is dominated by prodromal pain in the distribution of the involved nerves. Subsequently, vesicles develop that rupture and frequently become confluent. The lesions may involve the skin or mucosa of any of the branches of the trigeminal nerve and are characteristic in their unilateral distribution that stops at the midline. A cytologic smear of the vesicle fluid will exhibit the viral cytopathic effect common to both the HSV and the herpes zoster virus. Occasionally, it may be difficult to differentiate zoster from a zosteriform eruption of recurrent intraoral herpes simplex. Immunofluorescent staining of a cytologic smear for varicella zoster may be required to differentiate these lesions (1). Immunocompromised patients may exhibit an atypical pattern of involvement.

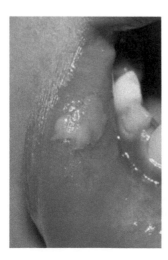

FIGURE 12 Traumatic ulcer. This child traumatized her anesthetized lower lip by chewing on it. The irregular ulcer is covered by a yellowish fibrinous membrane. The history and irregular appearance aid in distinguishing it from an aphthous lesion.

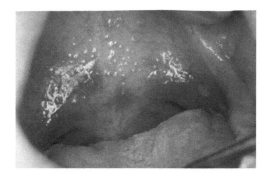

FIGURE 13 Crohn's disease. This individual has Crohn's disease affecting the gastrointestinal tract. These ulcers of the soft palate mucosa, although clinically aphthous-like in appearance, exhibit granulomatous inflammation consistent with Crohn's disease.

Treatment, Complications, and Prognosis

Oral antiviral medications are effective treatment for herpes zoster. The addition of oral corticosteroids is effective in reducing the morbidity of postherpetic neuralgia, which may produce pain outlasting the clinical lesions by months or more.

CANDIDAL STOMATITIS

Candida species are common commensal inhabitants of the oral cavity that may produce disease when predisposing factors shift the balance in the favor of the opportunistic organism. Common predisposing factors include antibiotic therapy, steroid therapy, xerostomia, and immunodeficiency. The lesions produced by overgrowth of Candida on the mucosal surface range from white or red lesions to combination of red and white lesions. Acute pseudomembraneous candidiasis (thrush) (Fig. 14) exhibits white, curd-like lesions that are easily wiped off. Atrophic candidiasis exhibits a red mucosal surface secondary to epithelial atrophy and mucosal inflammation (Figs. 15 and 16). Angular cheilitis (Perleche) is a localized inflammatory lesion, frequently associated with candidal and bacterial infection involving the angles of the mouth (Fig. 17), which exhibits erythema, fissuring, and crusting.

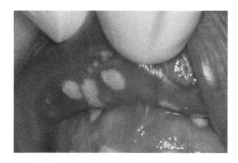
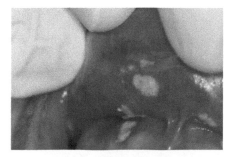

FIGURE 14 Acute pseudomembraneous candidiasis. This adult female developed candidiasis secondary to the extended use of oral topical steroids. She complained of generalized low-grade mucosal discomfort and an unpleasant taste in her mouth. The white colonies of Candida species, which consist of mattes of fungal pseudohyphae and desquamated epithelial debris, are easily wiped from the mucosal surface. The mucosa underlying the fungal colonies may be erythematous and may even bleed slightly. This was not the case in this patient, as the two posterior colonies of the upper lip mucosa in the left-hand figure revealed an intact mucosal surface when removed.

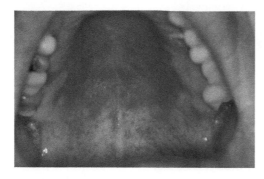

FIGURE 15 Erythematous candidiasis. This adult male complained of burning and low-grade discomfort when eating. A fungal culture was strongly positive for typical candidal colonies with 24 hours of incubation. The lesion cleared in several days with chlotrimazole troches.

Differential Diagnosis

Pseudomembranous candidiasis is the most common form of oral candidiasis. It is generally accompanied by rather mild symptoms of burning and altered taste. Atrophic candidiasis is associated with a greater degree of burning discomfort and frequently is associated with antibiotic use. Orally inhaled steroids also predispose to the development of oral candidiasis. Lesions that may resemble acute pseudomembraneous candidiasis include traumatic lesions (Fig. 18), erythema migrans, (Figs. 19–21), and pseudomembrane-covered aphthae, which are quite painful (Fig. 10). Pyostomatitis vegetans (Fig. 22), the oral mucosal lesion associated with ulcerative colitis, may superficially resemble pseudomembraneous candidiasis; however, the lesions cannot be wiped off the surface. Atrophic candidiasis must be differentiated from erythroplakia (Fig. 23).

Treatment, Complications, and Prognosis

Depending on the severity of the disease process, topical or systemic antifungal therapy may be used. Angular cheilitis is treated with topical antifungal agents. Identification and correction of any local or systemic predisposing factors (long-term antibiotics, steroids, diabetes, and immunosuppression) is important to prevent recurrence of the disease process (19).

ERYTHEMA MIGRANS

Erythema migrans is also referred to as stomatitis areata migrans. When it occurs on the tongue, its most common location, it is referred to as geographic tongue (Fig. 24). Although typically asymptomatic, it may occasionally produce a mild burning sensation, particularly in response to highly seasoned foods. It presents as an erythematous zone

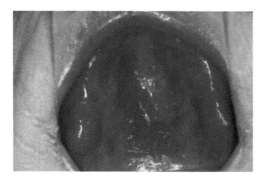

FIGURE 16 Erythematous candidiasis. This edentulous 68-year-old female complained of a sore mouth. The mucosa beneath her maxillary complete denture was erythematous and tender. She wore her denture continuously and attended to very little denture hygiene. The lesion cleared in response to topical antifungal therapy of both the mucosa and the denture base material (soaking the denture in nystatin suspension).

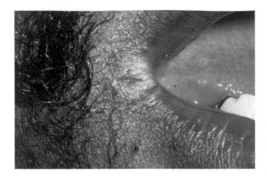

FIGURE 17 Angular cheilitis. This young adult male complained of painful cracking and fissuring at the angles of his mouth for the past two weeks. The lesions healed in seven days with topical antifungal therapy.

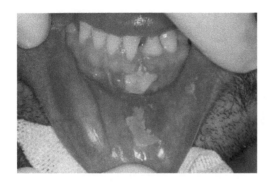

FIGURE 18 Chemical burn. This adult male placed aspirin tablets in the mandibular vestibule to relieve tooth discomfort. The clinical history is important in differentiating these lesions from acute pseudomembranous candidiasis, which is not usually difficult.

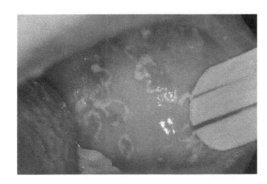

FIGURE 19 Acute pseudomembraneous candidiasis. This adult female complained of a burning mouth. These lesions of acute pseudomembraneous candidiasis bear a striking resemblance to erythema migrans (Figs. 20 and 21).

partially surrounded by a raised, serpiginous white line at the junction with uninvolved tissue. The lesions change patterns over time. The histopathology is highly suggestive of psoriasis. The cause of erythema migrans is unknown.

Differential Diagnosis

When erythema migrans occurs on the dorsum of the tongue, the clinical appearance is usually sufficiently distinctive to identify it on a clinical basis. It may cause confusion, however, when it involves sites other than the dorsal tongue (Fig. 20). In these cases, it must be differentiated from pseudomembraneous candidiasis (Fig. 21), erythroplakia, and lichenoid mucositis.

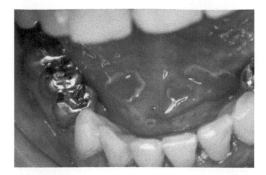

FIGURE 20 Erythema migrans. At sites other than the typical dorsal tongue location, erythema migrans may cause differential diagnostic confusion if one is not familiar with this clinical presentation. Red lesions in a high-risk site for oral cancer (floor of mouth) should be viewed with suspicion. In this case, the clinical features are typical, consisting of an erythematous, atrophic zone partially surrounded by a raised, serpiginous white line. If there is doubt, a biopsy should be performed. *Source*: Courtesy of Charles Dunlap, DDS.

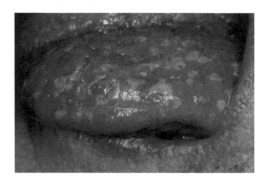

FIGURE 21 Erythema migrans. This is an unusual presentation of erythema migrans in its usual location on the dorsal tongue. The patient, an adult male microbiologist, reported that over the years it was repeatedly confused with pseudomembraneous candidiasis.

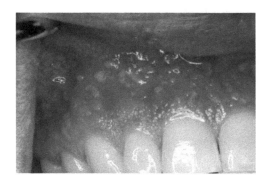

FIGURE 22 Pyostomatitis vegetans. This 49-year-old male with ulcerative colitis exhibits multiple yellowish-white plaques of the oral mucosa histologically consistent with pyostomatitis vegetans, the oral mucosal lesions of ulcerative colitis. *Source*: Courtesy of Bruce Barker, DDS.

Treatment, Complications, and Prognosis

Asymptomatic erythema migrans is not usually a clinical management problem. On the occasions when it is symptomatic, topical steroids are effective. The treatment goal should be to resolve the symptoms rather than eliminate the lesions.

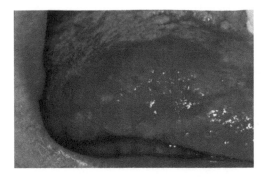

FIGURE 23 Erythroplakia. This 75-year-old male presented with a three-month history of discomfort involving the lateral border of his tongue. The lesion was nonindurated, exhibited a loss of the normal papillary surface and was mildly tender to palpation. A diagnostic biopsy was performed immediately and was diagnostic for squamous cell carcinoma.

COXSACKIE VIRUS STOMATITIS

Coxsackie virus infection may be associated with stomatitis secondary to multiple oral mucosal vesicles that rupture, forming shallow ulcers. Herpangina and hand, foot, and mouth disease are caused by specific strains of the Coxsackie virus. In both, the typical lesions are associated with flu-like symptoms.

Differential Diagnosis

The oral lesions of herpangina are few in number and usually involve the posterior area of the oral cavity, frequently the soft palate and adjacent tissues (Fig. 25). The lesions of hand, foot, and mouth disease are usually found in the more anterior parts of the mouth (Fig. 26). The fragile vesicles ulcerate rapidly and heal without scarring in less than two weeks. Coxsackie virus infection may occur in schoolchildren in epidemics, so there

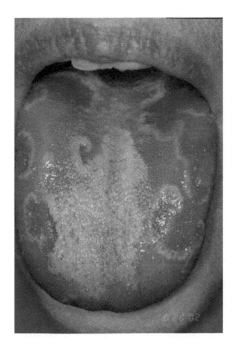

FIGURE 24 Erythema migrans. Also referred to as stomatitis areata migrans or a geographic tongue when it occurs on the dorsal tongue, its most common location. Although usually asymptomatic, it may cause a mild burning sensation. Frequent observation will demonstrate its changing pattern.

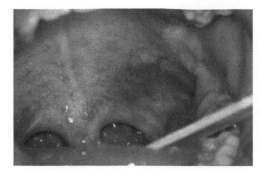

FIGURE 25 Herpangina. This individual complained of a sore throat and a low-grade fever. Note the posterior location in the oral cavity. The erythematous zone on the left soft palate contains three intact vesicles in a linear arrangement.

may be a known history of contact with an infected individual. Primary herpetic gingivostomatitis is associated with lesions more diffusely distributed throughout the mouth and usually exhibits a painful erythematous gingivitis. Recurrent aphthous stomatitis is not preceded by vesicles and is unassociated with systemic symptoms.

Treatment, Complications, and Prognosis

Treatment is supportive and symptomatic. Coxsackie virus infections are usually self-limiting and are typically unassociated with significant complications.

EROSIVE LICHEN PLANUS

Lichen planus is a chronic immunologically mediated mucocutaneous disease. Although the cause of lichen planus is unknown, the tissue manifestation is a dense infiltrate of T-lymphocytes within the lamina propria at the epithelial–connective tissue interface that damage the basal epithelial cell layer (20). The oral mucosal lesions of lichen planus appear in several forms. The most common presentation is the reticular form, which generally produces no symptoms. The erosive variant is associated with zones of erosion and ulceration within the reticulated areas that may produce significant morbidity (Fig. 27). Desquamative gingivitis (Fig. 28) is frequently seen in lichen planus. The lesions of erosive lichen planus are seen most frequently on the buccal mucosa, usually bilaterally.

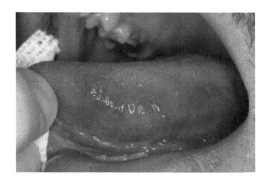

FIGURE 26 Hand, foot, and mouth disease. In contrast to herpangina, which is usually associated with lesions in the posterior oral cavity, the lesions of hand, foot, and mouth disease are usually confined to the anterior oral cavity. These lesions on the lateral tongue consist of painful ulcerations. This young adult also exhibited lesions of the skin of the hands and feet.

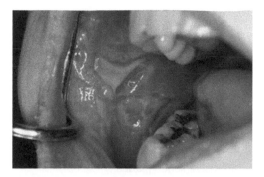

FIGURE 27 Erosive lichen planus. This middle-aged female exhibited bilateral painful lesions of erosive lichen planus as well as desquamative lesions of the gingiva. Note the central stellate ulcer covered with a yellowish fibrinous membrane surrounded by radiating white striae (of Wickham). There were no skin lesions of lichen planus. The therapeutic goal was to reduce pain and discomfort. Therapy consisted of a short burst of systemic corticosteroids in conjunction with topical steroids. The ulcerations healed within 10 days, leaving asymptomatic white striae.

Differential Diagnosis

Lichenoid lesions clinically identical to erosive lichen planus may be seen in lichenoid drug reactions (Fig. 29), chronic hepatitis C infection (Fig. 30), graft-versus-host disease, and lupus erythematosus. Direct immunofluorescent examination of lesions of lichen planus exhibits immunoreactants for fibrinogen in a continuous shaggy-appearing deposit along the basement membrane zone. Histologically, premalignant epithelial lesions may simulate the histology of lichen planus (lichenoid dysplasia). Chronic ulcerative stomatitis (CUS) should be included in the clinical differential diagnosis of erosive lichen planus. DIF in CUS reveals the presence of stratified epithelium-specific antinuclear antibodies (21,22).

Treatment, Complications, and Prognosis

In contrast to lichen planus of the skin, oral mucosal lichen planus exhibits a more chronic course, with exacerbation and remission of disease activity. The disease may last for years, with few patients experiencing complete remission. Depending on the severity of the

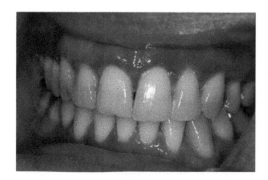

FIGURE 28 Desquamative gingivitis in lichen planus. This is the typical clinical appearance of desquamative gingivitis, a clinical reaction pattern that is seen in a number of disease processes, including lichen planus, mucous membrane pemphigoid, and pemphigus vulgaris. *Source*: Photo Credit: Bruce Barker, DDS.

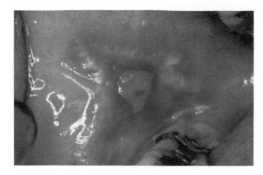

FIGURE 29 Lichenoid drug reaction. Note the central irregular ulceration covered by a yellowish fibrinous membrane surrounded by a peripheral erythematous, eroded zone and radiating white striae (of Wickham). This lesion represents a lichenoid drug reaction to a thiazide diuretic, a class of drug often associated with such reactions. This lesion is clinically identical to erosive lichen planus.

disease process, topical or systemic corticosteroids are effective (23). The therapeutic goal should be to provide relief of symptoms while minimizing the untoward effects of treatment. There are reports in the literature that erosive lichen planus predisposes to the development of squamous cell carcinoma. This controversy is clouded by the finding of epithelial dysplastic lesions with a lymphocytic infiltrate mimicking the histologic appearance of lichen planus. It is possible that these lichenoid dysplasias were misinterpreted as lichen planus. Until this issue is resolved, it is prudent to consider that there may be a predisposition, albeit small, to malignant transformation in erosive lichen planus, and prudent to provide appropriate clinical management of these patients.

MUCOUS MEMBRANE PEMPHIGOID

MMP is a chronic autoimmune mucocutaneous disease in which autoantibodies directed at structural proteins of the hemidesmosome destroy the epithelial–connective tissue attachment at the level of the basement membrane, producing a subepithelial separation (24,25). The protein targets of the autoantibodies include BP-1, BP-2, and laminin-5 (epiligrin), all components of the epithelial anchoring apparatus. MMP is a generalized term for a group of closely related disease processes (26). The term "oral mucous membrane pemphigoid" is used if the lesions are confined to the oral mucosa (Fig. 31). The term "cicatricial pemphigoid" is applied to patients with involvement of the ocular mucosa, which produces scarring and may result in blindness. The term "bullous pemphigoid" is

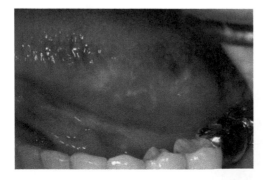

FIGURE 30 Lichenoid stomatitis in chronic hepatitis C. This red and white lesion at a high-risk site like the lateral border of the tongue was sensitive to spicy food and was highly suspicious for a premalignancy. A biopsy showed a lichenoid mucositis without dysplasia. Note the central erythematous area surrounded by white, radiating striae, the typical "lichenoid" clinical appearance. *Source*: Courtesy of Stacy Mullins, DDS.

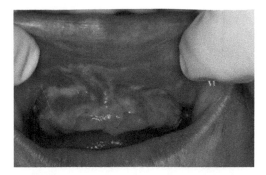

FIGURE 31 Mucous membrane pemphigoid. Middle-aged edentulous adult female with history of stomatitis of six months duration involving the upper and lower alveolar ridges. Observe the broad, confluent, ulcerated pseudomembrane-covered zones extending from the crest of the alveolar ridge to the reflection of the labial vestibule. An ophthalmologic workup was negative for ocular mucosal disease involvement. Direct immunofluorescence findings showed IgG and C3 deposits at the basement membrane zone. *Source*: Courtesy of Charles Dunlap, DDS.

applied if there is involvement of the skin. Both cicatricial and bullous pemphigoid may be associated with oral mucosal lesions. MMP is commonly seen in middle-aged females.

Differential Diagnosis

Erosive lichen planus, MMP, and pemphigus vulgaris (PV) may have similar clinical features. All may present with desquamative gingivitis (Fig. 32). Frequently in MMP, a gentle stream of air blown tangentially at the surface of the involved gingival mucosa will balloon up the epithelium (Fig. 33). They may be differentiated by DIF testing. In MMP, DIF exhibits a smooth linear deposit of immunoreactants (C3 and IgG) along the basement membrane zone. The Nikolsky sign is positive (Fig. 34). Primary herpes simplex is a febrile illness that exhibits an acute onset of vesicles.

Treatment, Complications, and Prognosis

Depending on the severity of the disease process, topical or systemic corticosteroids may be used. The therapeutic goal should be to provide relief of symptoms while minimizing

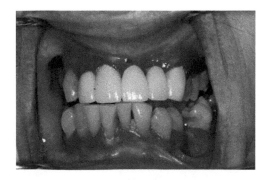

FIGURE 32 Desquamative gingivitis in mucous membrane pemphigoid. Note the gingival erythema and erosion. Desquamative gingivitis is a clinical reaction pattern that is seen in a number of disease processes, including lichen planus, mucous membrane pemphigoid, and pemphigus vulgaris.

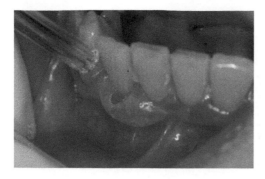

FIGURE 33 Desquamative gingivitis in mucous membrane pemphigoid. Note the epithelial separation produced by directing a gentle stream of air at the involved gingiva. This is a sign frequently seen in mucous membrane pemphigoid.

the untoward effects of treatment. Involvement of the ocular mucosa in cicatricial pemphigoid produces scarring and may result in blindness. The lesions may remain localized to the gingiva for a period but generally progress to involve adjacent areas. Treatment of the early lesions may prevent progression of the disease process.

DESQUAMATIVE GINGIVITIS

"Desquamative gingivitis" is a term used to describe a clinical reaction pattern that may be seen in a number of disease processes. It refers to a clinical condition in which the gingiva exhibits atrophy, erosion, and ulceration and possibly a positive Nikolsky sign (27,28). The term is used in a nonspecific manner, as are the terms "leukoplakia" and "erythroplakia," which refer to white and red lesions, respectively, which cannot be attributed to any specific disease process. The designation "desquamative" refers to the separation of the epithelium from the connective tissue.

Differential Diagnosis

The differential diagnosis of desquamative gingivitis includes erosive lichen planus (Fig. 28), lichenoid drug reaction, MMP (Fig. 32), and PV (Fig. 37). Often, a positive Nikolsky sign (Figs. 33 and 37) may be demonstrated. The Nikolsky sign indicates mucosal fragility and is seen in diseases with defective epithelial attachment and cell adhesion. In MMP, it is often possible to cause a large flap of gingival epithelium to balloon up (Fig. 33) by blowing a gentle, tangential stream of low-pressure air on an eroded gingival surface. This is surprisingly well tolerated by the patient. Gingival erosive lesions are best treated

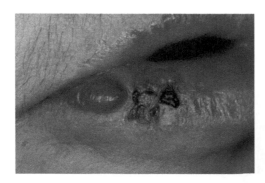

FIGURE 34 Mucous membrane pemphigoid. Positive Nikolsky sign was observed on the lower lip after retraction to facilitate oral examination. Note the adjacent, collapsed, crusted bulla. *Source*: Courtesy of Charles Dunlap, DDS.

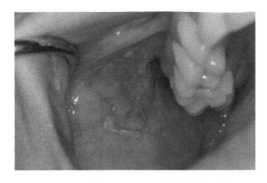

FIGURE 35 Pemphigus vulgaris. The lesions of pemphigus vulgaris typically exhibit a posterior location in the oral cavity. Note the collapsed intraepithelial bullae on the buccal mucosa and the lack of keratotic striae that would be typical of erosive lichen planus.

topically, using a custom flexible tray of the type used for topical fluoride application for dental caries prevention but extended to cover the gingival soft tissues. Linear IgA disease may present as desquamative gingivitis (29).

Treatment, Complications, and Prognosis
Please refer to the discussion of the individual disease processes that often present as desquamative gingivitis (erosive lichen planus, MMP, and PV).

PEMPHIGUS VULGARIS

PV is a chronic autoimmune mucocutaneous disease in which autoantibodies directed at structural proteins of the desmosome destroy the inter-epithelial cell attachments, producing acantholysis and subsequent suprabasal, intraepithelial bullae (30,31). The targets of the autoantibodies are the transmembrane glycoproteins desmoglein 1 and 3. PV is one member of a group of diseases characterized by autoimmune attack on the desmosomal attachment apparatus. Other members of the group include pemphigus foliaceus, vegetans, and erythematosus, which are less severe than PV. In the early stages, PV may be confined to the oral mucosa. In fact, oral mucosal lesions may be the presenting sign of the disease. The typical patient profile is an older adult. There is a higher incidence in certain populations sharing specific histocompatibility antigens, such as Ashkenazi Jews. Drug-induced pemphigus has been reported secondary to a number of drugs, including penicillamine, phenobarbital, and rifampin. Paraneoplastic pemphigus also occurs in conjunction with non-Hodgkin's lymphoma and chronic lymphocytic leukemia

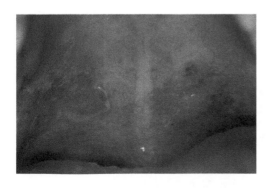

FIGURE 36 Pemphigus vulgaris. This 31-year-old female complained of a six-month history of oral mucosal discomfort. Note the posterior soft palate location of the collapsed, fragile intraepithelial bullae. *Source*: Courtesy of Bruce Barker, DDS.

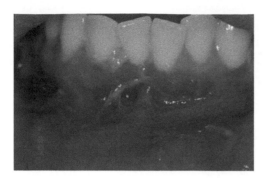

FIGURE 37 Pemphigus vulgaris with desquamative gingivitis. This adult female had a six-month history of desquamative lesions of the gingival and soft palate. In contrast to collapsed bullae of mucous membrane pemphigoid, which frequently billow up in response to a tangential stream of low-pressure air (Fig. 33), the bullae of pemphigus vulgaris are much more fragile and the epithelium simply piles up and desquamates in response to the air stream. *Source*: Courtesy of Charles Dunlap, DDS.

and a number of other neoplasms. PV most frequently involves the more posterior areas of the oral cavity (Fig. 35) such as the soft palate (Fig. 36).

Differential Diagnosis

The intraepithelial location of the bullae in PV makes them fragile and short-lived. They quickly rupture to form secondary eroded lesions. Acantholytic keratinocytes, termed "Tzanck cells," may be seen in exfoliative cytologic smears of bullous lesions. PV, erosive lichen planus, and MMP may have similar clinical features and all may present with desquamative gingivitis. They may be differentiated by DIF testing. In PV, DIF exhibits reteform, net-like deposit of immunoreactants (IgG) outlining the periphery of the epithelial cells in the spinous layer. In contrast to the collapsed bullae of MMP, which frequently billow up in response to a stream of low-pressure air, the bullae of PV are much more fragile and the epithelium simply piles up and desquamates in response to the air stream (Fig. 37).

Treatment, Complications, and Prognosis

Management of PV requires systemic corticosteroids, usually in combination with steroid-sparing immunosuppressive agents such as azathioprine. In addition to the clinical response, the effectiveness of therapy may be monitored with measurement of circulating

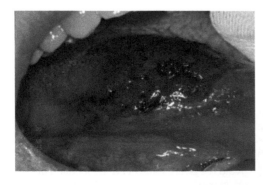

FIGURE 38 Erythroplakia. Toluidine Blue vital staining of the lesion shown in Figure 23. The areas of blue uptake represent areas of DNA concentration and were used to guide the selection of an appropriate biopsy site.

autoantibody titers. Prior to the advent of immunosuppressive therapy, PV was associated with a dismal prognosis with mortality as high as 80% secondary to infection and electrolyte disturbances. Although the mortality rate is currently much lower, the major causes of death in PV are now related to complications of the treatment (long-term corticosteroids).

ERYTHROPLAKIA

The World Health Organization defines erythroplakia as a red patch that cannot be attributed to any specific disease process (Fig. 23). The significance of erythroplakia is that there is a greater than 90% chance that the lesion will contain a high-grade (premalignant) epithelial dysplasia (32).

Differential Diagnosis

Erythroplakia must be included in the differential diagnosis of any red lesion that cannot be identified as a specific disease process. Areas of erythroplakia that contain white areas (speckled erythroplakia) should be treated like erythroplakia. Vital staining with Toluidine Blue dye can be useful in identifying the most appropriate site for a biopsy (Fig. 38).

Treatment, Complications, and Prognosis

All erythroplakic lesions should be treated with a high index of suspicion and receive a timely diagnosis by early biopsy. A red or red-and-white lesion that cannot be attributed to any specific disease process, especially in a high-risk site, has a strong likelihood of harboring a high-grade epithelial dysplasia.

ACUTE NECROTIZING ULCERATIVE GINGIVITIS

Necrotizing ulcerative gingivitis (NUG) is a fusospirochetal infection that occurs frequently in individuals with depressed systemic immunity states (HIV infection and infectious mononucleosis) and in those under psychologic stress (33–35). Historically, NUG has been referred to as Vincent's infection and "trench mouth."

Differential Diagnosis

In NUG, the interdental papillae undergo necrosis beginning at the tips and extending toward the crest of the dental alveolar bone. As a result of the soft-tissue necrosis, the interdental gingival papillae exhibit a "punched out" blunted, crateriform area covered by a fibrinonecrotic membrane (Fig. 39). The gingiva are exquisitely sensitive and often exhibit spontaneous bleeding. A fetid odor accompanies the soft-tissue necrosis. There may be associated systemic symptoms of fever, malaise, and lymphadenopathy. Primary herpetic gingivostomatitis also presents with exquisitely sensitive gingiva, but there is neither necrosis nor the characteristic fetid oral odor (36). Primary herpes simplex also involves the nonkeratinized oral mucosa, while NUG is confined to the gingiva.

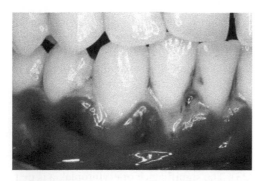

FIGURE 39 Necrotizing ulcerative gingivitis. This HIV-positive adult male presented with multiple, punched-out necrotic lesions of the interdental papillae. The gingivae were exquisitely painful. A fetid odor accompanied the necrotic lesions. On the third tooth from the lower left, the fusospirochetal infection has extended from the gingival mucosa into the periodontal ligament (necrotizing ulcerative periodontitis) *Source*: Courtesy of Department of Periodontics, School of Dentistry, University of Missouri, Kansas City, Missouri.

Treatment, Complications, and Prognosis

NUG generally responds to initial therapy of debridement, antimicrobial oral rinses, and antibiotic therapy (37). When the process heals, the altered gingival anatomy resulting from tissue loss through necrosis creates anatomic forms that predispose to recurrence of NUG and to the development of chronic periodontitis. NUG may progress from gingival soft-tissue involvement to produce loss of periodontal attachment (necrotizing ulcerative periodontitis) and may extend to involve the adjacent oral soft tissues (necrotizing ulcerative stomatitis). Extension of the infectious process through the soft tissues to the facial skin is termed "Noma" (cancrum oris).

ERYTHEMA MULTIFORME

EM is an acute, widely distributed hypersensitivity reaction associated with circulating immune complexes that are deposited in the basement membranes of the superficial vessels of the skin and mucosa. Subsequent complement activation produces vasculitis and thrombosis, leading to tissue ischemia and necrosis of the adjacent epithelium. The intensity of the skin and mucosal reaction varies from a localized minimal erythematous

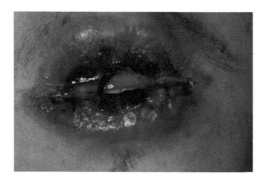

FIGURE 40 Erythema multiforme. Young adult male with rapid onset of generalized oral ulceration accompanied by typical target lesions of the skin. Note the hemorrhagic, encrusted lips, a feature frequently seen in erythema multiforme.

response to frank epithelial necrosis. Commonly identified precipitating factors include infections (herpes simplex, *Mycoplasma pneumoniae*) and medications (sulfonamides, barbiturates, and penicillin)—"drugs and bugs." Based on the intensity and severity of the hypersensitivity response, EM is classified into minor and major forms, with Stevens–Johnson syndrome (Chapter 22) and toxic epidermal necrolysis representing progressively more severe involvement, morbidity, and associated mortality. A multiday prodrome of fever, malaise, and headache precedes development of the mucocutaneous lesions. The classic skin lesion of EM is a concentric erythematous lesion described as resembling a target or bulls-eye. Oral mucosal lesions vary from focal aphthous-like involvement to diffuse areas of erythema, bulla formation, and ulceration (Fig. 6). Bullae collapse rapidly, leaving pseudomembrane-covered surfaces. The lips often appear hemorrhagic and crusted (Fig. 40).

Differential Diagnosis

EM is often described as a diagnosis of exclusion. Biopsy with DIF examination may be useful in excluding other disease processes with a similar clinical appearance, as well as in providing additional supportive findings. DIF reveals a perivascular deposition of immunoreactants (IgM and C3) around superficial blood vessels. Association of the lesions with a medication or an infection is supportive. An exfoliative cytologic spear can help rule out primary herpes.

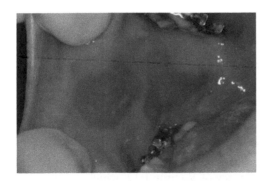

FIGURE 41 Contact stomatitis to nickel in orthodontic wire. This individual tolerated the placement of metal brackets on the teeth for an extended period. Shortly after inserting a nickel-containing orthodontic wire into the brackets, these painful erythematous patches arose on the buccal mucosa. The lesions cleared after removal of the wire. The metal brackets remained in place. *Source*: From Ref. 38.

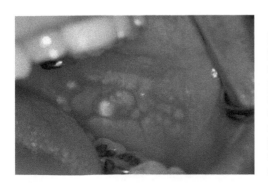

FIGURE 42 Contact allergy to cinnamon flavoring. This adult male chewed of cinnamon-flavored chewing gum and complained of a long-standing soreness of his buccal mucosa. Note the irregular ulcers, covered by fibrinous membranes, surrounded by white areas. The lesion completely healed within two weeks after withdrawal of the gum. *Source*: Courtesy of Charles Dunlap, DDS.

Treatment, Complications, and Prognosis
Identification and elimination of precipitating factors is key in the successful treatment of EM. EM may occur following herpetic infection in some patients. Preventing recurrent herpetic infections by judicious use of sunscreens to reduce ultraviolet exposure will assist in preventing secondary EM. For mild cases of EM, treatment may be symptomatic and supportive. The effectiveness of systemic corticosteroids is controversial. Severe cases may require hospitalization.

ALLERGIC CONTACT STOMATITIS

Allergic contact reactions are seen much less frequently on the oral mucosa than on the skin. A wide variety of substances may produce allergic contact stomatitis, including foods, additives, mouthwash, chewing gum, candy, and dental materials. Substances that are not directly allergenic may act as haptens to elicit an allergic response.

Differential Diagnosis
Erythema and burning are frequent clinical symptoms in acute contact stomatitis (Fig. 41). The lesions of chronic forms of contact stomatitis frequently exhibit a white component (38,39) in addition to the erythema (Fig. 42). Either form may exhibit erosion or ulceration. History is important in identifying a potential contact irritant.

Treatment, Complications, and Prognosis
Identification and elimination of the allergen controls the disease process. Corticosteroids may be useful to reduce symptoms.

GLOSSITIS
Glossitis may be associated with a number of conditions, ranging from metabolic to infectious conditions.

PERNICIOUS ANEMIA

Pernicious anemia is associated with atrophic gastritis. The marked loss of gastric parietal cells results in a deficiency of intrinsic factor, which is required to transport Vitamin B12 across the intestinal mucosa. The resulting deficiency of Vitamin B12, which is necessary

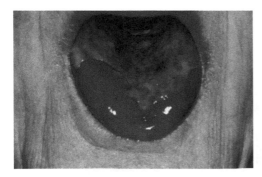

FIGURE 43 Pernicious anemia. This elderly female complained of a painful tongue. The mucosa of the anterior portion of the tongue was severely atrophic and totally devoid of lingual papillae. Posteriorly, the mucosa was extensively ulcerated and covered with a fibrinous membrane.

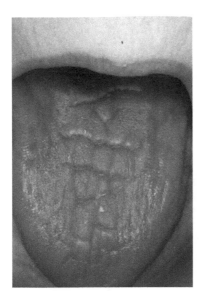

FIGURE 44 Iron deficiency anemia. This adult female complained of a sensitive tongue. Her hemoglobin level was 6.2 g/dL. There is extensive atrophy of the papillae of the dorsal tongue producing a shiny appearance. *Source*: Courtesy of Charles Dunlap, DDS.

for DNA synthesis, produces a megaloblastic anemia. The papillae of the dorsal tongue undergo atrophy, resulting in a red, smooth surface, which produces symptoms of pain and burning (Fig. 43).

Differential Diagnosis

A similar clinical appearance of the tongue mucosa may be seen in Vitamin B complex deficiencies and iron deficiency anemia (Fig. 44), which are also frequently associated with angular cheilitis. Since both Vitamin B12 and folate deficiencies exhibit macrocytic hyperchromic anemia, it is necessary to perform serum folate and B12 determinations in order to distinguish between them. Atrophic candidiasis (Fig. 45) may also produce a sensitive, erythematous, depapillated lingual mucosal surface.

Treatment, Complications, and Prognosis

The treatment of pernicious anemia involves intramuscular administration of Vitamin B12. The atrophic gastritis associated with pernicious anemia predisposes these patients to gastric carcinoma.

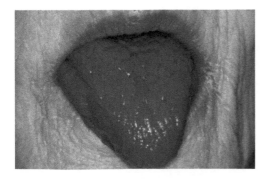

FIGURE 45 Atrophic candidiasis. This 67-year-old female with a fissured tongue complained of a two-month history of a painful, sensitive, red tongue. There is mild atrophy of the lingual papillae. Fungal culture was positive for candidal organisms. Her symptoms cleared and appearance of her tongue returned to her normal fissured appearance with the use of clotrimazole troches. *Source*: Photo courtesy of Bruce Barker, DDS.

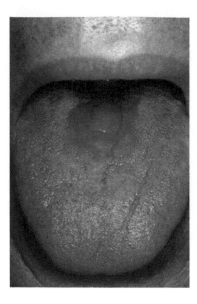

FIGURE 46   Central papillary atrophy. Also referred to as median rhomboid glossitis, this was long believed to be a developmental condition. It is now recognized as a form of erythematous candidiasis appearing as a well-demarcated zone of erythema in the midline of the dorsal tongue with a smooth or lobulated surface. The lesion is typically asymptomatic and frequently resolves with antifungal therapy.

IRON DEFICIENCY ANEMIA

Iron deficiency anemia is a common anemia in females. In addition to the clinical signs and symptoms of anemia, the papillae of the dorsal tongue undergo atrophy, resulting in a red, smooth surface, which produces symptoms of pain and burning (Fig. 44). Iron deficiency anemia is frequently associated with angular cheilitis.

Differential Diagnosis

In addition to the clinical symptoms of anemia, iron deficiency produces a microcytic, hypochromic anemia. Serum iron is low. Total iron-binding capacity is elevated. A similar clinical appearance of the tongue mucosa may be seen in Vitamin B complex deficiencies and pernicious anemia (Fig. 43). Atrophic candidiasis (Fig. 45) may also produce a sensitive, erythematous, depapillated lingual mucosal surface. In severe xerostomia, the tongue may exhibit atrophy of the lingual papillae and erythema that is frequently secondary to atrophic candidiasis. Central papillary atrophy is a localized form of depapillation secondary to candidiasis (Fig. 46).

Treatment, Complications, and Prognosis

Iron deficiency may be secondary to inadequate intake/absorption, increased loss, or increased demand. Treatment involves identification and correction of the underlying cause and iron supplementation. Individuals with the Plummer–Vinson syndrome (iron deficiency anemia, esophageal webs, and atrophic glossitis) are at increased risk for squamous carcinoma of the upper aerodigestive tract.

VITAMIN B DEFICIENCY

Deficiencies of the Vitamin B complex are unusual in developed countries but may be seen in individuals with underlying disease processes, especially those with eating disorders, malabsorption syndromes, and alcoholism. The papillae of the dorsal tongue undergo atrophy, resulting in a red, smooth surface, which produces symptoms of pain and burning.

Differential Diagnosis
A similar clinical appearance of the tongue mucosa may be seen in iron deficiency anemia (Fig. 44) and in pernicious anemia (Fig. 43). Folic acid deficiency produces a megaloblastic anemia. Atrophic candidiasis (Fig. 45) should be excluded.

Treatment, Complications, and Prognosis
The glossitis resolves with replacement therapy.

HERPETIC GLOSSITIS

Herpetic infections in immunocompromised patients often produce atypical clinical findings in contrast to those in immunocompetent individuals. Herpetic geometric glossitis is associated with an exquisitely tender and painful tongue exhibiting longitudinal furrows, frequently with cross-hatched branches (41).

Differential Diagnosis
Fissured tongue is a common anatomic variant of the lingual mucosa, which exhibits multiple, often anastomosing, but asymptomatic fissures.

Treatment, Complications, and Prognosis
Immunocompromised individuals with painful longitudinal furrows of the tongue should receive empiric oral acyclovir (1000 mg/day in five divided doses) treatment, while awaiting HSV-I culture results. Acyclovir-resistant forms of herpetic geometric glossitis have not been reported.

REFERENCES

1. Neville BW, Damm DD, Allen CM, et al. Oral and Maxillofacial Pathology. 2nd ed. Philadelphia, PA: WB Saunders Co., 2002.
2. Regezi JA, Sciubba JJ, Jordan RCK. Oral Pathology, Clinical Pathologic Correlations. 4th ed. St. Louis, MO: WB Saunders Co., 2003.
3. Sapp JP, Eversole LR, Wysocki GP. Contemporary Oral and Maxillofacial Pathology. 2nd ed. St. Louis, MO: Mosby, 2004.
4. Wood NK, Goaz PW. Differential Diagnosis of Oral and Maxillofacial Lesions. 5th ed. St. Louis, MO: Mosby, 1997.
5. Coleman GC, Flaitz CM, Vincent SD. Differential diagnosis of oral soft tissue lesions. Tex Dent J 2002; 119(6):484–488, 490–492, 494–503.
6. Flaitz CM. Differential diagnosis of oral mucosal lesions in children and adolescents. Adv Dermatol 2000; 16:39–79.
7. Nikitakis NG. Oral soft tissue lesions: a guide to differential diagnosis. Part II: Surface alterations. Braz J Oral Sci 2005; 4(13):707–715.
8. Vincent SD, Finkelstein MW. Differential diagnosis of oral ulcers. In: Coleman GC, Nelson JF, eds. Principles of Oral Diagnosis. St. Louis, MO: Mosby, 1993:328–351.
9. Huber MA. Herpes simplex type-1 virus infection. Quintessence Int 2003; 34(6):453–467.
10. Samonis G, Mantadakis E, Maraki S. Orofacial viral infections in the immunocompromised host (review). Oncol Rep 2000; 7(6):1389–1394.

11. Casiglia JM. Recurrent aphthous stomatitis: etiology, diagnosis, and treatment. Gen Dent 2002; 50 (2):157–166.
12. Porter SR, Hegarty A, Kaliakatsou F, et al. Recurrent aphthous stomatitis. Clin Dermatol 2000; 18 (5):569–578.
13. Porter SR, Leao JC. Review article: oral ulcers and its relevance to systemic disorders. Aliment Pharmacol Ther 2005; 21(4):295–306.
14. Rogers RS III. Recurrent aphthous stomatitis: clinical characteristics and associated systemic disorders. Semin Cutan Med Surg 1997; 16(4):278–283.
15. Scully C, Gorsky M, Lozada-Nur F. The diagnosis and management of recurrent aphthous stomatitis: a consensus approach. J Am Dent Assoc 2003; 134(2):200–207.
16. Letsinger JA, McCarty MA, Jorizzo JL. Complex aphthosis: a large case series with evaluation algorithm and therapeutic ladder from topicals to thalidomide. J Am Acad Dermatol 2005; 52(3 Pt 1):500–508.
17. Bell J. Amlexanox for the treatment of recurrent aphthous ulcers. Clin Drug Invest 2005; 25(9):555–566.
18. Kerr AR, Ship JA. Management strategies for HIV-associated aphthous stomatitis. Am J Clin Dermatol 2003; 4(10):669–680.
19. Akpan A, Morgan R. Oral candidiasis. Postgrad Med J 2002; 78(922):455–459.
20. Lodi G, Scully C, Carrozzo M, et al. Current controversies in oral lichen planus: report of an international consensus meeting. Part 1. Viral infections and etiopathogenesis. Oral Surg Oral Med Oral Path Oral Radiol Endod 2005; 100(1):40–51.
21. Lewis JE, Beutner EH, Rostami R, et al. Chronic ulcerative stomatitis with stratified epithelium-specific antinuclear antibodies. Int J Dermatol 1996; 35(4):272–275.
22. Lorenzana ER, Rees TD, Glass M, et al. Chronic ulcerative stomatitis: a case report. J Periodontol 2000; 71(1):104–111.
23. Gonzalez-Moles MA, Scully C. Vesiculo-erosive oral mucosal disease - Management with topical corticosteroids: (1) Fundamental principles and specific agents available. J Dent Res 2005; 84(4): 294–301.
24. Bagan J, Muzio LL, Scully C. Mucosal disease series. Number III. Mucous membrane pemphigoid. Oral Dis 2005; 11(4):197–218.
25. Parisi E, Raghavendra S, Werth VP, et al. Modification to the approach of the diagnosis of mucous membrane pemphigoid: a case report and literature review. Oral Surg Oral Med Oral Path Oral Rad Endod 2003; 95(2):182–186.
26. Chan LS, Ahmed AR, Anhalt GJ, et al. The first international consensus on mucous membrane pemphigoid: definition, diagnostic criteria, pathogenic factors, medical treatment, and prognostic indicators. Arch Dermatol 2002; 138(3):370–379.
27. Robinson NA, Wray D. Desquamative gingivitis: a sign of mucocutaneous disorders—a review. Aust Dent J 2003; 48(4):206–211.
28. Scully C, Porter SR. The clinical spectrum of desquamative gingivitis. Semin Cutan Med Surg 1997; 16(4):308–313.
29. O'Regan E, Bane A, Flint S, et al. Linear IgA disease presenting as desquamative gingivitis – a pattern poorly recognized in medicine. Arch Otolaryngol Head Neck Surg 2004; 130(4): 469–472.
30. Black M, Mignogna MD, Scully C. Number II - pemphigus vulgaris. Oral Dis 2005; 11(3) :119–130.
31. Scully C, Challacombe SJ. Pemphigus vulgaris: update on etiopathogenesis, oral manifestations, and management. Crit Rev Oral Biol Med 2002; 13(5):397–408.
32. Reichart PA, Philipsen HP. Oral erythroplakia - a review. Oral Oncology 2005; 41(6):551–561.
33. Cobb CM. HIV-associated periodontal disease. Northwest Dent 1993; 72(5):25–28.
34. Enwonwu CO, Falkler WA, Idigbe EO. Oro-facial gangrene (noma/cancrum oris): pathogenetic mechanisms. Crit Rev Oral Biol Med 2000; 11(2):159–171.
35. Rowland RW. Necrotizing ulcerative gingivitis. Ann Periodontol 1999; 4(1):65–73.
36. Klotz H. Differentiation between necrotic ulcerative gingivitis and primary herpetic gingivostomatitis. N Y State Dent J 1973; 39(5):283–294.
37. Horning GM, Cohen ME. Necrotizing ulcerative gingivitis, periodontitis, and stomatitis: clinical staging and predisposing factors. J Periodontol 1995; 66(11):990–998.
38. Dunlap CL, Vincent SK, Barker BF. Allergic reaction to orthodontic wire; report of a case. JADA 1989; 118(4):449–50.

39. Allen CM, Blozis GG. Oral mucosal reactions to cinnamon-flavored chewing gum. J Am Dent Assoc 1988; 116(6):664–667.
40. Miller RL, Gould AR, Bernstein ML. Cinnamon-induced stomatitis venenata, clinical and characteristic histopathologic features. Oral Surg Oral Med Oral Pathol 1992; 73(6):708–716.
41. Cohen PR, Kazi S, Grossman ME. Herpetic geometric glossitis: a distinctive pattern of lingual herpes simplex virus infection. South Med J 1995; 88(12):1231–1235.

33

Pharyngitis/Tonsillitis

Brian T. Andrews, Henry T. Hoffman, and Douglas K. Trask
Department of Otolaryngology-Head and Neck Surgery, University of Iowa College of Medicine, Iowa City, Iowa, U.S.A.

INTRODUCTION

Pharyngitis and adenotonsillitis are two of the most common diagnoses in primary care medicine, accounting for 15% of all outpatient medical appointments (1). This discussion will consider pharyngitis to include all inflammatory conditions of the pharynx, including the tonsils and adenoids. Adenotonsillitis is the term for inflammation of these pharyngeal subunits and is often used interchangeably with pharyngitis. Although pharyngitis most commonly results from infection, many systemic diseases may manifest themselves with similar signs and symptoms (Table 1). Discriminating between infectious and other causes of pharyngeal inflammation may be difficult and may delay appropriate treatment options.

DEFINITION

Inflammation of the pharynx is termed pharyngitis, regardless of the etiology. The pharynx is a fibromuscular tube connecting the nose and the oral cavity from above to the larynx and esophagus below. The pharynx functions as a conduit and is shared by the respiratory and digestive tracts. It is divided into three anatomic substructures: the nasopharynx, the oropharynx, and the hypopharynx.

The nasopharynx begins anteriorly at the choana with its superior limit at the skull base and the inferior limit at the soft palate. The adenoids are an aggregation of lymphoid tissue located on the posterior wall of the nasopharynx between the openings of the Eustachian tubes laterally (Fig. 1). Gerlach's tonsils are an aggregate of lymphoid tissue adjacent to the Eustachian tube openings. The anterior extent of the oropharynx is the glossopalatine arch, also termed the anterior tonsillar pillar. The superior limit of the oropharynx is the soft palate and the inferior limit is the tongue base. The palatine tonsils lie in a triangular space formed by the glossopalatine arch anteriorly and the pharyngopalatine arch posteriorly. The lingual tonsils are located on the posterior tongue base. Waldeyer's ring is the lymphatic tissue network composed of the adenoids, Gerlach's tonsils, palatine tonsils, and lingual tonsils. The hypopharynx is the segment of the upper aerodigestive tract that lies between the oropharynx superiorly and the esophagus and larynx inferiorly. The substructures of the hypopharynx are the postcricoid area anteriorly, the paired pyriform sinuses laterally, and the posterior pharyngeal wall.

The normal mucosal lining of the nasopharynx is ciliated pseudostratified respiratory epithelium. The oropharynx and hypopharynx are lined by a nonkeratinizing, stratified squamous epithelium. The mucosa and submucosa of the pharynx covers the superior, middle, and inferior constrictor muscles that represent the major muscular structures of the pharynx. Other minor muscles in the pharynx are the palatopharyngeus, the salpingopharyngeus, and the stylopharyngeus, as well as muscles of the soft palate. The pharynx is innervated by the pharyngeal plexus derived from CN IX and CN X.

CLINICAL MANIFESTATIONS

Symptoms of pharyngitis depend on the etiology. Sore throat is the most common symptom associated with pharyngitis and represents the third most common complaint encountered in office-based medicine (2,3). Dysphagia, odynophagia, ear pain, fever, and malaise are other associated symptoms. Airway obstruction presents less commonly. Noninfectious inflammatory conditions may cause a similar constellation of symptoms without fever and malaise. Less frequently encountered symptoms include globus sensation, voice changes, snoring, nasal congestion, and frequent throat clearing (4). Neoplasms occurring within the

TABLE 1 Etiology of Pharyngitis/Adenotonsillitis

I. Infection
  A. Bacterial
    1. *Streptococcus*
    2. *Arcanobacterium haemolyticum*
    3. *Neisseria gonorrhea*
    4. *Corynebacterium diphtheriae*
    5. *Bordetella pertussis*
    6. *Treponema pallidum*
    7. *Fusobacterium necrophorum*
    8. *Mycobacterium (tuberculosis, avium, intracellulare, kansasii, scrofulaceum)*
    9. Other bacterium (Mycoplasm, Francisella, Chlamydia, Anaerobes)
  B. Viral
    1. Adenovirus
    2. "Common cold" viruses (rhinovirus, coronavirus, parainfluenza virus, and influenza virus)
    3. Epstein–Barr virus
    4. Cytomegalovirus
    5. Coxsackie virus
    6. Herpes simplex virus
    7. Measles
    8. Human immunodeficiency virus
    9. Other viruses
  C. Fungal
    1. Candidiasis
    2. Aspergillosis
    3. Other mycosis
II. Neoplasms
  A. Hematological cancer
  B. Epithelial cell cancer
  C. Salivary cancer
III. Inflammatory/autoimmune disease
  A. Wegener's granulomatosis
  B. Sarcoidosis
  C. Crohn's disease
  D. Extraesophageal reflux disease
  E. Pemphigus
  F. Bullous pemphigoid
  G. Cicatricial pemphigoid
  H. Epidermolysis bullosa
  I. Stevens–Johnson syndrome
  J. Behçet's disease
IV. Iatrogenic
  A. Radiation
  B. Medications
V. Nutritional
  A. Vitamin deficiency
  B. Dehydration

pharynx produce similar symptoms but complaints are typically unilateral, in contrast to infectious or inflammatory conditions, which are bilateral. Dehydration and acute weight loss secondary to dysphagia occur with pharyngitis of any cause. Chronic progressive weight loss over several months is common in neoplastic etiologies. Cervical lymphadenopathy may be present with either infectious or neoplastic etiologies.

Erythema of the pharyngeal mucosa is the hallmark physical exam finding of pharyngitis. Tonsillar enlargement in patients with recurrent pharyngitis may be present.

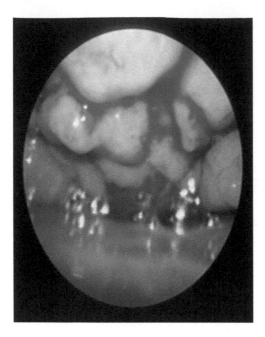

FIGURE 1 Normal adenoid tissue in the nasopharynx.

Tonsil size is commonly graded on a scale of one to four, with grade 1 tonsils being contained within the tonsillar pillars and grade 4 tonsils touching at the midline of the oropharynx (Fig. 2). Normal tonsils are often cryptic and may contain debris within the crypts, called tonsilliths. The adenoid bed may also be enlarged when viewed with mirror examination or through nasal endoscopy. The adenoid tissue contains more folds than crypts when compared with the palatine tonsils. A whitish-gray exudate covering the pharyngeal mucosa may result from sloughing epithelial cells (Fig. 3). Mucosal changes such as ulceration, petechiae, or maculopapules are common in noninfectious etiologies and warrant further examination.

PATHOGENESIS

Infection — Bacterial

Epidemiology.   At birth, the upper respiratory tract is colonized with multiple organisms and the normal bacterial flora is established. It consists primarily of Gram-positive aerobic organisms and anaerobic organisms. Infectious pharyngitis represents a change in this normal flora.

    Streptococcus.   *Streptococcus* species are Gram-positive cocci bacteria arranged most commonly in chains. They are ubiquitous inhabitants of the oral and nasal cavities. Members of this bacterial family are classified as either α-hemolytic or β-hemolytic, based on characterizations observed when grown on blood agar cultures. β-hemolytic streptococci are further classified based on carbohydrates found on their cell membranes. These are called Lancefield groups and consist of groups A though G.

    Group A β-Hemolytic *Streptococcus*.   *Streptococcus pyogenes*, also called group A β-hemolytic streptococcus (GABHS), is the most common pathogen in acute bacterial pharyngitis. It represents 5% to 10% of all infectious causes of pharyngitis in adults and 15% to 30% in children. GABHS is transmitted by aerosolized droplets or direct contact. GABHS has several virulence factors that contribute to its pathogenesis, including secreted

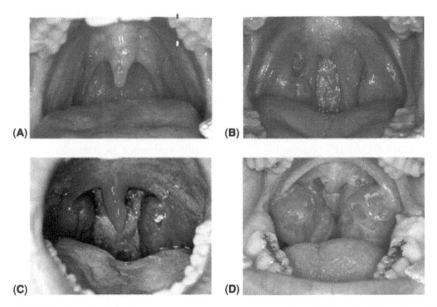

FIGURE 2 (**A**) Tonsillar hypertrophy grade-I tonsils. (**B**) Grade-II tonsils. (**C**) Grade-III tonsils. (**D**) Grade-IV tonsils ("kissing tonsils").

enzymes such as streptolysin O, streptolysin S, DNAase, hyaluronidase, and exotoxins A, B, and C.

Concern exists about the overuse of antibacterials in treating symptoms of infectious pharyngitis. Several scoring systems have been developed to limit the use of antibiotics to those patients with high probability of GABHS pharyngitis or other bacterial causes. Systems developed by Walsh (GABHS exposure, cervical nodes, pharyngeal exudates, temperature >101°F, and cough) and Centor (fever, cervical nodes, pharyngeal exudate, and absence of cough) have been employed to restrict antibiotic use to persons with bacterial etiologies and not viral causes. Unfortunately, long-term study of these systems has not strongly supported their clinical use.

Throat swab and culture remains the gold standard for diagnosis and has a sensitivity of approximately 90%. A rapid antigen detection test can be performed for faster analysis. This test uses an enzyme immunoassay to detect streptococcal carbohydrate antigens found

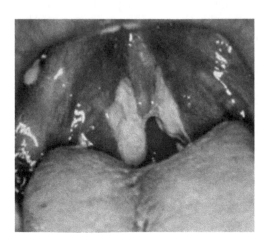

FIGURE 3 Acute pharyngitis and tonsillitis with an exudate covering the tonsils bilaterally.

on throat swabs. The sensitivity of this test is only 80% to 90%, but it is highly specific. Most cultures grown from patients with negative rapid strep tests will remain negative. Despite this information, most primary-care physicians advocate culture when rapid screens are negative. Newer optical immunoassays have been developed but their clinical superiority over previous enzyme immunoassays remains debatable. Asymptomatic carriers of GABHS with viral pharyngitis will test positive no matter what method is used, limiting any test's clinical usefulness.

Oral penicillin, or I.M. penicillin for noncompliant patients, is advocated by some as first-line treatment of GABHS pharyngitis (5). Antibiotic resistance is common in the bacteria found in the oropharynx, although extremely rare in GABHS. Most otolaryngologists use the broader-spectrum amoxicillin or amoxicillin/clavulanic acid as their first-line antibiotic of choice despite this knowledge (6). Second-line antibiotics include erythromycin, clindamycin, cephalexin, azithromycin, and clarithromycin. Cephalosporin may be slightly more effective at eliminating pharyngeal carrier states. Tonsillectomy is recommended for recurrent tonsillitis, and several surgical criteria have been suggested to limit unnecessary morbidity. The Paradise criteria advocate tonsillectomy following seven infections in one year, five infections/year for two years, or three infections/year for three years, and it is the most clinically recognized standard of care.

Treatment is directed at avoiding the long-term sequelae of GABHS in conjunction with alleviating acute localized symptoms. Peritonsillar abscess, scarlet fever, poststreptococcal glomerulonephritis, and acute rheumatic fever (carditis, polyarthritis, subcutaneous nodules, erythema marginatum, and chorea) are the most significant complications of GABHS. These conditions arise when antibodies directed against GABHS surface antigens cross-react with host tissues, resulting in localized tissue damage. Steroids and immunomodulators may be helpful in suppressing these conditions, but treatment is often supportive, because no curative measure exists. The routine use of antibacterials in acute pharyngitis is thought to have greatly decreased the incidence of these GABHS-related complications.

Other Streptococcus Species. *Streptococcus pneumoniae* as well as Streptococci group C and G are other common pathogens in the pharynx. Streptococci groups B, D, E, and F are less common but maintain a minor role in the etiology of bacterial pharyngitis. Symptoms of pharyngitis resulting from these organisms are similar to GABHS. Treatment strategies parallel those identified for GABHS. Acute poststreptococcal glomerulonephritis may arise in these patients similar to those with GABHS pharyngitis, but rheumatic fever has not been documented.

Arcanobacterium haemolyticum. *A. haemolyticum* causes approximately 1% to 5% of all cases of bacterial pharyngitis. It is an anaerobic Gram-positive rod transmitted by direct contact or respiratory droplets and is most commonly isolated from young adults. Pathogenesis of this organism results from the secretion of exotoxins such as phospholipase D and hemolysin. Signs and symptoms are similar to other infectious etiologies, with two unique features: A patchy, whitish-gray exudate is present on the pharyngeal mucosa and an erythematous, maculopapular skin rash similar to that of scarlet fever may be present. The rash usually begins on the extremities and spreads to the trunk sparing the face, palms, and soles. It typically lasts at least 48 hours and resolves spontaneously. Diagnosis is made by throat swab and culture. A negative rapid strep test in a young adult with a skin rash should raise suspicion. Resistance to antibiotics is increasing for this organism and current recommendations for first-line therapy include erythromycin, amoxicillin, and amoxicillin/clavulanic acid in place of penicillin. Second-line options include clindamycin, vancomycin, cephalexin, and gentamicin.

Corynebacterium diphtheriae. *C. diphtheriae* is a Gram-positive bacillus and is the infectious etiology of diphtheria. Three strains of *C. diphtheriae* exist: gravis, intermedius, and mitis, listed in order of decreasing severity. The incidence of diphtheria has been greatly reduced by widespread vaccination programs, and it is seldom encountered clinically in modern medicine.

Its pathogenicity has two distinct phenomena. Initially, colonization and proliferation of the bacterium in the oropharynx causes local tissue invasion. Subsequently, an exotoxin is released, which inhibits elongation factor-2 proteins in surrounding host cells, resulting in cell death. It is transmitted by direct mucosal contact or aerosolized particles. Symptoms of diphtheria include fever, lethargy, dysphagia, and odynophagia. The classic physical exam finding is a grayish exudate, or pseudomembrane, extending from the oropharynx to the larynx. When the exudate is removed, a bleeding submucosa is revealed. Cervical adenopathy is usually present and may cause a "bull neck" presentation. Airway obstruction may occur in severe cases. Diagnosis is made by throat swabs and culture. Coinfection with GABHS is common, and patients should be treated for both.

Treatment of suspected diphtheria should begin empirically, because delays may result in unnecessary comorbidities. A secure airway is the number one priority and elective intubation may be required. Administration of diphtheria antitoxin should be performed once an adequate airway is secured. The role of antibiotics in acute infection is debatable; they may serve solely to reduce the incidence of a carrier state. Antibiotics of choice include erythromycin and clindamycin. Alternatively, penicillin G, tetracycline, rifampin, and clindamycin may be used. The diphtheria vaccine has greatly decreased the incidence of this disease in developed countries. The vaccine is most commonly given as a triad, combining diphtheroid toxin, tetanus toxin, and pertussis, and it is ideally given in the first year of life. A booster is recommended every 10 years. Complications of diphtheria include myocarditis, motor neuritis, and acute renal failure.

Diphtheria is discussed in greater detail in Chapter 11.

Bordetella pertussis. *B. pertussis* is a Gram-negative coccobacillus that causes whooping cough. Whooping cough derives its name from the loud inspiratory sound made by infected persons. It is transmitted by direct mucosal contact or aerosolized particles. Clinically, it is divided into three stages. The catarrhal stage (7–14 days) symptoms are similar to any upper respiratory infection. The paroxysmal stage (two to four weeks) follows and is associated with the hallmark cough that is pathognomonic for this disease. The convalescent stage (one to two weeks) results in slow improvement of symptoms. *B. pertussis* produces an endotoxin as well as agglutinogens that necrose the oropharyngeal epithelium, resulting in mucosal slough and exudate formation. Treatment is supportive; antibiotics have limited use in treating this organism. Immunization has been effective in nearly eliminating this disease in developed countries, but it is still prevalent in lower socioeconomic classes and underdeveloped nations.

Neisseria gonorrhea. *N. gonorrhea* is a Gram-negative diplococci bacterium. Symptoms associated with pharyngeal infection include sore throat, fever, dysphagia, and odynophagia. A sexual history suggestive of orogenital contact should lead a clinician to further investigation. This organism most typically causes a whitish-yellow exudate to form over the tonsils and usually spares the pharyngeal walls. Diagnosis is made by pharyngeal swab and Gram stain revealing Gram-negative, bean-shaped diplococci. Cultures are used to confirm suggestive smears. Treatment of *N. gonorrhea* consists of single-dose ceftriaxone with or without oral doxycycline. Concomitant treatment for *Chlamydia trachomatis* should be administered, because cultures are not as sensitive for this organism and coinfections are common (40–50%). Azithromycin is the first-line treatment for *C. trachomatis*. Doxycycline, ofloxacin, or erythromycin may be used alternatively.

Please see Chapter 11 for a more detailed discussion of gonorrhea.

Treponema pallidum.   *T. pallidum* is the bacterial spirochete that causes syphilis. It is transmitted to the oropharynx by direct contact with mucosal surfaces, usually through orogenital sexual contact. Although presentation of acute syphilitic pharyngitis is rare, chronic pharyngitis in the presence of a suggestive sexual history should raise suspicion. Acute syphilitic pharyngitis is painless, and infected persons may progress to manifest symptoms of fever, sore throat, malaise, cervical adenopathy, and headache. Red maculopapular patches on the pharyngeal wall may be present and tonsil hypertrophy is common. A similar rash is seen on the palms and soles during secondary syphilis. Darkfield microscopy can be used to detect Treponema species and a Warthin–Starry stain can differentiate Treponema species. Rapid plasma reagin (RPR) is the most common serological screening test for syphilis. If the RPR is positive, fluorescent treponemal antibody absorption (FTA-ABS) or microhemagglutination assays for antibodies to *T. pallidum* (MHA-TP) should be performed for confirmation. Treatment consists of benzathine penicillin, tetracycline, or doxycycline.

Syphilis is discussed in greater detail in Chapter 15.

Fusobacterium necrophorum.   *F. necrophorum* is an anaerobic Gram-negative bacillus. It is a small component of the normal oral flora. *F. necrophorum* is the etiological agent of Lemierre Syndrome (LS). LS is a rare complication of acute *F. necrophorum* pharyngitis and is characterized by thrombophlebitis of the internal jugular vein and the associated propagation of multiple septic emboli. Symptoms include fever, lymphadenopathy, neck pain, dysphagia, and swelling, which may persist after initial pharyngeal symptoms resolve. Diagnosis is made clinically and confirmed with a computed tomography (CT) scan with contrast showing thrombosis of the internal jugular vein. Septic emboli may involve the lungs, kidneys, spleen, visceral organs, or extremities, necessitating a full body CT scan with contrast for adequate assessment. Intravenous antibiotics are the treatment of choice. Historically, ligation of the internal jugular vein was advocated, but no clinical data supports this practice and it is rarely performed today. The use of anticoagulation is controversial. No controlled studies have identified supportive evidence for the use of heparin or other anticoagulation but several case reports and small studies have shown a benefit.

Mycobacterium.   *Mycobacterium* is a Gram-negative acid-fast staining bacillus. Several species of this bacterium exist. The most familiar pathogen is *Mycobacterium tuberculosis*. Other species include *Mycobacterium avium, Mycobacterium intracellulare, Mycobacterium kansasii*, and *Mycobacterium scrofulaceum*. Mycobacterium species commonly infect the lungs, but pharyngeal involvement secondary to pulmonary expectorant exposure is possible. Clinically, the tonsils and pharynx may appear erythematous and mucosal surfaces may be ulcerated.

Cervical adenopathy may also be present, especially in cases where *M. scrofulaceum* is the infecting organism. Scrofula is an old-fashioned term used to describe neck manifestations of tuberculosis (TB). Laryngeal involvement may also be present. Diagnosis is made by performing acid-fast smears of sputum or tissues suspected of involvement. Cultures are often difficult to obtain and may take weeks to grow. Treatment of TB should be tailored to accommodate the specific antibiotic resistance profile. Isoniazid and rifampin used in combination is the first-line treatment option. Many physicians advocate triple therapy and may add ethambutol, streptomycin, or pyrazinamide. Treatment should be continued for 9 to 12 months and patients should be followed up with yearly chest X rays to monitor disease progression. A vaccine, Bacille Calmette–Guerin (BCG), is offered in many European countries but is not available in the United States. Its clinical usefulness is debatable since vaccinated persons can no longer use PPD skin testing to monitor for new or active TB infection. Mycobacterial diseases are discussed in more detail in Chapter 12.

Other Bacteria.   Many other species of bacteria play a minor role in the incidence of infectious pharyngitis. Some additional pathogens include *Yersinia enterocolitica, Mycoplasma pneumoniae, Francisella tularensis*, and *Chlamydia pneumoniae*. These entities are rare, self-limiting, and typically responsive to broad-spectrum antibiotics.

Infection—Viral

Adenovirus.   Adenovirus is the most common cause of viral pharyngitis. It is a double-stranded DNA virus. Serotypes 3, 4, and 7 are frequently associated with viral pharyngitis. It is transmitted by either respiratory droplets or direct contact. School-aged children are most commonly affected. The classic presentation includes fever, sore throat, coryza, and red eyes. Adenovirus is cytolytic to the epithelial cells it invades and induces a localized inflammatory response in the surrounding tissues. Nasopharyngeal swabs can be obtained for viral cultures and a negative monospot test should be confirmed. It is usually self-limiting and lasts five to seven days. Treatment is supportive. Severe morbidity and mortality are rare and only seen in patients with altered immune function. Complications of adenovirus infection include keratoconjunctivitis (pink eye), acute hemorrhagic cystitis/nephritis, and gastroenteritis. Ribavirin has been advocated in several case reports when systemic infection occurs.

Upper Respiratory Viruses.   Pharyngitis is a frequent component of the common cold. It may be caused by several upper respiratory viruses. Rhinovirus is the most common pathogen. Others viruses include parainfluenza virus, influenza virus, and coronavirus. The common cold will occur in any age group but extremes of age, immunosuppressed, and immunocompromised persons are most susceptible. The average healthy adult experiences cold-like symptoms at least twice a year. Transmission of viral particles occurs by inhaling respiratory particles or from direct contact. Signs and symptoms of viral pharyngitis are similar to those of bacterial pharyngitis. The incidence of laryngeal involvement is more common with viral infection when compared with bacterial infection and may help distinguish between the two etiologies. Other upper respiratory complaints include rhinorrhea, postnasal drip, nasal congestion, hoarseness, and cough. When associated with the influenza virus, gastrointestinal (GI) complaints such as stomach cramping and diarrhea are common.

Specific identification of the offending viral pathogen is not necessary, because symptoms are usually self-limiting and last approximately one week. There is no cure for the common cold or the flu, so treatment is targeted at symptom palliation. Some studies have demonstrated that zinc and vitamin C may decrease the length of viral-associated symptoms. Amantadine may decrease the duration of symptoms resulting from influenza virus infection when taken early in the prodromal stage.

Epstein-Barr Virus.   Epstein–Barr virus (EBV) is the causative agent of infectious mononucleosis. EBV is a double-stranded DNA virus in the herpesvirus family. It is transmitted by direct contact or by aerosolized viral particles. The virus infects B lymphocytes, and symptom manifestation consists of the triad of fever, lymphadenopathy, and pharyngitis. A white exudate on the tonsils is characteristic of EBV infection, and a skin rash may occur in patients treated with antibiotics, especially amoxicillin. Other symptoms include hepatosplenomegaly, hepatomegaly, encephalitis, pericarditis, and autoimmune hemolytic anemia. In rare cases, patients may present to an otolaryngologist with airway obstruction or cranial nerve palsies.

Diagnosis is made by the presence of heterophil antibodies detected on a monospot test. IgM antibodies to EBV viral capsid antigens can be screened if monospot tests are negative. Treatment for EPV is supportive, and symptoms may last for weeks to months. Splenomegaly is present in approximately 50% of infected patients and hepatomegaly is present in an additional 10% to 20%. Infected persons should be counseled to avoid contact sports for two to four months because of the risk of solid organ injury or rupture. In severe cases of mononucleosis, glucocorticoids may be used to diminish tonsillar hypertrophy and lymphadenopathy that may compromise the airway.

EBV is discussed in further detail in Chapter 10.

Cytomegalovirus.   Cytomegalovirus (CMV) is a double-stranded DNA virus in the herpesvirus family. CMV presents similarly to EBV and patients are commonly misdiagnosed with mononucleosis when acutely infected. CMV is transmitted by direct contact of mucosal surfaces, blood transfusion or organ transplant, maternal breast milk consumption, and rarely by aerosolized viral particles. Symptoms predominantly include fever, lymphadenopathy, and less commonly pharyngitis. Ulceration of the pharynx or esophagus may be present in severe cases, especially in immunocompromised patients with human immunodeficiency virus (HIV). CMV infection during pregnancy may result in fetal hearing loss, visual impairment, and diminished mental and/or motor capabilities.

Diagnosis is made by a rise in CMV antibody titers and a negative monospot test. Enzyme-linked immunosorbent assay (ELISA) antibody tests for CMV IgM antibodies are also available. Treatment is typically supportive because most cases are self-limiting. Ganciclovir has excellent activity against CMV and may be required in cases of severe infections, debilitated patients, and immunosuppressed or immunocompromised persons. Acyclovir, valacyclovir, famciclovir, cidofovir, and foscarnet may also be used.

Coxsackie Virus.   Coxsackie viruses are members of the enterovirus genus and are further divided into coxsackie A viruses and coxsackie B viruses. Coxsackie A viruses are important pathogens in the head and neck because they cause herpangina and hand-foot-and-mouth disease. There are 24 serotypes of coxsackie A viruses. Coxsackie viruses are spread by direct contact or fecal oral contamination. Diagnosis is made clinically although serological tests are available. ELISA IgM assays, cell cultures, and polymerase chain reaction (PCR) tests are all available.

Herpangina is caused by coxsackie A serotypes 2, 3, 4, 5, 6, 8, and 10. It is characterized by the presence of gray-white papulovesicles found on the structures of the oropharynx. These papulovesicles are surrounded by erythematous halos and progress to become ulcerative lesions. Lesions are usually present for five to seven days and resolve spontaneously. Hand-foot-and-mouth disease is most frequently caused by serotype 16. Patients present with ulcerated vesicles surrounded by erythematous halos. Oral lesions are usually the first to appear and are most commonly found on the tongue, palatal, buccal, and gingival mucosa. The oropharynx is rarely affected. Skin lesions appear one to two days after the oral lesions are present. They form as a maculopapular lesion surrounded by a red halo and are more common on the hands than the feet. Lesions usually resolve spontaneously in 5 to 10 days.

Oral lesions are often painful and may require symptomatic relief. Viscous lidocaine mouth rinses or mouthwashes containing combinations of bismuth, benadryl, carafate, or steroids may palliate localized symptoms. Acyclovir may reduce the duration of symptoms when prescribed during initial presentation.

Herpes Simplex Virus.   Herpes simplex virus (HSV) is a DNA virus with two distinct subtypes: HSV-1 and HSV-2. Classically, HSV-1 occurs more frequently in the head and neck regions and HSV-2 occurs more commonly in the genitourinary regions, but either virus may be detected in either location. The virus is transmitted by direct contact with infected mucus or saliva. Gingivostomatitis and pharyngitis are the most common head and neck symptoms of acute infection and may be accompanied by nonspecific complaints of fever, malaise, myalgia, and lymphadenopathy. Vesicular lesions on an erythematous base are the classic finding on physical exam. These most frequently are present at the vermillion borders and may be triggered by ultraviolet light exposure, hormonal changes, or stress. These lesions are often termed "cold sores." Lesions are less commonly present on the buccal mucosa, tonsils, and pharyngeal walls. The acute infection lasts 7 to 10 days and both lesions and symptoms resolve spontaneously. The virus is then thought to lie dormant in the dorsal root ganglion, and periodic reactivation of the virus results in recurrent infections.

Historically, diagnosis can be made by taking a vesicular scraping and performing a Tzanck smear, which is accurate in approximately 60% to 75% of infected patients. Viral cultures can also be grown and take approximately 48 hours for adequate inoculation and incubation. More recently, PCR techniques have replaced older techniques for rapid detection and viral subtyping. Antivirals such as acyclovir, valacyclovir, and famciclovir are used for treatment of herpes outbreaks. These drugs are most commonly taken orally, but a topical option is available for orolabial lesions and may decrease viral shedding. These medications are effective at limiting duration of symptoms but do not cure patients of the virus. These same medicines, used in a preventative fashion, prolong symptom-free disease recurrence in approximately 50% of infected patients.

Please refer to Chapter 10 for a more detailed discussion of herpes simplex.

Measles. Measles is single-stranded RNA virus in the paramyxovirus family. The incidence of this disease has been greatly reduced by the institution of vaccination programs in most developed countries. Rare cases of vaccine failure can occur and not all persons accept immunization recommendations. This disease is transmitted by direct contact of aerosolized particles. Symptoms usually begin one to two weeks after exposure and consist of cough, coryza, conjunctivitis, pharyngitis, lymphadenopathy, and fever. Mucosal lesions consisting of gray-white spots surrounded by an erythematous base are the hallmark physical exam finding and are referred to as Koplik's spots. Shortly after these initial presenting symptoms develop, a maculopapular rash begins on the head and neck and progresses toward the extremities. Diagnosis is clinical in most cases. The virus can be cultured if needed, and serological tests are available. Treatment is supportive and symptoms are self-limiting, lasting around two weeks. Bacterial superinfections should be treated accordingly. Vaccination for disease prevention is currently recommended and commonly given as a triad with mumps and rubella.

Human Immunodeficiency Virus. HIV is a retrovirus that infects CD4+ lymphocytes and monocytes. It is transmitted by sexual contact, blood transfusions, needle-stick injuries, maternal/fetal transmission across the placenta, and maternal breast milk consumption. Acute prodromes of HIV infection include fever, malaise, cervical lymphadenopathy, and pharyngitis. Initial presentation is often confused with infectious mononucleosis and diagnosis is often delayed. These symptoms are usually self-limiting and resolve in approximately 7 to 10 days. Opportunistic infections with diseases such as HSV, CMV, and candida are the hallmark of this infection as CD4+ counts plummet.

There are several tests available for HIV. The most commonly used are ELISA and immunoblotting (Western blots). PCR techniques and viral cultures are also used and may be more sensitive than traditional ELISA and Western blot assays. Newer tests utilize buccal mucosal swabs in place of serum. Treatment of HIV itself consists of multiple antiviral regimens combined in a "cocktail" protocol. Treatment of coinciding opportunistic infections is performed as indicated, and preventative medications are often used when CD4+ counts are decreased. Symptomatic relief with topical anesthetics or special mouthwashes containing combinations of steroids, carafate, benadryl, and Maalox may be beneficial when symptoms of pharyngitis persist.

HIV is discussed in detail in Chapter 16.

Infection—Fungal

Candidiasis. *Candida albicans* is a common organism found in the oral cavity flora that causes candidiasis in certain clinical situations. Candida has a capsule and forms true hyphae and pseudohyphae. It adheres to mucosal surfaces and is capable of superficial mucosal invasion. Factors that contribute to oral candida proliferation include uncontrolled diabetes mellitus, antibiotic therapy, and any condition that causes immunosuppression. Clinical features of candidiasis include white, cheesy plaques that can be wiped off with a tongue blade. The tongue and buccal mucosa are frequently infected, but tonsillar and pharyngeal lesions are not uncommon and may extend to the esophagus and larynx. Superficial infections are often painless and self-limiting. Deep infections can cause ulcerative lesions that are painful. Diagnosis is made by epithelial scrapings and KOH preparations demonstrating budding yeast and hyphae under light microscopy. Cultures may be obtained if needed. Treatment of oral candidiasis often begins with correction of underlying causes, such as stopping or changing antibiotics or better blood sugar control when possible. Nystatin suspension rinses and clotrimazole troches are often the first line of therapy for superficial infections. More severe infection should also be treated with oral fluconazole and may require several weeks of therapy for complete resolution.

Other Mycoses.   Infection of the tonsils and pharynx with other fungal elements is rare but may occur. Aspergillosis, Histoplasmosis, and Cryptococcus are the most common of these rare infections. Symptoms are similar to those seen with candidiasis. Diagnosis is made by cultures, and treatments are directed at the offending organism. Aggressive oral antimycotics are commonly employed.

Inflammatory/Autoimmune

Pemphigus.   Pemphigus is a rare disease that affects mucosal membranes. Although the term pemphigus may be erroneously used interchangeably with the condition bullous pemphigoid, it is a separate entity warranting a separate discussion. Pemphigus is characterized by vesicular lesions and bulla. There are multiple subtypes, with pemphigus vulgaris and pemphigus foliaceus being the most common (7). Other subtypes include pemphigus vegetans, pemphigus erythematosus, pemphigus herpetiformis, paraneoplastic pemphigus, drug-induced pemphigus, and IgA pemphigus. Although it is a disease of all ages, it typically occurs between the ages of 30 and 60. Pemphigus affects males and females equally. There is no known ethnic predilection. Its pathogenesis stems from an autoimmune mechanism in which circulating antibodies target keratinocyte cell surfaces. Cell-to-cell adhesion is disrupted and antibody complexes activate the complement cascade, creating local tissue damage. The cause of this autoimmune antibody formation is unknown, but it may be related to genetic factors or other autoimmune disorders.

Clinically, intermittent vesicles or bullae are produced that erupt, creating ulcerative lesions followed by complete resolution and remission. Nikolsky's sign is performed by the clinician rubbing unaffected areas of skin to precipitate skin sloughing. This test can be used to differentiate pemphigus from bullous pemphigoid and other blistering skin disorders. Diagnosis is made by direct immunofluorescence (DIF) microscopy of biopsies taken from affected areas or indirect immunofluorescence (IDIF) staining of a patient's serum. Histopathological specimens demonstrate intradermal blistering in which basal layer cells are separated from one another. Immunoblotting, immunoprecipitation, and ELISA are newer tests performed to detect PD.

Treatments are targeted to reduce autoantibody production and decrease local inflammatory response. Azathioprine combined with prednisone is the most commonly used regimen, although other immunomodulating drugs have been described with some success. Antibiotics may be necessary if secondary bacterial infections are suspected in the pharynx.

Bullous Pemphigoid. Bullous pemphigoid (BP) is an autoimmune disorder consisting of cutaneous vesiculobullous lesions that appear in areas of a previous rash. Oral mucosal lesions are rare sequelae. In contrast to pemphigus, BP rarely affects persons under age 60. No racial or gender predilection has been identified. Mucosal membranes are involved in approximately 50% to 60% of cases and the oropharynx is the most common location of mucosal involvement. Diagnostic testing is similar to that for pemphigus: tissue biopsies of lesions are used for DIF staining or serum is screened for autoimmune antibodies with IDIF staining. Immunoprecipitation, immunoblotting, and ELISA are also available. Histologically, a subepidermal blister is seen. The basement membrane is thickened but remains attached to underlying connective tissues. This is the distinguishing characteristic between bullous pemphigoid and pemphigus. Treatment consists of corticosteroids when necessary; however, outbreaks are usually self-limiting and often resolve spontaneously in the absence of intervention.

Other "Blistering" Diseases. Cicatricial pemphigoid (CP), Stevens–Johnson syndrome (SJS), and epidermolysis bullosa (EB) are rare causes of pharyngitis that deserve mentioning. CP is a rare, chronic blistering disease that involves the oral mucosa in nearly all patients; lesions may extend to the oropharynx in a significant number of persons. Blisters, ulcers, erosions, and scarring are demonstrated clinically. Diagnosis is made by tissue biopsy and immunostaining microscopy. Steroids and other immunosuppressants are used for supportive treatment.

SJS is an immune-complex–mediated hypersensitivity thought to arise from drug exposure, infection, or malignancy. Drugs associated with SJS include penicillin, sulfas, phenytoin, carbamazepine, and barbiturates. Infectious etiologies include viruses, bacteria, fungi, and protozoa. Erythematous vesicular skin lesions progress to bulla. Mucosal lesions in the oral cavity and pharynx are also common. Biopsy is used for histological identification. Treatment involves identifying, and when possible, eliminating the offending etiology. Skin and mucosal lesions generally resolve but SJS is fatal in 10% to 15% of patients. Please see Chapter 22 for a detailed discussion of SJS.

EB is a rare disorder characterized by skin and mucosal blister formation in response to mechanical trauma. The majority of cases are genetically inherited, although spontaneous cases are possible. Several forms of EB have been described, including EB simplex, EB junctional, and EB dystrophic, in order of decreasing incidence. The pathophysiology of this disease results from IgG autoantibodies targeting anchoring fibrils of collagen in the base membrane of the skin and mucosal surfaces. Shearing forces result in the rupture of bulla, leaving raw, painful submucosal exposure resulting in scar formation. Diagnosis is made by tissue biopsy. Preventative strategies are best; otherwise, treatment is supportive.

Wegener's Granulomatosis. Wegener's granulomatosis (WG) is an autoimmune disease characterized by granulomatous vasculitis in the respiratory tract and the kidneys. The vasculitis most commonly affects small arteries and veins, where it forms granulomas. Patients typically present to an otolaryngologist with sinus complaints such as drainage, pressure, and congestion. Mucosal ulceration may occur on the nasal septum and warrants a biopsy if WG is suspected. Primary involvement of the tonsils or pharynx is rare, but these areas may be inflamed secondary to post nasal drainage. The epidemiology, pathogenesis, diagnosis, treatment, and prognosis are discussed in more detail in Chapter 8.

Sarcoidosis. Sarcoidosis is an autoimmune disorder of unknown etiology. It affects multiple organ systems and is characterized by an accumulation of T-lymphocytes and mononuclear phagocytes causing noncaseating epithelioid granulomas. Its appearance in the oropharynx mimics that of infectious adenotonsillitis. Sarcoid frequently involves the epiglottis when head and neck manifestations are present. Tonsillar involvement is rare but has been described in case reports and results in tonsillar hypertrophy and erythema. The epidemiology, pathogenesis, diagnosis, treatment, and prognosis are discussed in more detail in Chapter 6.

Crohn's Disease.   Crohn's disease is an inflammatory disease of the GI tract, of unknown etiology. It is characterized by mucosal ulceration that extends through all layers of the digestive tract wall and is not limited to any one area of the GI system from mouth to anus. Approximately 10% of patients with Crohn's disease have pharyngeal involvement. Most commonly, ulcerative lesions are seen on the pharyngeal walls. The epidemiology, pathogenesis, diagnosis, treatment, and prognosis are discussed in more detail in Chapter 20.

Behçet's Disease.   Behçet's disease (BD) is a rare disorder of unknown etiology that affects mucocutaneous tissues, the eyes, and the genitourinary system. The classic triad of oral aphthous ulcers, uveitis, and genital ulcers is pathognomonic for BD. It may progress to involve the GI, pulmonary, renal, and central nervous systems, as well. Symptoms include malaise, fever, anorexia, and weight loss. Sore throat, dysphagia, and odynophagia are often present at acute presentation. BD is commonly misdiagnosed as pharyngitis or tonsillitis at initial presentation, resulting in a delay in appropriate treatment. Please refer to Chapter 3 for discussion of the epidemiology, pathogenesis, diagnosis, treatment, and prognosis of BD.

Extraesophageal Reflux Disease.   The presence of refluxed gastric contents represents a noxious stimulant to the pharyngeal mucosa and is a frequent cause of pharyngitis. Approximately 4% to 10% of patients seen by an otolaryngologist will have extraesophageal reflux disease (EERD) (8). Symptoms include globus sensation, cough, hoarseness, dysphagia, throat clearing, and persistent sore throat. The pathophysiology of EERD may be a result of direct acid-peptic exposure to the pharynx, mediated by vagal reflux, stimulating constant throat clearing and cough, or alternatively related to cricopharyngeal dysfunction (9).

On physical exam, the mucosa is often erythematous and edematous. Posterior pharyngeal wall cobblestoning and lingual tonsillar hypertrophy are often present in pediatric patients. Edema and erythema of the posterior glottis are the most common physical exam findings and may extend to the arytenoids, aryepiglottic folds, or postcricoid area. Pseudosulcus of the true vocal cords is highly indicative of EERD. Twenty-four-hour pH dual probe esophageal monitoring is the gold standard test in the diagnosis of EERD; however, the diagnosis is often made clinically with treatment started empirically.

Treatment consists of lifestyle and diet modification, weight loss, and pharmacotherapy. Proton pump inhibitors (PPIs) are the drug of choice. Mild cases may be treated with once-a-day medications taken one hour prior to the largest meal of the day, but b.i.d. therapy is often required. Patients treated empirically with good results may consider undergoing a trial of treatment cessation to confirm the continued presence of EERD, and pharmacotherapy should be restarted if symptoms return. H2 blockers (cimetidine, famotidine, and ranitidine) are less effective but may provide benefit in some patients. Patients whose symptoms persist after adequate therapeutic trials of PPIs, with ongoing EERD proven by a pH probe study, should be referred for consideration of a fundoplication procedure. The prognosis for symptom improvement is excellent, although globus sensation symptoms may persist for months after treatment implementation. Laryngopharyngeal reflux is a distinct entity from EERD and is more likely to respond to twice-a-day PPI therapy.

Radiation.   Radiation therapy, with or without chemotherapy, has become the primary treatment for oropharyngeal cancer. Primary treatment of head and neck neoplasms with radiation most commonly ranges from 60 to 70 Gy. Radiation exposure greater than 5 Gy may induce some degree of acute and/or chronic pharyngitis in nearly all patients (10). Furthermore, it affects the function of the major and minor salivary glands, reducing salivary outflow and increasing salivary viscosity.

Dysphagia and odynophagia are common symptoms, with swelling and airway obstruction occurring less frequently. Dehydration, malnutrition, and weight loss are common in severely affected patients without a secondary means of alimentation. Treatment is symptomatic. Appropriate hydration, in addition to the use of salivary substitutes and sucralfate, is recommended acutely. Salivary flow may be increased chronically with cholinergic drugs such as pilocarpine. Mouthwashes containing combinations of carafate, aluminum hydroxide, diphenhydramine, and nystatin can be useful for symptomatic relief. Superinfections with bacteria or fungi such as candida are common and should be managed accordingly. Oral or systemic glucocorticords may provide short-term relief of symptoms in severe manifestations of radiation pharyngitis.

The prognosis for symptom resolution is guarded at best, although improvement of symptoms up to one year following treatment is common. Predicting those who will experience severe symptoms from those with milder manifestations is not possible. The term "radiation recall" has been used to describe the return of symptoms in post-radiation-therapy patients who are undergoing chemotherapy. Its etiology is unknown and its treatment is similar to that of acute radiation therapy.

Periodic Fever, Aphthous Stomatitis, Pharyngitis, and Cervical Adenitis. The symptom complex of periodic fever, aphthous stomatitis, pharyngitis, and cervical adenitis (PFAPA) is a rare but well-described cause of recurrent pharyngitis and adenotonsillitis. Intermittent high-grade fevers up to 40°C are common; these last for three to five days and recur every 26 to 30 days. It affects young children in their first decade of life, without ethnic predilection. Its etiology is not yet understood and the diagnosis is made clinically. Most patients will have a rise in IgD titers at the time of presentation. Treatment is symptomatic. Glucocorticoids are used to control intermittent fevers, aphthous ulcers, and lymphadenopathy at the onset of presentation. Tonsillectomy has been therapeutic in a small number of patients. Cimetidine, acetaminophen, ibuprofen, antibiotics, aspirin, acyclovir, and colchicines have all been used with variable success in a small number of patients (11). The disease is self-limiting and the prognosis is excellent.

Neoplasm

Although neoplasms are not a cause of acute or chronic pharyngitis, tumors arising in the oropharynx often present with signs and symptoms that most commonly indicate an infectious etiology. Patients treated for infectious pharyngitis, who do not improve, warrant further investigation to identify a possible neoplasm. Common presenting symptoms of oropharyngeal cancer include unilateral sore throat, dysphagia, odynophagia, weight loss, and otalgia. On physical exam, an asymmetric pharyngeal mass is the hallmark clinical finding and warrants further investigation (Fig. 4). The mass may be ulcerative, fungating, or mucosal covered and detectable only by palpation. Cervical adenopathy is present with advanced disease that has metastasized to the locoregional lymph nodes. Risk factors for oropharyngeal cancer include tobacco and alcohol abuse. The human papilloma virus has a role in a subset of oropharyngeal tumors.

The majority of oropharyngeal cancers are epithelial in origin. Squamous cell cancer is the most common tumor. Adenocarcinoma and verrucous carcinoma may also arise in the oropharynx. Hematological neoplasms such as lymphoma are also found in the oropharynx and are discussed in more detail in Chapter 17. Rarely, minor salivary glands can give rise to carcinomas such as mucoepidermoid and adenoid cystic carcinoma arising in the pharynx. Tissue biopsy is necessary for pathological diagnosis and is supplemented with imaging studies (CT scans, magnetic resonance imaging, and/or positron emission

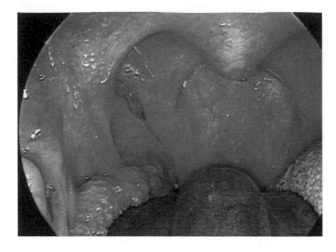

FIGURE 4 Tonsillar neoplasm—a squamous cell cancer lesion is seen in the right tonsillar fossa.

tomography) for metastatic evaluation. Treatment is dependent upon proper tumor identification. Radiation, chemotherapy, and surgery may be used individually or in combination, depending on the type of tumor and extent of disease.

SUMMARY

Pharyngitis and adenotonsillitis may be the initial manifestation of many focal and systemic diseases. Although the vast majority of these patients have an acute infectious process, other systemic diseases need to be ruled out. Delay in diagnosis may result in unnecessary morbidity and mortality.

REFERENCES

1. Thompson LDR, Wenig BM, Kornblut AD. Pharyngitis. In: Bailey BJ, Calhoun KH, Derkay CS, et al., eds. Head and Neck Surgery-Otolaryngology. Vol. 1. 3rd ed. Philadelphia, PA: Lippincott-Raven, 2001:543–554.
2. Cummings CW, Flint PW, Haughey BH, et al. Anatomy. In: Cummings CW, Flint PW, Haughey BH, et al., eds. Otolaryngology-Head and Neck Surgery. 4th ed. Philadelphia, PA: Mosby, Inc., 2005:4135–4165.
3. Bisno AL. Acute pharyngitis. N Engl J Med 2001; 344(3):205–211.
4. Huovinen P. Causes, diagnosis and treatment of pharyngitis. Compr Ther 1990; 16(10):59–65.
5. Gilbert DN, Moellering RC, Eliopoulos GM, et al. The Sanford Guide to Antimicrobial Therapy 2005. 35th ed. Hyde Park, VT: Antimicrobial Therapy. Inc., 2005.
6. Fairbanks DNF. Pocket Guide to Antimicrobial Therapy in Otolaryngology - Head and Neck Surgery. 12th ed. Alexandria, VA: American Academy of Otolaryngology- Head and Neck Surgery Foundation, Inc., 2005.
7. Kirtschig G, Wojnarowska F. Autoimmune blistering diseases: an up-date of diagnostic methods and investigations. Clin Exp Dermatol 1994; 19(2):97–112.
8. Wong RK, Hanson DG, Waring PJ, et al. ENT manifestations of gastroesophageal reflux. Am J Gastroenterol 2000; 95(8 suppl):S15–S22.
9. Rival R, Wong R, Mendelsohn M, et al. Role of gastroesophageal reflux disease in patients with cervical symptoms. Otolaryngol Head Neck Surg 1995; 113(4):364–369.
10. Epstein JB, Schubert MM. Oropharyngeal mucositis in cancer therapy. Review of pathogenesis, diagnosis, and management. Oncology (Williston Park) 2003; 17(12):1767–1779.
11. Thomas KT, Feder HM Jr, Lawton AR, et al. Periodic fever syndrome in children. J Pediatr 1999; 135 (1):15–21.

34

Dysphagia

Apurva Thekdi
Department of Surgery, Division of Otolaryngology-Head and Neck Surgery, University of California, San Diego, California, U.S.A.

INTRODUCTION

The true incidence of dysphagia in the general population remains unknown to date. The incidence has been described in select patient populations, and its prevalence in the general population can be inferred to be significant. A review of nursing home residents demonstrated that 30% to 40% have clinical evidence of dysphagia. Another well-studied population is those suffering stroke. Studies have shown that 30% to 40% of stroke patients will demonstrate symptoms of severe dysphagia, and as many as 20% will die from aspiration pneumonia in the first year (1). Given the number of new cerebrovascular events yearly, this is a significant number.

A single swallow consists of a series of complex neuromuscular events that must occur in a coordinated fashion. This complexity lends itself to dysfunction. The central control processors for swallowing are located in the brainstem, adjacent to the areas controlling such basic functions as respiration, core body temperature, and blood pressure. They are located dorsally in the brainstem, within and adjacent to the nucleus of the tractus solitarius as well as in the ventral region near the nucleus ambiguous (2). They lie adjacent to both sensory and motor nuclei of the vagus nerve, underlying this nerve's importance in swallowing physiology. The swallow reflex does not function in isolation, however, as Sasaki and Suzuki described, alterations in these reflex activities by a host of physiologic changes, including hypercapnia, hypoxia, and sedation, can dramatically alter it.

Dysphagia can be broadly divided into two distinct entities, oropharyngeal dysphagia and esophageal dysphagia. These will be treated separately in this chapter.

OROPHARYNGEAL DYSPHAGIA

Cerebrovascular Disease

Cerebrovascular disease is the most common disorder causing neurogenic oral and oropharyngeal dysphagia (3). Swallowing disorders have been reported in 27% to 50% of patients suffering from CVAs (4). The incidence is not limited to severe strokes, because even patients with mild-to-moderate strokes have a poorer long-term outcome directly attributable to their swallowing disorder (5). Given the complex neurophysiology associated with swallowing, a wide range of stroke locations can result in dysphagia. The gamut of cerebrovascular events, from major occlusive events to multiple small-vessel ischemic areas due to diabetes and chronic hypertension, to almost imperceptible brainstem infarcts, can result in oropharyngeal dysphagia. The extent of resulting cerebral ischemia defines the clinical presentation of the disorder. It is obvious that large occlusive ischemic events will result in a more severe dysphagia due to insults at multiple areas controlling swallowing physiology. Patients with brainstem strokes usually present with the most difficult to rehabilitate swallowing disorders. The deficits related to the strokes can often be predicted based on the site of the lesion.

Cortical strokes usually result in significant oral dysphagia, as well. Left-sided hemispheric strokes tend to produce a greater degree of oral dysfunction than other sites. This type of deficit results in a greater risk of aspiration due to poor control of the food bolus in the mouth and early spill to the pharynx. Patients with a dominant hemisphere CVA also often exhibit drooling due to an apparent "swallow apraxia" (6). Right-sided hemispheric strokes tend to produce a dysphagia characterized by apparently normal oral propulsion with a delayed pharyngeal response, resulting in the presence of the bolus in the pharynx without laryngeal closure. The resultant dysphagia is usually silent, and therefore, more insidious. Of the previously listed brainstem strokes, the lateral medullary syndrome produces the most dramatic dysphagia.

Neuromuscular Disorders

Many neuromuscular diseases cause dysphagia; in fact, the presenting symptom is often dysphagia. This is not surprising, considering the complex neuromuscular coordination required to execute a normal swallow. Although stroke patients develop sudden dysphagia, patients with other degenerative and nondegenerative neuromuscular diseases have a more insidious onset of dysphagia. Motor neuron diseases causing bulbar palsy or pseudobulbar palsy usually develop a progressive dysphagia and dysarthria with little upper or lower extremity involvement. Patients with myopathies must be identified early, because they have potentially treatable disorders.

Amyotrophic lateral sclerosis (ALS) has an incidence of around two per 100,000 with a usual age of onset in the sixth decade, although earlier onset is not uncommon. The incidence in men is slightly greater than in women. The typical symptom profile on onset is that of progressive, painless weakness. The symptoms that prompt evaluation by a physician are usually slurred speech or dysphagia. At least three-fourths of ALS patients will develop significant dysphagia before requiring ventilatory support, and detailed questioning will usually reveal that all patients have some dysphagia (7). The diagnosis requires the presence of both lower and upper motor neuron signs and progression of the disorder. Electromyography is an invaluable tool in the diagnosis. Tongue fasciculations at rest are almost pathognomonic for ALS; however, a thorough neurologic workup must be performed to exclude other disorders or neoplasms.

The inflammatory myopathies include dermatomyositis, polymyositis, and inclusion body myositis. These three disorders are characterized by inflammation and degeneration of skeletal muscle tissue and are thought to be autoimmune-mediated disorders. Although related in etiology, each has a characteristic clinical presentation. Dermatomyositis affects both children and adults. It is characterized by a patchy, discolored rash on the face, neck, shoulders, upper chest, elbows, knees, knuckles, and back that precedes muscle weakness. The most common symptom is a severe proximal muscle weakness, producing difficulty standing up, climbing stairs, lifting objects, and raising the arms above shoulder level. Dysphagia occurs in approximately one-third of all patients. Polymyositis also has as its most common symptom a proximal muscle weakness, although there is also a variable degree of involvement of the distal musculature and no associated rash. Dysphagia is equally common in polymyositis as in dermatomyositis. The dysphagia is primarily a result of increased pharyngeal transit time (8). Treatment for both polymyositis and dermatomyositis is with immunosuppressives such as prednisone, azathioprine, methotrexate, and intravenous immunoglobulin. Inclusion myositis is very similar to polymyositis in that it is characterized by a slow and relentless progressive weakness. Symptoms usually begin after the age of 50 and are also associated with more atrophy and a greater involvement of distal musculature than in polymyositis. Current treatment for inclusion body myositis is supportive because it is unresponsive to immunosuppressive drugs. These conditions are discussed further in Chapter 1.

Duchenne muscular dystrophy (DMD) is the most common childhood form of muscular dystrophy. The typical age of onset is two to six years. The early signs of DMD include frequent falling, difficulty getting up, and a waddling gait. The disease first affects the pelvic muscles, upper arms, and upper legs. By the age of 12, virtually all patients suffer dysphagia; by the age of 18, severe dysphagia and aspiration are common. The dysphagia of DMD is characterized by pronounced oral and pharyngeal muscular weakness. Oculopharyngeal muscular dystrophy (OPMD) is characterized by a gradual onset of dysphagia, ptosis, and facial weakness. OPMD is an autosomal-dominant disorder with an age of onset in the fourth and fifth decade. Dysphagia is often the presenting symptom. Patients with OPMD have poor pharyngeal peristalses, poor upper esophageal sphincter (UES) relaxation, and low lower esophageal sphincter (LES) pressures. Cricopharyngeal myotomy or UES dilation may be effective in temporarily improving dysphagia in these patients; however, the long-term prognosis is unchanged after intervention (9). Spinal muscular atrophies (SMAs) comprise a group of neuromuscular disorders with varied clinical presentations, most of which occur early in childhood. Over one-third of patients with SMAs suffer from dysphagia.

Myasthenia gravis (MG) is characterized by the gradual progression of weakness over several weeks to months. The weakness tends to progress throughout the day and is worsened with physical exertion. MG is an autoimmune disorder in which antibodies to acetylcholine receptors bind to the receptors on the postsynaptic membrane of the neuromuscular junction, causing internalization and degradation of the receptors. Dysphagia is the presenting sign in 6% to 15% of adult patients (10). Bulbar and facial muscles are often affected and those patients with bulbar involvement typically have worse dysphagia and often aspirate. Treatment initially consists of medication with Mestinon (pyridostigmine), an acetylcholinesterase inhibitor, and possibly thymectomy. As disease progresses, some patients are offered plasmapheresis. Swallowing function varies as muscle function varies, so patients should be encouraged to eat early in the day and after medication.

Parkinson's disease is a progressive degenerative disorder caused by the degeneration of dopamine-containing neurons in the substantia nigra. The resulting disorder is characterized by rigidity and resting tremor. The rigidity is caused by simultaneous contraction of agonist and antagonist muscle groups that are usually coordinated to produce fine muscle movements. The resulting dysphagia is a result of poor bolus transport during the oral phase, early spill into the pharynx, and a prolonged pharyngeal transit time. The frequent pneumonias caused by aspiration are one of the most common causes of death in patients with Parkinson's disease (11). Other manometric abnormalities include poor UES relaxation, open LES, delayed transport, and tertiary contractions (12). Treatment with dopaminergic agents for Parkinson's disease can improve the dysphagia, but as the disease progresses, medication becomes less and less effective.

Progressive supranuclear palsy (PSP) is a progressive degenerative extrapyramidal disease that often mimics Parkinson's disease. The age of onset is typically one to two decades younger than in Parkinson's patients. Other differentiating characteristics include bilateral supranuclear ophthalmoplegia and lack of response to dopaminergic agents. PSP patients usually suffer from a worse dysphagia than Parkinson's patients do. Unfortunately, no treatment is effective at improving this.

Iatrogenic Causes of Dysphagia

Chemotherapy and radiation therapy are becoming mainstays in the treatment of head and neck cancer. The mucosa of the oropharyngeal swallowing tract is lined with cells with rapid turnover, providing a prime target for cytotoxic chemotherapeutic agents and radiation. Irradiation induces the mitotic death of the basal cells of the mucosa. With traditional radiotherapy, there is a two-week delay before the onset of symptoms. Once the radiotherapy is completed, there is complete reepithelization within two to three weeks, resulting in significant symptomatic improvement. Late complications of radiotherapy include destruction of salivary gland tissue and fibrosis of connective tissue, resulting in trismus, poor pharyngeal motility, and UES dysfunction. The chemotherapeutics implicated in oropharyngeal mucositis are the antimetabolites, in particular, 5-fluorouracil, methotrexate, and the purine antagonists. The maintenance of swallowing, especially in the setting of gastrostomy feeding, throughout treatment is imperative in order to prevent mucosal adhesions in the hypopharynx and proximal esophagus. Amifostine is an organic thiophosphate protecting normal tissues from free radicals produced by RT and/or chemotherapy. Prospective studies have demonstrated its cytoprotective effect in the oropharyngeal mucosa (13).

ESOPHAGEAL DYSPHAGIA

Systemic Sclerosis

Systemic sclerosis is a disorder of the small arteries, resulting in proliferation of fibrosis affecting the skin and multiple end organs. There are two subtypes of systemic sclerosis, diffuse and limited cutaneous. Diffuse cutaneous systemic sclerosis is characterized by rapid progression with skin involvement proximal to the elbows and knees. There is usually the early onset of Raynaud's phenomenon and early visceral involvement. Limited cutaneous systemic sclerosis is characterized by a stable course and involvement limited to the skin of the face and extremities distal to the elbows and knees. The CREST (calcinosis, Raynaud's, esophageal dysmotility, sclerodactyly, and telangiectasias) variant is a form of the limited cutaneous subset.

Esophageal symptoms occur in 50% to 80% of patients (14), making them the third most common symptoms after skin and Raynaud's phenomenon. Typical symptoms include heartburn in up to three-fourths of patients and dysphagia in up to one-half of patients. Esophageal involvement is not correlated with skin symptoms, age of onset, duration of symptoms, or presence of Raynaud's. Patients with diffuse cutaneous systemic sclerosis tend to have worse symptoms.

The pathophysiology of systemic sclerosis is one of arteriolar sclerosis and a resultant patchy muscle atrophy and fibrosis. There also appears to be neural dysfunction that often precedes the smooth-muscle fibrosis. This eventually leads to a fibrotic, aperistaltic esophagus. The proximal striated muscle of the esophagus is uninvolved (15).

The most reliable diagnostic features of systemic sclerosis are manometric. Approximately 80% of patients will have a decreased amplitude of peristalsis in the distal esophagus as well as a decreased LES pressure. This is in distinction to primary achalasia, in which the LES pressure is elevated. Peristalsis in the proximal esophagus and UES pressures are preserved in systemic sclerosis.

The treatment of systemic sclerosis is primarily symptomatic. Proton pump inhibitors are very effective at reducing the incidence of erosive esophagitis and heartburn symptoms. The role of antireflux surgery is limited, considering the poor peristalsis in the distal esophagus.

Mixed Connective Tissue Disease

Mixed connective tissue disease (MCTD) is a relatively rare syndrome with clinical features that overlap with systemic sclerosis, systemic lupus erythematosus, idiopathic inflammatory myopathies, and rheumatoid arthritis (Chapter 1). The typical clinical features are Raynaud's phenomenon, polyarthritis, myalgias, swelling of the hands, and esophageal dysfunction. Unlike systemic sclerosis, patients with MCTD may respond to corticosteroids. The primary clinical esophageal symptoms are heartburn and regurgitation, occurring in 24% to 48% of patients (16). Oropharyngeal dysphagia and/or esophageal dysphagia are common symptoms. Barium esophagram studies show findings similar to those in systemic sclerosis, mainly diminished esophageal peristalsis, and a dilated esophagus. Modified barium swallow studies may show oropharyngeal dysfunction similar to that seen in patients with polymyositis. Manometry is similar to systemic sclerosis; however, the LES pressures are usually not as diminished.

Sjögren's Syndrome

Sjögren's syndrome is an autoimmune inflammatory disorder characterized by the destruction of the salivary and lacrimal glands, resulting in xerostomia and keratoconjunctivitis. Sjögren's syndrome can be a primary disorder or it can present in association with other autoimmune disorders. Autoantibodies anti-Ro and anti-La are found in 60% and 40%, respectively, of patients with Sjögren's. The histologic findings are consistent with the pathophysiology of an autoimmune disease directed at salivary and lacrimal tissue. Classically, a lymphocytic infiltrate is seen with acinar atrophy and hypertrophy of the ductal epithelial cells. Diagnosis is usually made through the biopsy of minor salivary gland tissue in the lower lip. The incidence of dysphagia in these patients has been reported as being anywhere from 32% to 92%. Although the exact mechanism of the dysphagia is unknown, it has been postulated that it is related to the lack of saliva acting as a lubricant. Manometric findings in Sjögren's patients are typically normal. Careful barium esophagrams can detect a subtle proximal esophageal web in up to 10% of patients (17). Treatment is directed at increasing salivary output. See Chapter 2 for further discussion of Sjögren's syndrome.

Diabetes Mellitus

Gastrointestinal (GI) symptoms such as nausea, vomiting, and diarrhea are relatively common in diabetes mellitus. Population-based studies in Australia have shown that esophageal symptoms are also more common in diabetics than in nondiabetic control patients (18). The underlying pathophysiology is presumed to be a neuropathy; there is a progressive axonal atrophy and segmental demyelination of the parasympathetic fibers in the esophagus. The most typical motility abnormality is ineffective peristalsis. In addition, diabetics suffer gastroparesis and delayed gastric emptying, resulting in increased gastroesophageal reflux. Complicating matters, diabetics suffer from sensory neuropathy in the esophagus; electrical stimulation in the esophagus has revealed reduced or absent cortical responses in diabetics studied, implying markedly reduced sensation (19). This correlates with the "silent" acid reflux disease found in diabetics.

Approximately one-third of diabetics have esophageal manometric abnormalities. The most common findings are diminished LES pressures and decreased amplitude of peristaltic waves in the distal esophagus. Other findings seen are multiple simultaneous contractions and multipeaked contractions. Aperistalsis is very rare (20).

Crohn's Disease

Crohn's disease is a systemic inflammatory disorder affecting the entire GI tract. Although Crohn's disease most commonly affects the distal alimentary tract, esophageal involvement does occur. One study of patients without esophageal symptoms showed evidence of esophageal involvement in 5% by upper endoscopy (21). The typical findings are small, punctuate ulcerations in the esophageal mucosa. Rarely, fissures may form leading to fistula formation with adjacent organs. When patients are symptomatic, the typical symptoms are dysphagia, odynophagia, and epigastric discomfort. See Chapter 20 for further discussion of Crohn's disease.

Chagas' Disease

Carlos Chagas described the tropical parasitic infection caused by *Trypanosoma cruzi* initially in 1909, while working in a remote area collecting bugs for malaria research. The protozoan *T. cruzi* is endemic to Central and South America and constitutes a significant public health concern in much of South America. The life cycle of *T. cruzi* involves transmission to humans from the feces of an insect vector. The acute phase is characterized by fever, malaise, and generalized lymphadenopathy. In many individuals, it is not recognized as Chagas' disease during this phase. Of infected individuals, only approximately 10% to 30% progress to the chronic phase (22). Esophageal histology reveals a hypertrophic muscular layer and a significant decrease in the number of ganglion cells in Auerbach's plexus.

The dysphagia that occurs with Chagas' disease can occur anywhere from weeks to years following infection. Initially, the dysphagia is intermittent; however, as the disease progresses, it becomes persistent and more severe. Regurgitation, aspiration with pneumonia, and weight loss are common. Roberto Dantas described esophageal motor abnormalities as documented by barium esophagram or manometry in 25% of asymptomatic individuals (23). These findings typically consist of dysrhythmic contractions in early phases. As the disease progresses, the manometric findings show decreasing peristaltic amplitudes and eventually aperistalsis, which is the hallmark of this disease. Radiographically, barium swallows show a dilated atonic esophagus, similar to that seen in primary achalasia. The diagnosis can be confirmed by serology; however, false positives can occur in patients with collagen vascular disease, leishmaniasis, malaria, and syphilis (24). Treatment of the acute disease, even when recognized, is successful in eradicating the organism less than 50% of the time. Typically, benznidazole and nifurtimox are used. Treatment of the esophageal disease is similar to that of primarily achalasia, namely, pneumatic dilation and chemical (botulinum toxin) or surgical myotomy.

Cutaneous Bullous Diseases

Many cutaneous disorders have associated esophageal involvement. The more common of these disorders include epidermolysis bullosa, cicatricial pemphigoid (CP), lichen planus, and pemphigus vulgaris. Epidermolysis bullosa is a relatively rare cutaneous disease mediated by circulating IgG antibodies directed against type VII collagen. Clinically, patients develop intradermal blistering lesions with scarring at sites of trauma (hands and feet are most common). The proximal third of the esophagus, consisting of stratified squamous epithelium, is at risk. Strictures can occur due to concentric scarring from large blisters. Treatment is dilation. There is reported treatment of severe cases by colonic interposition free tissue grafting, to replace the stratified squamous epithelium of the proximal third of the esophagus (25).

Bullous pemphigoid (BP) is another autoimmune blistering disease, which generally affects patients over the age of 60. It is the most common of the bullous cutaneous lesions. CP is a related, more heterogenous disease. In both diseases, autoantibodies to proteins in the basement membrane are the causative agents. Oral involvement is 40% in BP and reaches up to 100% in CP. As in epidermolysis bullosa, there is a very real risk of esophageal webs and strictures due to cicatricial scarring. Treatment for BP and CP is with corticosteroids; symptomatic strictures should be dilated.

REFERENCES

1. Scmidt EV, Smirnov VE, Ryabova VS. Results of the seven-year prospective study of stroke patients. Stroke 1988; 19(8):942–949.
2. Jean A. Brainstem organization of the swallowing network. Brain Behav Evol 1984; 25(2–3): 109–116.
3. Buchholz DW. Dysphagia associated with neurological disorders. Acta Otorhinolaryngol Belg 1994;48(2):143–155.
4. Mann G, Hankey GJ, Cameron D. Swallowing disorders after acute stroke: prevalence and diagnostic accuracy. Cerebrovasc Dis 2000; 10(5):380–386.
5. Smithard DG, O'Neill PA, Parks C, et al. Complications and outcome after acute stroke. Does dysphagia matter? Stroke 1996; 27(7):1200–1204; erratum in: Stroke 1998; 29(7):1480–1481.
6. Cook IJ. Normal and disordered swallowing: new insights. Baillieres Clin Gastroenterol 1991; 5(2):245–267.
7. Mayberry JF, Atkinson M. Swallowing problems in patients with motor neuron disease. J Clin Gastroenterol 1986; 8(3 Pt 1):233–234.
8. Dalakas MC. Polymyositis, dermatomyositis and inclusion-body myositis. N Eng J Med 1991; 325 (21):1487–1498.
9. Fradet G, Pouliot D, Robichaud R, et al. Upper esophageal sphincter myotomy in oculopharyngeal muscular dystrophy: long-term clinical results. Neuromuscul Disord 1997; 7(suppl 1):S90–S95.
10. Grob D. Myasthenia gravis. A review of pathogenesis and treatment. Arch Intern Med 1961; 108:615–638.
11. Lieberman AN, Horowitz L, Redmond P, et al. Dysphagia in Parkinson's disease. Am J Gastroenterol 1980; 74(2):157–160.
12. Leopold NA, Kagel MC. Pharyngo-esophageal dysphagia in Parkinson's disease. Dysphagia 1997; 12(1):11–20.
13. Buntzel J, Glatzel M, Kuttner K, et al. Amifostine in simultaneous radiochemotherapy of advanced head and neck cancer. Semin Radiat Oncol 2002; 12(1 suppl 1):4–13.
14. Abu-Shakra M, Guillemin F, Lee P. Gastrointestinal manifestations of systemic sclerosis. Semin Arthritis Rheum 1994; 24(1):29–39.
15. Treacy WL, Baggenstoss AH, Slocumb CH, et al. Scleroderma of the esophagus. A correlation of histologic and physiologic findings. Ann Intern Med 1963; 59:351–356.
16. Marshall JB, Kretschmar JM, Gerhardt DC, et al. Gastrointestinal manifestations of mixed connective tissue disease. Gastroenterology 1990; 98(5 Pt 1):1232–1238.
17. Kjellen G, Fransson SG, Lindstrom F, et al. Esophageal function, radiography, and dysphagia in Sjögren's syndrome. Dig Dis Sci 1986; 31(3):225–229.
18. Bytzer P, Talley NJ, Leemon M, et al. Prevalence of gastrointestinal symptoms associated with diabetes mellitus: a population-based survey of 15,000 adults. Arch Intern Med 2001; 161(16): 1989–1996.
19. Kamath MV, Tougas G, Fitzpatrick D, et al. Assessment of the visceral afferent and autonomic pathways in response to esophageal stimulation in control subjects and in patients with diabetes. Clin Invest Med 1998; 21(3):100–113.
20. Holloway RH, Tippett MD, Horowitz M, et al. Relationship between esophageal motility and transit in patients with type I diabetes mellitus. Am J Gastroenterol 1999; 94(11):3150–3157.
21. Alcantara M, Rodriguez R, Potenciano JL, et al. Endoscopic and bioptic findings in the upper gastrointestinal tract in patients with Crohn's disease. Endoscopy 1993; 25(4):282–286.
22. Miles MA. The discovery of Chagas disease: progress and prejudice. Infect Dis Clin North Am 2004;18(2):247–260.
23. Dantas RO, Deghaide NH, Donadi EA. Esophageal manometric and radiologic findings in asymptomatic subjects with Chagas' disease. J Clin Gastroenterol 1999; 28(3):245–248.
24. Kirchhoff LV. American trypanosomiasis (Chagas' disease) – a tropical disease now in the United States. N Engl J Med 1993; 329(9):639–644.
25. Elton C, Marshall RE, Hibbert J, et al. Pharyngogastric colonic interposition for total oesophageal occlusion in epidermolysis bullosa. Dis Esophagus 2000; 13(2):175–177.

35

Hoarseness and Laryngeal Paralysis

Gayle E. Woodson
Department of Surgery, Division of Otolaryngology, Southern Illinois University, Springfield, Illinois, U.S.A.

INTRODUCTION

Hoarseness is an extremely common yet varied symptom. An abnormal voice may sound raspy, breathy, or weak, or the pitch may be inappropriate. Often when a patient complains of hoarseness, the voice actually sounds normal but fatigues too quickly or requires too much effort. All of these symptoms indicate a problem with sound production within the larynx. Sometimes voice production is normal, but the sound is altered by abnormal resonance. For example, a peritonsillar abscess can cause a "hot potato voice," and a patient with a cold sounds hyponasal. Thus, the first task in diagnosing acute hoarseness is to define the precise nature of the problem. Is the problem in the larynx, the resonators, or the articulators? And exactly what is preventing production of a normal voice?

Diagnosis of a voice disorder entails two components: establishing the mechanism by which the voice is disrupted and then determining the etiology of the pathology. Table 1 lists mechanisms for hoarseness. Identifying the mechanism, however, does not always reveal the etiology. For example, evaluation may reveal that hoarseness is due to nodules on the vocal folds. The etiology of vocal nodules is most often voice abuse, and the vast majority of vocal nodules respond to speech therapy. Rarely, though, a nodule on the vocal fold is caused by rheumatoid arthritis (RA). In a patient with known RA, a vocal nodule can immediately be considered to be rheumatoid (see Chapter 1 for detailed discussion of RA manifesting in the head and neck). In a patient without known arthritis, a rheumatoid etiology would not be considered in the differential diagnosis until the patient fails to respond to a trial of voice therapy. Another issue is that more than one etiology may conspire in the genesis of a laryngeal pathology. For example, mucosal disruption due to a systemic illness such as pemphigoid can make a patient more susceptible to the ill effects of voice overuse or gastroesophageal reflux.

The three most common causes of acute hoarseness are upper respiratory infection, vocal abuse, and gastroesophageal reflux. Such problems generally resolve within two to six weeks. Vocal symptoms that persist beyond this time require investigation. Chronic hoarseness is most often due to chronic laryngitis, with causative factors that include acid reflux, voice abuse, smoking, allergies, and old age. Systemic illnesses are rarely found to be the cause of hoarseness. Although many systemic illnesses have the potential to affect the voice by impairing mucosal vibration or vocal fold motion, hoarseness is not often the presenting sign. Nevertheless, systemic illness does have a place in the differential diagnosis of hoarseness or laryngeal paralysis, but only when common causes are excluded or when the patient is already known to have a systemic disease. The following systemic diseases are known to adversely affect the voice.

WEGENER'S GRANULOMATOSIS

Wegener's granulomatosis is an autoimmune vasculitis that affects the respiratory tract and kidneys. Ocular involvement occurs in up to 50% of patients, and some patients present

TABLE 1 Mechanisms of Hoarseness

Mucosal inflammation/edema
Mass lesions of the vocal fold
Mechanical limitation of vocal fold motion
Laryngeal paralysis
Neuromotor dysfunction
Psychogenic factors

with epistaxis and/or chronic sinusitis. The larynx is involved in 6% to 25% of cases, usually with exophytic granulation tissue in the subglottis and sometimes the vocal folds. The inflammation can progress to subglottic stenosis.

There is a male predominance and onset is most common in the fifth and sixth decades. The classic criteria for diagnosis of Wegener's include necrotizing granuloma of the upper or lower respiratory tract and focal, necrotizing glomerulonephritis with fibrinoid necrosis and thrombosis of capillary loops. More recently, the diagnosis is established by disease in at least two organ systems, with positive biopsy in at least one. Tissue biopsy is the most reliable means of diagnosis but may be obscured by necrosis. anti-nuclear antibody (ANA) may be positive, but anti-nuclear cytoplasmic antibody (C-ANCA) is a more sensitive serologic test. Not infrequently, Wegener's is suspected as the cause of isolated idiopathic subglottic stenosis, but biopsies and serologic testing are negative.

Primary treatment of Wegener's granulomatosis is pharmacologic. Steroids are usually effective. Second-line therapy includes cytotoxic drugs. Medical therapy may keep the disease in check, but often the disease progresses. In systemic disease, death results from pulmonary and/or renal failure. Laryngeal stenosis may require endoscopic excision to relieve airway obstruction but may be complicated by scarring, with further voice impairment and recurrent obstruction (Fig. 1). Tracheotomy is an alternate way of relieving obstruction. Surgical management of stenosis and scarring may be attempted when there is no active disease, but it may be complicated by reactivation (1).

Wegener's granulomatosis is discussed in detail in Chapter 8.

RHEUMATOID ARTHRITIS

RA, discussed at length in Chapter 1, is a symmetric autoimmune polyarticular arthritis. It also affects nonarticular structures. Patients may have vasculitis, pulmonary fibrosis, and inflammatory changes in ligaments, tendons, and fascia.

Of patients with RA, 25% to 30% have cricoarytenoid arthritis, with symptoms of hoarseness, globus, odynophagia, and pain with speaking or coughing. If the joints become fixed in an adducted position, the airway can be severely obstructed. Cricoarytenoid

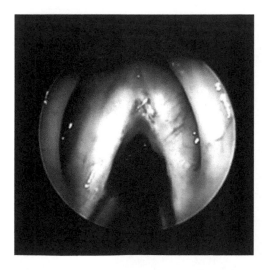

FIGURE 1 Glottic and subglottic stenosis in a patient with Wegener's granulomatosis.

arthritis may also occur in patients with other rheumatoid diseases such as Sjögren's syndrome or systemic lupus erythematosus (SLE). Laryngoscopy in cricoarytenoid arthritis reveals inflammation of the overlying mucosa and limited vocal-fold mobility. Diagnosis is established by palpation during direct laryngoscopy, which can demonstrate mechanical restriction of joint motion. Computed tomography (CT) imaging often demonstrates erosion of the cricoarytenoid joint, with surrounding soft-tissue edema. Cricoarytenoid arthritis may be asymptomatic because many RA patients have cricoarytenoid joint abnormalities on CT but no laryngeal problems (2). Tracheotomy is often required for acute airway obstruction; however, cricoarytenoid arthritis usually responds dramatically to steroid treatment.

A less common laryngeal manifestation is the rheumatoid nodule: a focal submucosal inflammatory infiltrate on the membranous vocal fold (Fig. 2). Rheumatoid nodules are characteristically seen as subcutaneous lesions in other parts of the body in 20% of patients. They occur on the vibratory edge of the vocal fold and can cause significant hoarseness (3). Simple endoscopic excision is effective, but recurrence has been reported (4).

SYSTEMIC LUPUS ERYTHEMATOSUS

SLE is a common autoimmune connective-tissue disease affecting 1 in 1000. It is much more prevalent in young females, with a female-to-male incidence of 9:1. It affects many organ systems. Skin rash is a very common presentation, typically appearing in the malar areas following sun exposure. Oral ulcerations develop in 40% of patients. Other systemic manifestations include myocarditis, nephritis, pneumonitis, and central nervous system (CNS) involvement.

Laryngeal involvement is rare in SLE, but hoarseness in the presence of characteristic signs and symptoms should raise suspicion of possible SLE. The cause of hoarseness in SLE patients is varied. One review of 97 SLE patients with laryngeal

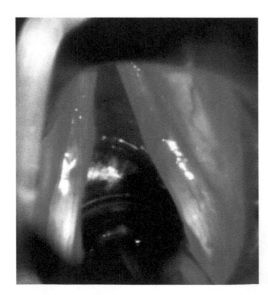

FIGURE 2 Rheumatoid nodule on left vocal fold with reactive changes on right vocal fold.

involvement found laryngeal edema in 28% and laryngeal paralysis in 11% (5). Less frequent involvement includes epiglottitis, subglottic stenosis, and rheumatoid nodules. Some patients develop stridor due to inflammatory lesions in the larynx and trachea. Biopsy of active lesions may aid in diagnosis by demonstrating mononuclear inflammation and immunofluorescent nuclear staining.

The clinical course of SLE is unpredictable. Treatment primarily consists of steroids. Please see Chapter 1 for discussion in detail of SLE.

AMYLOIDOSIS

This disease damages tissues by the accumulation of abnormal fibrillar substance. Amyloidosis is an idiopathic disease that may be either primary or secondary to multiple myeloma. The abnormal depositions may be local or diffuse, and may involve more than one organ system. The peak incidence is from 60 to 65 years, but it occurs as early as the third decade. Systemic disease is equally common in men and women, but there is a slight male predominance for disease localized in the head and neck. Amyloidosis can occur in practically any organ and commonly affects the kidneys, heart, nerves, gastrointestinal tract, skin, and lungs. Death is usually caused by kidney or heart failure.

Laryngeal amyloid is almost always localized and not systemic. Amyloid may be most frequently in the supraglottis, followed by glottis, and subglottis (6). One-third of patients may also have tracheal involvement. Symptoms of laryngeal involvement include hoarseness, stridor, globus, and dysphagia. Hemoptysis is rare. Laryngeal amyloidosis accounts for less than 1% of all benign laryngeal lesions.

On endoscopic exam, laryngeal lesions have a waxy, gray to yellow-orange appearance, with rubbery or firm texture. Sometimes the epiglottis is massively enlarged (3). Figure 3 depicts massive enlargement of the false vocal fold. Subglottic involvement can also project into the lumen and restrict the airway. Diagnosis can only be established by biopsy. With hematoxylin-eosin stain, amyloid is an extracellular, amorphous, pink material. Classic apple-green birefringence is seen with Congo red stain under polarized light. Electron microscopy shows linear, nonbranching fibrils in β-pleated sheets.

There is no specific treatment for amyloidosis. When it is secondary to multiple myeloma, the primary disease is managed pharmacologically by melphalan and prednisone. Systemic amyloidosis, however, can progress to death, despite control of the myeloma.

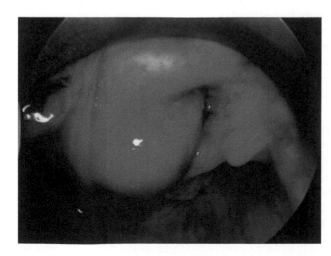

FIGURE 3 Laryngeal sarcoidosis involving epiglottis and left false vocal fold. Tip of laryngoscope is elevating the epiglottis.

Local symptoms of laryngeal amyloidosis can be managed by endoscopic excision, or less commonly, by open surgery. Total removal is often not possible and the disease typically recurs, requiring frequent surgery, or ultimately tracheotomy to relieve obstruction. Scarring from surgical excision can cause permanent airway or voice impairment.

PEMPHIGUS AND PEMPHIGOID

Pemphigus and pemphigoid are autoimmune diseases that produce blistering of skin and/or mucosa. In pemphigus, intraepithelial blistering is caused by destruction of desmogleins that connect epithelial cells. Its most common variant, pemphigus vulgaris, begins with ulcerating lesions in the mouth, as the outer epithelium of the blister sloughs. Later, skin is also involved. In pemphigoid, the basement membrane is attacked, resulting in subepithelial blisters. Mucosal involvement nearly always begins in the mouth and can spread as far caudal as the larynx. It does not involve the subglottis or trachea (7). Pemphigoid is a subepithelial blistering disease that affects skin and mucous membranes, including the nose and larynx (8).

Diagnosis is established by immunofluorescence to detect the antibodies causing the lesions. Biopsy is often negative because it shows nonspecific necrosis, particularly in the center of ulcerated lesions. Serology is sometimes helpful. Before the advent of drug treatment, pemphigus vulgaris was fatal in 99% of cases, but with treatment including dapsone, steroids, and azathioprine, mortality is 5% to 15%. The mucosal lesions of pemphigus and pemphigoid generally respond well to medical management, but untreated lesions may become infected and cause scarring sufficient to obstruct the airway.

RELAPSING POLYCHONDRITIS

Relapsing polychondritis is discussed in detail in Chapter 7. It is a chronic multisystem inflammation of cartilage (9). It may affect all types of cartilage including elastic cartilage of ears and nose, hyaline cartilage of joints, and tracheobronchial cartilage. About one-half of patients have airway involvement. The female-to-male ratio is 3:1. Peak onset is in the fourth to fifth decades. It occurs predominantly in Caucasians but occasionally in other races. Relapsing polychondritis can also affect other tissues such as the eyes, blood vessels, heart, and inner ear. It most often presents with sudden onset of auricular pain and erythema that spare the lobule, accompanied by fever and lethargy. Acute episodes resolve within 5 to 10 days, but recurrent bouts of inflammation are common, with progressive permanent destruction of the cartilage (Fig. 4).

Diagnosis is based primarily on the history and physical because biopsy usually shows nonspecific necrosis. A biopsy of perichondrium at the edge of the lesion may occasionally document the early stage of inflammation. Biopsy is indicated to exclude other conditions such as Wegener's granulomatosis. Conclusive diagnosis requires three of six features: bilateral auricular chondritis, nonerosive seronegative arthritis, nasal chondritis, ocular inflammation, respiratory tract chondritis, and audiovestibular damage.

Symptoms of laryngeal involvement include hoarseness, throat pain, and pain on phonation. Progressive loss of laryngeal cartilage impairs the airway and may cause emergent airway obstruction (Fig. 4).

Steroids provide dramatic response, but side effects limit long-term use. Other drugs that can be effective include dapsone, azathioprine, cyclophosphamide, cyclosporine, and penicillamine. Plasma exchange is also used. Surgical reconstruction of the airway is not effective, and the efficacy of tracheotomy is limited due to diffuse collapse of the trachea. Airway disease can progress to death from pneumonia or obstructive respiratory failure.

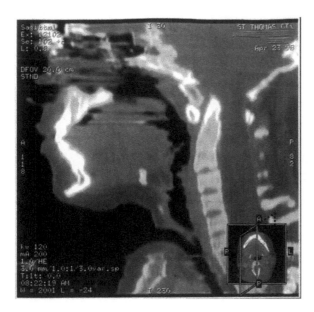

FIGURE 4   Resorption of laryngeal and tracheal cartilage, with granulation tissue over tracheotomy tract.

SARCOIDOSIS

This is an idiopathic chronic granulomatous disease that occasionally affects the larynx. Peak onset is from the age of 20 to 40 years. There is a higher incidence in African Americans, Puerto Ricans, and Scandinavians, and it is sometimes familial. The pathogenesis of sarcoidosis is unknown. One theory is that it results from a mycobacterial infection. It is usually systemic, most commonly including the lungs and hilar lymph nodes. Isolated local involvement is rare, so head and neck manifestations are virtually always in the context of disease in other sites. A review of 2319 patients seen at the Mayo Clinic for sarcoidosis found head and neck involvement in 9% of cases. Of these, the eyes and lacrimal system were involved in 40%, the nose in 13%, and the larynx in 6% (10). Symptoms of laryngeal involvement include hoarseness, dysphagia, stridor, and dyspnea.

On physical examination, supraglottic involvement appears as a pale and diffusely enlarged, sometimes nodular epiglottis. Vocal fold involvement appears as pale submucosal masses. Histopathologic examination of these lesions reveals characteristic granulomas. However, biopsy does not definitively establish the diagnosis, because many other conditions can produce granuloma. Laryngeal lesions require treatment only if symptomatic. Epiglottic lesions that cause dyspnea may be debulked endoscopically. Repeat surgery may be necessary. Vocal fold lesions may also impair the airway, and if so, they should be removed endoscopically; however, if the only symptom of a vocal fold lesion is hoarseness, surgery should be approached with caution. Postoperative scarring and tissue loss can further impair the voice, potentially causing severe dysphonia. Alternative management is intralesional steroid injections repeated at intervals (11).

Detailed discussion of sarcoidosis can be found in Chapter 6.

VIRAL NEUROPATHY

Viral neuropathy of the vagus or recurrent laryngeal nerve is believed to be a common cause of chronic cough, hoarseness, and/or laryngospasm, much as facial nerve palsy is attributed to viral illness. Patients report a flu-like illness, usually with severe coughing and

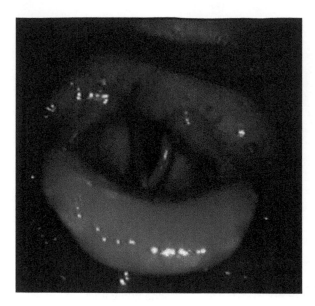

FIGURE 5 Acute laryngeal paralysis with herpetic vesicles in laryngeal and pharyngeal mucosa.

hoarseness, and examination may show unilateral laryngeal weakness or paralysis. In most cases, coughing and spasm resolve within six months, but the vocal fold weakness persists. There is little medical evidence for viral infection as a common cause of laryngeal paralysis; however, there are anecdotal reports of elevations of varicella-zoster immunoglobulin G levels in association with acute laryngeal paralysis. Mucosal lesions consistent with a herpetic infection have been noted in a patient with acute onset of laryngeal paralysis (Fig. 5) (12).

NEUROFIBROMATOSIS

Also known as Von Recklinghausen's disease, neurofibromatosis is an autosomal-dominant hereditary disorder that causes CNS tumors and cutaneous neurofibromata. The most common manifestation of this disease that is encountered in the practice of otolaryngology is the acoustic neuroma. Occasionally, a lesion involves the larynx (13). Figure 6 depicts a very large lesion in the posterior glottis of an infant. Treatment is difficult because complete removal of such a lesion in the larynx is usually not possible without total laryngectomy, and recurrence is common with partial removal.

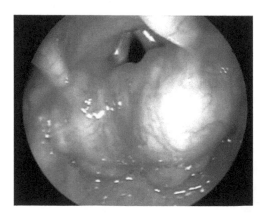

FIGURE 6 Large neurofibroma of the posterior glottis in an infant.

REFERENCES

1. Lebovics RS, Hoffman GS, Leavitt RY, et al. Management of subglottic stenosis in patients with Wegener's granulomatosis. Laryngoscope 1992; 102(12 Pt 1):1341–1345.
2. Brazeau-Lamontagne L, Charlin B, Levesque RY, et al. Cricoarytenoiditis: CT assessment in rheumatoid arthritis. Radiology 1986; 158(2):463–466.
3. Woo P, Mendelsohn J, Humphrey D. Rheumatoid nodules of the larynx. Otolaryngol Head Neck Surg 1995; 113(1):147–150.
4. Friedman BA. Rheumatoid nodules of the larynx. Arch Otolaryngol 1975; 101(6):361–363.
5. Teitel AD, MacKenzie CR, Stern R, et al. Laryngeal involvement in systemic lupus erythematosus. Semin Arthritis Rheum 1992; 22(3):203–214.
6. Lewis JE, Olsen KD, Kurtin PJ, et al. Laryngeal amyloidosis: a clinicopathologic and immunohistochemical review. Otolaryngol Head Neck Surg 1992; 106(4):372–377.
7. Hale EK, Bystryn JC. Laryngeal and nasal involvement in pemphigus vulgaris. J Am Acad Dermatol 2001; 44(4):609–611.
8. Whiteside OJ, Martinez Devesa P, Ali I, et al. Mucous membrane pemphigoid: nasal and laryngeal manifestations. J Laryngol Otol 2003; 117(11):885–888.
9. McCaffrey TV, McDonald TJ, McCaffrey LA. Head and neck manifestations of relapsing polychondritis: review of 29 cases. Otolaryngology 1978; 86(3 Pt 1):473–478.
10. Neel HB III, McDonald TJ. Laryngeal sarcoidosis: report of 13 patients. Ann Otol Rhinol Laryngol 1982; 91(4 Pt 1):359–362.
11. Krespi YP, Mitrani M, Husain S, et al. Treatment of laryngeal sarcoidosis with intralesional steroid injection. Ann Otol Rhinol Laryngol 1987; 96(6):713–715.
12. Wu CL, Linne OC, Chiang CW. Herpes zoster laryngis with prelaryngeal skin erythema. Ann Otol Rhinol Laryngol 2004; 113(2):113–114.
13. Holt GR. E.N.T. manifestations of Von Recklinghausen's disease. Laryngoscope 1978; 88(10): 1617–1632.

36

Cervical Adenitis and Pain

Phillip K. Pellitteri
Geisinger Health System, Danville, Pennsylvania, U.S.A.

INTRODUCTION

Systemic disease presenting with or manifesting signs and symptoms in the head and neck will frequently do so in the cervical regions. This discussion focuses on systemic diseases that result in cervical adenitis, with or without pain, as an initial or hallmark finding. The majority of these disorders occur as a consequence of inflammatory etiologies, often masquerading as a more benign process. It is therefore important to recognize that these clinical findings may represent a more serious illness, warranting timely diagnosis.

INFLAMMATORY DISORDERS

Systemic disease resulting from an inflammatory process may be separated into those disorders which have infectious etiologies and those resulting from noninfectious processes.

INFECTIOUS DISEASES

Mycobacterial Infection

The incidence of mycobacterial infections has undergone a varied course over the past 50 years. For an approximate 30-year period following 1950, the incidence in mycobacterial infection declined annually in excess of 5%. This was followed by a paradoxical sharp increase at the rate of approximately 20% during the late 1980s and early 1990s, due to multiple factors such as acquired immunodeficiency syndrome (AIDS), drug resistance, and population influx from endemic areas. With improved awareness, prevention, and drug therapy, the incidence has continued to decline from the late 1990s into the current 2000s.

Definition. Mycobacteria are nonmotile, non–spore-forming aerobic bacilli that resist decolorization by acids, thus the term "acid-fast" bacilli. The classically described mycobacterial infections were caused by *Mycobacterium tuberculosis*. Infections affecting the head and neck may be the result of *M. tuberculosis* or nontuberculous (atypical) mycobacteria.

Epidemiology. During the mid to late 1980s, the incidence of cervical mycobacterial disease was noted to rise, largely due to the increase in Asian and Hispanic immigrant populations into the American cities as well as the increase in patients infected with human immunodeficiency virus (HIV) manifesting immunodeficiency (AIDS). With heightened awareness, prevention, and improved public hygiene, the incidence into the current century has continued to decline since the mid 1990s. Currently, those at risk for mycobacterial disease include third-world immigrants and patients with immunodeficiency disorders but may also include the young, particularly with respect to atypical mycobacterial infection.

Clinical Manifestations. The head and neck manifestations of mycobacterial disease are broad in spectrum. In addition to the cervical lymph nodes, affected head and neck regions include the middle ear, nasal cavity and paranasal sinuses, oral cavity, pharynx, larynx, and salivary tissue.

The cervical lymph nodes represent the most common extrapulmonary site of involvement by mycobacterial infection (1). It is important to differentiate between tuberculous and atypical disease–induced cervical adenitis, as the clinical scenario and management are different.

Cervical adenitis caused by tuberculosis is noted to involve the supraclavicular and posterior nodal groups. The majority (greater than 80%) of patients with cervical tuberculosis do not have pulmonary disease and few patients present with the typical constitutional sequelae of fever, night sweats, hemoptysis, and weight loss.

In contrast, patients with atypical cervical mycobacterial infection present with isolated lymphadenitis involving submandibular and submental groups (Fig. 1). These patients almost never present with constitutional symptoms. Affected nodes may become densely adherent to the subcutaneous and cutaneous tissues, resulting in skin necrosis manifested by erythema and fluctuance (Fig. 2).

Diagnosis. Patients at risk for or suspected of having *M. tuberculosis* infection should have a chest X ray and a PPD skin test. Chest radiographs have a low yield of positive findings (less than 20%), whereas a positive PPD may be noted in up to 96% of those infected, provided the patient is not immunocompromised (2). In the event that a patient with HIV demonstrates immunocompromise, a skin reaction of 5 mm (as opposed to 10 mm) on PPD testing is deemed to be positive; this occurs in up to 40% of patients with HIV (3). In order to secure a definitive diagnosis, fine needle aspiration of a suspected lymph node may be performed. Although the initial smear may be positive for acid-fast bacilli in only 20% of patients, the presence of granulomatous inflammatory changes raises the suspicion of tuberculosis. A definitive culture may be obtained after six to eight weeks' incubation.

Atypical mycobacterial disease is suspected in patients unresponsive to medical therapy with a documented smear demonstrating acid-fast bacilli. In the absence of proven acid-fast positivity, material from curettage from a necrotic skin lesion may be used for further histologic examination and culture (Fig. 3).

Treatment. Cervical tuberculosis is a medically treated disease. Treatment is aimed at both systemic and local manifestations of the disorder. With a confirmed diagnosis, multiple-drug antimicrobial therapy is initiated. A four-drug regimen consisting of rifampin, ethambutol, isoniazid, and pyrazinamide is recommended, with the addition of streptomycin as an alternative. This schedule is continued for six months, sometimes with the deletion of ethambutol and/or pyrazinamide after two months. Pregnancy precludes the use of drug therapy until after delivery. Surgical nodal excision may be carried out to secure the diagnosis in the event a node remains enlarged following antimicrobial therapy or in the second or third trimester of pregnancy.

In contrast to tuberculous disease, atypical mycobacterial infection is frequently resistant to multidrug medical therapy. Causative organisms inducing drug resistance include *Mycobacterium avium-intracellulare*, *Mycobacterium scrofulaceum*, *Mycobacterium*

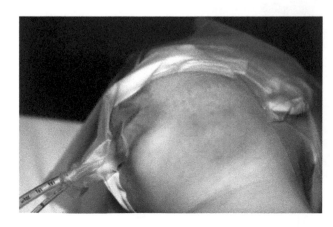

FIGURE 1 Atypical mycobacterial infection involving submental lymph node in a child. *Source*: Photo courtesy of Dr. Edward Wood.

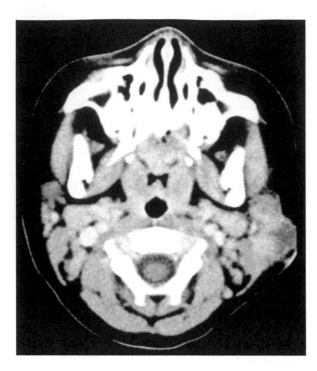

FIGURE 2 Axial computed tomography image demonstrating necrotic lymph node in a patient with atypical mycobacterial infection. *Source*: Photo courtesy of Dr. Edward Wood.

simiae, Mycobacterium chelonei, and *Mycobacterium fortuitum.* It is due to this resistance that atypical cervical infections are primarily treated with nodal excision, prior to capsular rupture, if possible (4). In the presence of skin necrosis and soft-tissue breakdown, curettage or excision of necrotic tissue is advocated.

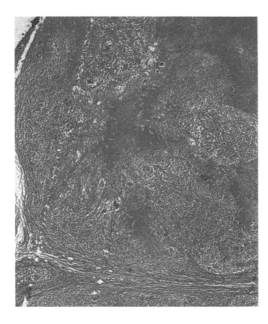

FIGURE 3 Mycobacterial infection in a lymph node with demonstration of caseating granulomata.

Complications and Prognosis. Complications related to cervical mycobacterial infections are few. Uncommonly, soft-tissue breakdown may occur to the extent that wide debridement is required, resulting in significant fibrosis and scarring. In the immuno-competent patient, response to therapy is generally favorable, with a low incidence of recrudescence. Immunocompromised patients may respond slowly or not at all to therapy and are at risk for recurrence. Mycobacterial infections are discussed in more detail in Chapter 12.

Cat-Scratch Disease

Cat-scratch disease, first described in 1931, has received little notoriety in the head and neck literature, despite the fact that 50% of patients present with cervical lymphadeno-pathy. The most extensive reports are noted in the pediatric literature, where it accounts for a sizable proportion of unilateral lymphadenopathy in children and adolescents (5).

Definition. Cat-scratch disease has been alternatively termed cat-scratch fever, benign lymphoreticulosis, or nonbacterial lymphadenitis. The cardinal feature of the disease is a subacute regional granulomatous lymphadenitis that follows a relatively mild clinical course. The etiologic agent is a pleomorphic gram-negative bacillus.

Epidemiology. Cat-scratch disease has a worldwide distribution, without gender or racial predilection. It is primarily a disease of children and adolescents, although nearly 25% of patients with the disease are over 30 years of age.

Pathogenesis. The causative bacillus is transmitted by direct contact from a cat scratch, bite, or lick. A history of exposure to a cat with identification of a primary inoculation site is obtained in the majority of patients affected.

Clinical Manifestations. The primary lesion develops as an erythematous, nonpruritic pustule 7 to 12 days following the inoculation. Lymphadenitis generally develops two to four weeks following inoculation and is located proximal to the inoculation site. The three most common regions affected by lymphadenitis include the axillary, cervical, and inguinal areas. Cervical adenitis, occurring in nearly 50% of patients, is typically noted in the upper cervical, submandibular, and nodal basins (Fig. 4). Most commonly, a single nodal basin will be involved, although multiple nodes within the group will be enlarged. Suppuration with acute tenderness, accompanied by fever, may occur in up to 30% of patients. Nodal enlargement generally resolves over two to three weeks but may persist for up to two years.

Most patients will experience mild constitutional symptoms such as malaise, headache, and fever. Atypical clinical manifestations occur in approximately 5% of patients, the most common of which is Parinaud's oculoglandular syndrome (6). This constellation of findings consists of granulomatous conjunctivitis with preauricular adenitis. The primary lesion occurs after rubbing the eye after holding a cat. The remaining atypical presentations are very rare, accounting for about 1% to 2% of all cases. These include central nervous system (CNS) involvement with encephalitis, myelitis, and radiculopathy. Encephalitis in children may induce seizure or coma. Other rare manifestations encountered include thrombocytopenic purpura, osteomyelitis, and hepatosplenomegaly.

Diagnosis. The diagnostic criteria for the identification of cat-scratch disease include history of cat exposure and inoculation, regional lymphadenitis, identification of gram-negative coccobacilli in aspirated material by Warthin–Starry stain, and histologic characteristics of cat-scratch disease on excisional biopsy (Figs. 5 and Fig. 6). Other causes

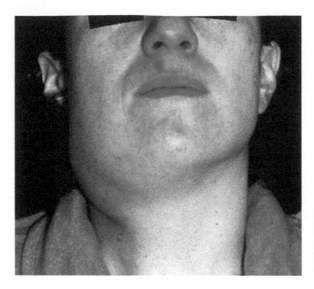

FIGURE 4 Patient with cervical lymphadenopathy secondary to cat-scratch disease. *Source*: Photo courtesy of Dr. Edward Wood.

of cervical lymphadenopathy should be excluded. The differential diagnosis should include nonspecific bacterial adenitis, lymphogranuloma venereum, mycobacterial infection, mononucleosis, tularemia, syphilis, toxoplasmosis, fungal disease, and neoplasms of the lymphoreticular system.

Treatment. Therapy is supportive, without any known specific antimicrobial treatment of benefit. Analgesics and warm compresses, especially for suppuration, appear to offer the most relief. Needle aspiration of suppurative nodes is helpful. Nodal excision is usually not necessary and potentially results in a draining sinus tract.

Complications and Prognosis. Complications resulting from cat-scratch disease are rare. The disorder most commonly follows a benign and self-limited course with near-universal recovery. Severe disease may result in significant suppuration of nodal groups that may require surgical drainage and debridement.

Cat-scratch disease is discussed in further detail in Chapter 11.

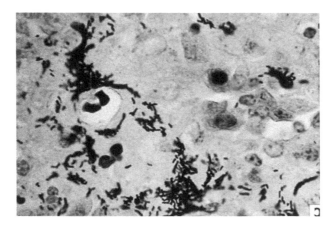

FIGURE 5 Gram-negative coccobacilli demonstrated by Warthin–Starry stain in needle aspirate from lymph node affected by cat-scratch disease. *Source*: Photo courtesy of Dr. Edward Wood.

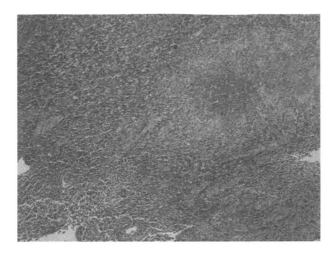

FIGURE 6 Histologic section from aspirate obtained from lymph node affected by cat-scratch disease. *Source*: Photo courtesy of Dr. Robert Brown.

Lyme Disease

Lyme disease was first described as a clinical entity in 1977 as a consequence of a clustering of children in Lyme, Connecticut, who were thought to be infected with juvenile arthritis (7). It became apparent that the disease was a multisystem illness that affected skin, CNS, lymphatics, joints, and heart.

Definition.   The etiologic agent isolated from patients with Lyme disease is the spirochete, *Borrelia burgdorferi*, found in the tick *Ixodes dammini*. Clinically, the infection is similar to syphilis in its multisystem involvement, stages and clinical course, and masquerade of other disorders.

Epidemiology.   Lyme disease is the most common vector-borne infection in the United States. The deer tick *I. dammini* serves as the intermediate host vector for the Borrelia organism. Nymphal ticks both acquire and pass the organism by horizontal transmission to the white-footed mouse. Adult ticks carrying the organism then occupy their preferred host, the white tail deer, which is not involved in the life cycle of the spirochete. Human infection generally occurs when nymphal ticks feed, between the months of May and July. Adult ticks will transmit the spirochete when they feed, in the autumn season. People of all ages and both genders may be affected. The Northeast United States demonstrates rates of disease higher than that of the western part of the country and Europe.

Pathogenesis.   Following inoculation by the tick, the spirochete spreads locally in the skin in the majority of patients, resulting in erythema migrans. It is at this point that the spirochete may be recovered and cultured from the skin lesion more readily than at any subsequent stage. During the second stage of the illness, the spirochete will spread to the lymph and blood, resulting in widespread systemic dissemination and the subsequent constellation of multiorgan symptoms characterizing the disorder.

Clinical Manifestations.   Lyme disease occurs in stages, manifesting different clinical signs/symptoms at each stage. The typical patient experiencing the untreated course of illness develops erythema migrans (stage I); followed by meningitis or facial palsy (stage II); followed months and perhaps years later by arthritis (stage III) (8). It is now known that specific symptoms do not always occur in a specific stage and that both symptoms and stage of infection may vary significantly from patient to patient.

The cervical lymphadenitis resulting from the spirochete generally occurs in stage I of early infection, generally regional in distribution relative to the inoculation site. It may be accompanied by fever and malaise. Disseminated infection during stage II is characterized most commonly by skin, CNS, and musculoskeletal symptoms. Annular rash, headache, and migratory arthralgias characterize this stage of infection. Patients are generally quite ill with severe weakness, fatigue, and discomfort. Late dissemination results in organ system sequestration of the spirochete with periods of quiescence and relapsing symptoms. It is at this point in stage II that differing proportions of patients will experience meningitis, cranial and/or peripheral neuropathies, and cardiac rhythm disturbances. Late stage II of the disease is characterized by relapsing arthralgias leading to frank intermittent episodes of arthritis in early stage III of the process.

Diagnosis.   Because of the difficulty in securing reliable culture material, serology represents the most effective modality for diagnosis.

Treatment.   Oral antimicrobials directed against the spirochete, generally doxycycline, are the treatment of choice for early or localized infection. Intravenous antibiotics (Ceftriaxone) are generally reserved for patients with neurologic abnormalities, excluding facial palsy.

Complications and Prognosis.   Timely treatment with appropriate antibiotics is usually curative, but longer courses of therapy are often required later in the illness. Some patients may not respond to treatment completely, resulting in recrudescent symptoms, or in the event of facial palsy, incomplete return of function.

Syphilis

Syphilis is a sexually transmitted disease resulting from infection by the spirochete *Treponema pallidum*. It is the oldest documented venereal disease, dating back to the 1400s. A more detailed discussion of syphilis appears in Chapter 15.

Epidemiology.   The United States has seen cyclic rises in the incidence of syphilis since nearly eliminating the disease in the late 1950s. Since 1990, the rate of primary and secondary syphilis has decreased nearly 90% to 2.5 cases per 100,000 people. Of the cases, 80% are reported to the Centers for Disease Control (CDC) and there appears to be a regional predilection for the Southeast (9). The rate of congenitally acquired syphilis has also undergone a decline similar to primary/secondary infection since the early 1990s where it occurs in approximately 14 per 100,000 births nationally (10).

Pathogenesis.   The infection by the spirochete occurs through contact of the lesion with traumatized or abraded mucous membrane or epidermis. This contact is most commonly associated with sexual transmission, with the exception of congenital syphilis. The risk of infection following sexual contact with a person with the disease is nearly 50%.

Clinical Manifestations.   The clinical course of syphilis is separated into stages: primary, secondary, latent, and tertiary. Each stage has a characteristic set of clinical entities associated with infection, and not all patients go on to develop tertiary syphilis.

The head and neck, as well as systemic manifestations of syphilis are myriad. With reference to the topic of discussion, regional (cervical) lymphadenopathy generally occurs early in infection, during the primary stage of syphilis. This stage is characterized by the chancre, an ulcerated painless lesion noted at the site of inoculation. In the instance of oral inoculation, the chancre will appear within the oral mucosa accompanied by firm, nontender lymphadenopathy in the upper cervical or submandibular nodal basins. With spontaneous resolution of the chancre, lymphadenopathy clears and generally does not recur unless associated with the benign gummata of tertiary syphilis.

Other head and neck manifestations of infection include sensorineural hearing loss in otosyphilis; chancres of the oral cavity in primary syphilis and pharynx in secondary syphilis; laryngeal chancres; mucous patches or gummata encompassing the full spectrum of stages associated with syphilitic infection; and numerous effects of congenital syphilis such as palatal defects, saddle nose deformities, and congenital deafness.

Systemic manifestations may involve multiple organs and are predicated on the clinical stage. Serious and disabling systemic involvement is usually associated with tertiary syphilis. The stage is characterized by organ system symptom complexes divided into neurosyphilis, cardiosyphilis, and benign gummatous syphilis. Neurosyphilis is characterized by meningeal signs, possibly with cranial nerve involvement; meningovascular syphilis and associated CNS ischemia and stroke; parenchymatous neurosyphilis associated with the classic sensory ataxia; and autonomic dysfunction of tabes dorsalis (11,12). Cardiosyphilis occurs as a consequence of spirochete invasion of the coronary vessels and aorta, leading to endarteritis obliterans. Involvement of the aortic root produces scarring and necrosis of the aortic wall media, resulting in aneurysm formation. Benign gummatous syphilis is characterized by destructive lesions (gummata) that affect soft tissue and bone throughout the body. These lesions represent an intense inflammatory response to the spirochete.

Diagnosis.   Studies established for diagnosis are separated into four categories, based in part upon their utility and distinct stages of the disease or with specific clinical manifestations. Dark field examination is used when spirochetes are plentiful and may be obtained from lesions. These include chancres, mucous patches, or fluid from FNA of enlarged lymph nodes. The use of fluorescent antibodies amplifies the utility of dark field examination. Serologic tests for the spirochete include venereal disease research laboratory test (VDRL), rapid plasma reagent test (RPR), unheated serum reagent test (USR), and toluidine red unheated serum test (TRUST), all of which are nontreponemal studies. These tests measure antibody response to treponemal particles and are somewhat nonspecific because other illnesses may cause release of similar antigens. Despite this, these tests may be used to follow treatment response. These tests are not positive following eradication of the disease.

Treponemal tests use the spirochete itself as the antigen and are used to complement the nontreponemal studies in establishing the diagnosis. These include the fluorescent treponemal antibody absorption test (FTA-ABS) and the microhemagglutinin-treponema pallidum test (MHA-TP). Both of these tests remain positive even following disease elimination; therefore, they cannot be used to measure response to treatment.

Treatment.   Parenteral penicillin G is the treatment of choice for syphilis. Dosing schedule and duration of administration vary with the stage and the severity of clinical disease.

Complications and Prognosis.   Untreated syphilis may be associated with significant lifelong disability. Progression of disease into a latent phase or tertiary syphilis occurs in approximately one-third of patients in each category. Untreated tertiary syphilis is associated with serious neurologic and/or cardiovascular complications. Appropriate and timely treatment is successful in the majority of patients diagnosed.

Tularemia

Tularemia is a zoonosis caused by *Francisella tularensis*, a small gram-negative bacillus. It is most commonly contracted by humans through bites of insects and through handling of infected animals, e.g., rabbits, hares, or muskrats. The clinical form infecting humans is ulceroglandular, with an ulcerative lesion on the skin and regional lymphadenitis.

Epidemiology. Although tularemia may be common in endemic areas, the variation in incidence is wide. Highest incidence in endemic areas occurs in the summer months, although the consumption of infected frozen meat will allow for an increase in winter months.

Pathogensis. Inoculation by insect or ingestion of infected meat represents the mode of transmission in humans. The inoculation site, skin or through mucosa, produces a tender ulcerative lesion accompanied by tender lymphadenopathy.

Clinical Manifestations. In patients primarily affected with head and neck disease, a primary ulcer is frequently not present. The only sign of illness may be a cervical mass, with or without general symptoms of infection. In other areas of the body, the inoculation site on skin results in an ulcerative lesion.

Diagnosis. The diagnosis of tularemia is based on paired antibody agglutination titers. Biopsy specimens of affected lymph nodes will show abscess formation with caseating necrosis. In the latter stages of the disease, the histologic picture will demonstrate granulomatous inflammation similar to mycobacterial infection or sarcoid.

Treatment. Treatment of the infection consists of tetracycline or streptomycin. Surgical drainage of abscessed lymph nodes may be necessary. The majority of patients respond favorably to treatment.

Kawasaki Disease

Mucocutaneous lymph node syndrome, or Kawasaki disease, is an acute febrile syndrome noted predominately in children less than 10 years of age.

Epidemiology. The entity, first recognized in Japanese children, demonstrates a predilection for Japanese children or American children with a Japanese background. American cases reported to the CDC indicate that the yearly incidence of Kawasaki disease is three times higher in Asian American children than in black children and more than six times higher in Asian American children than in white children, all under the age of eight, per 100,000. The incidence of the disease is higher in boys and associated with more serious complication in males.

Pathogenesis. The causative entity of the disease is unknown, although an infectious agent is suspected. There is no evidence that the disease is transmissible from person to person. Rickettsia-like bodies have been found in the tissues of some patients, although serologic tests have been negative for Rickettsia.

Clinical Manifestations. The disease is characterized by an early presentation of oropharyngeal inflammation, septic appearance with fever, and cervical adenitis. The appearance of a generalized rash with desquamation occurring over the trunk, with increased cervical adenopathy, follows the early signs. Coronary artery aneurysms and other cardiovascular complications, including coronary thrombosis, myocarditis, pericardial effusions, dysrhythmias, and mitral valve disease, may occur. Aneurysm development may occur in up to 20% of patients.

Diagnosis. Clinical manifestations noted above comprise the predominant criteria required for diagnosis in the absence of another known disease process. A thrombocytosis with elevated peripheral white cell count are associated laboratory findings.

Treatment. The administration of high-dose intravenous gamma globulin plus aspirin appears effective in preventing coronary artery aneurysm formation. This therapy has not been completely effective in eliminating all cardiovascular abnormalities, particularly those involving the coronary arteries.

Please see Chapter 9 for a more detailed discussion of Kawasaki disease.

Human Immunodeficiency Virus

Infection with HIV is often heralded by presenting signs and symptoms involving systems of the head and neck. Hence, otolaryngologists must remain cognizant of this when evaluating patients whose findings may constitute those attributable to HIV infection, for which there is no definitive cure. HIV is discussed in greater detail in Chapter 16.

Definition. HIV infection induces a disabling of T-cell immunocompetency, resulting in a constellation of findings associated with AIDS. Infection may be fulminant in susceptible individuals, accompanied by the full spectrum of AIDS or, alternatively, may pursue a chronic, minimally symptomatic course with appropriate maintenance therapy.

Epidemiology. Patient groups at greatest risk for infection with HIV and development of AIDS include intravenous drug users through contaminated needles and homosexuals engaging in unprotected sexual contact. Heterosexual contact with infected individuals, placental transmission from infected females, and previous blood transfusion–/health worker–related exposure constitute the remaining groups at risk.

Pathogenesis. The etiologic agent in the syndrome is a retrovirus, directed against T-cell–mediated immunity, which results in a susceptibility to develop a broad range of opportunistic infections and a variety of malignancies.

Clinical Manifestations. The systemic manifestations and those related to the head and neck are numerous. In general, they are associated with a specific immuno-deficient disorder caused by the retroviral infection: disseminated mycobacterial infection, cytomegalovirus infection, disseminated fungal infection, *Pneumocystis carinii* pneumonia (PCP), Kaposi's sarcoma, and Hodgkin's and non-Hodgkin's lymphoma, to name several.

Relative to the topic of discussion in this chapter, HIV-related cervical lymphadenopathy is prevalent in persons infected with the virus, occurring in 20% or more of these patients and especially early in infection. In most cases, this proves to be reactive adenitis, as acute HIV infection will often present with persistent generalized lymphatic enlargement (13). The typical constitutional signs and symptoms of fever, malaise, weight loss, and night sweats is commonly accompanied by the development of posterior cervical adenopathy, which is nontender. Less commonly, enlarged cervical nodes may occur as a consequence of a HIV-induced opportunistic infection or neoplasm such as *M. tuberculosis*, cryptococcus, coccidioidomycosis, Kaposi's sarcoma, or lymphoma. Subacute enlarging cervical nodes may progress to necrosis or abscess because of the immunodeficient status of the patient.

Other head and neck manifestations include parotid gland enlargement, oropharyngeal candidiasis, nasopharyngeal neoplasms (Kaposi or lymphoma), oral ulcerations, and oral hairy leukoplakia. Nontender parotid gland enlargement may be a heralding sign of HIV infection (14) and may be uni- or bilateral. Enlargement is most often attributable to the benign lymphoepithelial cyst, which is characterized by uni- or multilocular cyst masses, similar to the benign lymphoepithelial lesion found in Sjögren's syndrome. In contrast to the Sjögren's lesion, the cysts noted in HIV infection are thought to originate from ductal pressure induced by intraparotid lymph node hyperplasia associated with generalized lymphadenopathy (15). Please see Chapter 2 for detailed discussion of Sjögren's syndrome.

Diagnosis. The definitive diagnosis of HIV infection is made with the detection of retroviral antibodies in serum by the enzyme-linked immunosorbent assay (ELISA) test. This is followed by a Western Blot analysis to confirm the presence of retroviral proteins. Fine-needle-aspiration biopsy of cervical lymphadenopathy may be helpful in establishing the diagnosis but a negative result does not imply the absence of HIV-induced pathology.

Treatment.   Treatment is systemically directed with the intent of strengthening and maintaining the immune system. Optimizing the nutritional status of the patient is important in sustaining immunocompetency. Chemotherapy in the form of specific antimicrobial, antifungal, and/or antiviral therapy is directed against the opportunistic entity as indicated. Multidrug therapy is generally required, especially for mycobacterial infection. Neoplastic disease may require multimodality therapy, primarily chemotherapy and radiation. Surgical therapy for Kaposi's sarcoma or squamous cell carcinoma may become necessary. Azidothymidine (AZT) remains a mainstay in the maintenance therapy for chronic HIV infection in order to reduce the retroviral burden and optimize immunocompetence.

Prognosis.   HIV infection and AIDS-related illness remains a universally incurable disease. With improved retroviral drug therapy, patients may remain minimally symptomatic or asymptomatic for longer periods of time as the latent stage of the virus is lengthened. Acute fulminant infection may still quickly overcome the immune system, resulting in overwhelming opportunistic infections in susceptible individuals.

Mononucleosis

Infectious mononucleosis (IM) is a systemic, benign, self-limiting infectious lymphoproliferative disease, primarily caused by the Epstein–Barr virus (EBV). This disease is discussed in more detail in Chapter 10.

Epidemiology.   The disease primarily affects adolescents and young adults; however, it may occur in all age groups and has no gender predilection.

Pathogenesis.   Infection with EBV has been implicated in 85% to 95% of all episodes of IM. EBV is a DNA virus of the family *Herpes viride*. Other microorganisms associated with IM syndrome include cytomegalovirus, *Toxoplasma gondii*, rubella, hepatitis A virus, and certain adenoviruses. The infection is passed on by close personal contact (salivary and respiratory inhalation) with an infected individual.

Clinical Manifestations.   Clinical manifestations of mononucleosis vary considerably from patient to patient. Constitutional symptoms including fever, myalgia, malaise, and anorexia are initial complaints. Acute exudative pharyngotonsillitis is accompanied by tender cervical lymphadenopathy, especially in the posterior cervical chain. Hepatosplenomegaly is a part of the systemic presentation.

Diagnosis.   The diagnosis is confirmed by serologic testing. Paul-Bunnell heterophile agglutination test detects heterophil agglutinins to sheep red blood cells in the serum of patients with IM. A titer of 1:112 or more is considered diagnostic. The Mono Spot test uses horse erythrocytes for antibody detection and is more sensitive. The differential diagnosis of cervical adenitis from IM ranges from acute inflammatory reactive lymphadenopathy to lymphoma (16).

Treatment.   Therapy for IM is supportive including rest, hydration, and antipyretics.

Complications and Prognosis.   In general, the clinical course of IM is self-limited with a favorable prognosis for the majority of patients. Rarely, complications such as airway obstruction, splenic rupture, or cranial neuropathy may develop and can be life threatening.

NONINFECTIOUS DISORDERS

Sarcoidosis

Sarcoidosis is a chronic systemic granulomatous disease of unknown etiology, characterized by the presence of noncaseating granulomas in any organ system of the body. Involvement of the head and neck is noted in 10% to 15% of patients (17). Please see Chapter 6 for a detailed discussion of sarcoidosis.

Epidemiology.   Sarcoid has a slight female preponderance and occurs in all age groups, although more commonly in young adults.

Pathogenesis.   An etiology for sarcoid has not been established. Hallmark pathologic findings for the disorder include noncaseating granulomata consisting of modules of epithelioid histiocytes surrounded by a mixed inflammatory infiltrate (Fig. 7). Intracytoplasmic inclusions, asteroid and Schaumann bodies, can be seen. Special stains for a multiplicity of microorganisms are noted to be negative.

Clinical Manifestations.   Any organ system may be affected by sarcoid, but pulmonary and cutaneous involvement are typically noted. Otolaryngologic signs and symptoms include cervical lymphadenopathy (occurring in 50% of patients affected with head and neck disease), pharyngotonsillitis, nasal discharge and epistaxis, and salivary gland enlargement. Concurrent involvement of the uveal tract and parotid gland, "uveo-parotid fever" or "Heerfordts syndrome," may be accompanied by facial nerve palsy.

Diagnosis.   The differential diagnosis of sarcoid includes mycobacterial infection, fungal disease, and cat-scratch syndrome. The confirmation of sarcoid is usually secured with a demonstration of the typical histologic characteristics on tissue biopsy in the absence of an identifying infectious agent. The recommended evaluation of patients with suspected sarcoid includes chest radiographs, PPD with anergy panel, serum profile including liver function studies, erythrocyte sedimentation rate (ESR), and angiotensin

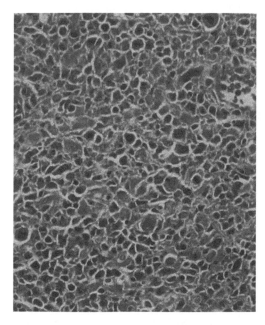

FIGURE 7   Infectious mononucleosis in a lymph node demonstrating cytologic atypia that may be mistaken for malignant lymphoma.

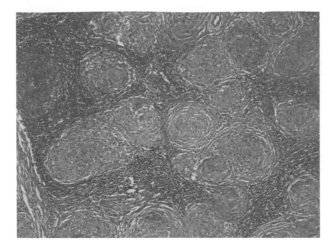

FIGURE 8 Histologic section from lymph node affected by sarcoidosis demonstrating non-caseating granulomas. *Source*: Photo courtesy of Dr. Robert Brown.

converting enzyme (ACE) levels. Although the ESR is elevated in most patients with sarcoid, it is nonspecific. The ACE level is elevated in the majority (80%) of patients with sarcoid but may be elevated in other rare granulomatous entities (Gaucher's disease and leprosy) and is not pathognomonic. However, when the clinical suspicion for sarcoid is high, elevation in ACE will support the diagnosis of the disease. Further, the ACE level will indicate the activity of the disease and thus may serve to assess treatment response.

Treatment. Therapy for sarcoid, especially for early-stage asymptomatic disease, is usually not necessary, because the disorder frequently undergoes spontaneous remission. Patients with more advanced disease, such as those with symptomatic pulmonary involvement, are treated with systemic corticosteroids; the majority responds favorably to treatment.

Prognosis. Most patients (70%) experience spontaneous resolution or successful treatment of disease. A small percentage of patients progress to advanced multisystem disease, leading to restrictive pulmonary disease and respiratory failure.

Nodular Fasciitis

Nodular fasciitis, sometimes known as pseudosarcomatous fasciitis, is a non-neoplastic proliferation of fibroblasts affecting soft tissue. Although not a classic systemic illness, it may affect any area of the body and can occur in the head and neck in as many as 20% of patients.

Epidemiology. There is no gender predominance in nodular fasciitis and the disorder commonly occurs in the third to fifth decades of life. Paradoxically, involvement of the head and neck, usually the neck, is more common in infants and children than in adults.

Pathogenesis. The disorder arises from the superficial fascial layers presenting in subcutaneous areas. There is no known etiologic agent, although a traumatic incident may induce the proliferative process.

Clinical Manifestations. A solitary painless mass in the area of involvement is the only clinical finding. The proliferative process may also affect deeper connective tissue layers arising within deep fascia or muscle.

Diagnosis. The diagnosis is established with tissue biopsy–usually incisional or excisional. The most important aspect of the diagnostic workup is the elimination of the possibility of a sarcoma. Histologically, the lesion is unencapsulated, with a proliferation of plump-appearing fibroblasts arranged in whorled fascicles (18).

Treatment. Local excision is the treatment of choice, with less than 5% of patients developing a recurrence. Spontaneous remission may occur in some patients.

Prognosis. The outcome for all patients is universally good.

Tangier Disease

Tangier disease is an autosomal-recessive disorder of lipoprotein metabolism that results in the deposition of xanthomatous cells in lymph nodes, tonsils, palate, spleen, and liver.

Epidemiology. The disorder was initially observed on Tangier Island in the Chesapeake Bay area of the United States. There appears to be gender predilection with the disease occurring in all age groups.

Pathogenesis. Tangier disease results in a deficiency of high-density lipoproteins and low levels of apoproteins. The metabolic imbalance ultimately results in deposition of clear xanthomatous cells throughout involved tissue.

Clinical Manifestations. Enlargement of involved tissues, including lymph nodes, is the presenting sign. Involvement of the tonsils demonstrates enlargement with a yellow appearance resembling pharyngotonsillitis. Cervical adenopathy is nontender.

Diagnosis. Tissue biopsy establishes the diagnosis. Histologically, multifocal deposition of clear cells is noted in the involved tissues.

Treatment. In general, no specific treatment is warranted unless symptoms occur. Significant tonsillar enlargement may require tonsillectomy.

Prognosis. The prognosis is good; however, coronary atherosclerosis is common in patients over 40 years of age.

NON-INFLAMMATORY DISORDERS

Non-inflammatory processes that may result in cervical lymph node enlargement and/or pain include neoplasms of the lympho-reticular system, such as lymphoma and leukemia, and neuromusculoskeletal disorders such as fibromyalgia and reflex-sympathetic dystrophy.

The constellation of signs and symptoms demonstrated by these entities is large and varied, warranting a discussion for each, which is beyond the scope of this chapter.

SUMMARY

Cervical adenitis, with or without pain, may represent the heralding sign of systemic disease. Although some of the causative entities may be self-limited and benign in course, others involve disorders that, if not recognized, may progress to serious illness. It is important that otolaryngologists remain vigilant so that these disease processes may be recognized when presenting initially in the head and neck.

REFERENCES

1. Al-Serhani AM. Mycobacterial infection of the head and neck: presentation and diagnosis. Laryngoscope 2001; 111(11 Pt 1):2012–2016.

2. Williams RG, Douglas-Jones T. Mycobacterium marches back. J Laryngol Otol 1995; 109(1): 5–13.
3. Manelpe AH, Lee KC. Tuberculous infections of the head and neck. Cur Opin Oto/HNS 1998; 6:190.
4. Rahal A, Abela A, Arcand PH, et al. Nontuberculous mycobacterial adenitis of the head and neck in children: experience from a tertiary care pediatric center. Laryngoscope 2001; 111(10): 1791–1796.
5. Carithers HA, Carithers CM, Edwards RO Jr. Cat-scratch disease: its natural history. JAMA 1969; 207(2):312–316.
6. Spires JR, Smith RJ. Cat-scratch disease. Otolaryngol Head Neck Surg 1986; 94(5):622–627.
7. Steere AC, Malawista SE, Snydman DR, et al. Lyme arthritis: an epidemic of oligoarticular arthritis in children and adults in three Connecticut communities. Arthritis Rheum 1977; 20(1):7–17.
8. Steere AC, Bartenhagen NH, Craft JE, et al. The early clinical manifestations of Lyme disease. Ann Intern Med 1983; 99(1):76–82.
9. Cates W Jr, Rothenberg RB, Blount JH. Syphilis control. The historic context and epidemiologic basis for interrupting sexual transmission of *Treponema pallidum*. Sex Transm Dis 1996; 23(1): 68–75.
10. Division of STD Prevention. Sexually transmitted disease surveillance, 1999, Atlanta, Centers for disease control and prevention (CDC), US Dept of Health and Human Services, 2000.
11. Wilcox RR, Godwin PG. Nerve deafness in early syphilis. Br J Vener Dis 1971; 47(6): 401–406.
12. Holmes MD, Brant-Zawadzki MM, Simon RP. Clinical features of meningovascular syphilis. Neurology 1984; 34(4):553–556.
13. Ellison E, LaPuerta P, Martin SE. Supraclavicular masses: results of a series of 309 cases biopsied by fine needle aspiration. Head Neck 1999; 21(3):239–246.
14. Kim MK, Alvi A. Common head and neck manifestations of AIDS. AIDS patient care STDS 1999; 13(11):641–644.
15. Sperling NM, Lin PT. Parotid disease associated with human immunodeficiency virus infection. Ear Nose Throat J 1990; 69(7):475–477.
16. Som PM, Brandwein MS, Silvers A. Nodal inclusion cysts of the parotid gland and parapharyngeal space: a discussion of lymphoepithelial, AIDS-related parotid, and branchial cysts, cystic Warthin's tumors and cysts in Sjögren's syndrome. Laryngoscope 1995; 105(10):1122–1128.
17. Salvador AH, Harrison EG Jr, Kyle RA. Lymphadenopathy due to infectious mononucleosis: its confusion with malignant lymphoma. Cancer 1971; 27(5):1029–1040.
18. McCaffrey TV, McDonald TJ. Sarcoidosis of the nose and paranasal sinuses. Laryngoscope 1983; 93 (10):1281–1284.
19. Cohen JP, Lachman LJ, Hammerschlag PE. Reversible facial paralysis in sarcoidosis. Confirmation by serum angiotensin-converting enzyme assay. Arch Otolaryngol 1983; 109(12):832–835.
20. DiNardo LJ, Wetmore RF, Potsic WP. Nodular fasciitis of the head and neck in children. A deceptive lesion. Arch Otolaryngol Head Neck Surg 1991; 117(9):1001–1002.
21. Schoenberg BS, Schoenberg DG. Eponym: tangerine tonsils in Tangier: high-density lipoprotein deficiency. South Med J 1978; 71(4):453–454.

37

Dermatologic Signs of Systemic Disease

Antoanella Bardan and Tissa Hata
Department of Medicine, Division of Dermatology, University of California, San Diego, California, U.S.A.

INTRODUCTION

Changes in the skin are often the first and most easily identifiable signs of systemic disease. This is especially true in the head and neck area. This chapter will discuss the cutaneous signs of Cowden's disease, Muir-Torre syndrome (MTS), Peutz-Jeghers syndrome (PJS), hereditary hemorrhagic telangiectasia (HHT), Stevens-Johnson syndrome (SJS), Hansen's disease, and glucagonoma in the area of the head and neck.

COWDEN'S SYNDROME

DEFINITION

Cowden syndrome (CS), also known as multiple hamartoma syndrome or Cowden disease, was first described by Lloyd and Dennis in 1963 (1) as a multisystem disorder with characteristic mucocutaneous lesions and abnormalities of the breast, thyroid, and gastrointestinal tract. They named the disorder after their first patient, Rachel Cowden, who died due to breast cancer. CS is a rare genetic disorder with an autosomal-dominant pattern of inheritance and variable expressivity. Characteristic lesions present in nearly all patients with CS include trichilemmomas on the face, acral keratoses on the hands, and oral papillomas of the mouth. Benign and malignant neoplasms of the breast and thyroid occur in up to two-thirds of patients. Intestinal tract hamartomatous polyps are seen in more than one-half of patients (2).

EPIDEMIOLOGY

CS is estimated to affect 1 in 200,000 individuals and has a strong female predominance. More than 150 cases have been reported in the literature and the majority of patients have been Caucasian. CS may be more common than has actually been reported, due to its variable expressivity and often subtle clinical findings (3).

PATHOGENESIS

Germline mutations in *PTEN*, a gene mapped to chromosome 10q22-23, have been found in most cases of CS (4). *PTEN* consists of nine exons spanning 100 kb of DNA and encodes a dual specificity phosphatase, which acts as a tumor-suppressor gene. Tissues capable of proliferation, such as epidermis, thyroid, and breast epithelium, and the oral and gastrointestinal mucosa are affected by disruption of this gene. *PTEN* mutations have also been observed in patients with Bannayan-Riley-Ruvalcaba (BRR) syndrome (characterized by hamartomatous polyps of the small and large intestine), and Lhermitte-Duclos disease (LDD), characterized by hamartomatous overgrowth of the cerebellar ganglion cells. This region was also found to be frequently deleted in thyroid tumors, and somatic mutations spanning this region are commonly found in glioblastoma, breast cancers (in association with CS), and advanced prostate cancer.

CLINICAL MANIFESTATIONS

Almost all patients with CS have characteristic mucocutaneous lesions that most often begin to appear in their second and third decades of life, although the age of onset of the skin signs varies from 4 to 75 years of age. The most frequently found cutaneous lesions are facial papules, which present as skin-colored or yellowish-tan verrucous papules that can resemble common warts and histologically reveal trichilemmomas or nonspecific hair follicle proliferations. These papules can be very numerous and can coalesce around facial orifices and ears (Fig. 1). The oral lesions present as 1 to 3 mm skin-colored papules, which can coalesce to form a characteristic cobblestone pattern (Fig. 2), or can be so extensive that they involve the entire oral cavity, including the tongue. Involvement of the mucosa is seen in over 80% of patients and usually follows the development of the facial lesions. Other cutaneous findings in CS include lipomas, hemangiomas, xanthomas, vitiligo, neuromas, café-au-lait spots, periorificial and acral lentigines, and acanthosis nigricans (2).

Although nearly every internal malignancy has been reported in association with CS, breast cancer is the most frequent and most serious complication, occurring in approximately 25% to 36% of female patients with CS. Men with germline *PTEN* mutations are also at risk of developing breast carcinomas. Fibrocystic disease of the breast and fibroadenomas is seen in 75% of women with CS.

Thyroid disease, including goiter, benign adenomas, fetal adenomas, thyroglossal duct cysts, and follicular adenocarcinoma, occurs in approximately two-thirds of patients with CS.

Other extracutaneous manifestations of CS include multiple hamartomatous polyps, which can be found anywhere in the gastrointestinal tract; benign ovarian cysts; leiomyomas of the uterus; and less frequently, teratomas, transitional cell carcinomas, and cervical cancer. Craniomegaly occurs in 80% of patients and is the most common skeletal manifestation of the disease. Ocular abnormalities are rare and include angioid streaks, cataracts, and myopia.

DIAGNOSIS

The diagnosis of CS is made according to the operational criteria established by the 2000 International CS Consortium (Table 1). CS overlaps with several other hamartomatous

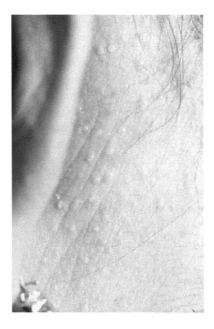

FIGURE 1   Postauricular trichilemmomas in a patient with Cowden syndrome. Courtesy of Dr. Terence O'Grady, University of California San Diego.

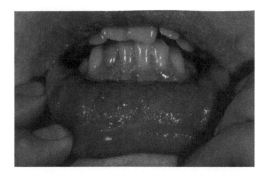

FIGURE 2 Trichilemmomas coalescing to form the characteristic cobblestone pattern on the oral mucosa of a patient with Cowden syndrome. Courtesy of Dr. Terence O'Grady, University of California San Diego.

syndromes, including BRR and LDD. LDD was once considered a distinct entity, but it is now thought to be a neurologic manifestation of CS, due to reports of mutations in the *PTEN* gene in patients with LDD. BRR has also been reported to have mutations in the *PTEN* gene, explaining the significant clinical overlap seen between BRR and CS, but lacks the high penetrance of cancer seen with CS.

Biopsy of the skin lesions to confirm the diagnosis of trichilemmomas is necessary, since their clinical appearance is nonspecific. The differential diagnosis of multiple facial trichilemmomas includes benign warts, angiofibromas, multiple fibrofolliculomas, and multiple basal cell cancers. Less commonly, the facial papules seen in CS can be mistaken for syringomas, steatocystomas, or even neurofibromas.

TREATMENT

The facial papules of CS respond variably to 5-fluorouracil, oral retinoids, curettage, laser ablation, cryosurgery, dermabrasion, or surgical excision, but the effects are temporary and often unsatisfactory. Thyroid function studies, thyroid scanning and/or ultrasound,

TABLE 1 International Cowden Syndrome Consortium Operational Criteria, 2000

Pathognomonic criteria	Major criteria	Minor criteria
Facial trichilemmomata	Breast carcinoma	Mental retardation
Acral keratoses	Nonmedullary thyroid cancer	Gastrointestinal disorder
Papillomatous papules	Macrocephaly	Hamartomata
Mucosal lesions	Lhermitte-Duclos disease	Other thyroid lesions
–	Endometrial carcinoma	Fibrocystic breast disease

Diagnosis in an individual can be established by any of the following:
1. Mucocutaneous lesions alone:
    Six or more facial papules, of which three or more must be trichilemmomas, or
    Cutaneous facial papules and oral mucosal papillomatosis, or
    Oral mucosal papillomatosis and acral keratoses, or
    Six or more palmoplantar keratoses
2. Two major criteria *but* one must include macrocephaly or Lhermitte-Duclos disease
3. One major and three minor criteria
4. Four minor criteria

Diagnosis for a patient with a family history of Cowden syndrome can be established by:
1. Any pathognomonic criterion
2. Any major criterion
3. Two minor criteria

complete blood count, urinalysis, mammography, chest radiography, pap smear, and uterine ultrasound should be performed as baseline studies in all patients and followed up periodically as indicated.

COMPLICATIONS AND PROGNOSIS

Complications of CS are a consequence of carcinoma development and are seen more frequently when diagnosis is delayed. A good prognosis depends on the early diagnosis and subsequent appropriate screening.

SUMMARY

Mucocutaneous lesions (trichilemmomas, acral keratoses, oral papillomas, and sclerotic fibromas) are the most important markers for CS since they are present in nearly all patients and frequently precede the development of internal disease. Early diagnosis of CS can lead to earlier detection and more effective treatment of the associated neoplasms.

*M*UIR-TORRE SYNDROME

DEFINITION

MTS consists of unusual cutaneous sebaceous neoplasms, keratoacanthomas (KAs), and internal malignancies. It was described independently by Muir (5) and Torre (6) in 1967. Their two patients had several internal malignancies and multiple KA-like lesions or multiple tumors of sebaceous origin.

EPIDEMIOLOGY

MTS is inherited in an autosomal-dominant manner; it has a high degree of penetrance and variable expressivity. Over 200 cases of MTS have been reported. MTS is seen in males more than in females, with a 3:2 male to female ratio, and the median age at diagnosis is 55 years. The sebaceous neoplasms precede or are concurrent with visceral malignancies in 41% of patients and occur after diagnosis of internal malignancy in 59% of patients (7).

PATHOGENESIS

MTS is part of the Lynch cancer family syndrome II, a subset of the hereditary nonpolyposis colorectal cancer syndromes and is caused by a mutation in the *MSH2* gene, a DNA mismatch-repair gene located on chromosome 2p. Mutations of another mismatch-repair gene, *MLH1*, located on chromosome 3p, have also been reported in MTS. Mutations in these DNA repair genes lead to tumor formation due to microsatellite instability.

CLINICAL MANIFESTATIONS

The defining features of MTS are at least one sebaceous adenoma, epithelioma, or carcinoma (excluding sebaceous hyperplasia and nevus sebaceous of Jadassohn) and at least one visceral cancer (7). Sebaceous tumors, of which sebaceous adenomas are most common, are usually located in the head and neck region and are often periocular. Sebaceous adenomas present as yellow papules or nodules and can be solitary or multiple (Fig. 3). Sebaceous carcinomas can be ocular or extraocular, both of which share a high risk of metastases to regional lymph nodes, bones, and viscera. Periocular sebaceous carcinomas can present as chronic blepharoconjunctivitis, recurrent chalazions, carbuncles, or painless nodules on the inner eyelid and are usually not associated with an underlying internal malignancy. However, because many patients with MTS have a sebaceous gland carcinoma, any sebaceous carcinoma must be considered as a possible marker for this syndrome.

KAs are seen in approximately 25% of patients with MTS and can also be solitary or multiple. KAs present as erythematous papules or nodules that arise within a few weeks and often have a central keratotic plug (Fig. 4).

The most commonly observed malignancies are colorectal carcinomas, which can be seen in more than 60% of patients and are usually located proximal to or at the splenic flexure, unlike colorectal cancer seen in the general population. The second most common site is the genitourinary tract, representing close to a quarter of all primary cancers in patients with MTS. Other cancers reported in patients with MTS include breast carcinomas, hematologic malignancies, head and neck cancers, lung carcinoma, chondrosarcoma, and neoplasms of the small intestine. More than one-third of patients with MTS have two or three visceral malignancies.

DIAGNOSIS

The diagnosis of MTS is based on the presence of a cutaneous sebaceous adenoma, sebaceous epithelioma, basal cell epithelioma with sebaceous differentiation, KA with sebaceous differentiation, or sebaceous carcinoma, and at least one visceral malignancy, in the absence of another probable cause (Table 2). The cutaneous sebaceous adenoma is probably the most sensitive marker for MTS, but any sebaceous neoplasm except sebaceous hyperplasia or nevus sebaceous of Jadassohn should raise the possibility of MTS. Multiple primary malignancies, especially if low grade, as well as multiple KAs, should prompt consideration of MTS. Seboacanthoma, a type of sebaceous adenoma, may be specific to this syndrome. Additionally, it has been suggested that cystic sebaceous

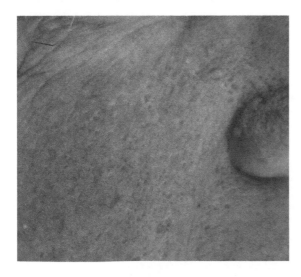

FIGURE 3 Multiple skin-colored, pearly papules representing sebaceous adenomas and carcinomas in a patient with Muir-Torre syndrome. Courtesy of Dr. Daniel Synkowski, University of California San Diego.

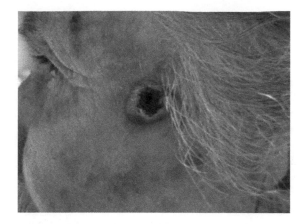

FIGURE 4 Keratoacanthoma. Erythematous nodule with heaped-up borders and a central crateriform ulceration.

tumors, many of which exhibit the microsatellite instability characteristic to this syndrome, may be a marker for the mismatch-repair defect seen in MTS.

TREATMENT

Sebaceous adenomas and sebaceous epitheliomas can be treated with excision, cryosurgery, or curettage. Mohs micrographic surgery is recommended for lesions of sebaceous carcinoma. Oral retinoids may prevent the formation of new sebaceous neoplasms in patients with MTS.

Complete and regular examinations for gastrointestinal and genitourinary cancer are recommended, and some suggest annual colonoscopy beginning at age 25. Women should have routine gynecologic examinations consisting of yearly breast and pelvic examinations and Pap smears, supplemented by endometrial aspiration or biopsy and transvaginal ultrasound as needed starting at age 30.

COMPLICATIONS AND PROGNOSIS

Visceral malignancies in MTS are low grade, and surgical removal of primary tumors and even metastases can be curative. Although many patients with MTS have metastatic

TABLE 2 Diagnostic Criteria for MTS

Group A	Group B	Group C
Sebaceous adenoma	Visceral malignancy	Multiple keratoacanthomas
Sebaceous epithelioma		Multiple visceral malignancies
Sebaceous carcinoma		Family history of MTS
Keratoacanthoma with sebaceous differentiation		
Diagnosis requires one criterion from Group A and Group B, or all three from Group C, in absence of predisposing factors such as extensive radiotherapy or AIDS		

Abbreviation: MTS, Muir-Torre syndrome.

disease, the cancers in many of these patients display a nonaggressive course. The median survival rate at 12 years after diagnosis is approximately 50%. Patients can live 25 to 30 years after resection of their first visceral neoplasms. Interestingly, a study evaluating microsatellite instability in tumor tissue of patients with MTS showed that patients who exhibited this finding had earlier onset of colorectal cancers and almost three times as many visceral cancers, but had significantly prolonged survival after visceral cancer diagnosis.

SUMMARY

MTS is likely more common than is reported. Identification of patients with MTS is important since all affected family members are at risk for developing visceral malignancies. Sebaceous adenomas, epitheliomas, and carcinomas, as well as any difficult to classify sebaceous neoplasm, should be viewed as a possible marker of MTS. Molecular genetic studies may facilitate the diagnosis of MTS.

*P*EUTZ-JEGHERS SYNDROME

DEFINITION

PJS consists of mucocutaneous hyperpigmentation and hamartomatous polyps of the gastrointestinal tract. PJS was described by Peutz in 1921. Hutchinson described the cutaneous findings present in this syndrome in 1896, but it was not until 1949 that Jeghers proposed their diagnostic significance.

EPIDEMIOLOGY

PJS affects men and women equally and has been described in many ethnic groups. Its prevalence is approximately 1:200,000 (8). It has an autosomal-dominant pattern of inheritance with variable penetrance. It is estimated that 25% to 50% of cases are due to sporadic mutations.

PATHOGENESIS

PJS is caused by a mutation in the *LKB1* (also known as *STK11*) gene, a serine threonine kinase, which has been mapped to chromosome 19p13.3 and is thought to be a tumor-suppressor gene. *LKB1* is a multifunctional kinase, which has been found to play a role in chromatin remodeling, cell cycle arrest, Wnt signaling, cell polarity, and energy metabolism. Mutations of this gene may interfere with its function as a tumor suppressor, but the signaling mechanisms that lead to PJS-related malignancies are not yet well understood (9).

CLINICAL MANIFESTATIONS

The mucocutaneous lesions of PJS consist of hyperpigmented (dark brown to black), round, 1 to 5 mm macules distributed on the central part of the face, lips, and oral mucosa (Fig. 5). Hyperpigmented macules may also be seen on the dorsal hands, feet, perianal area,

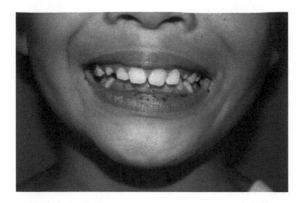

FIGURE 5 Multiple mucosal lentigines in a patient with Peutz-Jeghers
syndrome. Courtesy of Dr. Lawrence
Eichen field, University of California,
San Diego

and periumbilical skin. The macules can be present at birth or arise early in life. The
cutaneous lesions can fade with time, but the mucosal hyperpigmentation remains. The
hyperpigmented macules in PJS can be distinguished from freckles by their mucosal
involvement and the fact that they are commonly present at birth. The mucocutaneous
lesions in PJS precede the gastrointestinal manifestations. The median time to presentation
with polyps is 11 years of age, but the age of onset varies greatly. There are reported cases
of patients presenting with polyposis at birth, but this is very rare. Extraintestinal polyposis
may develop and can involve the nares, pelvis, bladder, and lungs. Although the rate of
neoplastic potential of the intestinal lesions is low, 48% of patients with PJS have been
reported to develop intestinal and extraintestinal malignancies that include neoplasms of
the colon, esophagus, rectum, stomach, small intestine, breast, pancreas, ovaries, cervix,
testicles, and uterus.

DIAGNOSIS

Clinical diagnosis of PJS is based on the mucocutaneous findings and the histologic
appearance of the polyps, which exhibit a unique microscopic morphology, with mucosa
interdigitating with smooth muscle fibers to form a characteristic arborizing pattern. A
definite diagnosis of PJS can be established by the presence of histopathologically
confirmed hamartomatous polyps and two of the following clinical criteria: family history,
hyperpigmentation, and small bowel polyposis. A probable diagnosis is based on the
clinical findings in the absence of histologic confirmation of hamartomatous polyps. To
confirm the diagnosis, genetic testing may be used, as screening for the *LKB1* mutation is
commercially available.

The differential diagnosis of PJS includes juvenile polyposis (polyposis without the
hyperpigmented macules), Cronkhite-Canada syndrome (polyposis and cutaneous
hyperpigmentation, but no mucosal lentigines), and Laugier-Hunziker syndrome
(mucocutaneous hyperpigmentation without gastrointestinal polyps).

TREATMENT

The mucocutaneous hyperpigmented macules seen in PJS are benign, and treatment is for
cosmetic purposes only. Large or symptomatic gastrointestinal polyps should be removed
and screening stool studies, radiologic studies, upper endoscopy, and colonoscopy are
recommended for any adolescent or adult suspected of having PJS. Patients also need to be

monitored regularly for extraintestinal malignancies with abdominal ultrasounds, annual breast exams, pelvic exams, and testicular exams, beginning at adolescence.

COMPLICATIONS AND PROGNOSIS

The polyps in PJS are benign hamartomas and have a low rate of malignant transformation, but because the polyps progress with age, they can lead to recurrent abdominal pain, bleeding, anemia, intussusception, and obstruction. Patients with PJS are susceptible to a multitude of internal malignancies, including tumors of the gastrointestinal tract, pancreas, testicles, ovaries, cervix, and uterus; aggressive screening protocols as mentioned above are recommended to decrease morbidity and mortality.

SUMMARY

PJS is an autosomal-dominant disorder characterized by hyperpigmented macules distributed on the central part of the face and intestinal polyps, which are commonly seen years after the cutaneous lesions. Patients with PJS are at higher risk for developing internal malignancies and should be appropriately screened.

*H*EREDITARY HEMORRHAGIC TELANGIECTASIA

DEFINITION

HHT, also known as Osler-Weber-Rendu disease, is a fairly common autosomal-dominant condition characterized by telangiectases of the dermis and mucous membranes and visceral arteriovenous malformations (AVMs). HHT was first reported in 1864 by Sutton and was named in 1909 by Hanes, who first described its histologic features. The triple eponymous title, Osler-Weber-Rendu, draws its name form Henri Rendu, Sir William Osler, and Frederick Weber, who published remarkably descriptive and accurate case reports of the disease at the turn of the last century (10).

EPIDEMIOLOGY

HHT has a wide ethnic and geographic distribution, with a prevalence of more than 1 in 10,000 people (11). It is inherited as an autosomal-dominant disease and now appears to be much more common than previously reported.

PATHOGENESIS

To date, mutations in two genes have been linked to HHT, accounting for most but not all clinical cases. Mutations of the *ENG* gene, localized to the long arm of chromosome 9 (9q33-q34.1), cause HHT1; mutations of the gene encoding activin receptor-like kinase 1, *ALK1* (also known as *ACVRL1*), localized on the long arm of chromosome 12 (12q11-q14), cause HHT2. It is not clear whether genotype-phenotype correlations can be established in HHT, but there may be a higher prevalence of pulmonary AVMs in HHT1.

ENG and *ALK1* encode receptor proteins, which are members of the transforming growth factor-beta (TGF β) superfamily. Therefore, HHT is caused by a disturbance in the

TGF β signaling pathway, which is an important pathway involved in cellular proliferation, differentiation, adhesion, and migration. However, the exact mechanism of how a disturbance of this pathway leads to HHT remains unclear.

CLINICAL MANIFESTATIONS

HHT is characterized by skin, mucosal membrane, and visceral telangiectasias, recurrent epistaxis, and visceral hemorrhages. The recurrent epistaxis is usually the first and most common sign of the disease. The lesions seen on physical exam are small, dark red telangiectases, with ill-defined borders and stellate appearance, occurring most commonly on the face, lips, tongue, palms, and fingers (Fig. 6). The telangiectasias seen on the skin and mucous membranes actually represent small AVMs, which explains their propensity to bleed. Visceral AVMs are found mostly in the lungs, central nervous system (CNS), upper gastrointestinal tract, and liver. The number and location of telangiectasias and AVMs vary widely between individuals and within the same family. The external, visible signs (telangiectasias and frequent nose bleeds) often do not manifest until the second or third decade of life. Internal AVMs in the brain, spinal cord, and lungs are thought to be largely congenital lesions and may present suddenly and with serious complication soon after birth or at an early age. If recognized, the underlying AVM is usually treatable.

DIAGNOSIS AND TREATMENT

Individuals with HHT should receive an initial workup at the time of diagnosis, followed by preventive care and surveillance. Recommended workup for patients with HHT includes complete blood count (CBC), evaluation for stool occult blood, brain magnetic resonance imaging to evaluate for cerebral AVMs, contrast echocardiography to screen for pulmonary shunting followed by chest computed tomography to evaluate pulmonary AVMs if shunting is found, and evaluation for liver involvement by listening for bruits on physical exam. Patients with evidence of pulmonary shunting should be placed on prophylactic antibiotics to prevent infected emboli. Pulmonary and cerebral AVMs are treated using transcatheter embolization, while treatment for symptomatic liver

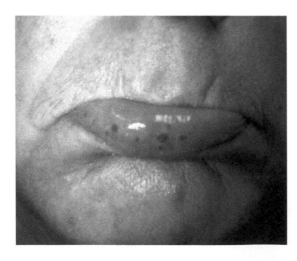

FIGURE 6 Matted telangiectasias on the lip of a patient with hereditary hemorrhagic telangiectasia. Courtesy of Dr. Terence O'Grady, University of California San Diego.

involvement consists of liver transplantation due to the high risk of liver infarction with embolization. Skin lesions usually require no treatment except for cosmetic reasons. Mild epistaxis is usually managed conservatively. Careful laser ablation is an effective treatment for moderate epistaxis; severe epistaxis can be treated by septal dermoplasty using split thickness skin grafts. Anemia secondary to gastrointestinal bleeding or epistaxis can usually be treated with iron supplementation. Additionally, patients with HHT should avoid medications that interfere with normal coagulation.

Given the complexity of care required for patients with HHT, multidisciplinary teams specializing in the treatment of these patients are ideal and usually consist of ear, nose, and throat (ENT) surgeons, interventional radiologists, pulmonologists, neuroradiologists, neurosurgeons, medical geneticists, genetic counselors, cardiologists, gastroenterologists, hematologists, and sometimes neurologists and pediatricians.

Individuals at risk for HHT should undergo evaluation to determine whether they are carriers of the disease. DNA testing is available and can be performed in relatives of patients with HHT.

COMPLICATIONS AND PROGNOSIS

Common complications in patients with HHT include upper and lower gastrointestinal bleeding, paradoxical emboli, and neurologic deficits. Underdiagnosed pulmonary and CNS AVMs can lead to severe complications and death. Prognosis in patients who are diagnosed early and followed up regularly by a specialized HHT multidisciplinary team is good. Patients with liver, pulmonary, and CNS involvement have a poorer prognosis.

SUMMARY

HHT is a relatively common, underdiagnosed autosomal-dominant disorder of AVMs and telangiectases, often first suspected in children with repeated epistaxis. Telangiectasias are often seen on the lips. AVMs are commonly found in the gastrointestinal tract, lungs, and brain, and can also be found in other organs. Mutations of *ENG* and *ALK1* are responsible for most cases of HHT; DNA testing is available. Preventive care and surveillance are very important for patients with HHT.

*S*TEVENS-JOHNSON SYNDROME

DEFINITION

SJS was first described in 1922 by two American physicians, Stevens and Johnson, who reported an acute mucocutaneous syndrome characterized by severe purulent conjunctivitis, severe stomatitis, extensive mucosal necrosis, and skin lesions of erythema multiforme (EM) in two young boys. SJS was later designated EM major by Bernard Thomas in 1950, but this designation is not currently accepted, as SJS and EM are now considered distinct disorders.

SJS is a rapidly progressive mucocutaneous eruption usually preceded by a respiratory illness, characterized by severe erosions of at least two mucosal surfaces with variable skin involvement ranging from erythematous macules to bullae and skin necrosis, and accompanied by fever, lymphadenopathy, and toxicity (12).

EPIDEMIOLOGY

The precise incidence of SJS is not known, due to clinical and histologic overlap with toxic epidermal necrolysis (TEN) and resulting confusion over the exact definition of these two disorders. The estimated incidence of SJS is 0.8 cases per million inhabitants with a peak incidence in the second decade of life and the majority of patients being children. Spring and summer peaks have been observed and there seems to be no sex or racial predilection.

PATHOGENESIS

There are many reported causes of SJS, but drugs represent the most common association. Among the most frequent offenders are nonsteroidal anti-inflammatory drugs (NSAIDs), sulfonamides, anticonvulsants, penicillins, doxycycline, and tetracyclines. In contrast to EM, infectious causes are not as frequently implicated (12). Other reported causative factors include fungal and viral infections, X-irradiation, and inflammatory bowel disease.

The mechanism through which NSAIDs, sulfonamides, and anticonvulsants may lead to SJS involves accumulation of arene oxides due to a deficiency in epoxide hydrolase in susceptible individuals (13). Genetic differences in the detoxification of drugs may be responsible and several enzymes have been implicated, including those responsible for acetylation and arene hydroxylation. Mucosal lesions follow ingestion of the drug by 14 to 56 days in drug-associated SJS, and drugs administered a few days prior to the onset of SJS are usually not implicated.

The pathogenesis of SJS in infectious-related disease remains unknown. Auto-antibodies to desmoplakin I and II, causing cell separation through disruption in the keratin cytoskeleton, have been detected in patients with SJS, but it is not known if these autoantibodies are primarily involved in the pathogenesis of SJS or merely play a role in the evolution of the disease.

CLINICAL MANIFESTATIONS

Most patients with SJS have a distinct prodrome of an upper respiratory illness with fever, sore throat, rhinitis, malaise, vomiting, and diarrhea 1 to 14 days prior to the mucocutaneous eruption. Two or more mucosal sites must be involved to make the diagnosis of SJS. The oral mucosa is always involved with extensive superficial necrosis of the lips and mouth, leading to hemorrhagic crusts and followed by denudation of the mucosa and severe stomatitis (Fig. 7). Purulent conjunctivitis with photophobia can be seen. Anal and genital mucosa, and less commonly the esophagus, respiratory epithelium, and nasal mucosa can also be involved.

Most patients with SJS have skin lesions in addition to the mucosal involvement. The skin lesions usually start as red macules and may be limited to a few targetoid lesions or may evolve rapidly into widespread dusky-red macules, which can become confluent.

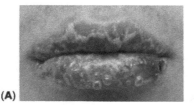
(A)

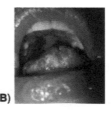
(B)

FIGURE 7 Extensive mucosal necrosis of the lips (**A**) and severe stomatitis (**B**) in a patient with Stevens-Johnson syndrome. Courtesy of Dr.

The lesions are usually tender and the patient is usually unable to eat or drink. Patients with SJS appear acutely ill and may have generalized lymphadenopathy or even hepatosplenomegaly. Arthralgias, hepatitis, nephritis, myocarditis, and gastrointestinal bleeding are occasionally seen.

An elevated erythrocyte sedimentation rate (ESR) is found in all patients with SJS; leukocytosis can be seen in more than one-half of patients. Other laboratory abnormalities include eosinophilia, elevated liver enzymes, leukopenia, proteinuria, and microscopic hematuria.

DIAGNOSIS

The diagnosis of SJS is made clinically, based on the characteristic prodrome of a respiratory illness followed by mucocutaneous necrosis involving at least two mucous membranes. Patients with widespread cutaneous necrosis can be difficult to classify, leading to confusion when trying to separate SJS from TEN, especially since the same factors can precipitate both. All forms of SJS have overlapping features with TEN, but most consider the condition to be SJS if two or more mucosal sites are involved. To distinguish SJS from EM, a skin biopsy showing extensive areas of epidermal necrosis can be helpful, as this should only be seen in SJS and TEN, but not in EM.

TREATMENT

Admission to a burn or intensive care unit can result in significant reduction in morbidity and mortality. Treatment is supportive and includes fluid and electrolyte imbalance corrections, strict monitoring of urinary output, caloric replacement, prevention of secondary infections, good skin and ophthalmologic care, and physical therapy. If there are large areas of denudation, the use of biological dressings or skin equivalents is recommended. Corticosteroids have been used to treat SJS in the past, but there are no clinical trials demonstrating efficacy, and recent retrospective studies suggest corticosteroids may adversely affect morbidity and mortality. Intravenous immunoglobulin (IVIG) has shown some promise when recently studied in nonblinded, nonplacebo-controlled clinical trials. Days with fever were reduced by 50%, but the general course of the disease was not influenced compared to historical controls.

COMPLICATIONS AND PROGNOSIS

SJS usually lasts four to six weeks and can be complicated by electrolyte imbalance, dehydration, secondary infections, and severe pneumonitis. Large areas of denudation can cause scarring leading to contractures. Ocular complications include corneal scarring, pseudomembrane formation leading to immobility of the eyelids, and lacrimal duct scarring. Lesions of the oral mucosa usually heal without complications. Esophageal or anal involvement can lead to strictures, and vaginal or urethral mucosal lesions can cause stenosis.

SJS can cause significant morbidity; the mortality rate is as high as 30% (12). If appropriate symptomatic treatment is given, the morbidity and mortality rates are lower (14).

SUMMARY

SJS is a severe illness with significant morbidity and mortality. It is characterized by an abrupt onset of mucocutaneous necrosis of at least two mucosal sites with variable skin involvement, following a characteristic prodrome of a respiratory illness. Most commonly, SJS is drug-induced, but many causative factors have been implicated. Treatment consists of supportive care and discontinuation of the offending agent; administration of corticosteroids or IVIG is controversial and not evidence-based.

Please see Chapter 22 for further discussion of SJS.

Hansen's disease

DEFINITION

The first written descriptions of leprosy, also known as Hansen's disease, date back to 600 *BC* in India and 200 *BC* in China. During the Middle Ages, leprosy reached epidemic proportions in Europe and was once worldwide in distribution. Now, leprosy is seen mainly in tropical and subtropical regions of Asia, Africa, and Central and South America. Leprosy is a slowly progressive, chronic infectious disease caused by the bacillus *Mycobacterium leprae*, an intracytoplasmic parasite of macrophages and Schwann cells.

EPIDEMIOLOGY

At the beginning of 2005, the global registered prevalence of leprosy was close to 300,000 (15). This number has fallen every year in the past decade, presumably due to availability and impact of multidrug therapy (MDT). The Indian subcontinent has the largest number of patients with leprosy; in the Americas, the highest incidence is seen in Brazil.

Men and women are affected equally, but the lepromatous form of leprosy is seen twice as frequently in men as in women. Leprosy can affect all ages and is spread through close or intimate contact. The bacillus is spread via nasal or oral droplets and, less often, from eroded skin. The incubation period ranges from months to decades, but is usually less than five years.

PATHOGENESIS

The bacillus *M. leprae* is a very small, slightly curved, acid-fast rod. It is an obligate intracellular parasite and it primarily affects the skin and peripheral nerves as it lives within macrophages and Schwann cells. *M. leprae* grows optimally at 35°C, and therefore has a preference for cooler areas of the body such as the nose, ears, and testicles.

The majority of exposed individuals do not develop disease. Susceptibility and type of response appear to correlate with specific human leukocyte antigen (HLA) types. For example, patients with HLA DR-2 and DR-3 are more likely to develop tuberculoid leprosy, and those with HLA DQ1 usually develop the lepromatous form. Humoral immunity is increased in forms that are associated with low cell-mediated immunity, such as lepromatous leprosy. A Th1 predominance is seen in patients with tuberculoid leprosy, while lepromatous leprosy is associated with a Th2 predominance (16).

CLINICAL MANIFESTATIONS

Leprosy has a wide spectrum of clinical presentations involving primarily the skin and nervous system. Due to involvement of peripheral nerves, which can become enlarged and palpable, cutaneous lesions of leprosy exhibit hypesthesia or anesthesia. Some peripheral nerves are more commonly affected, partly due to their superficial location. Branches of the facial nerve, the ulnar and radial nerves, the common peroneal nerve, and the posterior tibial nerve are commonly involved. Decreased sensation to pain and temperature and neurotrophic changes can also be noted on exam.

Historically, leprosy was divided into four types: lepromatous, which occurs in patients with depressed cell-mediated immunity; tuberculoid, occurring in patients with intact cell-mediated immunity; dimorphous; and indeterminate. The more recent and commonly accepted classification of leprosy is also based on polar forms and similarly reflects the underlying host immunity as measured by the T-lymphocyte and antibody responses to *M. leprae*, with lepromatous leprosy at one end, tuberculoid leprosy at the other end, and three types of borderline leprosy in-between.

Lepromatous leprosy, the form with the least cell-mediated immunity, has the greatest number of bacilli and is characterized by poorly defined, widespread, symmetric erythematous macules, papules, and nodules initially. The most common sites of involvement are the face, buttocks, and lower extremities. Involvement of the face can lead to leonine facies due to diffuse infiltration with the *M. leprae* bacilli (Fig. 8). Later signs include infiltration of the ear lobes, saddle nose, madarosis, ichthyosis of the lower extremities, and stocking-glove peripheral neuropathy. In severe cases, ocular symptoms develop due to infiltration of facial and trigeminal nerve branches (17).

Borderline leprosy is characterized by more asymmetric lesions that range in severity depending on which pole (lepromatous or tuberculoid) the patient is closer to.

Tuberculoid leprosy can present with only few skin lesions characterized by erythematous to hypopigmented plaques with raised borders, associated anesthesia, hypesthesia, alopecia, and unilateral trophic changes.

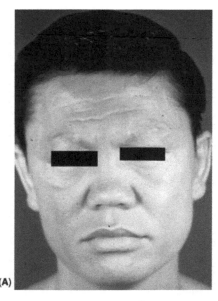 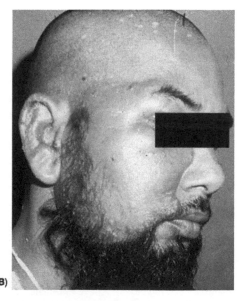

(A)   (B)

FIGURE 8 Diffuse infiltration of the face presenting as confluent indurated plaques on the face leading to madarosis in a patient with Hansen's disease (**A**). Reversal reaction in a patient undergoing treatment for Hansen's disease (**B**).

DIAGNOSIS

Diagnosis is made based on the clinical presentation and acid-fast staining of isolated bacilli or histologic examination with special stains.

TREATMENT

MDT as recommended by the World Health Organization is a safe, effective, and easily administered therapy for leprosy (Table 3). After the first dose, patients are no longer infectious to others, and transmission of leprosy is interrupted. Patients who have completed the prescribed medication regimen are considered cured, and there are virtually no relapses. Treatment can lead to development of acute inflammatory reactions for which additional medications are often required. Type I or reversal reactions, which can occur in patients with any type of leprosy upon commencement of therapy, can be treated with prednisone (Fig. 8B). Type II reactions, which occur in patients with the lepromatous form of leprosy who are undergoing treatment and are caused by formation of immune complexes in association with an excessive humoral immunity reaction, can be treated with thalidomide.

COMPLICATIONS AND PROGNOSIS

Leprosy is now considered a curable disease with a good prognosis and excellent survival rates. Prognosis is excellent in patients treated early. Complications arise from chronic infection and subsequent neurologic sequelae caused by infiltration of peripheral nerves. Disfigurement and peripheral neuropathies are irreversible and can only be avoided through early diagnosis and treatment.

SUMMARY

Leprosy is a slowly progressive, chronic infectious disease caused by *M. leprae*. The lesions of leprosy have a predilection for peripheral nerves and skin. Leprosy is a serious health issue in developing countries, and early diagnosis followed by prompt therapy is paramount in the strategy to control this chronic infectious disease.

TABLE 3 World Health Organization Recommended Multidrug Therapy Regimens

Multibacillary leprosy (>5 lesions)	Paucibacillary leprosy (2–5 lesions)	Paucibacillary leprosy (single lesion)
Rifampicin: 600 mg once a month	Rifampicin: 600 mg once a month	Single dose of: Rifampicin: 600 mg
Dapsone: 100 mg daily	Dapsone: 100 mg daily	Ofloxacin: 400 mg
Clofazimine: 300 mg once a month and 50 mg daily	Duration = 6 mo	Minocycline: 100 mg
Duration = 12 mo	—	
Dose adjustments for children:	*10–14 yr old*	
<10 yr old	Rifampicin: 450 mg/mo	
Rifampicin: 300 mg/mo	Dapsone: 50 mg/day	
Dapsone: 25 mg/day	Clofazimine: 150 mg/mo and 50 mg every other day	
Clofazimine: 100 mg/mo and 50 mg twice/wk		

GLUCAGONOMA SYNDROME

DEFINITION

Glucagon-secreting tumors of the pancreatic islets (glucagonomas) produce a distinctive syndrome characterized by the development of prominent mucocutaneous findings, adult-onset diabetes mellitus, weight loss, and anemia (18). Becker initially described the constellation of symptoms associated with an islet tumor of the pancreas in 1942.

The cutaneous component of this syndrome, termed necrolytic migratory erythema (NME), was first described by Wilkinson in his report of a patient with pancreatic carcinoma in 1973. The full syndrome was finally described by Mallison in 1974 in his review of nine patients with glucagon-secreting tumors.

EPIDEMIOLOGY

Glucagonoma is an extremely rare syndrome estimated to affect 1 in 20,000,000 per year, with approximately 200 cases to date reported worldwide. Most patients typically present in their fifth or sixth decade, but it has been reported in patients ranging from 10 to 84 years of age. Glucagonoma appears to affect males and females in equal numbers.

PATHOGENESIS

Glucagonoma is caused by glucagons-secreting tumors of the pancreatic islet. Glucagon stimulates hepatic gluconeogenesis and inhibits glucose breakdown and glycogen synthesis. The development of diabetes results from the actions of glycogen, as well as the relative concentrations of insulin and glucagon, which determines the net effect of hepatic glucose production (19). Weight loss is the result of the catabolic effects of glucagon, and anemia, the result of suppression of bone marrow erythropoiesis, again by glucagon, itself. The etiology of NME by glucagon has not been well established, although normalization of glucagon levels postresection often results in clearance of the skin lesions. Fatty acid deficiency, zinc deficiency, hepatic impairment, and amino acid deficiency also have been found to be important factors in NME development.

CLINICAL MANIFESTATIONS

NME is the hallmark finding in glucagonoma syndrome. It is characterized by a polymorphous eruption that most commonly presents as scaly, erythematous papules and plaques with superficial erosions. The lesions typically are in a perioral distribution on the face (Fig. 9), but also involve the perineum, lower abdomen, thighs, buttocks, and less commonly the distal extremities. NME has been reported to be the presenting complaint in approximately two-thirds of patients with this tumor, but there are only rare cases of glucagonoma without NME ever occurring. Stomatitis, glossitis, dystrophic nails, and alopecia can also be seen. The eruption is frequently misdiagnosed as seborrheic dermatitis or intertrigo and can also resemble pemphigus foliaceus, acrodermatitis enteropathica, chronic mucocutaneous candidiasis, or psoriasis.

Weight loss has been reported to be the most common initial symptom of glucagonoma (71%), followed by NME (67%), and diabetes (38%) (19).

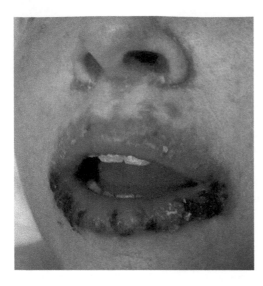

FIGURE 9 Perioral erythema and scale with superficial erosions and crusting characteristic of necrolytic migratory erythema. Courtesy of Dr. Kristina Callis, University of Utah.

DIAGNOSIS

The diagnosis of glucagonoma is made by three criteria: (*i*) an elevated serum glucagon level by radioimmunoassay; (*ii*) radiographically or histologically demonstrable neuroendocrine tumor; and (*iii*) characteristic clinical features (20). NME reportedly has been the single most consistent clinical finding that has led to diagnosis of glucagonoma. Other clinical features suggestive of glucagonoma include diabetes, weight loss, anemia, stomatitis, glossitis, dystrophic nails, and alopecia.

TREATMENT

Treatment of glucagonoma is typically through complete surgical resection of the glucagons-secreting tumor. If surgical resection is not a viable option, medical therapy with the somatostatin analogues octreotide and lanreotide has been reported. In very advanced cases, a variety of chemotherapeutic regimens have also been instituted.

COMPLICATIONS AND PROGNOSIS

The prognosis of glucagonoma is relatively good because the tumor is slow growing. Mean survival after diagnosis ranges from approximately three to seven years (20). The most common complications resulting in death in these patients are thromboembolism, sepsis, or gastrointestinal bleeding.

SUMMARY

Glucagonoma is a rare syndrome characterized by NME, weight loss, diabetes, and anemia, and NME is the most single consistent clinical finding leading to the diagnosis of glucagonoma. Awareness of this distinct skin eruption may allow for early diagnosis and better treatment, or even cure, of the underlying disorder.

REFERENCES

1. Lloyd KM II, Dennis M. Cowden's disease. A possible new symptom complex with multiple system involvement. Ann Intern Med 1963; 58:136-142.
2. Hildenbrand C, Burgdorf WH, Lautenschlager S. Cowden syndrome—diagnostic skin signs. Dermatology 2001; 202(4):362–366.
3. Eng C. Will the real Cowden syndrome please stand up: revised diagnostic criteria. J Med Genet 2000; 37(11):828–830.
4. Nelen MR, Padberg GW, Peeters EA, et al. Localization of the gene for Cowden disease to chromosome 10q22-23. Nat Genet 1996; 13(1):114–116.
5. Muir EG, Bell AJ, Barlow KA. Multiple primary carcinomata of the colon, duodenum, and larynx associated with kerato-acanthomata of the face. Br J Surg 1967; 54(3):191–195.
6. Torre D. Multiple sebaceous tumors. Arch Dermatol 1968; 98(5):549–551.
7. Schwartz RA, Torre DP. The Muir-Torre syndrome: a 25-year retrospect. J Am Acad Dermatol 1995; 33(1):90–104.
8. Schreibman IR, Baker M, Amos C, et al. The hamartomatous polyposis syndromes: a clinical and molecular review. Am J Gastroenterol 2005; 100(2):476–490.
9. Marignani PA. LKB1, the multitasking tumour suppressor kinase. J Clin Pathol 2005; 58(1): 15–19.
10. Pau H, Carney AS, Murty GE. Hereditary haemorrhagic telangiectasia (Osler-Weber-Rendu syndrome): otorhinolaryngological manifestations. Clin Otolaryngol Allied Sci 2001; 26(2): 93–98.
11. Bayrak-Toydemir P, Mao R, Lewin S, et al. Hereditary hemorrhagic telangiectasia: an overview of diagnosis and management in the molecular era for clinicians. Genet Med 2004; 6(4): 175–191.
12. Bastuji-Garin S, Rzany B, Stern RS, et al. Clinical classification of cases of toxic epidermal necrolysis, Stevens-Johnson syndrome, and erythema multiforme. Arch Dermatol 1993; 129(1): 92–96.
13. Sullivan JR, Shear NH. The drug hypersensitivity syndrome: what is the pathogenesis? Arch Dermatol 2001; 137(3):357–364.
14. Leaute-Labreze C, Lamireau T, Chawki D, et al. Diagnosis, classification, and management of erythema multiforme and Stevens-Johnson syndrome. Arch Dis Child 2000; 83(4):347–352.
15. http://www.who.int/lep/ (accessed September 2005).
16. Ramos-e-Silva M, Rebello PF. Leprosy. Recognition and treatment. Am J Clin Dermatol 2001; 2 (4):203–211.
17. Ramos-E-Silva M, Oliveira ML, Munhoz-da-Fontoura GH. Leprosy: uncommon presentations. Clin Dermatol 2005; 23(5):509–514.
18. Kahan RS, Perez-Figaredo RA, Neimanis A. Necrolytic migratory erythema. Distinctive dermatosis of the glucagonoma syndrome. Arch Dermatol 1977; 113(6):792–797.
19. Wermers RA, Fatourechi V, Wynne AG, et al. The glucagonoma syndrome: clinical and pathologic features in 21 patients. Medicine (Baltimore) 1996; 75(2):53–63.
20. Chastain MA. The glucagonoma syndrome: a review of its features and discussion of new perspectives. Am J Med Sci 2001; 321(5):306–320.

Index

ACAID, *See:* Anterior-chamber associated immune deviation
ACE, *See:* Angiotensin converting enzyme
Acetazolamide, 348
Acetylsalicylic acid (ASA), 383
'Acid-fast bacilli' (AFB), 170
Acquired immune deficiency syndrome (AIDS), 204, 230–250, 405–406, *See also* Human immunodeficiency virus
Acral keratoses, 545
ACS, *See:* Acute chest syndrome
Active pulmonary disease, 102
Acute anterior uveitis, 301
Acute bacterial otitis externa, 363
Acute chest syndrome (ACS), 289
Acute invasive fungal sinusitis, 191–193
  clinical manifestations, 191–192
  complications and prognosis, 193
  diagnosis, 192
  epidemiology, 193
  pathophysiology, 191
  treatment, 192–193
    Amphotericin B, 193
    antifungal therapy, 192
    Aspergillus, 193
    Casopofungin, 193
    external ethmoidectomy, 193
    itraconazole, 193
    surgical debridement, 192
    systemic antifungal therapy, 193
    transnasal endoscopic surgery, 193
Acute myelogenous leukemia (AML), 420
Acute otitis media, 407
Acute promyelocytic leukemia (AML), 254
Acute sudden hearing loss, 137
Acute uveitis, 64
Acyclovir, 128, 138, 142
Adalimumab, 71
Adamantiades-Behçet's disease, 27–40
  clinical manifestations, 29–35

[Adamantiades-Behçet's disease clinical manifestations]
    head and neck, 29–32: articular manifestations, 30; genital ulcers, 30; neurologic manifestations, 30; ocular manifestations, 30–32; oral ulcers, 30; skin manifestations, 30
  complications and prognosis, 38
  diagnosis, 35–36
    nonspecific tests, 35
    criteria for, 35
  differential diagnosis, 36
  epidemiology, 28
  histopathologic evaluation, 29
  pathergy in, 33
  pathogenesis, 28–29
    immune cross-reactivity, 28
  skin lesions in, 33
    acneiform/pustular lesions, 33
    erythema nodosum, 33
    pustular lesion, 33
    ulcerative lesion, 33
  systemic manifestations, 32–34
    articular, 32
    cutaneous, 32
    gastrointestinal, 34
    general manifestations, 32
    nervous system, 34
    pulmonary, 34
  treatment, 36–38
    anti–TNF-α therapy, 36
    antitumor necrosis factor-α (INF-α) therapy, 36
    Azathioprine, 36
    chlorambucil, 36
    corticosteroids, 36
    cyclophosphamide, 36
    cyclosporine, 36
    cytotoxics, 36
    infliximab, 36
    Interferon-α (IFN-α) therapy, 36
    Thalidomide, 36
  vulvar ulcerations in, 34
Adenopathy, 410, 501
AFB, *See* Acid-fast bacilli